Marijuana and Madnes

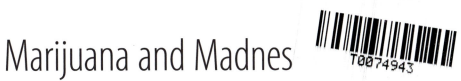

Marijuana and Madness

Third Edition

Edited by

Deepak Cyril D'Souza
Yale University School of Medicine

David J. Castle
University of Tasmania

Sir Robin M. Murray
Institute of Psychiatry

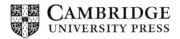
CAMBRIDGE
UNIVERSITY PRESS

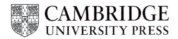
CAMBRIDGE
UNIVERSITY PRESS

Shaftesbury Road, Cambridge CB2 8EA, United Kingdom

One Liberty Plaza, 20th Floor, New York, NY 10006, USA

477 Williamstown Road, Port Melbourne, VIC 3207, Australia

314–321, 3rd Floor, Plot 3, Splendor Forum, Jasola District Centre, New Delhi – 110025, India

103 Penang Road, #05-06/07, Visioncrest Commercial, Singapore 238467

Cambridge University Press is part of Cambridge University Press & Assessment,
a department of the University of Cambridge.

We share the University's mission to contribute to society through the pursuit of
education, learning and research at the highest international levels of excellence.

www.cambridge.org
Information on this title: www.cambridge.org/9781009305433

DOI: 10.1017/9781108943246

First edition published 2004
Second edition published 2012
Third edition published 2023

Printed in Great Britain by Ashford Colour Press Ltd.

A catalogue record for this publication is available from the British Library.

Library of Congress Cataloging-in-Publication Data
Names: D'Souza, Deepak Cyril, editor. | Castle, David J., editor. | Murray, Robin M., 1944- editor.
Title: Marijuana and madness / edited by Deepak D'Souza, David Castle, Sir Robin Murray.
Description: Third edition. | Cambridge, United Kingdom ; New York : Cambridge University Press, 2023. |
    Includes bibliographical references and index.
Identifiers: LCCN 2022053404 (print) | LCCN 2022053405 (ebook) | ISBN 9781108837835 (hardback) |
    ISBN 9781009305433 (paperback) | ISBN 9781108943246 (epub)
Subjects: MESH: Marijuana Abuse–psychology | Marijuana Smoking–adverse effects | Cannabinoids–pharmacology |
    Mental Disorders–complications
Classification: LCC RC568.C2 (print) | LCC RC568.C2 (ebook) | NLM WM 276 | DDC 362.29/5–dc23/eng/20230118
LC record available at https://lccn.loc.gov/2022053404
LC ebook record available at https://lccn.loc.gov/2022053405

ISBN 978-1-009-30543-3 Paperback

Contents

Contributors

Arpana Agrawal, PhD
Washington University School of Medicine, USA

Ryan Bogdan, PhD
Washington University in St. Louis, USA

Mary Cannon, MD, PhD
RCSI University of Medicine and Health Sciences, Ireland

Andre Ferrer Carvalho, MD, PhD
Deakin University, Australia

David J. Castle, MD
University of Tasmania, Australia

Alexandra Chisholm, PhD
Icahn School of Medicine, USA

Sarah M. C. Colbert, PhD
Washington University School of Medicine, USA

Alexandria S. Coles, MSc
University of Toronto, Canada

David Copolov, MD, PhD
Monash University, Australia

Sam Craft, PhD
University of Bath, UK

H. Valerie Curran, PhD
University College London, UK

Marco De Toffol, MD
Veris Delli Ponti Scorrano Hospital, Italy

Brian Dean, PhD
Florey Institute of Neuroscience and Mental Health, Australia

Louisa Degenhardt, PhD
University of New South Wales, Australia

Marta Di Forti, MD, PhD
King's College London, UK

Elena Dragioti, PhD
Linköping University, Sweden

Deepak Cyril D'Souza, MD
Yale University School of Medicine, USA

Liana Fattore, PhD
CNR Institute of Neuroscience-Cagliari, Italy

Jacqueline-Marie Ferland, PhD
Icahn School of Medicine, USA

Tom P. Freeman, PhD
University of Bath, UK

Suhas Ganesh, MD
Yale University School of Medicine, USA

Tony P. George, MD, FRCPC
University of Toronto, Canada

Gabriella Gobbi, MD, PhD
McGill University, Canada

Michelle Murphy Green, MS
Indiana University, USA

Lisa-Marie Greenwood, PhD
Australian National University, Australia

Sinan Guloksuz, MD, PhD
Maastricht University Medical Center, The Netherlands

Wayne Hall, PhD
University of Queensland, Australia

Deborah Hasin, PhD
Columbia University, USA

Colm Healy, PhD
RCSI University of Medicine and Health Sciences,
Ireland

Cécile Henquet, PhD
Maastricht University, The Netherlands

Yasmin L. Hurd, PhD
Icahn School of Medicine, USA

Emma C. Johnson, PhD
Washington University School of Medicine, USA

Shubham Kamal, MBBS
Yale University School of Medicine, USA

Matcheri S. Keshavan, MD
Harvard Medical School, USA

Ashley E. Kivlichan, BS
University of Toronto, Canada

Rebecca Kuepper, PhD
Maastricht University, The Netherlands

Will Lawn, PhD
King's College London, UK

Grace Lethbridge, BHSc
McMaster University, Canada

F. Markus Leweke, MD MA
University of Sydney, Australia

Valentina Lorenzetti, PhD
Australian Catholic University, Australia

Ken Mackie, MD
Indiana University, USA

Paolo Marino, MD
King's College London, UK

Matteo Marti, PhD
University of Ferrara, Italy

Ashley M. Schnakenberg Martin, PhD
Yale University School of Medicine, USA

Kayleigh N. McCarty, PhD
VA Boston Healthcare System

Erin A. McClure, PhD
Medical University of South Carolina (MUSC), USA

Jane Metrik, PhD
Brown University School of Public Health, USA

Paul D. Morrison, MD, PhD
Argyll and Bute Hospital, UK

Robin M. Murray, MD
King's College London, UK

Jim van Os, MD, PhD
Utrecht University Medical Center, The
Netherlands

Sachin Patel, MD, PhD
Northwestern University, USA

Beth Patterson, BScN, BEd, MSc
McMaster University, Canada

Sarah E. Paul, MA
Washington University in St. Louis, USA

Godfrey D. Pearlson, MD
Yale University School of Medicine, USA

Jairo Vinícius Pinto, MD, PhD
University Hospital, Universidade Federal de Santa
Catarina, Brazil

Emmet Power, MB BCh
RCSI University of Medicine and Health Sciences,
Ireland

Rachel A. Rabin, PhD
McGill University, Canada

Rajiv Radhakrishnan, MD
Yale University School of Medicine, USA

Mohini Ranganathan, MD
Yale University School of Medicine, USA

Victoria Rodriguez, MD
King's College of London, UK

Cynthia E. Rogers, MD
Washington University School of Medicine, USA

Cathrin Rohleder, PhD
University of Sydney, Australia

Tiziana Rubino, PhD
University of Insubria, Italy

Tabea Schoeler, PhD
University of Lausanne, Switzerland

R. Andrew Sewell, MD†
Yale University School of Medicine, USA

Patrick D. Skosnik, PhD
Yale University School of Medicine, USA

Marco Solmi, MD, PhD
University of Ottawa, Canada

Nadia Solowij, PhD
University of Wollongong, Australia

Edoardo Spinazzola, MD
King's College London, UK

Suresh Sundram, MBBS, PhD
Monash University, Australia

Toral S. Surti, MD, PhD
Yale University School of Medicine, USA

Giulia Trotta, MD
King's College London, UK

Michael Van Ameringen, MD, FRCPC
McMaster University, Canada

Evangelos Vassos, MD
King's College London, UK

Nathan D. Winters, PhD
Vanderbilt University School of Medicine, USA

Erica Zamberletti, PhD
University of Insubria, Italy

Mauren Letícia Ziak, MD, MSc
Faculdade Pequeno Príncipe, Brazil

Preface

Since the first and second editions of *Marijuana and Madness* were published in 2004 and 2012, respectively, interest in cannabis, cannabinoids, and mental health has continued to grow. Since the last edition of this book, the landscape of cannabis has changed. The strength of cannabis has increased, with a number of highly potent forms of cannabis-derived products becoming available; cannabis laws have been liberalized in many jurisdictions; and the large-scale commercialization of cannabis has begun. In parallel, the science of the endocannabinoid system has advanced. Given the changes in legality, availability, and potency of cannabis, the adverse consequences of cannabis are likely to be seen more frequently in contemporary society than in studies conducted decades ago. Indeed, the topic has moved from being of interest mainly to specialists in psychosis and addiction to being a public mental health concern. The third edition of this book addresses these changes and more. The first edition had 13 chapters and the second edition had 21 chapters. This third edition has 32 chapters, with updates to core chapters from the first and second editions and a number of entirely new chapters. Consistent with the growing awareness of the consequences of cannabis exposure, the scope of the book has expanded beyond psychosis, to include bipolar disorder, depression, anxiety disorders, and cannabis use disorder.

The first part of the book covers the pharmacology of cannabis and the endocannabinoid system. Mackie reviews how cannabis works in the brain, followed by an overview of the endocannabinoid system (Winters and Patel), and synthetic cannabinoids (Fattore and Marti). These chapters set the stage for chapters addressing some of the most pressing concerns about the acute and chronic consequences of cannabis use.

Addressing the changing face of cannabis, Hasin provides an overview of the epidemiology of cannabis use and cannabis use disorder, followed by a review of the changing potency of cannabis (Freeman and Craft). Then, Hall and Degenhardt review the health policy implications of the relationship between cannabis and mental illness.

Any theory associating exposure to cannabis with long-term negative mental health consequences needs to have biological plausibility; that is, there needs to be a plausible underlying biological mechanism. If the endocannabinoid system is involved in adolescent brain development, then perturbation of this system at critical periods of brain development may have far reaching consequences. The impact of cannabis exposure on the adolescent brain is discussed in animals (Zamberletti and Rubino) and humans (Ferland et al.). Greenwood and colleagues review the short- and long-term effects of cannabis on cognition. As cannabis is being increasingly used by women during pregnancy, Paul et al. review the impact of prenatal cannabis exposure on neurodevelopment and behaviour.

The relationship between cannabis and anxiety (Lethbridge et al.), depression and suicidal behaviour (Gobbi), and bipolar disorder (Pinto and Ziak) is covered in the ensuing section, teasing apart cause and effect and considering implications for treatment.

Radhakrishnan et al. review the evidence on the relationship between cannabis and psychosis proneness. Going further, Spinazzola et al. discuss factors that might predispose cannabis using individuals to psychosis and suggest that the link between cannabis use and schizophrenia is unlikely to be just the result of a genetic predisposition, it is more likely the result of an interplay between genes and the environment. Martin-Schnakenberg and colleagues address experimental and other evidence showing that cannabis and cannabinoids are linked to positive, negative, and cognitive symptoms, as well as producing impairments in electrophysiological indices of information processing.

Extending the cannabis/psychosis theme, Power and colleagues address the important and contentious question in the field as to whether cannabis actually causes schizophrenia. Colbert and Johnson review genetic explanations for the link between cannabis and schizophrenia. Pearlson and Keshavan provide evidence suggesting the possibility of a cannabis associated psychosis subtype.

Beyond the hypothesis linking exposure to exocannabinoids such as cannabis to psychosis, there is emerging evidence that the endocannabinoid system may be altered in schizophrenia. Sundram et al. and Morrison review the post-mortem, animal and invivo evidence on the state of the endocannabinoid system in schizophrenia.

One of the vexing clinical conundrums is the discrepancy between the "benefits" of cannabis reported by users and the negative consequences on the course and expression of schizophrenia observed by clinicians. Ganesh et al. review the acute effects of cannabis and cannabinoids in people with psychotic illness, whilst Schoeler provides an overview of the impact of cannabis on the long-term course of schizophrenia.

Several new chapters addressing emerging issues relevant to cannabis use have been added. Trotta et al. review the growing interest in the association between cannabis exposure and violence, while a number of chapters focus on cannabis addiction. Curran and colleagues review the neurobiology, expression, and treatment of cannabis use disorder, and in related chapters Metrik and McCarty review the characteristics, course, and treatment of cannabis withdrawal syndrome, while Ganesh and Agrawal provide a synopsis of the genetics of cannabis addiction. In a clinically-focused chapter, Coles et al. address potential treatments for cannabis misuse in individuals with psychosis.

Given that cannabis is often used with tobacco, especially in Europe, understanding the relationship between the two is important. Rabin et al. review the interactions between cannabis and withdrawal. There is increasing recognition that people use cannabis to facilitate sleep, and that the endocannabinoid system may be involved in sleep; Skosnik and Surti assess the role of cannabis and the endocannabinoid system in sleep.

Lastly, beyond the recreational use of cannabis, there is increasing interest in the 'medical use' of cannabis. Leweke and Rohleder address the intriguing possibility that cannabidiol (CBD) may have beneficial effects in schizophrenia, while De Toffol and colleagues review the evidence on the 'medical use' of cannabis.

As editors, we are excited at the richness of the material provided to us by the contributors, all leaders in their field. We hope that readers will be likewise impressed at the progress that has been made in our understanding of the relationship between cannabis, cannabinoids, and neuropsychiatric disorders.

Chapter

1

How Cannabis Works in the Brain

Michelle Murphy Green and Ken Mackie

1.1 Introduction

The unique psychoactivity of cannabis has been appreciated for millennia. However, only in the past 50 years have we begun to understand how cannabis produces these effects. Cannabis contains many different molecules of unique classes and actions. Most of the characteristic psychoactivity of cannabis is a result of delta-9-tetrahydrocannabinol (THC), however additional constituents (such as cannabidiol (CBD)) of cannabis may either modify THC's psychoactivity or produce their own unique psychoactivity (Spindle et al., 2020). The primary target of THC and many other cannabis constituents is the endocannabinoid system. This interesting neuromodulatory system consists of receptors, endogenous cannabinoids (endocannabinoids), and the enzymes responsible for endocannabinoid synthesis and degradation (Howlett et al., 2002). THC interacts with the two major endocannabinoid receptors, CB1 and CB2, with most THC psychoactivity being caused by THC engagement of CB1 receptors. Thus, effects of THC will be determined by three-way interactions between THC, endocannabinoids, and cannabinoid receptors. Like all drugs, the effects of cannabis are determined in part by its route of administration and its pharmacokinetics, so different routes of cannabis consumption (e.g., inhaled versus edibles) may be expected to have divergent effects.

1.2 Distribution of the Endocannabinoid System throughout the Brain

An understanding of the actions of cannabis in the brain requires a thorough understanding of where CB1 receptors are found. CB1 receptors are embedded in the cell membrane. The CNS distribution of CB1 receptors was first characterized using autoradiography using the high affinity radioligand, CP-55,940 (Herkenham et al., 1991).

These findings were supported and extended by subsequent studies using immunohistochemistry with antibodies targeting the N- or C-terminal domains of CB1 (Egertova and Elphick, 2000; Tsou et al., 1998) and are consistent with *in situ* hybridization studies localizing CB1 mRNA (Matsuda et al., 1993). Studies using these different techniques identified high densities of CB1 receptors in the hippocampus, basal ganglia, and cerebellum, with moderate levels of the CB1 receptor expressed in the prefrontal cortex, amygdala, and hypothalamus. However, there are low levels of CB1 receptor expression in most thalamic and brainstem nuclei (Egertova and Elphick, 2000; Zou and Kumar, 2018). The high concentrations of CB1 receptors in cortical brain regions support the endocannabinoid system's role in regulating executive cognitive functions such as decision-making, learning, and memory, as well as psychomotor coordination. Additionally, the low levels of CB1 receptors in brain regions responsible for cardiovascular and respiratory functions may explain why consuming even very high amounts of cannabis is not lethal.

> CB1 receptors are widely distributed in the CNS, with higher levels found in brain areas that correspond with cannabis's effects, such as the cortex, basal ganglia, amygdala, hypothalamus, and cerebellum (Figure 1.1).

At the cellular level, endocannabinoid receptor expression differs between brain areas and among cell types. In neurons in the cortex and hippocampus, CB1 receptors are highly expressed in cholecystokinin (CCK) positive inter-neurons with lower expression in glutamatergic and other neurons. In the striatum, CB1 receptors are highly expressed in medium spiny neurons. Finally, in the cerebellum, CB1 receptors are expressed in parallel fibres, climbing fibres, and basket cells (Lu and Mackie, 2016). CB1 receptors

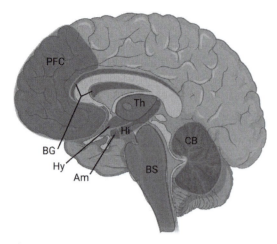

Figure 1.1 CB1 receptor distribution in CNS. High levels of CB1 receptors are found broadly throughout the brain, including in the cortex, basal ganglia, amygdala, hypothalamus, and cerebellum. Much lower levels are found in the thalamus and brainstem (see text for more details). [Created with BioRender.com].
PFC = prefrontal cortex; BG = basal ganglia; Hy = hypothalamus; Am = amygdala; Th = thalamus; Hi = hippocampus; BS = brainstem; CB = cerebellum. A black and white version of this figure will appear in some formats. For the colour version, please refer to the plate section.

are also expressed in some astrocytes (Han et al., 2012). Conversely, CB2 receptor expression is higher in activated microglia and pericytes, though CB2 may be expressed in a limited set of neurons and its level of expression modulated by pathological insults (Atwood and Mackie, 2010). Within neurons, the majority of CB1 receptors are pre-synaptic (axons and terminal), with lower levels of expression in cell bodies and dendrites (Marsicano and Lutz, 1999). In addition to being localized on the plasma membrane, CB1 may be expressed in some organelles, such as mitochondria (Benard et al., 2012). Not surprisingly, this localization of CB1 receptors plays an important role in determining how the endocannabinoid system regulates neuronal and network function in the brain.

1.3 What Does the Endocannabinoid System Do?

The endocannabinoid system functions via a complex and inter-related network of cannabinoid receptors, endogenous cannabinoids, and synthesizing and degrading enzymes. For the purposes of this chapter, we will now focus primarily on CB1 receptors as they are the most highly expressed and prevalent cannabinoid receptor in the brain and a major target of THC. CB1 receptors are G protein-couple receptors

(GPCR's) and primarily couple with the $G_{i/o}$ family of G proteins. Thus, upon activation, CB1 receptors inhibit adenylyl cyclase to attenuate cyclic AMP production. In addition, they activate various mitogen-activated protein kinases (MAPKs) and phosphatidylinositol-3-kinase (PI3K). Another major consequence of neuronal CB1 receptor stimulation is activation of inwardly rectifying potassium channels and an inhibition of several voltage-activate calcium channels (Howlett et al., 2002). A final consequence of CB1 activation can be the recruitment of beta-arrestins to the receptor, which might contribute to down-regulation of CB1 receptor signalling and/or the diversion of CB1 signalling toward new pathways. The consequence of neuronal CB1 receptor activation is often the inhibition of neuronal firing and neurotransmission. Although, since many CB1 receptors are expressed on GABAergic neurons, CB1 activation can increase network activity by decreasing inhibition.

CB2 receptors are also $G_{i/o}$ coupled receptors engaging similar signalling pathways as CB1 receptors. Both CB1 and CB2 receptors show the general characteristics of typical GPCRs (Kenakin, 2019), including several characteristics that are key to understanding the interactions between phytocannabinoids and endocannabinoids. The first is potency, the affinity of the interaction of the ligand with the receptor, relevant for both agonists and antagonists. The second is efficacy, the extent to which an agonist activates CB1 or CB2 receptor signalling. Since low efficacy agonists only exhibit partial agonism under some conditions, it is better to refer to ligands in term of efficacy rather than 'partial' or 'full' agonists as the latter designation is system-dependent. Negative efficacy (i.e., a decrease of a signalling pathway below basal levels) is seen with 'inverse agonists', such as the CB1 antagonist, rimonabant. The third is functional selectivity. Functional selectivity is a characterization of signalling pathways activated by a specific agonist. For example, an agonist might activate many pathways similarly (i.e., a 'balanced' agonist) or just a couple of pathways (i.e., a 'biased' agonist). The fourth is allosteric modulation. Allosteric modulators positively or negatively affect the signalling of a receptor by interacting at a site on the receptor distinct from the orthosteric site (the site where the canonical ligand for the receptor binds).

A major role for endocannabinoids is to activate CB1 receptors where they elicit several forms of retrograde signalling (Figure 1.2). The two best-known

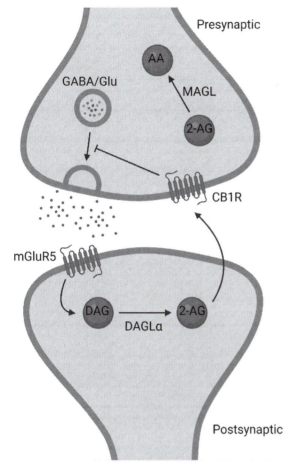

Presynaptic

GABA/Glu

Postsynaptic

Figure 1.2 Schematic of canonical retrograde signalling by the endocannabinoid system. Release of glutamate or depolarization of the post-synaptic neuron leads to synthesis of 2-AG, which diffuses retrogradely across the synapse. Released 2-AG engages and activates CB1 receptors to inhibit neurotransmitter release. 2-AG is primarily hydrolysed by MAGL to arachidonic acid and glycerol, which are reincorporated into membrane phospholipids, to terminate a cycle of retrograde signalling. [Created with BioRender. com]. A black and white version of this figure will appear in some formats. For the colour version, please refer to the plate section.

endocannabinoids are 2-archidonoylglycerol (2-AG) and anandamide (AEA). 2-AG appears to be the major endocannabinoid involved in retrograde signalling. 2-AG is primarily synthesized in post-synaptic dendrites from phosphatidyl inositol bisphosphate by the sequential action of phospholipase C and diacylglycerol lipase-α (DAGLα). When released into the synaptic cleft, 2-AG travels across the synapse to activate pre-synaptic cannabinoid receptors to inhibit neurotransmitter release. Subsequently, 2-AG is degraded by monoacylglycerol lipase (MAGL).

The endocannabinoid system utilizes retrograde signalling to inhibit neurotransmitter release at many synapses to regulate neuronal signalling and synaptic plasticity (Figure 1.3).

1.3.1 DSI/DSE

Depolarization-induced suppression of inhibition (DSI) and depolarization-induced suppression of excitation (DSE) are two short-term forms of synaptic plasticity relating to GABAergic and glutamatergic neurons, respectively. Since DSI and DSE have broadly similar mechanisms, we will discuss DSI and DSE together. DSI and DSE are triggered by strong post-synaptic depolarization of a neuron, and manifest as a transient inhibition of neurotransmitter release onto the depolarized neuron. DSI and DSE are mediated by depolarization-generated 2-AG traveling retrogradely across the synapse and activating pre-synaptic CB1 receptors, which, in turn, inhibit voltage-dependent calcium influx into the nerve terminal to depress calcium-dependent neurotransmitter release (Diana and Marty, 2004).

1.3.2 MSI/MSE

Metabotropic-induced suppression of inhibition (MSI) and metabotropic-induced suppression of excitation (MSE) are another two related forms of short-term synaptic plasticity. As opposed to DSI and DSE, which are mediated by calcium influx following depolarization, MSI and MSE are mediated by post-synaptic Gq/11-linked GPCRs. These receptors are activated by acetylcholine or glutamate (for example) released from surrounding cells and activation of the relevant Gq/11-linked GPCR activates phospholipase C (PLC). PLC produces diacylglycerol (DAG) that is hydrolysed to 2-AG via DAGLα. 2-AG is released into the synapse to activate pre-synaptic CB1 receptors and transiently inhibit neurotransmitter release (Mackie, 2008).

1.3.3 LTD

Unlike the previous two forms of endocannabinoid-mediated synaptic plasticity, long-term depression (LTD) differs in that it has a long-lasting effect on synaptic strength. LTD is induced by persistent low-frequency stimulation of glutamatergic pathways that release glutamate from neighbouring neurons. The

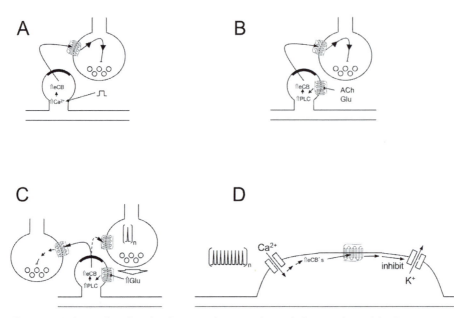

Figure 1.3 Endocannabinoid-mediated synaptic plasticity and control of neuronal excitability. Four major mechanisms by which endocannabinoids can affect neurotransmission and neuronal excitability (see text for more details). (A) DSI/DSE; (B) MSI/MSE; (C) LTD; (D) SSI.

glutamate then activates post-synaptic GPCRs via a signalling pathway similar to that in MSI and MSE to produce 2-AG, which decreases neurotransmitter release. Prolonged (e.g., 10 minutes) stimulation of CB1 receptors leads to long-term inhibition of neurotransmitter release. A hallmark of LTD is that the inhibition of neurotransmitter release continues after initial stimulation has ended and 2-AG is no longer being synthesized. LTD comes in two basic forms: heterosynaptic and homosynaptic. Heterosynaptic LTD is LTD occurring at synapses adjacent to the stimulated synapses. A classic example of this would be stimulation of hippocampal Schaeffer collaterals increasing local levels of 2-AG leading to LTD at adjacent CB1-containing inter-neurons. Homosynaptic LTD differs in that the LTD occurs at the same synapse that is being stimulated. This is often demonstrated at glutamatergic inputs into the nucleus accumbens or striatum. LTD is perhaps the most involved form of endocannabinoid-mediated synaptic plasticity and has been shown to play an important role in the maturation of cortical circuits (Itami et al., 2016).

1.3.4 SSI

In addition to being able to mediate synaptic plasticity in several forms, the endocannabinoid system is also capable of inhibiting neuronal excitability via slow self-inhibition (SSI). This process is most prevalent in cortical inter-neurons and cerebellar basket cells as well as some cortical principle cells. SSI is induced by repeated depolarization of a neuron, with a mechanism that involves increased intracellular calcium, 2-AG synthesis, stimulation of somatic CB1 receptors, and activation of inwardly rectifying potassium channels (Marinelli et al., 2008). SSI is an example highlighting that even low levels of CB1 receptors can have profound effects on neuronal excitability.

1.4 Cannabis Compounds

The cannabis plant contains over 420 chemical compounds, with more than 100 of these being classified as phytocannabinoids (Atakan, 2012). Phytocannabinoids are organic molecules synthesized by cannabis and (interestingly) by a few unrelated organisms. Phytocannabinoids typically contain a dihydrobenzopyran ring and a hydrophobic alkyl side chain (Figure 1.4). The best-known and well-researched of the phytocannabinoids are delta-9-tetrahydrocannabinol (THC) and cannabidiol (CBD). In addition, cannabis produces a number of related compounds such as delta-8-THC, tetrahydrocannabivarin (THCV), cannabinol (CBN), cannabigerol (CBG), and cannabichromene (CBC). These compounds have attracted substantial interest for their possible

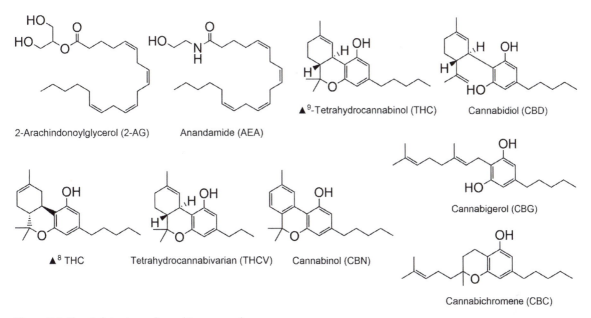

Figure 1.4 Chemical structures of cannabis compounds

biological or therapeutic actions. Cannabis also contains variable levels of a number of terpenes, the molecules that give different cannabis cultvars their distinctive aromas. However, our understanding of the impact of terpenes in the actions of cannabis on the brain is limited (Turner et al., 2017). Therefore, we will only focus on phytocannabinoids in this chapter.

> Phytocannabinoids are molecules synthesized by cannabis and are often capable of interacting with the endocannabinoid system. The best-known phytocannabinoids are THC and CBD.

Phytocannabinoids are synthesized in their acid forms (denoted by an 'A' after the three letter abbreviation, e.g., THCA) in the trichomes of the cannabis plant (Figure 1.5), with the female plant synthesizing greater quantities than the male plant. Both genetics and environment strongly influence the types and quantities of phytocannabinoids synthesized. The common pre-cursor to THC, CBD, and CBC is cannabigerolic acid (CBGA), which is synthesized from olivetolic acid and geranyl pyrophosphate (Figure 1.5). CBGA is metabolized by dedicated THC, CBD, and CBC synthases to yield the acidic versions of THC, CBD, and CBC, respectively.

Notably, the fidelity of these synthetic enzymes is not absolute, so CBD synthase may produce minor amounts of THC and so forth. The acidic forms of each cannabinoid undergo spontaneous decarboxylation (increased by gentle heating or light) to yield THC, CBD, and CBC. Under oxidizing conditions, THC will be degraded to cannabidiol. Further details on the synthesis of phytocannabinoids can be found in recent reviews by Gulck and Moller (2020) and Tahir et al. (2021).

THC was the third compound to be isolated from the cannabis plant and is responsible for the classic psychoactivity of cannabis (Gaoni and Mechoulam, 1964), while CBD was the second isolated compound and was discovered a year previously (Mechoulam and Shvo, 1963). THC and CBD are isomers with similar chemical structures. However, these compounds differ in that THC contains an intact dihydropyran ring while in CBD the ring is open, revealing a free hydroxyl group (Atakan, 2012). Importantly, these small structural differences result in completely different pharmacological properties that will be further explored in this chapter.

1.5 Pharmacokinetics

THC absorption and, hence, the impact of cannabis varies greatly depending upon its route of

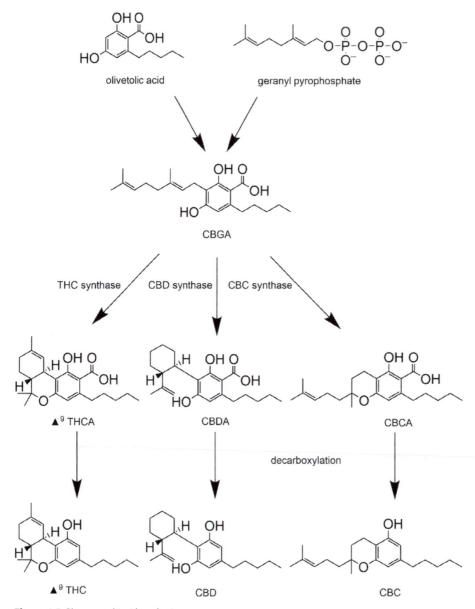

Figure 1.5 Phytocannabinoid synthesis

administration. The popularity of inhalation as a route of cannabis consumption is a consequence of THC volatilization following the heating of cannabis or cannabis extracts to above ~160°C. Inhalation, by vaping or smoking produces fast absorption into the bloodstream due to the lipophilicity of THC and the high surface area of the lungs. After inhalation of a single puff, THC is detected in plasma within seconds and reaches peak plasma concentration within 3–10 minutes (Huestis, 2007). Bioavailability of inhaled THC ranges between 10 and 35%, with differences influenced by regularity of use, depth of inhalation, duration of puff, and duration of breath holding. Conversely, oral administration produces a slower absorption with peak plasma concentrations being reached in 1–2 hours. Because of less efficient absorption in the intestines and significant first pass metabolism oral consumption of cannabis products decreases THC bioavailability to between 4 and 12% (Grotenhermen, 2003). Several other potential routes of administration include intravenous, transcutaneous, and rectal, with each having its own unique consequences on THC pharmacokinetics, but these alternative routes of administration are rarely used during recreational cannabis use.

Once in the body, THC is highly lipophilic and approximately 90% circulates bound to plasma proteins in blood (Sharma et al., 2012). THC rapidly crosses the blood–brain barrier and high quantities enter the brain (Amin and Ali, 2019). Because of its lipophilicity, THC accumulates in tissues with significant fat, notably adipose tissue. Adipose tissue also acts as a depot for long-term storage from which THC and its metabolites are absorbed from the blood stream and then slowly released. THC is initially metabolized by the liver via the P450 cytochrome system (primarily, CYP2C9). Hydroxylation of THC produces 11-OH-THC, which is slightly more potent than THC. Further oxidation (primarily by CYP2C9 and CYP3A4) produces 11-nor-9-carboxy-delta-8-tetrahydrocannabinol (THC–COOH), the primary inactive metabolite. Finally, THC–COOH undergoes glucuronidation to produce glucuronide conjugates which are subsequently excreted in faeces and urine (Lucas et al., 2018; Sharma et al., 2012). The preceding are the primary pathways and numerous less common degradative routes have been described, leading to a wide range of intermediate metabolites.

Because of efficient first pass metabolism, orally consumed THC yields much higher levels of 11-OH-THC and lower levels of THC than inhalation. This might account for some of the differences in psychoactivity ascribed to the oral versus inhaled routes of administration. Sex differences in THC pharmacokinetics have been reported, with females generally having faster onset, higher peak levels, and exposure for a given dose (Nadulski et al., 2005).

> After inhalation, THC is quickly absorbed into the bloodstream and peak plasma concentrations reached within minutes. Once in the body, THC is stored in adipose tissue and slowly released back into the bloodstream before excretion.

The pharmacokinetics of CBD share similarities with THC pharmacokinetics, however there are some differences. For example, following inhalation, CBD reaches peak plasma concentrations in about 3 minutes and its bioavailability ranges between 11 and 45%. As with THC, oral administration of CBD is less efficient that inhalation, and oral CBD is more slowly absorbed, with peak plasma concentrations reached 2–4 hours after consumption. Bioavailability has been reported to be between 13 and 19% (Millar et al., 2018) but is strongly affected by concurrent food consumption. CBD is degraded by pathways that are similar to THC's (though with some differences in the cytochrome P450s involved) and achieve plasma profiles similar to THC's. Of note, CBD inhibits degradation of THC to THC–COOH, thus substantial CBD consumption with THC may result in elevated THC levels and increased THC exposure.

1.6 Effect of Phytocannabinoids on CB1 and Other Receptors

Due to their structural differences, THC and CBD have varying and potentially counteracting interactions with CB1 receptors. Like the endocannabinoids, THC binds to the orthosteric site of the CB1 receptor. THC is a low efficacy agonist, thus, in cells with few CB1 receptors or poor coupling of CB1 receptors to signalling pathways, it acts as a partial agonist, stimulating downstream signalling pathways and inhibiting pre-synaptic neurotransmitter release. In contrast, the endocannabinoid 2-AG is a high efficacy agonist (though of low potency). (Of note, anandamide is a low efficacy agonist, with an efficacy similar to THC's.) Under these circumstances, THC may, thus, antagonize 2-AG signalling (Straiker and Mackie, 2005). Of note, even though THC may not be activating classical CB1 pathways such as inhibition of neurotransmitter release, it is still capable of desensitizing CB1 receptors (Straiker et al., 2018). However, the situation is quite different in cells with many CB1 receptors and/or efficient CB1 receptor coupling. Here, THC may mimic the effects of 2-AG and other efficacious agonists (Laaris et al., 2010). It is likely that the consequences of the inter-play between THC and 2-AG varies across brain regions and cell types, as research has found THC capable of both inhibiting and promoting endocannabinoid actions. It is interesting to speculate that the unique psychoactive profile of cannabis, compared to potent synthetic cannabinoids (i.e., so-called spice compounds, all of which appear to be highly efficacious agonists), is due to THC's subtle ability to enhance endocannabinoid

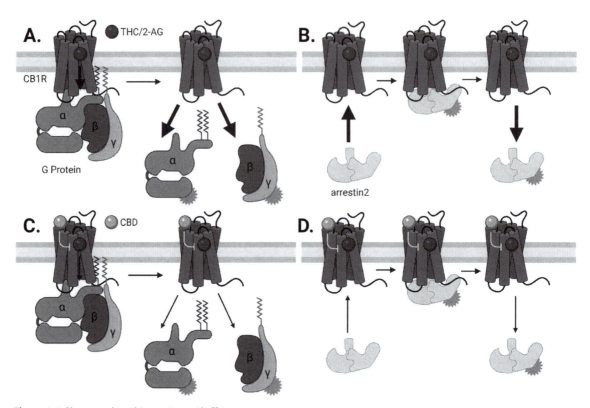

Figure 1.6 Phytocannabinoid Interactions with CB1 receptors.
(A) THC/2-AG effect on G-protein signalling. (B) THC/2-AG effect on arrestin2 recruitment and signalling. (C) CBD inhibiting THC/2-AG induced G-protein signalling. (D) CBD inhibiting THC/2-AG induced arrestin2 recruitment and signalling [created with BioRender.com]. A black and white version of this figure will appear in some formats. For the colour version, please refer to the plate section.

action in some cells while opposing it in others. This duality of action may also explain why even high doses of rimonabant only mildly reduce cannabis psychoactivity while fully ablating the autonomic effects of cannabis (Huestis et al., 2001, 2007). An additional factor that needs to be considered in understanding the differences between THC and endocannabinoid action on CB1 receptors are the kinetics. Much 2-AG is rapidly released, engages cannabinoid receptors, and then is rapidly degraded in a matter of seconds (Farrell et al., 2021). On the other hand, THC (and synthetic cannabinoid levels) rise on a much slower time scale (minutes to hours), resulting in prolonged engagement of the receptor by the cannabinoid.

> THC can act as a full or partial agonist at CB1 receptors, which may explain its complex behavioural effects. Conversely, as one of its targets, CBD is a negative allosteric modulator of CB1, inhibiting the effects of endogenous and exogenous cannabinoids.

Compared to THC's effects that appear primarily mediated by its interactions with the CB1 orthosteric site, CBD's effects on CB1 receptors are caused via indirect interaction(s) (Figure 1.6). CBD only has a low affinity for the CB1 orthosteric site and instead binds with relatively high affinity to an allosteric site, acting as a negative allosteric modulator. In this capacity it reduces the efficacy and potency of endogenous and exogenous cannabinoids. For example, CBD reduces the efficacy and potency of 2-AG and THC to recruit arrestin2 to CB1 receptors (Laprairie et al., 2015) as well as attenuating 2-AG-mediated inhibition of synaptic transmission (Straiker et al., 2018). For this reason, CBD does not produce the characteristic 'high' associated with cannabis use and may even limit the psychoactive effects of THC when they are administered concurrently (McPartland et al., 2015).

Interactions between CBD and THC are of immense public health importance. Concurrent CBD and THC can slow the metabolism of THC, leading to increased exposure. On the other hand, pre-clinical and some clinical evidence suggests that CBD may protect against some detrimental effects of cannabis. In the quest to increase THC content through selective breeding, the CBD content of recreational cannabis relative to THC content has decreased precipitously over the past 30 years (Dujourdy and Besacier, 2017; ElSohly et al., 2016). If CBD is indeed protective against some of the detrimental effects of THC (for example, on the developing brain), then there would be an incentive to understand what the minimally protective amount of CBD in cannabis is and how it is protective. Certainly, this is a topic that deserves further careful study.

In addition to CB1, CBD interacts with numerous other targets (as reviewed by de Almeida and Devi (2020)). Several clinical reports suggest that high doses (typically several 100 mg) of CBD are anxiolytic (as reviewed by O'Sullivan et al. (2021)). The target of CBD in this case, based on pre-clinical studies, appears to involve serotonin 5HT1A receptors and not CB1 receptors.

Another interesting effect of CBD is to decrease heroin craving in abstinent individuals with heroin use disorder. However, as this effect was observed with several hundred milligrams of CBD, it is unlikely that consumption of cannabis will deliver enough CBD to produce this effect.

Finally, CBD is beneficial in some forms of paediatric epilepsy through a currently unknown target. Efficacy is achieved at 10–20 mg/kg, doses that will be reached through the consumption of purified preparations of CBD and unlikely to be obtained via consumption of recreational cannabis preparations (Billakota et al., 2019).

Several other phytocannabinoids interact with CB1 receptors. Many of these are low efficacy agonists, such as delta-8-THC, and, thus, their pharmacology is similar to THC's pharmacology. However, an interesting exception is THCV. THCV is a potent orthosteric ligand for CB1, with low nanomolar affinity (McPartland et al., 2015). Interestingly, THCV's intrinsic efficacy is very low, so it behaves as a potent CB1 antagonist in many assays (McPartland et al., 2015). THCV is also a low efficacy agonist of CB2 receptors (McPartland et al., 2015). Because of this profile, THCV has attracted interest as a potential 'natural' antagonist of CB1 receptors that may not suffer from the psychiatric liability of rimonabant. THCV content of cannabis can be modified by selective breeding, though all high THCV strains currently available also contain significant levels of THC.

1.6.1 THC, CBD, and Inflammation

Neuroinflammation is thought to play a role in the pathogenesis of several psychiatric diseases. Interestingly, while the endocannabinoid system is broadly thought to be anti-inflammatory, some clinical (Da Silva et al., 2019) and substantial pre-clinical evidence suggests that consumption of THC or the attenuation of CB1 signalling (which might occur during chronic THC use) may cause or exacerbate neuroinflammation (Cutando et al., 2013; Zamberletti et al., 2015). In contrast, CB2 activation is generally anti-inflammatory, as is CBD. Whether THC-induced neuroinflammation contributes increased risk for psychiatric disorders with heavy cannabis use and if CBD ameliorates this risk deserves further study.

1.7 Conclusion

The psychoactivity of cannabis is mediated by complex interactions of phytocannabinoids with the endocannabinoid system in the brain. CB1 receptors are widely distributed throughout the brain, with higher levels found in regions whose functions cannabis is known to impact.

Conversely, low levels of CB1 receptors are found in brain regions spared by cannabis. The endocannabinoid system, consisting of endocannabinoids, cannabinoids receptors, and synthetic and degradative enzymes, broadly utilizes retrograde signalling to regulate neurotransmitter release at a number of synapses and influences several forms of synaptic plasticity. Cannabis contains several compounds that interact with the endocannabinoid system in different ways.

The best-known of these compounds are THC and CBD. THC directly engages CB1 receptors as a low efficacy agonist with complex interactions with the endocannabinoid system. In contrast, CBD interacts indirectly with CB1 receptors to act as a negative allosteric modulator. It is through these interactions with the endocannabinoid system in the brain that cannabis is able to produce its characteristic affects.

References

de Almeida, D. L., and Devi, L. A. (2020). Diversity of molecular targets and signaling pathways for CBD. *Pharmacol Res Perspect*, **8**, e00682.

Amin, M. R., and Ali, D. W. (2019). Pharmacology of medical cannabis. *Adv Exp Med Biol*, **1162**, 151–165.

Atakan, Z. (2012). Cannabis, a complex plant: Different compounds and different effects on individuals. *Ther Adv Psychopharmacol*, **2**, 241–254.

Atwood, B. K., and Mackie, K. (2010). CB2: A cannabinoid receptor with an identity crisis. *Br J Pharmacol*, **160**, 467–479.

Benard, G., Massa, F., Puente, N., et al. (2012). Mitochondrial CB(1) receptors regulate neuronal energy metabolism. *Nat Neurosci*, **15**, 558–564.

Billakota, S., Devinsky, O., and Marsh, E. (2019). Cannabinoid therapy in epilepsy. *Curr Opin Neurol*, **32**, 220–226.

Cutando, L., Busquets-Garcia, A., Puighermanal, E., et al. (2013). Microglial activation underlies cerebellar deficits produced by repeated cannabis exposure. *J Clin Invest*, **123**, 2816–2831.

Da Silva, T., Hafizi, S., Watts, J. J., et al. (2019). In vivo imaging of translocator protein in long-term cannabis users. *JAMA Psychiatry*, **76**, 1305–1313.

Diana, M. A., and Marty, A. (2004). Endocannabinoid-mediated short-term synaptic plasticity: Depolarization-induced suppression of inhibition (DSI) and depolarization-induced suppression of excitation (DSE). *Br J Pharmacol*, **142**, 9–19.

Dujourdy, L., and Besacier, F. (2017). A study of cannabis potency in France over a 25 years period (1992–2016). *Forensic Sci Int*, **272**, 72–80.

Egertova, M., and Elphick, M. R. (2000). Localisation of cannabinoid receptors in the rat brain using antibodies to the intracellular C-terminal tail of CB. *J Comp Neurol*, **422**, 159–171.

ElSohly, M. A., Mehmedic, Z., Foster, S., et al. (2016). Changes in cannabis potency over the last 2 decades (1995–2014): Analysis of current data in the United States. *Biol Psychiatry*, **79**, 613–619.

Farrell, J. S., Colangeli, R., Dong, A., et al. (2021). In vivo endocannabinoid dynamics at the timescale of physiological and pathological neural activity. *Neuron*, **109**, 2398–2403 e4.

Gaoni, Y., and Mechoulam, R. (1964). Isolation, structure, and partial synthesis of an active constituent of hashish. *J Am Chem Soc*, **86**, 1646–1647.

Grotenhermen, F. (2003). Pharmacokinetics and pharmacodynamics of cannabinoids. *Clin Pharmacokinet*, **42**, 327–360.

Gulck, T., and Moller, B. L. (2020). Phytocannabinoids: Origins and biosynthesis. *Trends Plant Sci*, **25**, 985–1004.

Han, J., Kesner, P., Metna-Laurent, M., et al. (2012). Acute cannabinoids impair working memory through astroglial CB1 receptor modulation of hippocampal LTD. *Cell*, **148**, 1039–1050.

Herkenham, M., Lynn, A. B., Johnson, M. R., et al. (1991). Characterization and localization of cannabinoid receptors in rat brain: A quantitative in vitro autoradiographic study. *J Neurosci*, **11**, 563–583.

Howlett, A. C., Barth, F., Bonner, T. I., et al. (2002). International union of pharmacology. XXVII. Classification of cannabinoid receptors. *Pharmacol Rev*, **54**, 161–202.

Huestis, M. A. (2007). Human cannabinoid pharmacokinetics. *Chem Biodivers*, **4**, 1770–1804.

Huestis, M. A., Boyd, S. J., Heishman, S. J., et al. (2007). Single and multiple doses of rimonabant antagonize acute effects of smoked cannabis in male cannabis users. *Psychopharmacology (Berl)*, **194**, 505–515.

Huestis, M. A., Gorelick, D. A., Heishman, S. J., et al. (2001). Blockade of effects of smoked marijuana by the CB1-selective cannabinoid receptor antagonist SR141716. *Arch Gen Psychiatry*, **58**, 322–328.

Itami, C., Huang, J. Y., Yamasaki, M., et al. (2016). Developmental switch in spike timing-dependent plasticity and cannabinoid-dependent reorganization of the thalamocortical projection in the barrel cortex. *J Neurosci*, **36**, 7039–7054.

Kenakin, T. (2019). Emergent concepts of receptor pharmacology. *Handb Exp Pharmacol*, **260**, 17–41.

Laaris, N., Good, C. H., and Lupica, C. R. (2010). Delta9-tetrahydrocannabinol is a full agonist at CB1 receptors on GABA neuron axon terminals in the hippocampus. *Neuropharmacology*, **59**, 121–127.

Laprairie, R. B., Bagher, A. M., Kelly, M. E., et al. (2015). Cannabidiol is a negative allosteric modulator of the cannabinoid CB1 receptor. *Br J Pharmacol*, **172**, 4790–4805.

Lu, H. C., and Mackie, K. (2016). An introduction to the endogenous cannabinoid system. *Biol Psychiatry*, **79**, 516–525.

Lucas, C. J., Galettis, P., and Schneider, J. (2018). The pharmacokinetics and the pharmacodynamics of cannabinoids. *Br J Clin Pharmacol*, **84**, 2477–2482.

Mackie, K. (2008). Signaling via CNS cannabinoid receptors. *Mol Cell Endocrinol*, **286**, S60–S65.

Marinelli, S., Pacioni, S., Bisogno, T., et al. (2008). The endocannabinoid 2-arachidonoylglycerol is responsible for the slow self-inhibition in neocortical interneurons. *J Neurosci*, **28**, 13532–13541.

Marsicano, G., and Lutz, B. (1999). Expression of the cannabinoid receptor CB1 in distinct neuronal subpopulations in the adult mouse forebrain. *Eur J Neurosci*, **11**, 4213–4225.

Matsuda, L. A., Bonner, T. I., and Lolait, S. J. (1993). Localization of cannabinoid receptor mRNA in rat brain. *J Comp Neurol*, **327**, 535–550.

McPartland, J. M., Duncan, M., Di Marzo, V., et al. (2015). Are cannabidiol and Delta(9)-tetrahydrocannabivarin negative modulators of the endocannabinoid system? A systematic review. *Br J Pharmacol*, **172**, 737–753.

Mechoulam, R., and Shvo, Y. (1963). Hashish. I. The structure of cannabidiol. *Tetrahedron*, **19**, 2073–2078.

Millar, S. A., Stone, N. L., Yates, A. S., et al. (2018). A systematic review on the pharmacokinetics of cannabidiol in humans. *Front Pharmacol*, **9**, 1365.

Nadulski, T., Pragst, F., Weinberg, G., et al. (2005). Randomized, double-blind, placebo-controlled study about the effects of cannabidiol (CBD) on the pharmacokinetics of Delta9-tetrahydrocannabinol (THC) after oral application of THC verses standardized cannabis extract. *Ther Drug Monit*, **27**, 799–810.

O'Sullivan, S. E., Stevenson, C. W., and Laviolette, S. R. (2021) Could cannabidiol be a treatment for coronavirus disease-19-related anxiety disorders? *Cannabis Cannabinoid Res*, **6**, 7–18.

Sharma, P., Murthy, P., and Bharath, M. M. (2012). Chemistry, metabolism, and toxicology of cannabis: Clinical implications. *Iran J Psychiatry*, **7**, 149–156.

Spindle, T. R., Cone, E. J., Goffi, E., et al. (2020). Pharmacodynamic effects of vaporized and oral cannabidiol (CBD) and vaporized CBD-dominant cannabis in infrequent cannabis users. *Drug Alcohol Depend*, **211**, 107937.

Straiker, A., Dvorakova, M., Zimmowitch, A., et al. (2018). Cannabidiol inhibits endocannabinoid signaling in autaptic hippocampal neurons. *Mol Pharmacol*, **94**, 743–748.

Straiker, A., and Mackie, K. (2005). Depolarization-induced suppression of excitation in murine autaptic hippocampal neurones. *J Physiol*, **569**, 501–517.

Tahir, M. N., Shahbazi, F., Rondeau-Gagne, S., et al. (2021). The biosynthesis of the cannabinoids. *J Cannabis Res*, **3**, 7.

Tsou, K., Brown, S., Sanudo-Pena, M. C., et al. (1998). Immunohistochemical distribution of cannabinoid CB1 receptors in the rat central nervous system. *Neuroscience*, **83**, 393–411.

Turner, S. E., Williams, C. M., Iversen, L., et al. (2017). Molecular pharmacology of phytocannabinoids. *Prog Chem Org Nat Prod*, **103**, 61–101.

Zamberletti, E., Gabaglio, M., Prini, P., et al. (2015). Cortical neuroinflammation contributes to long-term cognitive dysfunctions following adolescent delta-9-tetrahydrocannabinol treatment in female rats. *Eur Neuropsychopharmacol*, **25**, 2404–2415.

Zou, S., and Kumar, U. (2018). Cannabinoid receptors and the endocannabinoid system: Signaling and function in the central nervous system. *Int J Mol Sci*, **19**, 833.

The Function of the Endocannabinoid System

Nathan D. Winters and Sachin Patel

2.1 Introduction

The *Cannabis sativa* plant, also known as marijuana, is among the most widely used substances globally, with human use dating back to 500 BC (Ren et al., 2019). Largely used for its medicinal and psychotropic effects, the *Cannabis sativa* plant contains a plethora of bioactive compounds known as phytocannabinoids, of which >100 have been identified (Turner et al., 2017). Most notably among these are delta-9-tetrahydrocannabinol (THC) and cannabidiol (CBD). THC is the primary psychoactive constituent of *Cannabis* and is responsible for the 'high' experienced by *Cannabis* users. THC exerts its psychoactive effects through activation of type-1 cannabinoid (CB_1) receptors, which are a major component of the endogenous cannabinoid (endocannabinoid; eCB) system (ECS). CBD is non-psychoactive and exerts its effects through complex polypharmacology that engages a variety of different molecular targets (Ibeas Bih et al., 2015). Interestingly, the study of *Cannabis*-derived phytocannabinoid compounds pre-dates the discovery of the ECS – the structures and stereochemistry of THC and CBD were first described in 1960s (Gaoni and Mechoulam, 1964; Mechoulam and Shvo, 1963), whereas the first cannabinoid receptor (CB_1) was functionally described in 1988 (Devane et al., 1988) and cloned in 1990 (Matsuda et al., 1990). Indeed, the discovery of the ECS was largely born from efforts to identify the biological mechanism subserving the psychotropic effects of THC. Early hypotheses regarding the mechanism of THC posited that the highly hydrophobic nature of phytocannabinoid compounds led them to act by non-specifically disrupting cellular membrane properties (Lawrence and Gill, 1975). Later studies observed that the actions of THC and cannabimimetic compounds were stereoselective (Mechoulam et al., 1980), drove cellular responses characteristic of a G protein-coupled receptor (GPCR) (Howlett

and Fleming, 1984), and required active G_i proteins (Howlett et al., 1986), suggesting cannabinoids exerted their effects through a selective GPCR and this was later confirmed via the cloning of CB_1 (Matsuda et al., 1990). The discovery of the cannabinoid receptors has led to a rich and continuously expanding field of study describing the expansive functions of the ECS.

The ECS is a broadly expressed, lipid-derived neuromodulatory system that is comprised of the cannabinoid receptors (CB_1 and CB_2), the eCB ligands (2-arachidonoylglycerol, 2-AG; anandamide, AEA; other minor eCB ligands), and the enzymes responsible for the synthesis and breakdown of the eCB ligands. The ECS is heavily expressed in the central nervous system (CNS) and has a variety of functions in other tissues as well, including in the gastrointestinal tract, cardiovascular system, reproductive organs, and various immune cells, among others. For the purposes of this chapter, we will focus on eCB functions within the CNS. Generally, eCBs act as retrograde signalling molecules that diffuse from the post-synaptic compartments of neurons to activate pre-synaptic cannabinoid receptors that act to decrease neurotransmitter release probability (discussed in Section 2.4). Aside from canonical retrograde signalling at neuronal synapses, a myriad of additional functions of eCBs in the CNS have been described and continue to be discovered, such as receptors at non-synaptic sites, eCB interactions with additional (non-$CB_{1/2}$) targets, and eCB signalling in glial cells. These topics will be addressed later in this chapter.

2.2 Cannabinoid Receptors

There are two cannabinoid receptors, denoted CB_1 and CB_2. Both are seven-transmembrane, class A G protein-coupled receptors (GPCRs) that canonically couple to $G_{i/o}$ proteins (of note, CB_1 has been shown to couple to other G proteins in some contexts [Eldeeb et al., 2016; Finlay et al., 2017; Lauckner et al., 2005]). CB_1 is the predominant cannabinoid receptor in the CNS, although CB_2 is expressed at low levels also. CB_1 is the primary CNS target for THC, where it is a partial agonist. CBD acts as a negative allosteric modulator at CB_1 (Laprairie et al., 2015). These receptors generally act at pre-synaptic axon terminals to decrease neurotransmitter release probability by a number of defined biochemical mechanisms, such as inhibition of adenylate cyclase-cAMP signalling, inhibition of certain types of voltage-gated calcium channels, and activation of G protein-coupled, inward-rectifying potassium channels. A number of other signalling pathways may be recruited by these receptors as well. For example, CB_1 signalling can confer neuroprotective effects via recruitment of PI_3K/Akt/mTORC1 signalling in some brain areas (Blázquez et al., 2015). Details regarding diverse CB_1 signalling mechanisms have been reviewed in detail elsewhere (Haspula and Clark, 2020; Nogueras-Ortiz and Yudowski, 2016). These receptors are expressed at the terminals of both excitatory and inhibitory neurons and can, thus, play pivotal roles in regulating excitation–inhibition balance in a manner dependent on brain region. Cannabinoid receptors can also directly and indirectly modulate the release of a number of other neurotransmitters as well, such as acetylcholine, norepinephrine, and dopamine (Covey et al., 2017; Pertwee and Ross, 2002).

The apparent depth and complexity of cannabinoid receptor signalling in the CNS continues to expand with continuing research efforts. CB_1 interacts with a variety of other proteins that modulate its function and confer brain region-specific signalling modalities. For example, CB_1 can heterodimerize with a number of other GPCRs in the brain, such as the μ opioid (Hojo et al., 2008), dopamine D2 (Khan and Lee, 2014), and adenosine 2A receptors (Carriba et al., 2007; Moreno et al., 2018), among others. Other non-GPCR proteins that interact with and modulate CB_1 have been described as well, such as cannabinoid receptor interacting protein 1a (CRIP1a) (Niehaus et al., 2007). CB_1 has also been described to exhibit intracellular (i.e., non-plasma membrane) signalling mechanisms, most notably being the description of CB_1 on mitochondrial membranes, where it modulates bioenergetic metabolism in neurons (Bénard et al., 2012). A recent critical advance in our understanding of cannabinoid receptor function, particularly for novel therapeutic discovery at these receptors, is the recent determination of high-resolution structures of CB_1 and CB_2 in various ligand- and G protein-bound states via x-ray crystallography and cryo-electron microscopy methods (Hua et al., 2016, 2017, 2020; Li et al., 2019; Shao et al., 2016; Xing et al., 2020). These discoveries have revealed significant insights into the activation mechanisms of these receptors at atomic resolution and will likely facilitate the discovery of new therapeutic cannabinoid compounds (Congreve et al., 2020).

2.3 Endocannabinoids and Their Synthetic and Degradative Enzymes

Endocannabinoids (eCB) are lipid-derived signalling molecules that are naturally produced by cells and are the native ligands for the cannabinoid receptors. Unlike many other releasable signalling molecules, endocannabinoids are not stored in vesicles (and cannot be, due to their lipophilic nature), but rather are synthesized and released on-demand in response to various physiological stimuli. The primary eCB molecules are 2-arachidonoylglycerol (2-AG) and anandamide (AEA; also known as N-arachidonoylethanolamine). These endocannabinoids and the *Cannabis*-derived phytocannabinoids THC and CBD are depicted in Figure 2.1. A number of other minor eCB ligands exist as well, and have been reviewed elsewhere (Pertwee et al., 2010). 2-AG is a full agonist and AEA a partial agonist at the cannabinoid receptors. Aside from $CB_{1/2}$ receptors, eCBs engage a number of other targets as well, although reports of each ligand's activity at alternative targets are conflicting and vary greatly between assays and model systems. Other proposed targets of these ligands include transient receptor potential vanilloid 1 (TRPV1) (Petrosino et al., 2016; Zygmunt et al., 1999), GPR55 (Lauckner et al., 2008; Ryberg et al., 2007), peroxisome proliferator-activated receptors (PPARs) (O'Sullivan, 2007), K_v4 potassium channels (Gantz and Bean, 2017), $GABA_A$ receptors (Bakas et al., 2017), and others. In addition to their divergent pharmacology, each eCB also exhibits differential biosynthetic and metabolic pathways, discussed next.

2-AG is synthesized in a calcium-dependent manner by the enzyme diacylglycerol lipase (DAGL). DAGL is expressed post-synaptically in dendritic compartments and is stimulated by elevated levels of

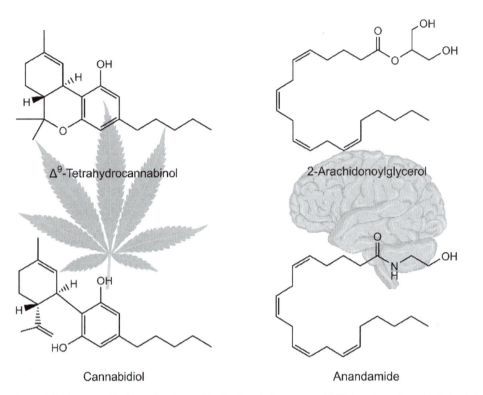

Figure 2.1 Phytocannabinoids and endocannabinoids: Chemical structures of (left) the primary *Cannabis*-derived phytocannabinoids, delta-9-tetrahydrocannabinol (THC) and cannabidiol (CBD) and (right) the major brain endocannabinoids, 2-arachidonoylglycerol (2-AG) and anandamide (AEA; also N-arachidonoylethanolamine).

calcium. Calcium elevations stimulating 2-AG synthesis can be derived from intracellular stores recruited by G_q-coupled GPCRs or through voltage-gated calcium channels and N-methyl D-aspartate (NMDA) receptors (Ohno-Shosaku et al., 2007) during periods of heightened neuronal activity. 2-AG is metabolized at its pre-synaptic site of action by monoacylglycerol lipase (MAGL). A number of other enzymes can metabolize 2-AG as well, albeit to a smaller extent, such as alpha–beta hydrolase domain-containing 2 and 6 (ABHD2/6) and cyclooxygenase 2 (COX-2). AEA synthesis is relatively more complex but is generally via the enzyme N-acylphosphatidylethanolamine-specific phospholipase D (NAPE-PLD). In contrast to 2-AG, AEA is metabolized post-synaptically by the intracellular enzyme fatty acid amide hydrolase (FAAH). Further details on eCB biosynthesis and degradation can be found in Cascio and Marini (2015). The precise mechanisms by which the eCB ligands are released after synthesis remain inconclusive. Passive diffusion of lipid molecules

through an aqueous medium would be entropically unfavourable, and thus alternative models for eCB transport across the synapse have been proposed. One such proposed model is transsynaptic transport by fatty acid-binding protein 5 (FABP5), which may be locally secreted by astrocytes (Haj-Dahmane et al., 2018). A definitive model for retrograde eCB transport and/or diffusion remains to be resolved.

2.4 Endocannabinoid Signalling at the Synapse

The general mechanisms of retrograde eCB signalling at synapses serve to confer control to post-synaptic cells in modulating the degree of pre-synaptic input they receive. eCB release is mediated by the mechanisms highlighted in Figure 2.2 and exists in both tonic (continuous) and phasic (activity-dependent) modes, and this varies by brain region, cell type, and neurotransmitter system. The general mechanisms of eCB regulation of the synapse are depicted in Figure 2.2.

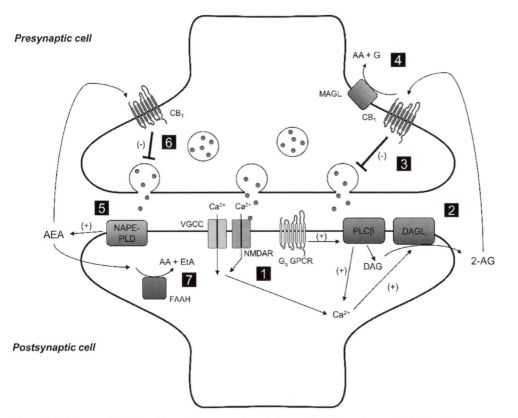

Figure 2.2 Endocannabinoid signalling at the synapse. General diagram depicting endocannabinoid signalling at a neuronal synapse. Some biochemical steps have been omitted for clarity. Grey circles represent glutamate. (1) Enhanced neuronal activity leads to calcium influx through VGCCs and NMDARs. Calcium elevations are also stimulated downstream of Gq GPCR stimulation of PLCβ. (2) Calcium stimulates DAG activity and 2-AG synthesis. 2-AG diffuses in a retrograde manner to activate pre-synaptic CB$_1$ receptors. (3) CB$_1$ activation inhibits neurotransmitter release. (4) 2-AG is metabolized to AA and G via MAGL. (5) AEA is synthesized by NAPE-PLD and then diffuses in a retrograde manner to activate pre-synaptic CB$_1$ receptors. (6) As is seen with 2-AG signalling, CB$_1$ activation inhibits neurotransmitter release. (7) AEA is metabolized to AA and EtA post-synaptically by FAAH.

AA, arachidonic acid; 2-AG, 2-arachidonoylglycerol; AEA, anandamide or N-arachidonoylethanolamine; EtA, ethanolamine; DAGL, diacylglycerol lipase; FAAH, fatty acid amide hydrolase; MAGL, monoacylglycerol lipase; NAPE-PLD, N-acylphosphatidylethanolamine-specific phospholipase D; NMDAR, N-methyl-D-aspartate receptor; PLCβ, phospholipase C beta. A black and white version of this figure will appear in some formats. For the colour version, please refer to the plate section.

Phasic eCB release most often involves 2-AG, whereas AEA canonically provides tonic regulation of synapses (although tonic 2-AG signalling exists as well [Marcus et al., 2020; Oubraim et al., 2021]). Furthermore, eCB-CB$_1$ signalling can also result in variable types of plasticity. Phasic eCB release often results in a form of short-term plasticity, termed depolarization-induced suppression of excitation (DSE) or inhibition (DSI), for glutamatergic or GABAergic synapses, respectively. In some contexts, activation of pre-synaptic cannabinoid receptors results in a much longer, sustained depression of neurotransmitter release, known as long-term depression (LTD). In contrast to conventional models, some mechanisms involving eCB *potentiation* of neurotransmitter release are beginning to emerge (see Piette et al., 2020 for review).

Much of the early literature on CNS eCB signalling highlights neuronally-produced eCBs acting on cannabinoid receptors on neuronal synapses. More recently, the known complexity of the ECS has vastly expanded as the critical functions of eCB signalling within glial cells have begun to emerge. eCB signalling has been identified as an important mechanism for bidirectional neuron-glia signalling, with both groups of cells expressing cannabinoid receptors and the molecular machinery to produce eCBs (Covelo et al., 2021). Of particular interest to eCB regulation at the synapse, astrocytic eCB signalling has emerged as an important regulator of neuronal synapses. CB_1 receptors have been identified on astrocytes, and astrocytes respond to eCBs by mobilizing calcium to drive gliotransmitter release, which can act on receptors present at the synapse (Navarrete and Araque, 2008). For example, activation of CB_1 receptors on astrocytes in the CA1 region of the hippocampus can potentiate glutamate release onto neurons via a mechanism involving pre-synaptic metabotropic glutamate receptor 1 (Navarrete and Araque, 2010). Other studies have and continue to identify similar signalling mechanisms, with the specific gliotransmission systems and synaptic effects varying by brain region. The behavioural functions of glial eCB signalling remain poorly understood. One recent study identified that CB_1 activation in the medial central amygdala (CeM) enhances synaptic GABA release and suppresses synaptic glutamate release, and activation of these astrocytes inhibits CeM neuron activity and suppresses the expression of learned fear (Martin-Fernandez et al., 2017). Future studies will further our understanding of glial eCB mechanisms in complex behaviours.

2.5 Physiological Functions of CNS Endocannabinoid Signalling

The complex mechanisms of eCB signalling in the CNS play pivotal roles in regulating a variety of behavioural and physiological functions, a select number of which are highlighted here:

- *Regulation of stress and anxiety*: eCB signalling is a critical mediator of the brain's response to stress, and deficiencies in eCB signalling are linked to anxiety and increased susceptibility to the negative effects of stress (Bluett et al., 2017). In rodent models, eCB levels in limbic brain areas, such as the amygdala and hypothalamus, change in response to stress exposure, generally with decreases in AEA and increases in 2-AG (Hill et al., 2010, 2017). AEA reduction plays a role in the initiation of a stress response, whereas mobilization of 2-AG is important for termination of the stress response (Hill and McEwen, 2010) and blockade of eCB signalling exacerbates stress-induced activation of the HPA axis (Patel et al., 2004). Pharmacological depletion or augmentation of eCB signalling can exacerbate or mitigate, respectively, anxiety-like behaviours in rodents (Bedse et al., 2017). Accordingly, there is

much interest in targeting the eCB system in the development of anxiolytic drugs (Patel et al., 2017). See Bedse et al. (2020) and Petrie et al. (2021) for further review of eCB regulation of stress and anxiety.

- *Regulation of pain*: It is well documented that administration of exogenous cannabinoids leads to analgesia (Walker and Huang, 2002), suggesting a role for eCB signalling in modulating pain. Indeed, eCBs modulate pain processing at several levels. Peripheral nociceptive neurons express cannabinoid receptors and both CB_1 and CB_2 receptors have been implicated in modulating peripheral pain processing (Agarwal et al., 2007; Guindon and Beaulieu, 2006; Guindon et al., 2007). The ECS is also present in the spinal cord (Nyilas et al., 2009) and can modulate spinal pain transmission – intrathecal injection of cannabinoids produces analgesia (Smith and Martin, 1992) and spinal cord eCB levels increase in neuropathic pain states (Garcia-Ovejero et al., 2009). Finally, eCBs exhibit supraspinal mechanisms of pain modulation as well. eCB signalling within several brain areas, including the periaqueductal grey and rostral ventromedial medulla, can promote analgesia via regulation of descending pain pathways (Palazzo et al., 2010). See Guindon and Hohmann (2009) and Finn et al. (2021) for further reviews of eCB regulation of pain.

- *Regulation of sleep*: THC has sleep-promoting effects (Feinberg et al., 1976) and improved sleep quality is often reported as a motive for cannabis use (Bonn-Miller et al., 2014), suggesting a role for the ECS in natural sleep regulation. Indeed, brain eCB levels exhibit diurnal fluctuations in rodents. AEA and 2-AG show an inverse relationship in this context, with AEA levels highest during the dark (wakeful) phase, and 2-AG levels highest during the light (sleeping) phase (Valenti et al., 2004). Consistent with this, augmenting 2-AG levels by pharmacological inhibition of MAGL promotes some sub-types of sleep (Pava et al., 2016). Similar observations have been made in humans as well – serum AEA levels were highest at waking and lowest before the onset of sleep in a small set of human subjects (Vaughn et al., 2010). Further studies in rodents have begun to identify eCB-mediated mechanisms modulating the activity of brain areas involved regulating sleep and circadian rhythmicity, such as the suprachiasmatic nucleus (Acuna-Goycolea et al., 2010; Hablitz et al., 2020), although how these mechanisms directly regulate sleep remains incompletely understood. See Kesner and Lovinger (2020) for further review of eCB regulation of sleep.

In addition to these highlighted functions, the ECS is involved in a variety of other behavioural functions as well, including (but not limited to) feeding behaviour (Watkins and Kim, 2015), learning and memory (Kruk-Slomka et al., 2017), and addiction (Parsons and Hurd, 2015).

2.6 Emerging Functions of Cannabinoid Receptors: Intracellular Signalling

Cannabinoid receptor functions have largely been attributed to receptors expressed on the plasma membrane. However, a recent and growing body of evidence supports a role of CB_1 receptor signalling in intracellular compartments, particularly at mitochondria (Bénard et al., 2012). CB_1 activation on mitochondria negatively regulates cellular respiration, and this effect has been linked to the amnesic effects of cannabinoids (Hebert-Chatelain et al., 2016). Surprisingly, mitochondrial CB_1 has been demonstrated to decrease synaptic release in some brain areas (Soria-Gomez et al., 2021), a function conventionally ascribed to plasma membrane cannabinoid

receptors. Of note, CB_2 receptors also exhibit intracellular localization in brain tissue (den Boon et al., 2012; note, this study does not specify mitochondria) and mitochondrial cannabinoid receptors have been reported in other tissues as well (Mendizabal-Zubiaga et al., 2016).

2.7 Conclusion

The ECS is a complex neuromodulatory signalling system that plays pivotal roles in brain physiology as well as in other peripheral tissues. Initially identified as the biological target for the psychotropic effects of *Cannabis*, the ECS has been the subject of a continuously growing field of research aimed at understanding its myriad physiological functions as well as identifying novel drugs targeting components of ECS. Ongoing efforts in ECS-targeted drug development include a wide range of strategies, ranging from novel receptor ligands to catabolic enzyme inhibitors, to boost tissue eCB levels. Further characterization of the complex biology of this system and ongoing therapeutic development efforts will likely be synergistic in better leveraging the ECS for the treatment of a wide range of disorders.

Acknowledgements

The authors of this chapter would like to thank Natalie Perez for graphic design assistance for Figure 2.1.

References

Acuna-Goycolea, C., Obrietan, K., and Van Den Pol, A. N. (2010). Cannabinoids excite circadian clock neurons. *J Neurosci*, **30**, 10061–10066.

Agarwal, N., Pacher, P., Tegeder, I., et al. (2007). Cannabinoids mediate analgesia largely via peripheral type 1 cannabinoid receptors in nociceptors. *Nat Neurosci*, **10**, 870–879.

Bakas, T., van Nieuwenhuijzen, P. S., Devenish, S. O., et al. (2017). The direct actions of cannabidiol and 2-arachidonoyl glycerol at

GABAA receptors. *Pharmacol Res*, **119**, 358–370.

Bedse, G., Hartley, N. D., Neale, E., et al. (2017). Functional redundancy between canonical endocannabinoid signaling systems in the modulation of anxiety. *Biol Psychiatry*, **82**, 488–499.

Bedse, G., Hill, M. N., and Patel, S. (2020). 2-Arachidonoylglycerol modulation of anxiety and stress adaptation: From grass roots to novel therapeutics. *Biol Psychiatry*, **88**, 520–530.

Bénard, G., Massa, F., Puente, N., et al. (2012). Mitochondrial CB1

receptors regulate neuronal energy metabolism. *Nat Neurosci*, **15**, 558–564.

Blázquez, C., Chiarlone, A., Bellocchio, L., et al. (2015). The CB1 cannabinoid receptor signals striatal neuroprotection via a PI3K/Akt/mTORC1/BDNF pathway. *Cell Death Differ*, **22**, 1618–1629.

Bluett, R. J., Báldi, R., Haymer, A., et al. (2017). Endocannabinoid signalling modulates susceptibility to traumatic stress exposure. *Nat Commun*, **8**, 14782.

Bonn-Miller, M. O., Boden, M. T., Bucossi, M. M., et al. (2014). Self-reported cannabis use characteristics, patterns and helpfulness among medical cannabis users. *Am J Drug Alcohol Abuse*, **40**, 23–30.

den Boon, F. S., Chameau, P., Schaafsma-Zhao, Q., et al. (2012). Excitability of prefrontal cortical pyramidal neurons is modulated by activation of intracellular type-2 cannabinoid receptors. *Proc Natl Acad Sci USA*, **109**, 3534–3539.

Carriba, P., Ortiz, O., Patkar, K., et al. (2007). Striatal adenosine A2A and cannabinoid CB1 receptors form functional heteromeric complexes that mediate the motor effects of cannabinoids. *Neuropsychopharmacology*, **32**, 2249–2259.

Cascio, M. G., and Marini, P. (2015). Biosynthesis and fate of endocannabinoids. *Handb Exp Pharmacol*, **231**, 39–58.

Congreve, M., de Graaf, C., Swain, N. A., et al. (2020). Impact of GPCR structures on drug discovery. *Cell*, **181**, 81–91.

Covelo, A., Eraso-Pichot, A., Fernández-Moncada, I., et al. (2021). CB1R-dependent regulation of astrocyte physiology and astrocyte-neuron interactions. *Neuropharmacology*, **195**, 108678.

Covey, D. P., Mateo, Y., Sulzer, D., et al. (2017). Endocannabinoid modulation of dopamine neurotransmission. *Neuropharmacology*, **124**, 52–61.

Devane, W. A., Dysarz, F. A., Johnson, M. R., et al. (1988). Determination and characterization of a cannabinoid receptor in rat brain. *Mol Pharmacol*, **34**, 605–613.

Eldeeb, K., Leone-Kabler, S., and Howlett, A. C. (2016). CB1 cannabinoid receptor-mediated increases in cyclic AMP accumulation are correlated with reduced Gi/o function. *J Basic Clin Physiol Pharmacol*, **27**, 311–322.

Feinberg, I., Jones, R., Walker, J., et al. (1976). Effects of marijuana extract and tetrahydrocannabinol on electroencephalographic sleep patterns. *Clin Pharmacol Ther*, **19**, 782–794.

Finlay, D. B., Cawston, E. E., Grimsey, N. L., et al. (2017). Gα_s signalling of the CB1 receptor and the influence of receptor number. *Br J Pharmacol*, **174**, 2545–2562.

Finn, D. P., Haroutounian, S., Hohmann, A. G., et al. (2021). Cannabinoids, the endocannabinoid system, and pain: A review of preclinical studies. *Pain*, **162**, S5–25.

Gantz, S. C., and Bean, B. P. (2017). Cell-autonomous excitation of midbrain dopamine neurons by endocannabinoid-dependent lipid signaling. *Neuron*, **93**, 1375–1387.

Gaoni, Y., and Mechoulam, R. (1964). Isolation, structure, and partial synthesis of an active constituent of hashish. *J Am Chem Soc*, **86**, 1646–1647.

Garcia-Ovejero, D., Arevalo-Martin, A., Petrosino, S., et al. (2009). The endocannabinoid system is modulated in response to spinal cord injury in rats. *Neurobiol Dis*, **33**, 57–71.

Guindon, J., and Beaulieu, P. (2006). Antihyperalgesic effects of local injections of anandamide, ibuprofen, rofecoxib and their combinations in a model of neuropathic pain, *Neuropharmacology*, **50**, 814–823.

Guindon, J., Desroches, J., and Beaulieu, P. (2007). The antinociceptive effects of intraplantar injections of 2-arachidonoyl glycerol are mediated by cannabinoid CB 2 receptors. *Br J Pharmacol*, **150**, 693–701.

Guindon, J., and Hohmann, A. (2009) The endocannabinoid system and pain. *CNS Neurol Disord – Drug Targets*, **8**, 403–421.

Hablitz, L. M., Gunesch, A. N., Cravetchi, O., et al. (2020). Cannabinoid signaling recruits astrocytes to modulate presynaptic function in the suprachiasmatic nucleus. *eNeuro*, 7, ENEURO.0081-19.2020.

Haj-Dahmane, S., Shen, R. Y., Elmes, M. W., et al. (2018) Fatty-acid-binding protein 5 controls retrograde endocannabinoid signaling at central glutamate synapses. *Proc Natl Acad Sci USA*, **115**, 3482–3487.

Haspula, D., and Clark, M. A. (2020) Cannabinoid receptors: An update on cell signaling, pathophysiological roles and therapeutic opportunities in neurological, cardiovascular, and inflammatory diseases. *Int J Mol Sci*, **21**, 7693.

Hebert-Chatelain, E., Desprez, T., Serrat, R., et al. (2016) A cannabinoid link between mitochondria and memory. *Nature*, **539**, 555–559.

Hill, M. N., Campolongo, P., Yehuda, R., et al. (2017). Integrating endocannabinoid signaling and cannabinoids into the biology and treatment of posttraumatic stress disorder. *Neuropsychopharmacology*, **43**, 80–102.

Hill, M. N., and McEwen, B. S. (2010). Involvement of the endocannabinoid system in the neurobehavioural effects of stress and glucocorticoids. *Prog Neuro-Psychopharmacology Biol Psychiatry*, **34**, 791–797.

Hill, M. N., McLaughlin, R. J., Bingham, B., et al. (2010). Endogenous cannabinoid signaling is essential for stress adaptation. *Proc Natl Acad Sci USA*, **107**, 9406–9411.

Hojo, M., Sudo, Y., Ando, Y., et al. (2008). μ-Opioid receptor forms a functional heterodimer with cannabinoid CB1 receptor:

Electrophysiological and fret assay analysis. *J Pharmacol Sci*, **108**, 308–319.

Howlett, A. C., and Fleming, R. M. (1984). Cannabinoid inhibition of adenylate cyclase. Pharmacology of the response in neuroblastoma cell membrane. *Mol Pharmacol*, **26**, 532–538.

Howlett, A. C., Qualy, J. M., and Khachatrian, L. L. (1986). Involvement of G(i) in the inhibition of adenylate cyclase by cannabimimetic drugs. *Mol Pharmacol*, **29**, 307–313.

Hua, T., Li, X., Wu, L., et al. (2020). Activation and signaling mechanism revealed by cannabinoid receptor-Gi complex structures. *Cell*, **180**, 655–665.

Hua, T., Vemuri, K., Nikas, S. P., et al. (2017). Crystal structures of agonist-bound human cannabinoid receptor CB$_1$. *Nature*, **547**, 468–471.

Hua, T., Vemuri, K., Pu, M., et al. (2016). Crystal structure of the human cannabinoid receptor CB1. *Cell*, **167**, 750–762.

Ibeas Bih, C., Chen, T., Nunn, A. V., et al. (2015). Molecular targets of cannabidiol in neurological disorders. *Neurotherapeutics*, **12**, 699–730.

Kesner, A. J., and Lovinger, D. M. (2020). Cannabinoids, endocannabinoids and sleep. *Front Mol Neurosci*, **13**, 125.

Khan, S. S., and Lee, F. J. S. (2014). Delineation of domains within the cannabinoid CB1 and dopamine D2 receptors that mediate the formation of the heterodimer complex. *J Mol Neurosci*, **53**, 10–21.

Kruk-Slomka, M., Dzik, A., Budzynska, B., et al. (2017). Endocannabinoid system: The direct and indirect involvement in the memory and learning processes – A short review. *Mol Neurobiol*, **54**, 8332–8347.

Laprairie, R. B., Bagher, A. M., Kelly, M. E., et al. (2015). Cannabidiol is a negative allosteric modulator of the cannabinoid CB1 receptor. *Br J Pharmacol*, **172**, 4790–4805.

Lauckner, J. E., Hille, B., and Mackie, K. (2005). The cannabinoid agonist WIN55,212-2 increases intracellular calcium via CB1 receptor coupling to Gq/11 G proteins. *Proc Natl Acad Sci USA*, **102**, 19144–19149.

Lauckner, J. E., Jensen, J. B., Chen, H.-Y., et al. (2008). GPR55 is a cannabinoid receptor that increases intracellular calcium and inhibits M current. *Proc Natl Acad Sci USA*, **105**, 2699–2704.

Lawrence, D. K., and Gill, E. W. (1975). The effects of Δ1 tetrahydrocannabinol and other cannabinoids on spin labeled liposomes and their relationship to mechanisms of general anesthesia. *Mol Pharmacol*, **11**, 595–602.

Li, X., Hua, T., Vemuri, K., et al. (2019). Crystal structure of the human cannabinoid receptor CB2. *Cell*, **176**, 459–467.

Marcus, D. J., Bedse, G., Gaulden, A. D., et al. (2020). Endocannabinoid signaling collapse mediates stress-induced amygdalo-cortical strengthening. *Neuron*, **105**, 1062–1076.e6.

Martin-Fernandez, M., Jamison, S., Robin, L. M., et al. (2017). Synapse-specific astrocyte gating of amygdala-related behavior. *Nat Neurosci*, **20**, 1540–1548.

Matsuda, L. A., Lolait, S. J., Brownstein, M. J., et al. (1990). Structure of a cannabinoid receptor and functional expression of the cloned cDNA. *Nature*, **346**, 561–564.

Mechoulam, R., Lander, N., Srebnik, M., et al. (1980). Stereochemical requirements for cannabinoid activity. *J Med Chem*, **23**, 1068–1072.

Mechoulam, R., and Shvo, Y. (1963). Hashish-I. The structure of cannabidiol. *Tetrahedron*, **19**, 2073–2078.

Mendizabal-Zubiaga, J., Melser, S., Bénard, G., et al. (2016). Cannabinoid CB1 receptors are localized in striated muscle mitochondria and regulate mitochondrial respiration. *Front Physiol*, **7**, 476.

Moreno, E., Chiarlone, A., Medrano, M., et al. (2018). Singular location and signaling profile of adenosine A2A-cannabinoid CB1 receptor heteromers in the dorsal striatum. *Neuropsychopharmacology*, **43**, 964–977.

Navarrete, M., and Araque, A. (2008). Endocannabinoids mediate neuron-astrocyte communication. *Neuron*, **57**, 883–893.

(2010). Endocannabinoids potentiate synaptic transmission through stimulation of astrocytes. *Neuron*, **68**, 113–126.

Niehaus, J. L., Liu, Y., Wallis, K. T., et al. (2007). CB1 cannabinoid receptor activity is modulated by the cannabinoid receptor interacting protein CRIP 1a. *Mol Pharmacol*, **72**, 1557–1566.

Nogueras-Ortiz, C., and Yudowski, G. A. (2016). The multiple waves of cannabinoid 1 receptor signaling. *Mol Pharmacol*, **90**, 620–626.

Nyilas, R., Gregg, L. C., Mackie, K., et al. (2009). Molecular architecture of endocannabinoid signaling at nociceptive synapses mediating analgesia. *Eur J Neurosci*, **29**, 1964–1978.

O'Sullivan, S. E. (2007). Cannabinoids go nuclear: Evidence for activation of peroxisome proliferator-activated receptors. *Br J Pharmacol*, **152**, 576–582.

Ohno-Shosaku, T., Hashimotodani, Y., Ano, M., et al. (2007). Endocannabinoid signalling triggered by NMDA receptor-mediated calcium entry into rat hippocampal neurons. *J Physiol*, **584**, 407–418.

Oubraim, S., Wang, R., Hausknecht, K. A., et al. (2021). Tonic endocannabinoid signaling gates synaptic plasticity in dorsal raphe nucleus serotonin neurons through peroxisome proliferator-activated receptors. *Front Pharmacol*, **12**, 1–14.

Palazzo, E., Luongo, L., Novellis, V., et al. (2010). The role of cannabinoid receptors in the descending modulation of pain. *Pharmaceuticals*, **3**, 2661–2673.

Parsons, L. H., and Hurd, Y. L. (2015). Endocannabinoid signalling in reward and addiction. *Nat Rev Neurosci*, **16**, 579–594.

Patel, S., Hill, M. N., Cheer, J. F., et al. (2017). The endocannabinoid system as a target for novel anxiolytic drugs. *Neurosci Biobehav Rev*, **76**, 56–66.

Patel, S., Roelke, C. T., Rademacher, D. J., et al. (2004). Endocannabinoid signaling negatively modulates stress-induced activation of the hypothalamic-pituitary-adrenal axis. *Endocrinology*, **145**, 5431–5438.

Pava, M. J., Makriyannis, A., and Lovinger, D. M. (2016). Endocannabinoid signaling regulates sleep stability. *PLoS ONE*, **11**, e0152473.

Pertwee, R. G., Howlett, A. C., Abood, M. E., et al. (2010). International union of basic and clinical pharmacology. LXXIX. Cannabinoid receptors and their ligands: Beyond CB1 and CB2. *Pharmacol Rev*, **62**, 588–631.

Pertwee, R. G., and Ross, R. A. (2002). Cannabinoid receptors and their ligands. *Prostaglandins Leukot Essent Fat Acids*, **66**, 101–121.

Petrie, G. N., Nastase, A. S., Aukema, R. J., et al. (2021). Endocannabinoids, cannabinoids and the regulation of anxiety. *Neuropharmacology*, **195**, 108626.

Petrosino, S., Schiano Moriello, A., Cerrato, S., et al. (2016). The anti-inflammatory mediator palmitoylethanolamide enhances the levels of 2-arachidonoyl-glycerol and potentiates its actions at TRPV1 cation channels. *Br J Pharmacol*, **173**, 1154–1162.

Piette, C., Cui, Y., Gervasi, N., et al. (2020). Lights on endocannabinoid-mediated synaptic potentiation. *Front Mol Neurosci*, **13**, 132.

Ren, M., Tang, Z., Wu, X., et al. (2019). The origins of cannabis smoking: Chemical residue evidence from the first millennium BCE in the Pamirs. *Sci Adv*, **5**, 1–8.

Ryberg, E., Larsson, N., Sjögren, S., et al. (2007). The orphan receptor GPR55 is a novel cannabinoid receptor. *Br J Pharmacol*, **152**, 1092–1101.

Shao, Z., Yin, J., Chapman, K., et al. (2016). High-resolution crystal structure of the human CB1 cannabinoid receptor. *Nature*, **540**, 602–606.

Smith, P. B., and Martin, B. R. (1992). Spinal mechanisms of $\Delta9$-tetrahydrocannabinol-induced analgesia. *Brain Res*, **578**, 8–12.

Soria-Gomez, E., Pagano Zottola, A. C., Mariani, Y., et al. (2021). Subcellular specificity of cannabinoid effects in striatonigral circuits. *Neuron*, **109**, 1513–1526.

Turner, S. E., Williams, C. M., Iversen, L., et al. (2017). Molecular pharmacology of phytocannabinoids. *Prog Chem Org Nat Prod*, **103**, 61–101.

Valenti, M., Viganò, D., Casico, M. G., et al. (2004). Differential diurnal variations of anandamide and 2-arachidonoyl-glycerol levels in rat brain. *Cell Mol Life Sci*, **61**, 945–950.

Vaughn, L. K., Denning, G., Stuhr, K. L., et al. (2010). Endocannabinoid signalling: Has it got rhythm? *Br J Pharmacol*, **160**, 530–543.

Walker, J. M., and Huang, S. M. (2002). Cannabinoid analgesia. *Pharmacol Ther*, **95**, 127–135.

Watkins, B. A., and Kim, J. (2015). The endocannabinoid system: Directing eating behavior and macronutrient metabolism. *Front Psychol*, **5**, 1506.

Xing, C., Zhuang, Y., Xu, T. H., et al. (2020). Cryo-EM structure of the human cannabinoid receptor CB2-Gi signaling complex. *Cell*, **180**, 645–654.

Zygmunt, P. M., Petersson, J., Andersson, D. A., et al. (1999). Vanilloid receptors on sensory nerves mediate the vasodilator action of anandamide. *Nature*, **400**, 452–457.

Chapter

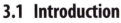

3

Synthetic Cannabinoids

Liana Fattore and Matteo Marti

3.1 Introduction

Since the discovery of the endogenous cannabinoid system as a neuromodulatory system composed of receptors, endogenous ligands, and enzymes responsible for their synthesis and degradation, synthetic cannabinoid agonists and antagonists have been developed, and some of them used to treat specific pathologic conditions. The therapeutic potential of synthetic cannabinoids is indeed still an open question (De Luca and Fattore, 2018). However, contrary to the first cannabinoid receptor agonists originally synthesized for their therapeutic potential, for example the cyclohexylphenol CP-55940 (Pfizer, 1974), the HU-210 compound (Hebrew University, 1988), the naphtoylindole WIN-55212-2 (Sterling-Winthropand, 1994), and the JWH-018 compound (Clemson University, 1994), the newest synthetic cannabinoids show full agonistic activity and high potency at cannabinoid type 1 (CB_1) and type 2 (CB_2) receptors. These new compounds are widely consumed for recreational purposes and abused worldwide. Accumulating case reports of acute and sometimes fatal intoxications associated with consumption of new synthetic cannabinoids reveal that this newest generation of synthetic cannabinoids are less likely to possess therapeutic potential and that adverse effects exceed the desired ones (Altintop, 2020; Sud et al., 2018). Yet, recreational use of synthetic cannabinoid agonists is part of a more general picture of substance use patterns and the drug market. Indeed, over the last decades, an incredibly high number of new psychoactive substances (NPS) have flooded the drug market as legal alternatives to common drugs of abuse.

Similar to many other different classes of NPS, new generations of synthetic cannabinoids have been sold on the global drug market as marijuana-like herbal mixtures since 2004, if not earlier (Dresen et al., 2010; Fattore and Fratta, 2011). Along with synthetic cathinones, cannabinoid designer drugs are the most popular classes of NPS that are posing a major risk to public health due to their harmful medical and psychiatric effects and abuse potential (Weinstein et al., 2017). Commonly known as 'Spice' (mostly in the EU), 'K2' (mostly in the US), 'Kronic' (mostly in Australia), or 'legal highs', these products are typically sprayed on vegetable mixtures, wrapped in sachets with the indication 'not for human consumption', and sold on websites and in specialized shops ('head shops') as marijuana-like compounds, incense, or potpourri (Seely et al., 2012). Recently, synthetic cannabinoids have been sold as 'e-liquids' and taken by vaping via electronic cigarettes (Angerer et al., 2019; Münster-Müller et al., 2020; Wu et al., 2021). Contrary to the natural plant that they are supposed to mimic, products containing synthetic cannabinoids cause frequent and severe negative effects that are not only dangerous but also quite unpredictable (see Box 3.1).

3.2 Pharmacological and Toxicological Effects

Some synthetic cannabinoid-containing herbal mixtures have been reported to induce effects similar to those obtained by smoking cannabis, including physical relaxation, changes in perception, and mild euphoria. Data from both animal and clinical studies indicate that these compounds produce an assortment of effects resembling Δ^9-THC intoxication but that the effects are more profound than with Δ^9-THC itself. This is likely because they are extremely potent full agonists of cannabinoid receptors, show higher potency and affinity for the CB_1 and CB_2 receptors (Basavarajappa and Subbanna, 2019), and induce more adverse and longer-lasting effects (Cohen and Weinstein, 2018; Palamar et al., 2017). Their agonistic activity at the CB_1 receptor is responsible for the reported high mood and feeling of well-being and

> **Box 3.1** Reasons for unpredictable effects of synthetic cannabinoids
>
> - Lack of standardization and quality controls during the manufacturing process.
> - The variety of chemicals they may contain (i.e., ingredients of the same brand can vary over time and across countries).
> - Unknown interactions with other substances present in the herbal mixture (i.e., the provided ingredient list, when present, is often incomplete or purposely misleading).
> - Adverse effects due to the presence of toxic substances such as brodifacoum (Riley et al., 2019; Fasih, 2021).
> - Inter- and intra-batch variations, both in terms of type and quantity of substances present, resulting in unintentional overdosing (Auwärter et al., 2009).
> - The presence of different synthetic cannabinoids in the same package (Langer et al., 2016) may increase the risk of enhancing their pharmaco-toxicological effects (Ossato et al., 2016).
> - Excipients and other additives in the mixture.

likely contributes to the energizing and disinhibiting effects reported by Spice users (Schifano et al., 2009).

Some synthetic cannabinoids have long half-lives and produce active metabolites that also have high affinity for CB_1 and CB_2 receptors (Brents et al., 2011, 2012) and which may induce tachyphylaxis (Wells and Ott, 2011). Sustained binding of metabolites to the CB_1 receptor is likely to account for their potency and long duration of pharmacologic effects and toxicity (Martinotti et al., 2017). Furthermore, the differential ability of synthetic cannabinoids to bind to other receptors (i.e., GPR55; Wang et al., 2020) or to activate G protein or β-arrestine pathways (Grafinger et al., 2021a, 2021b) could modulate their pharmaco-toxicological responses in diverse ways. Synthetic cannabinoids can also cause adverse drug–drug interactions with other substances of abuse as well as with therapeutic agents (Tai and Fantegrossi, 2017).

The first two synthetic cannabinoids identified at the end of 2008 as the main active (not declared) ingredients of an herbal blend were the C8 homolog of the non-classical cannabinoid CP-47497 (i.e., CP-47497-C8) and the naphthoylindole JWH-018 (Auwärter et al., 2009; Uchiyama et al., 2010). The latter is the same cannabimimetic compound originally synthesized by Dr John W. Huffman (JWH) in the 1980s during his search for therapeutically useful cannabinoid drugs. JWH-018 is at present the most studied and best characterized of the newer cannabinoid agonists, and its abuse potential has been demonstrated in animal studies (Cooper et al., 2021; Hiranita, 2015) and linked to its dopaminergic stimulant action (De Luca et al., 2015). Animal studies have also showed that repeated exposure to JWH-018 induces tolerance to its cataleptic and hypothermic

effects and transiently increases serotonin 5-HT_{1A} receptor responsiveness without affecting 5-HT_{2A} receptor responsiveness in male rats (Elmore and Baumann, 2018). JWH-018 also produces oxidative stress in human SH-SY5Y cells (Sezer et al., 2020) that could represent an underlying mechanism of its neurotoxicity. Similarly to the unrelated adamantylindazole compound AKB48, the psychostimulant effects induced by JWH-018 are likely to be mediated by both cannabinoid CB_1 and dopamine receptors and associated with an increased release of dopamine from the ventral striatum rather than through altered activity of the dopamine transporter (DAT) (Ossato et al., 2017). Together with its halogenated derivatives JWH-018-Cl and JWH-018-Br, JWH-018 has been shown to interfere with hippocampal transmission and memory mechanisms in mice, resulting in cognitive deficits (Barbieri et al., 2016); and to impair sensorimotor responses in mice (Bilel et al., 2020). Importantly, human metabolites of JWH-018 and JWH-073 have been shown to bind with high affinity to CB_2 receptors and to possess distinctive signalling properties (Rajasekaran et al., 2013).

Soon after the regulation of JWH-018, new further synthetic cannabinoids appeared on the market, including second generation compounds like the alkyl derivatives (e.g., AM-2201, MAM-2201, AM-694), the N-methylpiperidines compounds (e.g., AM-2233, AM-1220), and the benzoindoles (e.g., AM-679, RCS-4). A third generation of synthetic cannabinoid agonists include indazoles or benzimidazoles (e.g., AKB-48, 5F-AKB-48, FUBIMINA), molecules in which the carbonyl group is replaced with a carboxylic or carboxy-amide functional group (e.g., APICA, SDB-005) and quinolones (e.g., PB-22, 5F-PB-22,

BB-22). Subsequently, many other compounds appeared, and are continuing to appear, on the drug market, including MDMB-CHMICA that induces a spectrum of effects similar to other synthetic cannabinoids but with a particularly high incidence of adverse effects (Haden et al., 2017). In light of the evidence that fluorinate cannabinoid agonists such as 5F-ADBINACA, ABFUBINACA, and STS-135 induce a variety of serious pharmaco-toxicological actions that might explain their detrimental effects in users (Canazza et al., 2017), it has been suggested that fluorination can increase the power and/or effectiveness of these compounds (Canazza et al., 2016).

Importantly, representative synthetic cannabimimetic drugs from five different chemical groups, namely cyclohexylphenols (e.g., CP47497-C8), aminoalkylindoles (e.g., AM-2201, UR-144), 1-alkylindazoles (e.g., 5F-AKB-48, AM-2201-IC), tetramethylcyclopropyl indoles (e.g., XLR-11), and benzoylindoles (e.g., RCS-4), have been shown to possess genotoxic properties whereby they impact the stability of genetic material and cause chromosomal damage without causing gene mutations (Ferk et al., 2016; Koller et al., 2014, 2015). More recently, in vitro studies using human TK6 cells have revealed the mutagenic capacity of several synthetic cannabinoids belonging to different indole- and indazole-structures (Lenzi et al., 2020) as well as a strong cytotoxic potential for several synthetic cannabinoid agonists (Coccini et al., 2021; Gampfer et al., 2021). The CP-55940 compound, for example, has been found to induce apoptosis in a human skeletal muscle model via regulation of CB_1, but not CB_2, receptors and L-type Ca^{2+} channels (Tomiyama and Funada, 2021). Heavy use of synthetic cannabinoids has also been reported to induce DNA damage and increase oxidative stress and inflammatory processes (Guler et al., 2020).

3.3 Intoxication

According to an increasing number of case reports, many individuals present in emergency departments and intensive care units after using synthetic cannabinoids with a variety of manifestations, including central nervous system depression (some are deeply unconscious), seizures, confusion, psychomotor agitation, anxiety, and suicidal ideation (Besli et al., 2015; Thomas et al., 2012; Wells and Ott, 2011). Clinical studies have reported that, compared to placebo, synthetic cannabinoids can acutely affect specific cognitive functions and that, compared to both natural cannabis and non-cannabis users, non-intoxicated users perform differently in various affective and cognitive tasks (reviewed in Akram et al., 2019). Among the most frequent clinical consequences of synthetic cannabinoids use are cardiovascular effects, which may include hypertension, syncope, ischemic stroke, myocardial or cerebral infarction and thrombotic events. Cases of tachycardia following confirmed synthetic cannabinoid ingestion have also been reported (Lapoint et al., 2011), as have ECG changes. Notably, contrary to the beneficial effects of Δ^9-THC and other cannabinoid agonists on gastrointestinal diseases, acute gastric dilatation and hepatic portal venous gas have been reported after consumption of the newest synthetic cannabinoid agonists (Sevinc et al., 2015). Liver damage, hepatotoxicity, and kidney failure (Solimini et al., 2017; Zarifi and Vyas, 2017), as well as hyperthermia, hyperemesis, and rhabdomyolysis (Argamany et al., 2016; Sweeney et al., 2016), have also been reported after use of Spice/K2-containing products. Increased liver enzyme levels are commonly found (Yalçın et al., 2018).

Less is known about the long-term effects of the latest synthetic cannabinoids, although self-harm, self-mutilation, and self-inflicted burns have been reported (Escelsior et al., 2021; Meijer et al., 2014; Thomas et al., 2012). Chronic use of synthetic cannabinoid agonists may lead to impaired performance on working memory and other cognitive tasks (Cohen et al., 2017). After months of Spice use, halting speech, avoidant eye contact, and serious cognitive impairment have been observed (Benford and Caplan, 2011; Zimmermann et al., 2009). Tolerance and withdrawal have also been reported after eight months of daily consumption of Spice (Zimmermann et al., 2009).

Use of synthetic cannabinoids also impacts driving capacity, and numerous cases of users involved in traffic collisions have been reported, with drivers typically presenting with dilated pupils, failure of convergence of the eyes, low body temperature, and muscle rigidity (Karinen et al., 2015; Musshoff et al., 2014). Confusion, slurred speech, lack of coordination, lethargy, and body and eyelid tremor are also commonly observed in intoxicated drivers (Louis et al., 2014; Peterson and Couper, 2015). Depending on the specific compound, a blank stare, failure of horizontal gaze, and vertical gaze nystagmus may also be observed (Lemos, 2014). Worryingly, relatively low concentrations of synthetic cannabinoids can be sufficient to impair driving significantly (Kaneko, 2017; McCain et al., 2018). Findings from animal studies support the notion that driving under the influence of synthetic cannabinoids can be especially risky, as synthetic cannabinoids of different generations and chemical classes are capable of significantly altering sensorimotor functions (Bilel et al., 2019, 2020; Canazza et al., 2016, 2017; Morbiato et al., 2020; Ossato et al., 2015, 2016).

In terms of the induction of psychotic and psychotic-like phenomena, a double blind, placebo-controlled study showed that a moderate dose of JWH-018 induced dissociative (i.e., confusion, amnesia, derealization, depersonalization) and psychedelic effects (i.e. altered internal and external perception) in healthy subjects with no history of mental illness (Theunissen et al., 2022). There is also evidence that products containing new synthetic cannabinoid agonists may exacerbate previously stable psychotic symptoms in vulnerable individuals and trigger new-onset psychosis in individuals with no previous history of psychosis (Fattore, 2016; Hobbs et al., 2018; Peglow et al., 2012; Roberto et al., 2016). In psychiatric settings, it has been observed that synthetic cannabinoid users are typically more agitated and aggressive and showed more psychotic symptoms than cannabis users (van Amsterdam et al., 2015). A single-centre cross-sectional analysis of male patients diagnosed with synthetic cannabinoid-induced psychosis noted high rates of suicidal ideation, involuntary hospitalization, and poor inhibitory control (Altintas et al., 2016). Interestingly, a retrospective chart review showed that women using synthetic cannabinoids were significantly more agitated than men (Nia et al., 2019), suggesting a greater sensitivity to the effects of synthetic cannabinoids in females than in males. The enhanced vulnerability to psychosis found in synthetic cannabinoid users has been associated with abnormal white matter integrity, suggesting that the disturbed brain connectivity observed in adolescents and young adults who use synthetic cannabinoids may underpin the cognitive impairment and the increased risk of psychosis (Zorlu et al., 2016).

Management of acute intoxication with synthetic cannabinoids typically entails supportive care and intravenous fluids to treat fluid and electrolyte alterations (Hermanns-Clausen et al., 2013), although some symptom relief has been reported with benzodiazepines and the antipsychotics quetiapine (Cooper, 2016), haloperidol, and risperidone (Van der Veer and Friday, 2011). Antiemetics can be used to treat hyperemesis (Ukaigwe et al., 2014). Although psychotic symptoms typically resolve within five to eight days of hospitalization and/or antipsychotic treatment, in some cases they can persist well beyond acute intoxication and last up to five months (Hurst et al., 2011).

3.4 Who Uses Synthetic Cannabis?

Curiosity, availability, easy access, affordable cost, and perceived legality are among the most common reasons reported by first-time consumers for using synthetic cannabinoids. Most users smoke synthetic cannabinoids using a joint or a 'bong' (i.e., a water pipe). As they are not easily detected in routine urine and blood analyses, these compounds are particularly attractive to people undergoing drug testing in the workplace or substance use treatment programmes. Homeless or shelter residents and mentally ill persons are overrepresented amongst individuals presenting to public psychiatric emergency departments in the context of synthetic cannabis use (Joseph et al., 2017). Moreover, marijuana users can use synthetic cannabinoids to alleviate cannabis withdrawal (Gunderson et al., 2012).

Although gender- and sex-dependent differences in the prevalence of cannabis use disorders, patterns of cannabis use, and pharmacological effects have been consistently described in clinical and animal studies (Cooper and Craft, 2018; Fattore, 2013; Fattore and Fratta, 2010), relatively little is known about these parameters as they pertain to synthetic cannabinoid agonists (Fattore et al., 2020). That said, males are more likely than females to use synthetic cannabinoids (Castellanos et al., 2011; Forrester et al., 2011), but the differential vulnerability of males and females to their side-effects has been inconsistently reported (DAWN, 2012; Nia et al., 2018). Male users often smoke cigarettes, are binge alcohol drinkers, and use marijuana daily (Caviness et al., 2015; Egan et al., 2015; Gutierrez and Cooper, 2014). Female users are likely to initiate use of synthetic cannabinoids earlier than males (Vidourek et al., 2013), yet male–female differences in the use of synthetic cannabinoid agonists are less evident among users aged 12–34 years old (Palamar et al., 2015).

Adolescents represent the majority of users who share information and experiences about their consumption through online communities and drug forums (Miliano et al., 2018). In light of the effects of exogenous cannabinoids on brain neurodevelopment (see Chapters 7 and 8), use of synthetic cannabis in adolescence is particularly concerning. Pre-natal exposure also carries risks (see Chapter 25), and pregnant female users represent another very worrying group, placing the exposed foetus at an increased risk of neurodevelopmental disorders (e.g., schizophrenia, ADHD, autism) (Alexandre et al., 2020).

3.5 Conclusion

The synthetic cannabinoid agonists, like the JWH series, were initially synthesized for scientific purposes before the illegal drug market turned them into potent and dangerous recreational drugs. The newer synthetic cannabinoids do not seem to possess the therapeutic potential of THC or cannabidiol, nabilone, dronabinol, or nabiximols. Rather, acute intoxication with these agents can have serious psychiatric, cognitive, and medical consequences. Some of these adverse effects have been reported after consumption of cannabis plant (see Chapters 11, 12, and 14) while others, such as hypertension, emesis, seizures, agitation, aggressiveness, and hypokalaemia, are characteristic and usually not observed even after high doses of cannabis (Hermanns-Clausen et al., 2013). Also, as detailed in Chapters 14 and 17, there is a growing concern about the link between cannabis and psychotic disorders such as schizophrenia. One characteristic of this link is a dose–response relationship. Given that synthetic cannabinoids are more potent than THC or THC containing cannabis, it would be reasonable to assume that the link with psychosis might be amplified with synthetic cannabinoids. The newer synthetic cannabinoid agonists thus represent a serious concern for the medical and scientific community, at least until more information on their pharmacology, toxicology, and long-term effects is acquired.

Abbreviations

ABFUBINACA, (S)-N-(1-amino-3-methyl-1-oxobutan-2-yl)-1-(4-fluorobenzyl)-1H-indazole-3-carboxamide; ADHD, Attention Deficit and Hyperactivity Disorder; AKB48, N-(1-adamantyl)-1-pentyl-1H-indazole-3-carboxamide; AM-694, 1-(5-fluoropentyl)-3-(2-iodobenzoyl)indole; AM-679, (2-iodophenyl)(1-pentyl-1H-indol-3-yl)methanone; AM-1220, (1-((1-methylpiperidin-2-yl)methyl)-1H-indol-3-yl)(naphthalen-1-yl)methanone; AM-2201, [1-(5-fluoropentyl)-1H-indol-3-yl](naphthalen-1-yl)methanone; AM-2233, (2-iodophenyl)(1-((1-methylpiperidin-2-yl)methyl)-1H-indol-3-yl)methanone; APICA, N-(1-Adamantyl)-1-pentyl-1H-indole-3-carboxamide; BB-22, Quinolin-8-yl 1-(cyclohexylmethyl)-1H-indole-3-carboxylate; CB_1, Cannabinoid type 1 receptor; CB_2, Cannabinoid type 2 receptor; CP-55940, rel-2-((1R,2R,5R)-5-hydroxy-2-(3-hydroxypropyl)cyclohexyl)-5-(2-methyloctan-2-yl)pheno; CP-47497, rel-2-((1R,3S)-3-hydroxycyclohexyl)-5-(2-methyloctan-2-yl)phenol; DAT, Dopamine Transporter; ECG, Electrocardiogram; EU, European Union; Δ^9-THC, delta-9-tetrahydrocannabinol; EMCDDA, European Monitoring Centre for Drugs and Drug Addiction; FUBIMINA, [1-(5-Fluoropentyl)-1H-benzimidazol-2-yl](1-naphthyl)methanone; GPR55, G protein-coupled receptor 55; HU-210, (6aR,10aR)-9-(hydroxymethyl)-6,6-dimethyl-3-(2-methyloctan-2-yl)-6a,7,10,10a-tetrahydro-6H-benzo[c]chromen-1-ol; JWH-018, (1-(cyclohexylmethyl)-1H-indol-3-yl)(naphthalen-1-yl)methanone; MAM-2201, (1-(2-fluoropentyl)-1H-indol-3-yl)(4-methylnaphthalen-1-yl)methanone; MDMB-CHMICA, (methyl-2-[[1-(cyclohexylmethyl)indole-3-carbonyl]amino]-3,3-dimethylbutanoate); NPS, Novel Psychoactive Substances; PB-22, 1-Pentyl-1H-indole-3-carboxylic acid 8-quinolinyl ester; RCS-4, 2-(4-methoxyphenyl)-1-(1-pentyl-indol-3-yl)methanone; SDB-005, Naphthalen-1-yl 1-pentyl-1H-indazole-3-carboxylate; STS-135, N-(Adamantan-1-yl)-1-(5-fluoropentyl)-1H-indole-3-carboxamide; UR-144, (1-pentyl-1H-indol-3-yl)(2,2,3,3-tetramethylcyclopropyl)methanone; WIN-55212-2, (11R)-2-Methyl-11-[(morpholin-4-yl)methyl]-3-(naphthalene-1-carbonyl)-9-oxa-1-azatricyclo[6.3.1.04,12]dodeca-2,4(12),5,7-tetraene; WDR, World Drug Report; XLR-11, [1-(5-fluoropentyl)-1H-indol-3-yl](2,2,3,3-tetramethylcyclopropyl)methanone; 5F-ADBINACA, N-(1-amino-3,3-dimethyl-1-oxobutan-2-yl)-1-(5-fluoropentyl)-1H-indazole-3-carboxamide; 5-HT_{1A}, Serotonin sub-type 1A receptor; 5-HT_{2A}, Serotonin sub-type 2A receptor

References

Akram, H., Mokrysz, C., and Curran, H. V. (2019). What are the psychological effects of using synthetic cannabinoids? A systematic review. *J Psychopharmacol*, 33, 271–283.

Alexandre, J., Carmo, H., Carvalho, F., et al. (2020). Synthetic cannabinoids and their impact on neurodevelopmental processes. *Addict Biol*, 25, e12824.

Altintas, M., Inanc. L., Oruc, G. A., et al. (2016). Clinical characteristics of synthetic cannabinoid-induced psychosis in relation to schizophrenia: A single-center cross-sectional analysis of concurrently hospitalized patients. *Neuropsychiatr Dis Treat*, 12, 1893–1900.

Altintop, I. (2020). A 4-year retrospective analysis of patients presenting at the emergency department with synthetic cannabinoid intoxication in Turkey. *J Clin Psychopharmacol*, 40, 464–467.

van Amsterdam, J., Brunt, T., and van den Brink, W. (2015). The adverse health effects of synthetic cannabinoids with emphasis on psychosis-like effects. *J Psychopharmacol*, 29, 254–263.

Angerer, V., Franz, F., Moosmann, B., et al. (2019). 5F-Cumyl-PINACA in 'e-liquids' for electronic cigarettes: Comprehensive characterization of a new type of synthetic cannabinoid in a trendy product including investigations on the in vitro and in vivo phase I metabolism of 5F-Cumyl-PINACA and its non-fluorinated analog Cumyl-PINACA. *Forensic Toxicol*, 37, 186–196.

Argamany, J. R., Reveles, K. R., and Duhon, B. (2016). Synthetic cannabinoid hyperemesis resulting in rhabdomyolysis and acute renal failure. *Am J Emerg Med*, 34, 765.e1–2.

Auwärter, V., Dresen, S., Weinmann W., et al. (2009). 'Spice' and other herbal blends: Harmless incense or cannabinoid designer drugs? *J Mass Spectrom*, 44, 832–837.

Barbieri, M., Ossato, A., Canazza, I., et al. (2016). Synthetic cannabinoid JWH-018 and its halogenated derivatives JWH-018-Cl and JWH-018-Br impair novel object recognition in mice: Behavioral, electrophysiological and neurochemical evidence. *Neuropharmacology*, 109, 254–269.

Basavarajappa, B. S., and Subbanna, S. (2019). Potential mechanisms underlying the deleterious effects of synthetic cannabinoids found in spice/K2 products. *Brain Sci*, 9, 14.

Benford, D. M., and Caplan, J. P. (2011). Psychiatric sequelae of spice, k2, and synthetic cannabinoid receptor agonists. *Psychosomatics*, 52, 295.

Besli, G. E., Ikiz, M. A., Yildirim, S., et al. (2015). Synthetic cannabinoid abuse in adolescents: A case series. *J Emerg Med*, 49, 644–650.

Bilel, S., Tirri, M., Arfè, R., et al. (2019). Pharmacological and behavioral effects of the synthetic cannabinoid AKB48 in rats. *Front Neurosci*, 13, 1163.

Bilel, S., Tirri, M., Arfè, R., et al. (2020). Novel halogenated synthetic cannabinoids impair sensorimotor functions in mice. *Neurotoxicology*, 76, 17–32.

Brents, L. K., Gallus-Zawada, A., Radominska-Pandya, A., et al. (2012). Monohydroxylated metabolites of the K2 synthetic cannabinoid JWH-073 retain intermediate to high cannabinoid 1 receptor (CB1R) affinity and exhibit neutral antagonist to partial agonist activity. *Biochem Pharmacol*, 83, 952–961.

Brents, L. K., Reichard, E. E., Zimmerman, S. M., et al. (2011). Phase I hydroxylated metabolites of the K2 synthetic cannabinoid JWH-018 retain in vitro and in vivo cannabinoid 1 receptor affinity and activity. *PLoS ONE*, 6, e21917.

Canazza, I., Ossato, A., Trapella, C., et al. (2016). Effect of the novel synthetic cannabinoids AKB48 and 5F-AKB48 on 'tetrad', sensorimotor, neurological and neurochemical responses in mice. In vitro and in vivo pharmacological studies. *Psychopharmacology*, 233, 3685–3709.

Canazza, I., Ossato, A., Vincenzi, F., et al. (2017). Pharmaco-toxicological effects of the novel third-generation fluorinate synthetic cannabinoids, 5F-ADBINACA, AB-FUBINACA, and STS-135 in mice. In vitro and in vivo studies. *Hum Psychopharmacol*, 32, 3.

Castellanos, D., Singh, S., Thornton, G., et al. (2011). Synthetic cannabinoid use: A case series of adolescents. *J Adolesc Health*, 49, 347–349.

Caviness, C. M., Tzilos, G., Anderson, B. J., et al. (2015). Synthetic cannabinoids: Use and predictors in a community sample of young adults. *Subst Abus*, 36, 368–373.

Coccini, T., De Simone, U., Lonati, D., et al. (2021). MAM-2201, one of the most potent-naphthoyl indole derivative-synthetic cannabinoids, exerts toxic effects on human cell-based models of neurons and astrocytes. *Neurotox Res*, 39, 1251–1273.

Cohen, K., Kapitány-Fövény, M., Mama, Y., et al. (2017). The effects of synthetic cannabinoids on executive function. *Psychopharmacology*, 234, 1121–1134.

Cohen, K., and Weinstein, A. M. (2018). Synthetic and non-synthetic cannabinoid drugs and their adverse effects: A review from public health prospective. *Front Public Health*, 6, 162.

Cooper, Z. D. (2016). Adverse effects of synthetic cannabinoids: Management of acute toxicity and withdrawal. *Curr Psychiatry Rep*, **18**, 52.

Cooper, Z. D., and Craft, R. M. (2018). Sex-dependent effects of cannabis and cannabinoids: A translational perspective. *Neuropsychopharmacology*, **43**, 34–51.

Cooper, Z. D., Evans, S. M., and Foltin, R. W. (2021). Self-administration of inhaled delta-9-tetrahydrocannabinol and synthetic cannabinoids in non-human primates. *Exp Clin Psychopharmacol*, **29**, 137–146.

DAWN. (2012). The DAWN Report: Drug-Related Emergency Department Visits Involving Synthetic Cannabinoids; Substance Abuse and Mental Health Services Administration (SAMHSA), Center for Behavioral Health Statistics and Quality: Rockville, MD.

De Luca, M. A., Bimpisidis, Z., Melis, M., et al. (2015). Stimulation of in vivo dopamine transmission and intravenous self-administration in rats and mice by JWH-018, a Spice cannabinoid. *Neuropharmacology*, **99**, 705–714.

De Luca, M. A., and Fattore, L. (2018). Therapeutic use of synthetic cannabinoids: Still an open issue? *Clin Ther*, **40**, 1457–1466.

Dresen, S., Ferreirós, N., Pütz, M., et al. (2010). Monitoring of herbal mixtures potentially containing synthetic cannabinoids as psychoactive compounds. *J Mass Spectrom*, **45**, 1095–1232.

Egan, K. L., Suerken, C. K., Reboussin, B. A., et al. (2015). K2 and spice use among a cohort of college students in southeast region of the USA. *Am J Drug Alcohol Abuse*, **41**, 317–322.

Elmore, J. S., and Baumann, M. H. (2018). Repeated exposure to the 'spice' cannabinoid JWH-018 induces tolerance and enhances responsiveness to 5-HT1A receptor stimulation in male rats. *Front Psychiatry*, **9**, 55.

Escelsior, A., Belvederi Murri, M., Corsini, G. P., et al. (2021). Cannabinoid use and self-injurious behaviours: A systematic review and meta-analysis. *J Affect Disord*, **278**, 85–98.

Fasih, A. (2021). Lethal coagulopathy resulting from the consumption of contaminated synthetic cannabinoids: The story of a public health crisis. *J Public Health (Oxf)*, **43**, e1–e6.

Fattore, L. (2013). Considering gender in cannabinoid research: A step towards personalized treatment of marijuana addicts. *Drug Test Anal*, **5**, 57–61.

Fattore, L. (2016). Synthetic cannabinoids: Further evidence supporting the relationship between cannabinoids and psychosis. *Biol Psychiatry*, **79**, 539–548.

Fattore, L., and Fratta, W. (2010). How important are sex differences in cannabinoid action? *Br J Pharmacol*, **160**, 544–548.

Fattore, L., and Fratta, W. (2011). Beyond THC: The new generation of cannabinoid designer drugs. *Front Behav Neurosci*, 5, 60.

Fattore, L., Marti, M., Mostallino, R., et al. (2020). Sex and gender differences in the effects of novel psychoactive substances. *Brain Sci*, **10**, 606.

Ferk, F., Gminski, R., Al-Serori, H., et al. (2016). Genotoxic properties of XLR-11, a widely consumed synthetic cannabinoid, and of the benzoyl indole RCS-4. *Arch Toxicol*, **90**, 3111–3123.

Forrester, M. B., Kleinschmidt, K., Schwarz, E., et al. (2011). Synthetic cannabinoid exposures reported to Texas poison centers. *J Addict Dis*, **30**, 351–358.

Gampfer, T. M., Wagmann, L., Belkacemi, A., et al. (2021). Cytotoxicity, metabolism, and isozyme mapping of the synthetic cannabinoids JWH-200, A-796260, and 5F-EMB-PINACA studied by means of in vitro systems. *Arch Toxicol*, **95**, 3539–3557.

Grafinger, K. E., Cannaert, A., Ametovski, A., et al. (2021a). Systematic evaluation of a panel of 30 synthetic cannabinoid receptor agonists structurally related to MMB-4en-PICA, MDMB-4en-PINACA, ADB-4en-PINACA, and MMB-4CN-BUTINACA using a combination of binding and different CB1 receptor activation assays-Part II: Structure activity relationship assessment via a β-arrestin recruitment assay. *Drug Test Anal*, **13**, 1402–1411.

Grafinger, K. E., Vandeputte, M. M., Cannaert, A., et al. (2021b). Systematic evaluation of a panel of 30 synthetic cannabinoid receptor agonists structurally related to MMB-4en-PICA, MDMB-4en-PINACA, ADB-4en-PINACA, and MMB-4CN-BUTINACA using a combination of binding and different CB1 receptor activation assays. Part III: The G protein pathway and critical comparison of different assays. *Drug Test Anal*, **13**, 1412–1429.

Guler, E. M., Bektay, M. Y., Akyildiz, A. G., et al. (2020). Investigation of DNA damage, oxidative stress, and inflammation in synthetic cannabinoid users. *Hum Exp Toxicol*, **39**, 1454–1462.

Gunderson, E. W., Haughey, H. M., Ait-Daoud, N., et al. (2012). 'Spice' and 'K2' herbal highs: A case series and systematic review of the clinical effects and biopsychosocial implications of synthetic cannabinoid use in humans. *Am J Addict*, **21**, 320–326.

Gutierrez, K. M., and Cooper, T. V. (2014). Investigating correlates of synthetic marijuana and salvia use in light and intermittent smokers and college students in a predominantly Hispanic sample.

Exp Clin Psychopharmacol, **22**, 524–529.

Haden, M., Archer, J. R., Dargan, P. I., et al. (2017). MDMB-CHMICA: Availability, patterns of use, and toxicity associated with this novel psychoactive substance. *Subst Use Misuse*, **52**, 223–232.

Hermanns-Clausen, M., Kneisel, S., Szabo, B., et al. (2013). Acute toxicity due to the confirmed consumption of synthetic cannabinoids: Clinical and laboratory findings. *Addiction*, **108**, 534–544.

Hiranita, T. (2015). Self-administration of JWH-018 a synthetic cannabinoid in experimentally naïve rats. *J Alcohol Drug Depend*, **3**, e128.

Hobbs, M., Kalk, N. J., Morrison, P. D., et al. (2018). Spicing it up: Synthetic cannabinoid receptor agonists and psychosis: A systematic review. *Eur Neuropsychopharmacol*, **28**, 1289–1304.

Hurst, D., Loeffler, G., and McLay, R. (2011). Psychosis associated with synthetic cannabinoid agonists: A case series. *Am J Psychiatry*, **168**, 1119.

Joseph, A. M., Manseau, M. W., Lalane, M., et al. (2017). Characteristics associated with synthetic cannabinoid use among patients treated in a public psychiatric emergency setting. *Am J Drug Alcohol Abuse*, **43**, 117–122.

Kaneko, S. (2017). Motor vehicle collisions caused by the 'super-strength' synthetic cannabinoids, MAM-2201, 5F-PB-22, 5F-AB-PINACA, 5F-AMB and 5F-ADB in Japan experienced from 2012 to 2014. *Forensic Toxicol*, **35**, 244–251.

Karinen, R., Tuv, S. S., Øiestad, E. L., et al. (2015). Concentrations of APINACA, 5F-APINACA, UR-144 and its degradant product in blood samples from six impaired drivers compared to previous reported concentrations of other synthetic cannabinoids. *Forensic Sci Int*, **246**, 98–103.

Koller, V. J., Auwärter, V., Grummt, T., et al. (2014). Investigation of the in vitro toxicological properties of the synthetic cannabimimetic drug CP-47,497-C8. *Toxicol Appl Pharmacol*, **277**, 164–171.

Koller, V. J., Ferk, F., Al-Serori, H., et al. (2015). Genotoxic properties of representatives of alkylindazoles and aminoalkyl-indoles which are consumed as synthetic cannabinoids. *Food Chem Toxicol*, **80**, 130–136.

Langer, N., Lindigkeit, R., Schiebel, H. M., et al. (2016). Identification and quantification of synthetic cannabinoids in 'spice-like' herbal mixtures: Update of the German situation for the spring of 2016. *Forensic Sci Int*, **269**, 31–41.

Lapoint, J., James, L. P., Moran, C. L., et al. (2011). Severe toxicity following synthetic cannabinoid ingestion. *Clin Toxicol*, **49**, 760–764.

Lemos, N. P. (2014). Driving under the influence of synthetic cannabinoid receptor agonist XLR-11. *J Forensic Sci*, **59**, 1679–1683.

Lenzi, M., Cocchi, V., Cavazza, L., et al. (2020). Genotoxic properties of synthetic cannabinoids on TK6 human cells by flow cytometry. *Int J Mol Sci*, **21**, 1150.

Louis, A., Peterson, B. L., and Couper, F. J. (2014). XLR-11 and UR-144 in Washington state and state of Alaska driving cases. *J Anal Toxicol*, **38**, 563–568.

Martinotti, G., Santacroce, R., Papanti, D., et al. (2017). Synthetic cannabinoids: Psychopharmacology, clinical aspects, psychotic onset. *CNS Neurol Disord Drug Targets*, **16**, 567–575.

McCain, K. R., Jones, J. O., Chilbert, K. T., et al. (2018). Impaired driving associated with the synthetic cannabinoid 5F-Adb. *J Forensic*

Sci Criminol, **6**, 10.15744/2348-9804.6.105.

Meijer, K. A., Russo, R. R., and Adhvaryu, D. V. (2014). Smoking synthetic marijuana leads to self-mutilation requiring bilateral amputations. *Orthopedics*, **37**, 391–394.

Miliano, C., Margiani, G., Fattore, L., et al. (2018). Sales and advertising channels of new psychoactive substances (NPS): Internet, social networks, and smartphone apps. *Brain Sci*, **8**, 123.

Morbiato, E., Bilel, S., Tirri, M., et al. (2020). Potential of the zebrafish model for the forensic toxicology screening of NPS: A comparative study of the effects of APINAC and methiopropamine on the behavior of zebrafish larvae and mice. *Neurotoxicology*, **78**, 36–46.

Münster-Müller, S., Matzenbach, I., Knepper, T., et al. (2020). Profiling of synthesis-related impurities of the synthetic cannabinoid Cumyl-5F-PINACA in seized samples of e-liquids via multivariate analysis of UHPLC-MSn data. *Drug Test Anal*, **12**, 119–126.

Musshoff, F., Madea, B., Kernbach-Wighton, G., et al. (2014). Driving under the influence of synthetic cannabinoids ('Spice'): A case series. *Int J Legal Med*, **128**, 59–64.

Nia, A. B., Mann, C., Kaur, H., et al. (2018). Cannabis use: Neurobiological, behavioral, and sex/gender considerations. *Curr Behav Neurosci Rep*, **5**, 271–280.

Nia, A. B., Mann, C. L., Spriggs, S., et al. (2019). The relevance of sex in the association of synthetic cannabinoid use with psychosis and agitation in an inpatient population. *J Clin Psychiatry*, **80**, 18m12539.

Ossato, A., Canazza, I., Trapella, C., et al. (2016). Effect of JWH-250, JWH-073 and their interaction on 'tetrad', sensorimotor, neurological and neurochemical responses in mice. *Prog*

Neuropsychopharmacol Biol Psychiatry, **67**, 31–50.

Ossato, A., Uccelli, L., Bilel, S., et al. (2017). Psychostimulant effect of the synthetic cannabinoid JWH-018 and AKB48: Behavioral, neurochemical, and dopamine transporter scan imaging studies in mice. *Front Psychiatry*, **8**, 130.

Ossato, A., Vigolo, A., Trapella, C., et al. (2015). JWH-018 impairs sensorimotor functions in mice. *Neuroscience*, **300**, 174–188.

Palamar, J. J., Acosta, P., Calderón, F. F., et al. (2017). Assessing self-reported use of new psychoactive substances: The impact of gate questions. *Am J Drug Alcohol Abuse*, **43**, 609–617.

Palamar, J. J., Martins, S. S., Su, M. K., et al. (2015). Self-reported use of novel psychoactive substances in a US nationally representative survey: Prevalence, correlates, and a call for new survey methods to prevent underreporting. *Drug Alcohol Depend*, **156**, 112–119.

Peglow, S., Buchner, J., and Briscoe, G. (2012). Synthetic cannabinoid induced psychosis in a previously nonpsychotic patient. *Am J Addict*, **21**, 287–288.

Peterson, B. L., and Couper, F. J. (2015). Concentrations of AB-CHMINACA and AB-PINACA and driving behavior in suspected impaired driving cases. *J Anal Toxicol*, **39**, 642–647.

Rajasekaran, M., Brents, L. K., Franks, L. N., et al. (2013). Human metabolites of synthetic cannabinoids JWH-018 and JWH-073 bind with high affinity and act as potent agonists at cannabinoid type-2 receptors. *Toxicol Appl Pharmacol*, **269**, 100–108.

Riley, S. B., Sochat, M., Moser, K., et al. (2019). Case of brodifacoum-contaminated synthetic cannabinoid. *Clin Toxicol*, **57**, 143–144.

Roberto, A. J., Lorenzo, A., Li, K. J., et al. (2016). First-episode of synthetic cannabinoid-induced psychosis in a young adult, successfully managed with hospitalization and risperidone. *Case Rep Psychiatry*, **2016**, 7257489.

Schifano, F., Corazza, O., Deluca, P., et al. (2009). Psychoactive drug or mystical incense? Overview of the online available information on spice products. *Int J Cult Ment Health*, **2**, 137–144.

Seely, K. A., Lapoint, J., Moran, J. H., et al. (2012). Spice drugs are more than harmless herbal blends: A review of the pharmacology and toxicology of synthetic cannabinoids. *Prog Neuropsychopharmacol Biol Psychiatry*, **39**, 234–243.

Sevinc, M. M., Kinaci, E., Bayrak, S., et al. (2015). Extraordinary cause of acute gastric dilatation and hepatic portal venous gas: Chronic use of synthetic cannabinoid. *World J Gastroenterol*, **21**, 10704–10708.

Sezer, Y., Jannuzzi, A. T., Huestis, M. A., et al. (2020). In vitro assessment of the cytotoxic, genotoxic and oxidative stress effects of the synthetic cannabinoid JWH-018 in human SH-SY5Y neuronal cells. *Toxicol Res*, **9**, 734–740.

Solimini, R., Busardò, F. P., Rotolo, M. C., et al. (2017). Hepatotoxicity associated to synthetic cannabinoids use. *Eur Rev Med Pharmacol Sci*, **21**, 1–6.

Sud, P., Gordon, M., Tortora, L., et al. (2018). Retrospective chart review of synthetic cannabinoid intoxication with toxicologic analysis. *West J Emerg Med*, **19**, 567–572.

Sweeney, B., Talebi, S., Toro, D., et al. (2016). Hyperthermia and severe rhabdomyolysis from synthetic cannabinoids. *Am J Emerg Med*, **34**, 121.e1–2.

Tai, S., and Fantegrossi, W. E. (2017). Pharmacological and toxicological effects of synthetic cannabinoids and their metabolites. *Curr Top Behav Neurosci*, **32**, 249–262.

Theunissen, E. L., Reckweg, J. T., Hutten, N. R. P. W., et al. (2022). Psychotomimetic symptoms after a moderate dose of a synthetic cannabinoid (JWH-018): Implications for psychosis. *Psychopharmacology*, **239**, 1251–1261.

Thomas, S., Bliss, S., and Malik, M. (2012). Suicidal ideation and self-harm following K2 use. *J Okla State Med Assoc*, **105**, 430–433.

Tomiyama, K. I., and Funada, M. (2021). Synthetic cannabinoid CP-55,940 induces apoptosis in a human skeletal muscle model via regulation of CB1 receptors and L-type Ca^{2+} channels. *Arch Toxicol*, **95**, 617–630.

Uchiyama, N., Kikura-Hanajiri, R., Ogata, J., et al. (2010). Chemical analysis of synthetic cannabinoids as designer drugs in herbal products. *Forensic Sci Int*, **198**, 31–38.

Ukaigwe, A., Karmacharya, P., and Donato, A. (2014). A gut gone to pot: A case of cannabinoid hyperemesis syndrome due to K2, a synthetic cannabinoid. *Case Rep Emerg Med*, 167098.

Van der Veer, N., and Friday, J. (2011). Persistent psychosis following the use of Spice. *Schizophr Res*, **130**, 285–286.

Vidourek, R. A., King, K. A., and Burbage, M. L. (2013). Reasons for synthetic THC use among college students. *J Drug Educ*, **43**, 353–363.

Wang, X. F., Galaj, E., Bi, G. H., et al. (2020). Different receptor mechanisms underlying phytocannabinoid- versus synthetic cannabinoid-induced tetrad effects: Opposite roles of CB1 /CB2 versus GPR55 receptors. *Br J Pharmacol*, **177**, 1865–1880.

Weinstein, A. M., Rosca, P., Fattore, L., et al. (2017). Synthetic cathinone and cannabinoid designer drugs pose a major risk for public health. *Front Psychiatry*, **8**, 156.

Wells, D. L., and Ott, C. A. (2011). The 'new' marijuana. *Ann Pharmacother*, **45**, 414–417.

Wu, N., Danoun, S., Balayssac, S., et al. (2021). Synthetic cannabinoids in e-liquids: A proton and fluorine NMR analysis from a conventional spectrometer to a compact one. *Forensic Sci Int*, **324**, 110813.

Yalçın, M., Tunalı, N., Yıldız, H., et al. (2018). Sociodemographic and clinical characteristics of synthetic cannabinoid users in a large psychiatric emergency department in Turkey. *J Addict Dis*, **37**, 259–267.

Zarifi, C., and Vyas, S. (2017). Spice-y kidney failure: A case report and systematic review of acute kidney injury attributable to the use of synthetic cannabis. *Perm J*, **21**, 16–160.

Zimmermann, U. S., Winkelmann, P. R., Pilhatsch, M., et al. (2009). Withdrawal phenomena and dependence syndrome after the consumption of 'spice gold'. *Dtsch Artzebl Int*, **106**, 464–467.

Zorlu, N., Di Biase, A. M., Kalaycı, Ç. Ç., et al. (2016). Abnormal white matter integrity in synthetic cannabinoid users. *Eur Neuropsychopharmacol*, **26**, 1818–1825.

The Epidemiology of Cannabis Use and Cannabis Use Disorder

Deborah Hasin

4.1 Five Key Points

1. The prevalence of current cannabis use and of cannabis use disorder increases with age through adolescence, is highest in young adults, and then declines in older age groups.
2. Cannabis use and cannabis use disorder are more prevalent in males than in females across age groups, although the gender ratio may be changing in the most recent cohorts of youth in the United States.
3. Studies from seven countries show that the prevalence of cannabis use disorder among adult cannabis users is much higher than commonly assumed, ranging from 20 to 33% of users, depending on their frequency of use.
4. Time trends in the prevalence of adolescent and adult cannabis use do not always follow the same patterns.
5. Time trend studies show increases in the prevalence of adult cannabis use and (where measured) in cannabis use disorder in countries that have relaxed their legal restrictions on cannabis use, including the United States, Canada, and Uruguay.

Cannabis is among the most widely used psychoactive substances in the United States (Azofeifa et al., 2016; Carliner et al., 2017; Compton et al., 2016; Grucza et al., 2016b; Hasin et al., 2015b; Kerr et al., 2018) and in other countries (World Health Organization, 2021). While some individuals use cannabis without harm, others experience acute cognitive/motor impairments (Hasin and Aharonovich, 2020; Sofuoglu et al., 2010; Volkow et al., 2016), withdrawal (Livne et al., 2019), respiratory symptoms (Ghasemiesfe et al., 2018), vehicle crashes (Asbridge et al., 2012; Brady and Li, 2014; Hartman and Huestis, 2013; Hartman et al., 2015; Lenne et al., 2010; Li et al., 2012; Rogeberg and Elvik, 2016; Strand et al., 2016; Watson and Mann,

2016), other acute symptoms requiring emergency treatment (Bollom et al., 2018; Gajendran et al., 2020; Richards, 2018; Zhu and Wu, 2016), and cannabis use disorder (CUD) (Hasin et al., 2013, 2016). CUD is characterized by continuing cannabis use despite ongoing related problems, and is associated with substantial comorbidity and impairment (Gutkind et al., 2021; Hasin et al., 2016). Therefore, understanding the prevalence and time trends of cannabis use and cannabis use disorder in the general population is an important public health priority. Trends in perceived risk of cannabis use provide a context for the distributions and trends. This chapter reviews three main areas:

1. Measurement issues in epidemiologic studies of cannabis.
2. Recent prevalence estimates of cannabis use, CUD, CUD among users, and perceived risk.
3. Time trends in the prevalence of cannabis use, CUD, and perceived risk.

4.2 Measurement Issues

Cannabis Use. Cannabis use is measured in surveys by self-report, including interviews and self-administered questionnaires, ranging from single questions to complex modules. Advantages of self-report include the ability to query specific timeframes (e.g., prior 30 days, prior 12 months) and aspects of use (e.g., frequency). Disadvantages include potential under-reporting due to forgetting or social desirability. Frequency of use is most often queried, while measuring quantity or level of THC exposure is challenging for non-standardized substances such as cannabis.

Perceived Risk of Cannabis Use. Surveys measure perceived risk with general questions about how risky participants see hypothetical frequencies of use (e.g., trying cannabis once or twice or using daily). The risks are not defined, so how respondents understand the questions is not explicit. Users and non-users are all queried to gauge overall public perception of cannabis use and changes over time. Risk perception is inversely related to population prevalence of cannabis use, although this link has recently become weaker in US adolescents (Sarvet et al., 2018).

Cannabis Use Disorder (CUD). Substance use disorders comprise the main substance-related diagnoses in the psychiatric nomenclatures used to classify mental illnesses, including the tenth International Classification of Disease of the World Health Organization published in 1990 (ICD-10; (World Health Organization, 2016)) and the Diagnostic and Statistical Manuals (DSM) of the American Psychiatric Association DSM-IV (American Psychiatric Association, 1994) and DSM-5 (American Psychiatric Association, 2013). In the United States, DSM-IV and DSM-5 are used for research and clinical purposes. Clinical modifications (CM) of the ICD are used for large-scale medical record-keeping, billing, and reporting purposes, including ICD-9-CM (Centers for Disease Control and Prevention, 2015) and ICD-10-CM (Centers for Disease Control and Prevention, 2021), introduced in 2015.

Table 4.1 shows the CUD criteria across the systems. DSM-IV, ICD-10, ICD-9-CM, and ICD-10-CM include cannabis dependence, and a category termed 'abuse' in DSM-IV, ICD-9-CM, and ICD-10-CM, and 'harmful use' in ICD-10. Dependence and abuse/harmful use are commonly combined into one category, 'cannabis use disorder' (CUD) for prevalence and time trend estimates. In DSM-5, a single CUD category combines most DSM-IV criteria for cannabis dependence and abuse plus cannabis withdrawal and craving. CUD is measured using interviews, self-report measures, or (in electronic health record systems) by provider diagnoses. Issues in measuring CUD include under-reporting of symptoms due to stigma or forgetting and, among individuals who see cannabis as harmless, not recognizing the relationship of CUD symptoms to their cannabis use. Also, operationalization of criteria may influence reporting, for example, the degree of severity built into wording ('did you ever …' versus 'did you frequently …'). Despite these concerns, studies show that CUD diagnoses are reliable and valid (Denis et al., 2015; Grant et al., 2015b; Hasin et al., 2006, 2015a, 2020).

4.3 Prevalence, US Adults

The main sources of nationally representative US adult data are the yearly National Survey on Drug Use and Health (NSDUH) surveys (Substance Abuse and Mental Health Services Administration) and three national surveys conducted by the National Institute on Alcohol Abuse and Alcoholism (NIAAA) (Grant, 1996, 1997; Grant et al., 2003, 2014). The target populations are household residents. Participants were evaluated in their homes using structured interviews and self-administered questionnaires. Approximately 47,000 participants aged ≥18 were included yearly in the 2002–2019 NSDUH surveys. The three NIAAA-sponsored surveys included the National Longitudinal Alcohol Epidemiologic Survey (NLAES, 1992 [Grant, 1996, 1997]); the National Epidemiologic Survey on Alcohol and Related Conditions (NESARC, 2001–2002), conducted in 2001–2002 (Grant et al., 2004); and the NESARC-III, 2012–2013 (Grant et al., 2015a), with sample sizes ranging from ~36,000 to ~43,000.

4.3.1 NSDUH 2019 (Substance Abuse and Mental Health Services Administration, 2020)

Cannabis Use. Of adults age ≥18, 18.0% reported any past-year cannabis use. Rates were higher in adults aged 18–25 (35.4%) than those aged ≥26 (15.2%). Men had higher rates than women (21.2% versus 15.0%), with a narrower gender difference in younger adults (men, 36.5% versus women, 34.3%) than those aged ≥26 (men, 18.7% versus women, 12.1%), suggesting a narrower gender gap in more recent birth cohorts. Rates were 18.9% among Whites, 20.0% in Blacks, 20.4% in Native American and Alaska Natives (AIANs), 14.6% in NHOPI (Native Hawaiian or Other Pacific Islander), 7.9% in Asians, and 30.5% in those reporting two or more races. Among Hispanics, the rate was 15.2%. Rates ranged from 15.7% for those who had not completed high school to 21.5% for those with partial college education. Rates were higher for unemployed individuals (29.3%) than others (range, 12.6–21.0%).

Daily/Near-Daily Cannabis Use. Daily/near-daily cannabis use was reported by 3.9%, with a sharp age difference: 7.5% in those aged 18–25 versus 3.5% in those aged ≥26. Among cannabis users, 21.8% used daily/near-daily.

Perceived Risk. Perceiving great risk of harm from smoking marijuana once or twice a week was

Table 4.1 Diagnostic criteria for cannabis use disorder in DSM-IV, DSM-5, and ICD-10

	Cannabis Dependence DSM-IV	Cannabis Use Disorder DSM-5[1]	Cannabis Dependence (F1x.2) ICD-10[2]
Stem	A maladaptive pattern of cannabis use, leading to clinically significant impairment or distress, as manifested by three or more of the following occurring at any time in the same 12-month period.	A problematic pattern of cannabis use, leading to clinically significant impairment or distress, as manifested by at least two of the following occurring within a 12-month period.	Three or more of the following manifestations should have occurred together for at least one month or occurred together repeatedly within a 12-month period.
1.	Craving – Not included	Craving or a strong desire or urge to use cannabis	A strong desire or sense of compulsion to use cannabis (craving or compulsion)
2.	Persistent desire or unsuccessful attempts to cut down or control cannabis use	There is persistent desire or unsuccessful efforts to cut down or control cannabis use	Not included
3.	Cannabis often taken in larger amounts or over a longer period of time than intended	Cannabis often taken in larger amounts or over longer period than intended	Difficulties in controlling cannabis-taking behaviour in terms of onset, termination, or levels of use (*loss of control*)
4.	Important social, occupational ,or recreational activities given up or reduced because of cannabis use	Recurrent cannabis use resulting in a failure to fulfil major role obligations at work, school, or home	Progressive neglect of alternative pleasures and responsibilities because of cannabis use, or increased amount of time necessary to obtain or take cannabis or to recover from its effects
5.	A great deal of time is spent in activities necessary to obtain cannabis, use it, or recover from its effects	A great deal of time is spent in activities necessary to obtain cannabis, use it, or recover from its effects	Subsumed in the above criterion
6.	Cannabis use is continued despite knowledge of having a persistent or recurrent physical or psychological problem that is likely to have been caused or exacerbated by cannabis	Continued cannabis use despite having persistent or recurrent social or inter-personal problems caused or exacerbated by the effects of cannabis.	Persisting with cannabis use despite clear evidence of overtly harmful consequences
7.	Tolerance: as defined by either (a) a need for markedly increased amounts of cannabis to achieve the desired effects or (b) markedly diminished effect with continued use of the same amount of cannabis	Tolerance is defined by either of the following: (a) a need for markedly increased amounts of the substance to achieve intoxication or desired effect or (b) a markedly diminished effect with continued use of the same amount of the substance	Tolerance: such that increased doses of the psychoactive substances are required in order to achieve effects originally produced by lower doses
8.	Withdrawal not included	Withdrawal as manifested by either of the following: (a) the characteristic withdrawal syndrome for cannabis or (b) cannabis or a closely related substance is taken to	A physiological withdrawal state when cannabis use has ceased or been reduced, as evidenced by the characteristic withdrawal syndrome for the substance; or use of cannabis or a closely

Table 4.1 *(cont.)*

		Cannabis Dependence	Cannabis Use Disorder	Cannabis Dependence (F1x.2)
		DSM-IV	**DSM-5**[1]	**ICD-10**[2]
			relieve or avoid cannabis withdrawal symptoms	related substance with the intention of relieving or avoiding withdrawal symptoms
	9.	Not included in dependence	Important social, occupational, or recreational activities given up or reduced because of cannabis use	Not included in dependence
	10.	Not included in dependence	Recurrent cannabis use in situations in which it is physically hazardous	Not included in dependence
	11.	Not included in dependence	Cannabis use continued despite knowledge of having a persistent or recurrent physical or psychological problem caused or exacerbated by cannabis use	Not included in dependence
		DSM-IV Cannabis abuse	DSM-5 Cannabis abuse – no equivalent category	ICD-10 Cannabis harmful use[2] (F1x.2)
	Stem	A maladaptive pattern of cannabis use leading to clinically significant impairment or distress, as manifested by 1 or more of the following, occurring within a 12-month period.		Clear evidence that cannabis use was responsible for (or substantially contributed to):
	12.	Recurrent cannabis use in situations in which it is typically hazardous (e.g., driving)	see Row 10; now subsumed under DSM-5 Cannabis Use Disorder	Physical harm
	13.	Recurrent substance use which results in failure to fulfil major obligations at work, school, or home	see Row 4; now subsumed under DSM-5 Cannabis Use Disorder	Impaired judgment or dysfunctional behaviour leading to disability or consequences for inter-personal relationships
	14.	Recurrent substance-related legal problems (e.g., driving an automobile or operating a machine when impaired by substance use)	Not included	Not included
	15.	Cannabis use continued despite knowledge of having persistent or recurrent social or inter-personal problems caused or exacerbated by the effects of cannabis	See Row 11; similar criterion now subsumed under DSM-5 Cannabis Use Disorder	Psychological harm

[1] In DSM-5, the diagnosis of cannabis use disorder is further classified according to severity: two to three symptoms: mild; four to five symptoms: moderate; six or more symptoms: severe.
[2] World Health Organization (2016). International Statistical Classification of Diseases and Related Health Problems (10th ed.). Available: https://icd.who.int/browse10/2016/en (Last accessed 15 October 2021).

reported by 28.6%, with a lower rate in those aged 18-25 than ≥26 (15.0% versus 30.8%).

DSM-IV CUD. The rate of past-year CUD was 1.7%, higher in those aged 18–25 than in those aged ≥26 (5.8% versus 1.0%).

DSM-IV CUD among Individuals Who Used Cannabis. In NSDUH data from 2015 to 2016, the prevalence of CUD was studied among past-year daily/near-daily cannabis users, stratified by age group (Santaella-Tenorio et al., 2019). Risk was greater among adults aged 18–25 than aged ≥26 (31.8% versus 15.7%).

4.3.2 NESARC-III (2012–2013) (Hasin et al., 2015b)

Cannabis Use. Of adults aged ≥18, 9.5% reported any past-year cannabis use. The rate was highest in adults aged 18–29 (21.2%), and lower among those aged 30–34, 45–64, and ≥65 (10.1%, 5.9%, and 1.3%, respectively). Men had nearly twice the rate of women (12.3% versus 6.9%). Among non-Hispanics, rates were 9.4% in Whites, 12.7% in Blacks, 17.1% in AIANs, and 5.0% in Asians. In Hispanics, the rate was 8.4%. Rates differed little by education (range, 9.1–10.4%). Individuals in the lowest income category (USD $0–$19,999) had a higher rate (15.6%) than those with higher incomes (range, 5.9–9.8%).

DSM-5 CUD (Hasin et al., 2016). The rate of past-year CUD was 2.9.%. This was highest in adults aged 18–29 (7.5%) and lower in others (2.9%, 1.3%, and 0.3% in those aged 30–34, 45–64, and ≥65). Rates were higher in men than women (4.2% versus 1.7%). Among non-Hispanics, CUD prevalence was 2.7% in Whites, 4.6% in Blacks, 5.5% in AIANs, and 1.3% in Asians. In Hispanics, the rate was 2.8%. Rates were lowest among those with at least some college (2.5%) and highest among those with high school only (10.4%). Those in the lowest income category (USD $0–$19,999) had a higher prevalence (5.4%) than those with higher incomes (range, 1.5–2.8%).

DSM-IV CUD among Cannabis Users (Hasin et al., 2015b). Among cannabis users, the rate of DSM-IV CUD was 30.6%. Risk was greater for men than women (34.2% versus 24.6%) and among younger adults (35.4%) than others (range, 22.6–29.0%). Rates were higher among non-Hispanic Blacks and Hispanics (35.8% and 33.3%, respectively) than whites (28.9%), AIANs (31.9%), or Asians (26.0%). Rates were lowest among those with

some college (27.7%) and highest among those with high school only (35.0%). Those in the lowest income category (USD $0–$19,999) had a higher rate (34.6%) than others (range, 26.0–29.7%).

4.4 Prevalence, International Adults

Past-Year Use. Globally, cannabis is the most widely-used illicit substance (United Nations Office on Drugs and Crime, 2020). Presented here are estimates based on information from the United Nations Office on Drugs and Crime (UNODC) (United Nations Office on Drugs and Crime, 2021), with additional information from national studies and peer-reviewed articles. UNODC estimates that globally, in 2019, 4% of individuals age 15–64 used cannabis in the past year.

Africa and Asia. UNODC estimated the prevalence of past-year cannabis use in Africa as 6.4%. The UNODC estimate for Asia was 3% in India, 1.3% in Thailand, and 1.4% in Indonesia. In a meta-analysis of Asian countries (Naveed et al., 2020) the pooled CUD prevalence rate was 3.4%.

The Americas Other Than the United States. UNODC prevalence estimates for Central America and South America were 3.1% and 3.5%, respectively. Additional information from the Organization for Economic Cooperation and Development (OECD and The World Bank, 2020) provided the 2017 prevalence of past-year adult cannabis use in 16 Central and South American countries. These prevalences ranged from 1% in Bolivia, Ecuador, and Panama to 8% and 9% in Argentina and Uruguay, respectively, and 15% in Jamaica and Chile. In this region, the mean prevalence was 5% and the median was 3%.

Canada. UNODC indicated a past-year prevalence of cannabis use in Canadian adults of 25%, similar to a 2018 rate of 27.6% in a Canadian survey of adults aged 16–65 (Goodman et al., 2020).

Australia and New Zealand. UNODC reported a prevalence of 12.1% in this region. Additional information from a 2019 survey from the National Drug Strategy Household Surveys in Australia (Chan et al., 2021) showed a prevalence of past-year adult occasional use as highest in adults aged 18–24 (21.9%), and lower in successively older age groups, with the lowest prevalence (4.07%) among those aged 55–74. The prevalence of daily use followed a similar age pattern, ranging from 2.4% in those aged 18–24 to 0.83% in those aged 55–74.

Europe. UNODC indicated a prevalence of adult past-year cannabis use in Western and Central

Europe as ~7.8%. A review indicated prevalences of past-year adult cannabis use in 2014–2016 of 5% in Romania, 7.5% in Sweden, 10% in Bulgaria, 12% in Finland, 13% in Ireland, 13% in the United Kingdom, and 17% in Spain (Manthey, 2019). Population surveys in the United Kingdom indicated 2018 past-year prevalences of cannabis use of 7.1%, 8.4%, and 5.9% in England and Wales, Scotland, and Northern Ireland, respectively (Public Health England et al., 2021). In Ireland, the adult prevalence of cannabis use was 18.3% and the prevalence of CUD among users was 41.3% (Millar et al., 2021).

4.5 Prevalence, US Adolescents

The two main sources of nationally representative US adolescent data on cannabis use are the yearly NSDUH (age 12–17) and Monitoring the Future (MTF) surveys (National Institute on Drug Abuse, 2021; University of Michigan, 2021). The NSDUH survey methodology has already been described; youth aged 12–17 are included. Monitoring the Future surveys include a total of ~50,000 students yearly across 8th, 10th, and 12th grades (approximately 13, 15, and 17 years old) who participate in confidential self-administered surveys in schools. The MTF complex sample design provides national estimates of cannabis use and other health behaviours and conditions among school-attending adolescents (National Institute on Drug Abuse, 2021). Using consistent survey questions, MTF has collected data on cannabis use in all three grades since 1991.

4.5.1 NSDUH Youth (Substance Abuse and Mental Health Services Administration, 2020)

Past-Year Cannabis Use. In 2019, 13.2% reported past-year cannabis use. Among boys and girls, 13.0% and 13.4% reported past-year use; thus, youth prevalence was slightly higher in girls. Prevalence of use was 13.0% in Whites, 12.7% in Blacks, 17.9% in AIANs, 4.0% in Asians, 15.4% in those with two or more race/ethnic categories, and 15.2% in Hispanics.

Daily/Near-Daily Use. The prevalence of past-year daily/near-daily cannabis use was 1.1%; among these, 8.6% had daily/near-daily use.

Perceived Great Risk. Of youth, 22.6% perceived great risk in using cannabis once a month.

4.5.2 Monitoring The Future, 2019 (Johnston et al., 2020)

MTF provides separate information for 8th, 10th, and 12th graders, but not pooled across grades. The prevalence of any past-year cannabis use shows a clear ascending age gradient among 8th, 10th, and 12th graders (11.8%, 28.8%, and 35.7%), as does the prevalence of daily use (8th, 10th, and 12th graders: 1.3%, 4.8%, and 6.4%, respectively).

Perceived Great Risk. Perceived great risk in using cannabis regularly was higher in younger than older adolescents: 51.4% in 8th graders, 39.5% in 10th graders, and 30.5% in 12th graders.

4.6 Prevalence, International Adolescents

In UNODC reports (United Nations Office on Drugs and Crime, 2021), past-year cannabis use among students aged 15–17 was reported as 2.5% in Tunisia, 2.5% in Egypt, 5.0% in Morocco, 5.1% in Costa Rica, and 6.6% in El Salvador; and <1.0% among those aged 10–17 in India. Among students aged 15–16 in 34 European countries, the mean rate of past-year cannabis use was approximately 13%, with a range of 5.1% in Iceland to 23% in Czechia and Italy. By gender, 15% of boys and 11% of girls reported past-year cannabis use. In addition, pooled 2015 youth data from 20 European countries showed a mean prevalence of 12.11% (Benedetti et al., 2021) and a much lower prevalence of frequent use, 0.68%. In 2017 online surveys of youth aged 16–19, past-month use was reported by 12.7% in Canada and 10.3% in England (Wadsworth and Hammond, 2019), while perceived harm in use was reported by approximately 37% of youth in Canada and England. In Australia in 2019, 7.6% of youth aged 14–17 used cannabis once or twice to weekly in the past year, and 0.44% used daily (Chan et al., 2021).

4.7 Time Trends, United States

US Trends in Adult Cannabis Use. In NESARC surveys, between 2001–2002 and 2012–2013, the prevalence of cannabis use more than doubled, to 9.5% (Hasin et al., 2015b). NSDUH surveys from 2002 to 2014 (Azofeifa et al., 2016; Carliner et al., 2017; Compton et al., 2016) indicated that past-year cannabis use increased from 10.4% to 13.3%, as did past-year daily/near daily use and mean days used; and past-month use and daily/near daily use; 2007 was the year these increases began. NSDUH data show further increases in past-year use by 2019, to 18.0% (Substance Abuse and Mental Health Services Administration, 2020), reflecting a 75% increase since 2002. Additionally, cannabis or its metabolites in biological samples from drivers in fatal crashes increased significantly between 1999 and 2010 (Brady and Li, 2014), as did cannabis or metabolites in samples from pilots in fatal crashes since 2000 (McKay and Groff, 2016). Calls to poison exposure centres involving cannabis increased 150% from 2000 to 2017 (O'Neill-Dee et al., 2020).

US Trends in Perceived Risk. Between 2002–2014, the proportion of US adults perceiving no risk in cannabis use increased from 5.6% to 15.1%. Among users, perceiving no risk increased from 28.4% to 49.5% (Compton et al., 2016).

US Trends in Adult CUD. NLAES, NESARC, and NESARC-III data showed that the prevalence of past-year DSM-IV CUD increased from 1.2% to 1.5% from 1991–1992 to 2001–2002 (Compton et al., 2004), and to 2.9% by 2012–2013 (Hasin et al., 2015b). However, NSDUH surveys did not show an increase in DSM-IV CUD from 2002 to 2014, remaining at ~1.5% (Compton et al., 2016; Grucza et al., 2016b). Given these inconsistencies, NSDUH data from 2017 were re-examined with a proxy measure for DSM-5 CUD, which indicated an increase (Compton et al., 2019). Studies of large-scale electronic medical record databases that included ICD-9-CM CUD diagnoses (Centers for Disease Control and Prevention, 2015) provided additional information. These showed increases in prevalence from 2002 to 2009 in Veterans Administration patients (Bonn-Miller et al., 2012); from 2002 to 2011 (Charilaou et al., 2017) and from 1998 to 2014 (Singh, 2022) in national samples of hospital inpatients, and in inpatients from individual states between 1997 and 2014 (Shi, 2017).

US Trends in Youth Cannabis Use. In NSDUH 2002–2014 surveys, the prevalence of any past-year use among youth aged 12–17 decreased significantly, from 15.8% to 13.1% (Grucza et al., 2016a; Han et al., 2017), remaining stable in 2019 (13.2%) (Substance Abuse and Mental Health Services Administration, 2020). MTF surveys (Miech et al., 2021) showed that any past-year use was at its lowest in 1991 (6.2%, 23.9%, and 31.2% in 8th, 10th, and 12th graders, respectively), reached a high late in the 1990s (e.g.,

in 1999, 16.5%, 32.1%, and 37.8% in 8th, 10th, and 12th graders, respectively), and then decreased by 2020 in 8th and 10th graders (to 11.4% and 28.0%, respectively) while fluctuating from year to year in 12th graders (e.g., 35.2% in 2020). Of concern were increases in daily use, from a low in 1991 (0.2%, 0.8%, and 2.0% in 8th, 10th, and 12th graders, respectively) to 1.1%, 4.4%, and 6.9%, respectively, in 2020. An additional concern was a sharp increase in cannabis vaping, reported by 3.9%, 12.6%, and 14.0% of 8th, 10th, and 12th graders, respectively, in 2019 (Miech et al., 2020).

US Trends in Adolescent CUD. From 2002 to 2014, CUD prevalence in NSDUH participants aged 12–17 decreased from 4.3% to 2.3% (Grucza et al., 2016a; Han et al., 2017). In 2020, the prevalence was 2.8% (Substance Abuse and Mental Health Services Administration, 2020). The MTF did not assess CUD in adolescents.

4.8 Time Trends, International

Australia/New Zealand. In Australia, between 2001 and 2019 (Chan et al., 2021), the prevalence of cannabis use decreased among participants aged 14–39, with the sharpest decrease (21% to 8%) among those aged 14–17. In contrast, the prevalence of use increased among adults aged 40–54 (from 7.2% to 11.1%) and aged 55–74 (from 1.0% to 4.9%). Daily use also decreased among those aged 14–39 (from 2.5% to 0.44%) but increased from 1.1% to 2.2% among those aged 40–54, and from 0.01% to 0.83% among those aged 55–74.

United Kingdom (Public Health England et al., 2021). National surveys in England and Wales among those aged 16–59 showed a significant decrease in the prevalence of any past-year use from 1996 (9.5%) to 2018–2019 (7.6%). In Scotland, among those aged 16–64, the prevalence of use increased slightly between 2008/2009 and 2017/2018, from 7.7% to 8.4%. In Northern Ireland, the prevalence of use since 2008–2009 in those aged 15–64 was fairly stable, at around 5%.

Other Countries. UNODC (United Nations Office on Drugs and Crime, 2021) suggested an increase in the prevalence of adult cannabis use in several countries, including Belgium, France, Germany, the Netherlands, Norway, and Sweden, but not Italy and Spain. Across European secondary school students aged 15–16, the prevalence of past-year use has been stable since 2007 (~12.5%), although declines in this age group were found in countries with particularly high prevalence of use, for example, Czechia, France, and Spain. In South America, adult cannabis use increased in Argentina and Chile, but not in Bolivia or Columbia (United Nations Office on Drugs and Crime, 2021). Trends in two countries, Canada and Uruguay, are of particular interest because these countries legalized cannabis use. In Canada, which legalized use in 2018, cannabis use increased from 2018 to 2020. In Uruguay, which legalized use in 2013, the prevalence in adults increased from nearly zero in 2001 to about 12.5% in 2018, with greater increases from 2013 to 2018, and in students aged 13–17, from 8% in 2003 to 20% in 2018.

4.9 Discussion

This chapter indicates that the prevalence of cannabis use among adults varies widely across regions, countries, demographic characteristics, and time. However, prevalence is consistently highest among young adults. Gender differences are also found, with higher rates among males, although this may be changing in younger US cohorts. Across regions, prevalence rates of past-year use were lowest in Asian countries and some countries in Central and South America, and intermediate in Australia, New Zealand, and many European countries. The highest prevalences were found in recent surveys in North America, including the United States and Canada.

Less prevalence information was available on CUD, and rates varied even between US surveys, a finding attributed to differences in sensitivity of the diagnostic measures used (Compton et al., 2019). However, the demographic characteristics of those with past-year CUD were consistent across surveys, with a higher prevalence in younger adults and in men compared to women.

It is important to note the prevalence of CUD among cannabis users, commonly assumed to be low (10%) (Degenhardt and Hall, 2012; Hall and Degenhardt, 2009; Koob and Le Moal, 2001; Leung et al., 2020). However, this assumption is based on data almost 30 years old (Anthony et al., 1994). Since then, cannabis products have become more potent (Englund et al., 2017; Rigucci et al., 2016) and CUD definitions have been refined (Hasin et al., 2013). A recent meta-analysis of CUD prevalence among users in seven countries showed a pooled estimate of 22% (Leung et al., 2020) while, among frequent users, the risk of CUD was even greater, approximately one in three. This updated information about the risk for CUD among cannabis users is important to convey to clinicians, policymakers, and the public.

Across studies, the prevalence of adolescent past-year cannabis use varied widely, with two major US studies reporting overall prevalences of 13.2% in those ages 12–17 and prevalences ranging from 11.8 to 35.7% from grades 8 to 12 (modal ages 13–17). About 20% of US adolescents perceived risk in any cannabis use, while one-third to one-half perceived great risk in regular use. In other countries, prevalence was lowest in Asian and Central American countries, and intermediate in European countries. Some of this variation in prevalence was almost certainly due to true group differences, but methodological differences are also likely to account for some of the variability. These include inconsistencies in the age groups in the different studies, since the likelihood of cannabis use varies by age, and variation across survey sampling methods, measurement, and degree of confidentiality experienced by the participants.

Trends in prevalence differed markedly between US adolescents and adults. In US adults, cannabis use and CUD increased over the last decade during a time of increasingly permissive cannabis laws. The same was found in Canada and Uruguay during their post-legalization periods. In contrast, the prevalence of adolescent cannabis use has tended to decrease, although results across studies were less consistent than those for adults. Less information was available on adolescent CUD, but the decreases in adolescent CUD in NSDUH data were consistent with the decreases in rates of cannabis use in NSDUH and MTF.

The limitations of the data and findings presented in this chapter are many. These include inconsistencies in years covered, sample designs, age ranges, measures used, methods of collecting data (e.g., self-versus interviewer-administered), and adjustment methods used to produce representative findings. In addition, few surveys have covered medical as well as non-medical cannabis use, or types of cannabis products used (e.g., flower/plant versus concentrates), which affects potency. These latter features merit inclusion in all future large-scale epidemiologic studies of cannabis.

4.10 Conclusion

The prevalence of cannabis use and CUD varies widely by world region and by age. However, evidence is clear that prevalences have recently increased in North American adults. While stable rates or decreases were seen in adolescents, recent increases in daily use among users, and in vaping, warrant attention. As marketing intensifies after passage of recreational marijuana laws and as public attitudes toward cannabis continue to become more positive, further increases in use may be seen in adults and in some youth. Policymakers will need to address prevention in passing legislation, and in increasing treatment services to meet an increasing need. Some public education may prove useful as well. Such educational efforts should avoid exaggerated scare tactics, such as those of the mid-twentieth century, but instead provide a balanced picture that informs the public about potential pros and cons of cannabis use.

References

American Psychiatric Association. (1994). *Diagnostic and Statistical Manual of Mental Disorders*, 4th ed. Virginia: American Psychiatric Association.

(2013). *Diagnostic and Statistical Manual of Mental Disorders*, 5th ed. Virginia: American Psychiatric Association.

Anthony, J. C., Warner, L. A., and Kessler, R. C. (1994). Comparative epidemiology of dependence on tobacco, alcohol, controlled substances, and inhalants: Basic findings from the National Comorbidity Survey. *Exp Clin Psychopharmacol*, **2**, 244–268.

Asbridge, M., Hayden, J. A., and Cartwright, J. L. (2012). Acute cannabis consumption and motor vehicle collision risk: Systematic review of observational studies and meta-analysis. *BMJ*, **344**, e536.

Azofeifa, A., Mattson, M. E., Schauer, G., et al. (2016). National estimates of marijuana use and related indicators: National Survey on Drug Use and Health, United States, 2002–2014. *Morbid Mortal Week Rep (MMWR)*, **65**, 1–28.

Benedetti, E., Resce, G., Brunori, P., et al. (2021). Cannabis policy changes and adolescent cannabis use: Evidence from Europe. *Int J Environ Res Public Health*, **18**, 5174.

Bollom, A., Austrie, J., Hirsch, W., et al. (2018). Emergency department burden of nausea and vomiting associated with cannabis use disorder: US trends from 2006 to 2013. *J Clin Gastroenterol*, **52**, 778–783.

Bonn-Miller, M. O., Harris, A. H., and Trafton, J. A. (2012). Prevalence of cannabis use disorder diagnoses among veterans in 2002, 2008, and 2009. *Psychol Serv*, **9**, 404–416.

Brady, J. E., and Li, G. (2014). Trends in alcohol and other drugs detected in fatally injured drivers in the United States, 1999–2010. *Am J Epidemiol*, **179**, 692–699.

Carliner, H., Mauro, P. M., Brown, Q. L., et al. (2017). The widening gender gap in marijuana use prevalence in the U.S. during a period of economic change, 2002–2014. *Drug Alcohol Depend*, **170**, 51–58.

Centers for Disease Control and Prevention. (2015). *International Classification of Diseases*, 9th Revision, Clinical Modification (ICD-9-CM). Available at: www.cdc.gov/nchs/icd/icd9cm.htm (Last accessed 17 October 2021).

(2021). *International Classification of Diseases*, 10th Revision, Clinical Modification (ICD-10-CM). Available at: www.cdc.gov/nchs/icd/icd10cm.htm (Last accessed 17 October 2021).

Chan, G., Chiu, V., Sun, T., et al. (2021). Age-related trends in cannabis use in Australia. Findings from a series of large nationally representative surveys. *Addict Behav*, **123**, 107059.

Charilaou, P., Agnihotri, K., Garcia, P., et al. (2017). Trends of cannabis use disorder in the inpatient: 2002 to 2011. *Am J Med*, **130**, 678–687 e7.

Compton, W. M., Grant, B. F., Colliver, J. D., et al. (2004). Prevalence of marijuana use disorders in the United States: 1991–1992 and 2001–2002. *JAMA*, **291**, 2114–2121.

Compton, W. M., Han, B., Jones, C. M., et al. (2016). Marijuana use and use disorders in adults in the USA, 2002–14: Analysis of annual cross-sectional surveys. *Lancet Psychiatry*, **3**, 954–964.

(2019). Cannabis use disorders among adults in the United States during a time of increasing use of cannabis. *Drug Alcohol Depend*, **204**, 107468.

Degenhardt, L., & Hall, W. (2012). Extent of illicit drug use and dependence, and their contribution to the global burden of disease. *Lancet*, **379**, 55–70.

Denis, C. M., Gelernter, J., Hart, A. B., et al. (2015). Inter-observer reliability of DSM-5 substance use disorders. *Drug Alcohol Depend*, **153**, 229–235.

Englund, A., Freeman, T. P., Murray, R. M., et al. (2017). Can we make cannabis safer? *Lancet Psychiatry*, **4**, 643–648.

Gajendran, M., Sifuentes, J., Bashashati, M., et al. (2020). Cannabinoid hyperemesis syndrome: Definition, pathophysiology, clinical spectrum, insights into acute and long-term management. *J Invest Med*, **68**, 1309–1316.

Ghasemiesfe, M., Ravi, D., Vali, M., et al. (2018). Marijuana use, respiratory symptoms, and pulmonary function: A systematic review and meta-analysis. *Ann Intern Med*, **169**, 106–115.

Goodman, S., Wadsworth, E., Leos-Toro, C., et al. (2020). Prevalence and forms of cannabis use in legal vs. illegal recreational cannabis markets. *Int J Drug Policy*, **76**, 102658.

Grant, B. F. (1996). Prevalence and correlates of drug use and DSM-IV drug dependence in the United States: Results of the National Longitudinal Alcohol Epidemiologic Survey. *J Subst Abuse*, **8**, 195–210.

(1997). Prevalence and correlates of alcohol use and DSM-IV alcohol dependence in the United States: Results of the National Longitudinal Alcohol Epidemiologic Survey. *J Stud Alcohol*, **58**, 464–473.

Grant, B. F., Chu, A., Sigman, R., et al. (2014). *Source and Accuracy Statement: National Epidemiologic Survey on Alcohol and Related Conditions-III (NESARC-III)*. Rockville, MD: National Institute on Alcohol Abuse and Alcoholism. Available at: www .niaaa.nih.gov/sites/default/files/ NESARC_Final_Report_FINAL_ 1_8_15.pdf (Last accessed 10 October 2021).

Grant, B. F., Goldstein, R. B., Saha, T. D., et al. (2015a). Epidemiology of DSM-5 alcohol use disorder: Results from the National Epidemiologic Survey on Alcohol and Related Conditions III. *JAMA Psychiatry*, **72**, 757–766.

Grant, B. F., Goldstein, R. B., Smith, S. M., et al. (2015b). The Alcohol Use Disorder and Associated Disabilities Interview Schedule-5 (AUDADIS-5): Reliability of

substance use and psychiatric disorder modules in a general population sample. *Drug Alcohol Depend*, **148**, 27–33.

Grant, B. F., Moore, T. C., Shepard, J., et al. (2003). *Source and Accuracy Statement: Wave 1 National Epidemiologic Survey on Alcohol and Related Conditions (NESARC)*. Bethesda, MD: National Institute on Alcohol Abuse and Alcoholism.

Grant, B. F., Stinson, F. S., Dawson, D. A., et al. (2004). Prevalence and co-occurrence of substance use disorders and independent mood and anxiety disorders: Results from the National Epidemiologic Survey on Alcohol and Related Conditions. *Arch Gen Psychiatry*, **61**, 807–816.

Grucza, R. A., Agrawal, A., Krauss, M. J., et al. (2016a). Declining prevalence of marijuana use disorders among adolescents in the United States, 2002 to 2013. *J Am Acad Child Adolesc Psychiatry*, **55**, 487–494 e6.

(2016b). Recent trends in the prevalence of marijuana use and associated disorders in the United States. *JAMA Psychiatry*, **73**, 300–301.

Gutkind, S., Fink, D. S., Shmulewitz, D., et al. Psychosocial and health problems associated with alcohol use disorder and cannabis use disorder in U.S. adults. Drug Alcohol Depend. 2021 Dec 1;229 (Pt B):109137.

Hall, W., and Degenhardt, L. (2009). Adverse health effects of non-medical cannabis use. *Lancet*, **374**, 1383–1391.

Han, B., Compton, W. M., Jones, C. M., et al. (2017). Cannabis use and cannabis use disorders among youth in the United States, 2002–2014. *J Clin Psychiatry*, **78**, 1404–1413.

Hartman, R. L., Brown, T. L., Milavetz, G., et al. (2015) Cannabis effects on driving lateral control with and

without alcohol. *Drug Alcohol Depend*, **154**, 25–37.

Hartman, R. L., and Huestis, M. A. (2013). Cannabis effects on driving skills. *Clin Chem*, **59**, 478–492.

Hasin, D., Samet, S., Nunes, E., et al. (2006). Diagnosis of comorbid psychiatric disorders in substance users assessed with the Psychiatric Research Interview for Substance and Mental Disorders for DSM-IV. *Am J Psychiatry*, **163**, 689–696.

Hasin, D., Shmulewitz, D., Stohl, M., et al. (2020). Test–retest reliability of DSM-5 substance disorder measures as assessed with the PRISM-5, a clinician-administered diagnostic interview. *Drug Alcohol Depend*, **216**, 108294.

Hasin, D. S., and Aharonovich, E. (2020). Implications of medical and recreational marijuana laws for neuroscience research: A review. *Curr Behav Neurosci Rep*, 7, 258–266.

Hasin, D. S., Greenstein, E., Aivadyan, C., et al. (2015a) The Alcohol Use Disorder and Associated Disabilities Interview Schedule-5 (AUDADIS-5): Procedural validity of substance use disorders modules through clinical re-appraisal in a general population sample. *Drug Alcohol Depend*, **148**, 40–46.

Hasin, D. S., Kerridge, B. T., Saha, T. D., et al. (2016). Prevalence and correlates of DSM-5 cannabis use disorder, 2012–2013: Findings from the National Epidemiologic Survey on Alcohol and Related Conditions-III. *Am J Psychiatry*, **173**, 588–599.

Hasin, D. S., O'Brien, C. P., Auriacombe, M., et al. (2013). DSM-5 criteria for substance use disorders: Recommendations and rationale. *Am J Psychiatry*, **170**, 834–851.

Hasin, D. S., Saha, T. D., Kerridge, B. T., et al. (2015b). Prevalence of marijuana use disorders in the

United States between 2001–2002 and 2012–2013. *JAMA Psychiatry*, **72**, 1235–1242.

Johnston, L. D., Miech, R. A., O'Malley, P. M., et al. (2020). *Demographic Subgroup Trends among Adolescents in the Use of Various Licit and Illicit Drugs, 1975–2019.* Ann Arbor, MI: Institute for Social Research, University of Michigan. Available at: www.monitoringthefuture.org/pubs/occpapers/mtf-occ94.pdf (Last accessed 17 October 2021).

Kerr, W. C., Lui, C., and Ye, Y. (2018). Trends and age, period and cohort effects for marijuana use prevalence in the 1984–2015 US National Alcohol Surveys. *Addiction*, **113**, 473–481.

Koob, G. F., and Le Moal, M. (2001). Drug addiction, dysregulation of reward, and allostasis. *Neuropsychopharmacology*, **24**, 97–129.

Lenne, M. G., Dietze, P. M., Triggs, T. J., et al. (2010). The effects of cannabis and alcohol on simulated arterial driving: Influences of driving experience and task demand. *Accid Anal Prev*, **42**, 859–866.

Leung, J., Chan, G. C. K., Hides, L., et al. (2020). What is the prevalence and risk of cannabis use disorders among people who use cannabis? A systematic review and meta-analysis. *Addict Behav*, **109**, 106479.

Li, M. C., Brady, J. E., DiMaggio, C. J., et al. (2012). Marijuana use and motor vehicle crashes. *Epidemiol Rev*, **34**, 65–72.

Livne, O., Shmulewitz, D., Lev-Ran, S., et al. (2019). DSM-5 cannabis withdrawal syndrome: Demographic and clinical correlates in U.S. adults. *Drug Alcohol Depend*, **195**, 170–177.

Manthey, J. (2019). Cannabis use in Europe: Current trends and public health concerns. *Int J Drug Policy*, **68**, 93–96.

McKay, M. P., and Groff, L. (2016). 23 years of toxicology testing fatally injured pilots: Implications for aviation and other modes of transportation. *Accid Anal Prev*, **90**, 108–117.

Miech, R. A., Johnston, L. D., O'Malley, P. M., et al. (2021). *Monitoring the Future National Survey Results on Drug Use, 1975–2020: Volume I, Secondary School Students.* Ann Arbor, MI: Institute for Social Research, University of Michigan. Available at: www.monitoringthefuture.org/pubs/monographs/mtf-vol1_2020.pdf (Last accessed 17 October 2021).

Miech, R. A., Patrick, M. E., O'Malley, P. M., et al. (2020). Trends in reported marijuana vaping among US adolescents, 2017–2019. *JAMA*, **323**, 475–476.

Millar, S. R., Mongan, D., O'Dwyer, C., et al. (2021). Correlates of patterns of cannabis use, abuse and dependence: Evidence from two national surveys in Ireland. *Eur J Public Health*, **31**, 441–447.

National Institute on Drug Abuse. (2021). *Monitoring the Future.* Available at: www.drugabuse.gov/drug-topics/trends-statistics/monitoring-future (Last accessed 18 October 2021).

Naveed, S., Waqas, A., Chaudhary, A. M. D., et al. (2020). Prevalence of common mental disorders in south Asia: A systematic review and meta-regression analysis. *Frontiers in Psychiatry*, **11**, 573150.

O'Neill-Dee, C., Spiller, H. A., Casavant, M. J., et al. (2020). Natural psychoactive substance-related exposures reported to United States poison control centers, 2000–2017. *Clin Toxicol*, **58**, 813–820.

OECD and The World Bank. (2020). *Health at a Glance: Latin America and the Caribbean 2020.* Available at: www.oecd-ilibrary.org/content/publication/6089164f-en (Last accessed 22 October 2021).

Public Health England, Home Office, Welsh Government, The Scottish Government, Public Health Wales & Department of Health (Northern Ireland). (2021). *United Kingdom Drug Situation: Focal Point annual report.* Available at: www.gov.uk/government/publications/united-kingdom-drug-situation-focal-point-annual-report (Last accessed 22 October 2021).

Richards, J. R. (2018). Cannabinoid hyperemesis syndrome: Pathophysiology and treatment in the emergency department. *J Emerg Med*, **54**, 354–363.

Rigucci, S., Marques, T. R., Di Forti, M., et al. (2016). Effect of high-potency cannabis on corpus callosum microstructure. *Psychol Med*, **46**, 841–854.

Rogeberg, O., and Elvik, R. (2016). The effects of cannabis intoxication on motor vehicle collision revisited and revised. *Addiction*, **111**, 1348–1359.

Santaella-Tenorio, J., Levy, N. S., Segura, L. E., et al. (2019). Cannabis use disorder among people using cannabis daily/almost daily in the United States, 2002–2016. *Drug Alcohol Depend*, **205**, 107621.

Sarvet, A. L., Wall, M. M., Keyes, K. M., et al. (2018). Recent rapid decrease in adolescents' perception that marijuana is harmful, but no concurrent increase in use. *Drug Alcohol Depend*, **186**, 68–74.

Shi, Y. (2017). Medical marijuana policies and hospitalizations related to marijuana and opioid pain reliever. *Drug Alcohol Depend*, **173**, 144–150.

Singh, J. A. (2022). Time-trends in hospitalizations with cannabis use disorder: A 17-year U.S. national study. *Subst Abus*, **43**, 408–414.

Sofuoglu, M., Sugarman, D. E., and Carroll, K. M. (2010). Cognitive function as an emerging treatment target for marijuana addiction. *Exp Clin Psychopharmacol*, **18**, 109–119.

Strand, M. C., Gjerde, H., and Morland, J. (2016). Driving under the influence of non-alcohol drugs: An update. Part II: Experimental studies. *Forensic Sci Rev*, **28**, 79–101.

Substance Abuse and Mental Health Services Administration. (2020). *2019 NSDUH Detailed Tables*. Available at: www.samhsa.gov/data/report/2019-nsduh-detailed-tables (Last accessed 15 October 2021).

United Nations Office on Drugs and Crime. (2020). *UNODC World Drug Report 2020: Global Drug Use Rising; while COVID-19 Has Far Reaching Impact on Global Drug Markets*. Vienna: United Nations Office on Drugs and Crime.

(2021). *World Drug Report 2021*. Available at: www.unodc.org/res/wdr2021/field/WDR21_Booklet_3.pdf (Last accessed 17 October 2021).

University of Michigan. (2021). *Monitoring the Future*. Available at: www.monitoringthefuture.org/ (Last accessed 17 October 2021).

Volkow, N. D., Swanson, J. M., Evins, A. E., et al. (2016). Effects of cannabis use on human behavior, including cognition, motivation, and psychosis: A review. *JAMA Psychiatry*, **73**, 292–297.

Wadsworth, E., and Hammond, D. (2019). International differences in patterns of cannabis use among youth: Prevalence, perceptions of harm, and driving under the influence in Canada, England & United States. *Addict Behav*, **90**, 171–175.

Watson, T. M., and Mann, R. E. (2016). International approaches to driving under the influence of cannabis: A review of evidence on impact. *Drug Alcohol Depend*, **169**, 148–155.

World Health Organization. (2016). *International Statistical Classification of Diseases and Related Health Problems*, 10th ed. Available at: https://icd.who.int/browse10/2016/en (Last accessed 15 October 2021).

(2021). *Cannabis*. Available at: www.who.int/teams/mental-health-and-substance-use/alcohol-drugs-and-addictive-behaviours/drugs-psychoactive/cannabis (Last accessed 17 October 2021).

Zhu, H., and Wu, L. T. (2016). Trends and correlates of cannabis-involved emergency department visits: 2004 to 2011. *J Addict Med*, **10**, 429–436.

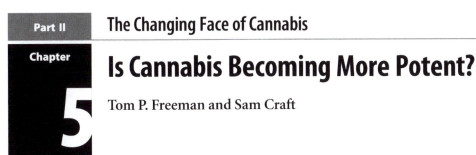

Chapter

5

Is Cannabis Becoming More Potent?

Tom P. Freeman and Sam Craft

5.1 What Is Cannabis Potency and Why Does It Matter?

The cannabis plant synthesizes cannabinoids such as delta-9-tetrahydrocannabinol (THC) and cannabidiol (CBD) in glandular trichomes, which are most abundant on the flowering tops of female plants. Within these glandular trichomes, a common pre-cursor (cannabigerolic acid) is either converted to THC acid (which can be decarboxylated to THC) or CBD acid (which can be decarboxylated to CBD) (Taura et al., 2007). This process is genetically determined such that cannabis plants fall into three distinct chemotypes: THC-dominant (producing high levels of THC and minimal CBD), mixed THC/CBD (producing moderate levels of THC and CBD), and CBD dominant (producing high levels of CBD and minimal THC) (De Meijer et al., 2003).

Cannabis potency refers to the total concentration of THC in cannabis products, including both THC and THC acid. THC acid is often abundant in cannabis products but is decarboxylated to THC by heat during consumption (for example, due to combustion or vaporization). The total concentration of THC can be estimated as follows: total THC = THC + 0.877 THC acid. In this chapter we use the terms 'cannabis potency', 'THC', and 'THC concentration' to refer to total THC concentration, in line with convention in the scientific literature. Similarly, we use 'CBD' and 'CBD concentration' to refer to total CBD (total CBD = CBD + 0.877 CBD acid).

THC is the primary intoxicating cannabinoid in cannabis, and causes dose-dependent increases in anxiety, psychotic-like experiences, and memory impairment (Curran et al., 2002; D'Souza et al., 2004). Cannabis potency is relevant for public health because most of the psychoactive effects of cannabis are driven by THC and the use of higher potency cannabis is associated with a greater dose of THC

consumed (Freeman et al., 2014; van der Pol et al., 2014). Although there is some evidence that people reduce their dose when using more potent cannabis products, this effect is only partial such that they still deliver higher doses of THC (Leung et al., 2021).

Studies investigating the long-term impact of different cannabis products have found evidence that higher potency products carry a greater risk of harm. Evidence is robust for cannabis use disorders, with several studies reporting that use of higher potency cannabis products is associated with a greater severity of symptoms compared to lower potency products (Craft et al., 2020; Freeman and Winstock, 2015; Hines et al., 2020). Moreover, national increases in cannabis potency in the United States and the Netherlands have been associated with a faster onset of first cannabis use disorder symptoms (Arterberry et al., 2019) and increased treatment admissions for cannabis in addiction services (Freeman et al., 2018).

In addition to cannabis use disorders, there is compelling evidence that use of higher potency cannabis products is associated with poorer outcomes related to psychosis. Daily use of high potency cannabis has been found to carry a five-fold increased risk of psychotic disorder in studies conducted in the United Kingdom (Di Forti et al., 2015) and a multisite study in Europe and Brazil (Di Forti et al., 2019). Moreover, variation in patterns of high potency cannabis use across Europe and Brazil were associated with adjusted incidence across sites (Di Forti et al., 2019). Daily use of higher potency cannabis products has also been found to be associated with an earlier onset of psychosis (Di Forti et al., 2014), increased risk of relapse to psychosis following a first episode, more relapses, shorter latency to relapse, and more intense psychiatric care (Schoeler et al., 2016). Overall, there is mounting evidence that cannabis potency may be an important factor in determining the risk of adverse outcomes from cannabis use.

Although other cannabinoids such as cannabidiol (CBD) may influence the effects of THC, evidence for this has been mixed (A. M. Freeman et al., 2019). Likewise, the therapeutic efficacy of CBD in psychiatric disorders is also mixed. Studies showing clinical benefits of CBD for disorders such as psychosis (Leweke et al., 2012; McGuire et al., 2018), anxiety (Bergamaschi et al., 2011; Zuardi et al., 2017), and addictions (Freeman et al., 2020; Hurd et al., 2019) have typically administered moderate-to-high doses of CBD (ranging from 300 mg to 100 mg, oral administration) while doses of CBD delivered during cannabis use would be considerably lower. However, monitoring CBD concentrations in cannabis may also be relevant for understanding the health effects of cannabis as a secondary consideration to THC.

5.2 How Has Cannabis Potency Changed over Time?

The most widely used cannabis product is herbal cannabis (or cannabis flower). Herbal cannabis refers to floral and foliar material from female cannabis plants, which are cut from the plant and dried to create a product ready for use. There are two distinct types of herbal cannabis: Seeded herbal cannabis (or traditional herbal cannabis/marijuana) refers to herbal cannabis that has been pollinated, with THC concentrations typically ranging from 2 to 6% (Potter et al., 2018). By contrast, sinsemilla (meaning 'without seeds') refers to herbal cannabis produced from unpollinated female plants, with THC concentrations typically ranging from 10 to 20%.

A systematic review and meta-analysis of studies reporting mean changes in THC and/or CBD concentrations over at least three annual time points (Freeman et al., 2021) estimated annual changes in THC and/or CBD within each study using random effects meta-regression. Next, these estimates were pooled in random effects models to estimate changes from all data available internationally. For all herbal cannabis samples, data on THC concentrations were available from 66,747 cannabis samples collected from 1970 to 2017 in the United States (Burgdorf et al., 2011; Chandra et al., 2019; ElSohly et al., 2016; Sevigny, 2013), United Kingdom (Pitts et al., 1990), Italy (Zamengo et al., 2014), and New Zealand (Poulsen and Sutherland, 2000). Meta-analysis of all herbal cannabis estimated an increase of 0.29% THC per year internationally (95% CI = 0.11–0.47, $p < 0.001$; Figure 5.1). These findings can be attributable to a shift toward market dominance of sinsemilla

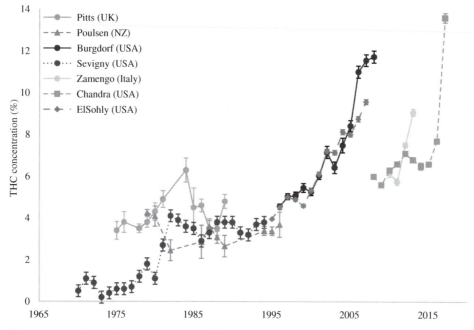

Figure 5.1 Mean (standard error) concentrations of delta-9-tetrahydrocannabinol (THC) in all herbal cannabis over time. Adapted from Freeman et al. (2021) under a CC BY-NC license.

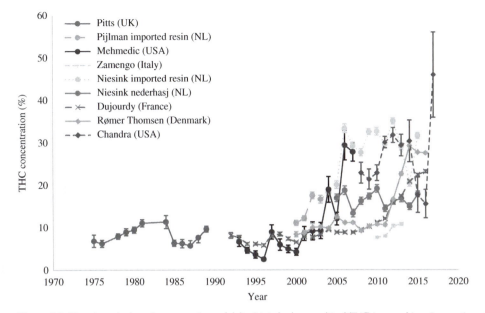

Figure 5.2 Mean (standard error) concentrations of delta-9-tetrahydrocannabinol (THC) in cannabis resin over time. Adapted from Freeman et al. (2021) under a CC BY-NC license.

relative to seeded herbal cannabis over time. There was limited evidence of changes in THC over time when analysing these different types of samples separately, with an estimated change of 0.17% (95% CI = −0.02–0.36, p = 0.079) for seeded herbal cannabis and 0.26% (95% CI = −0.09–0.61, p = 0.141) for sinsemilla. Meta-analysis of CBD concentrations found no evidence for changes over time in all herbal cannabis, with an estimated change of −0.01% per year (95% CI = −0.02–0.01, p = 0.280).

Another widely used cannabis product is cannabis resin (or hashish). Cannabis resin is produced by physically extracting trichomes from the cannabis plant using a range of methods such as sieving or rubbing the plant material to produce compressed blocks of cannabis plant material. Due to the wide range of approaches to cannabis resin production (including the cannabis plant material used and the method of extraction), THC concentrations can vary widely, from <1% to 30% (Potter et al., 2018). Cannabis resin often contains notable levels of CBD, which indicates the use of plant material that is not limited to THC-dominant chemotypes, as would be expected in landrace conditions (Potter et al., 2008) such as traditional 'kief' plants grown in Morocco.

A systematic review and meta-analysis (Freeman et al., 2021) included data from 17,371 cannabis resin samples collected from 1975 to 2017 in the United States (Chandra et al., 2019; Mehmedic et al., 2010), United Kingdom (Pitts et al., 1990), Netherlands (Niesink et al., 2015; Pijlman et al., 2005), France (Dujourdy and Besacier, 2017), Denmark (Rømer Thomsen et al., 2019), and Italy (Zamengo et al., 2014). Meta-analysis indicated an annual increase of 0.57% THC in cannabis resin each year (95% CI = 0.10–1.03, p = 0.017; Figure 5.2). It is notable that increases in the potency of cannabis resin were two-fold greater than those observed in all herbal cannabis. This may be attributable to a shift toward more efficient extraction methods, such as the use of icy water or dry ice, as exposing cannabis plant material to cold temperatures can increase the efficiency of extraction (EMCDDA, 2019). Additionally, there is some evidence that higher THC producing cannabis plants have been replacing traditional landrace kief plants in Morocco, resulting in higher potency cannabis resin trafficked to European drug markets (Chouvy and Afsahi, 2014). Meta-analysis of CBD concentrations found no evidence for changes over time in cannabis resin, with an estimated change of 0.03% per year (95% CI = −0.11–0.18, p = 0.651).

45

5.3 How Have Cannabis Products Changed and Diversified in New Legal Markets?

Over recent years there has been a major shift toward the liberalization of cannabis policy. At the time of writing, 21 US states (and Washington DC), Canada, and Uruguay have legalized cannabis for non-medical use, and more jurisdictions are expected to follow. The issue of potency features in much of the cannabis policy discourse, with proponents of legalization arguing that it provides better control over cannabis products and other market conditions (e.g., Meacher et al., 2019). Although monitoring data from the majority of newly-regulated retail markets are yet to emerge, the data currently available show a different picture, with upward trends in the potency of traditional products and the proliferation of new, highly potent products. In the US state of Washington, the first licensed retailer opened in 2014 and, since then, an inventory traceability system has tracked the cannabinoid content and price of all products sold at the retail (and wholesale) level. Unlike monitoring databases in other jurisdictions, this has been made available to researchers and currently these are the only systematically collected data in which legal cannabis markets can be monitored. Crudely comparing different analyses of these data, we can see that, between 2014 and 2017, the THC content of herbal cannabis increased from around 15% to over 21%, whilst the average CBD content remained at less than 0.5% (Davenport, 2021; Smart et al., 2017). Also, across this period, THC-dominant chemovars accounted for 99% of all cannabis flower sales (making up approximately 60% of all cannabis sales). By contrast, the average THC concentrations in seized illicit herbal cannabis in the United States was around 11% in 2014 and 14% in 2017 (with CBD concentrations also remaining at less than 0.5%) (ElSohly et al., 2021). Also, whilst the price of illicit cannabis has been increasing across Europe where cannabis is widely prohibited (T. P. Freeman et al., 2019), increases in the potency of legal cannabis have coincided with sharp reductions in price. Between 2014 and 2017, the price per 10 mg dose of cannabis flower in Washington State halved from approximately 0.6$ to approximately 0.3$ (Davenport, 2021).

Furthermore, consumers in legal markets are increasingly shifting away from flower products toward more potent cannabis extracts (or concentrates), which accounted for nearly 30% of all retail sales in Washington State in 2017 (Davenport, 2021). Extracts refer to a broad range of products which contain high concentrations of cannabinoids extracted from the cannabis plant using various extraction methods, including the use of solvents such as butane. On average these contain around 60% THC and they are typically consumed in ways which rapidly deliver high doses to the consumer (e.g., through a process known as 'dabbing', which involves placing cannabis extracts on a heated surface and inhaling the vapours). The effects of extracts are reported to be stronger and longer lasting compared to smoked cannabis (Loflin and Earleywine, 2014) and, although research in this area is in its infancy, there are early indications that these products are associated with increased health harms (Loflin and Earleywine, 2014; Meier, 2017). Extracts are also commonly sold as oils or liquids for vaporizers and, although the potency of these products has increased in recent years, vaporizers offer a steadier, less intense cannabis delivery system which may reduce the harms associated with smoking cannabis (Budney et al., 2015). Additionally, extracts containing higher/more balanced proportions of CBD are increasing in popularity, although these still only account for a small proportion (approximately 1%) of extract sales (Davenport, 2021).

Sales of cannabis infused edibles (and liquids) has also risen in legal markets, representing approximately 8% of all transactions in Washington State (Davenport, 2021; Smart et al., 2017). Rather than percentage of total weight, the cannabinoid content of edibles is typically measured in milligrams (mg) and, in most US states, THC content is currently limited to 5–10 mg per serving and 50–100 mg per product, while, in Canada, edibles are not permitted to contain more than 5–10 mg of THC per product. Despite these restrictions, and perhaps due to the delayed onset of intoxication, edibles have been associated with an increased risk of adverse events from overconsumption or problems with dosing (Barrus et al., 2016). Additionally, the prevalence of edibles is also increasing in illicit markets, and data from Canada show that the advertised THC content of edibles sold by illegal retailers often exceed the limits imposed in legal markets (Mahamad et al., 2020).

It should be noted that much of the potency data reported here refer to the labelled cannabinoid content, and concerns have been raised over the accuracy and reliability of cannabinoid labelling of legal products in US states (Jikomes and Zoorob, 2018; Vandrey et al., 2015). Also, data are taken primarily from the state of Washington and are not necessarily a reflection of all legal markets, and differences in regulations between jurisdictions are likely to influence the market response. Data from the first two months after cannabis legalization in Canada in 2018 show that the average potency of legal herbal cannabis was around 16%, which was markedly lower than the average of illicit herbal cannabis (around 21%) (Mahamad et al., 2020) and the average seen in Washington State (i.e., 21% in 2017). However, these are data from the early stages of a market in transition, and how potency and products change in Canada and beyond as legal markets become more established remains to be seen.

5.4 What Are the Methodological Limitations of Research on Cannabis Potency and How Can They Be Overcome?

There are some important methodological limitations to consider when interpreting data on cannabis potency. First, there is a potential risk of bias regarding the representativeness of samples tested. Such bias can be introduced in several ways. For example, studies on cannabis potency may be limited to specific regions where research was conducted and may not be generalizable outside of these areas. Furthermore, sampling methodology is an important potential source of bias. The majority of data come from police seizures and law enforcement methods may be biased (for example, certain types of people are more likely to be searched and particular regions of a country may experience greater law enforcement for drugs, such as in cities or in ports where trafficking occurs). Additionally, there may be differences in the type of product seized at the wholesale level when compared to the retail level. Concerns about representativeness can be overcome more readily in jurisdictions where cannabis sales are tolerated. For example, the Trimbos Institute in the Netherlands conducts the highest quality cannabis monitoring programme worldwide. Each year in January (to control for seasonal variation in potency), a randomized sample of national retail outlets are visited by

researchers to conduct test purchases of a range of cannabis products prior to analysis. This protocol has been followed for over 20 years, generating robust evidence on variation in cannabis products in the Netherlands (Niesink et al., 2015; Pijlman et al., 2005). The emergence of new legal markets in US states, Canada, Uruguay, and elsewhere may facilitate the monitoring of cannabis products by addressing potential sources of bias from sample representativeness. An alternative method that can be applied in jurisdictions where cannabis is illegal is to quantify the potency of cannabis samples obtained from people who use cannabis rather than police seizures (Freeman et al., 2014).

An additional methodological consideration is the use of different techniques and protocols for quantifying concentrations of THC and/or CBD, which may result in different laboratories producing varying estimates for the same sample. This can be overcome by following standardized protocols, such as recommended by the United Nations Office on Drugs and Crime (2009). Additionally, the use of control samples with known potencies (e.g., products from the Office of Medicinal Cannabis in the Netherlands) can be included in analysis in a blinded manner (Niesink et al., 2015). It is also important that cannabis samples are stored appropriately and analysed promptly, as prolonged storage and/or exposure to heat and/or light can speed conversion of THC to cannabinol, resulting in an underestimate of cannabis potency (Sevigny, 2013). Methodological concerns about the analytical technique and protocol are likely to be less problematic in studies where cannabis samples are analysed in academic or government laboratories. By contrast, risk of bias may be greater in commercial contexts such as testing of cannabis products in Washington State, where systematic variation has been detected across testing facilities (Jikomes and Zoorob, 2018).

A final limitation of research on cannabis potency is that it may not readily apply to all cannabis products, including newer and increasingly popular products such as edibles or liquid extracts used for vaping. As the market diversifies, there is an increasing need for standardized metrics. For example, the 5 mg standard THC unit (Freeman and Lorenzetti, 2020) applies to all cannabis products and methods of administration. This standard THC unit has been endorsed by the US National Institutes of Health (NIDA, 2021) and may facilitate monitoring of

Box 5.1 Definitions for different cannabis types and administration methods

Product/administration method	Definitions
Herbal cannabis	Dried floral and foliar material cut from female cannabis plants. The two main types are seeded herbal cannabis and sinsemilla (meaning 'without seeds').
Cannabis resin	Compressed blocks of extracted cannabis plant trichomes, also known as hashish.
Cannabis extracts	Highly concentrated cannabis products produced through various extraction methods, also known as concentrates.
Edibles	Cannabis infused foods or liquids for oral consumption.
Vaporizers	Electronic devices which heat cannabis into a vapor for inhalation.
Dabbing	Placing cannabis extracts on a heated surface (usually a metal plate, or 'dab rig') and inhaling the vapours.

cannabis products, particularly those for which the concept of potency does not readily apply.

5.5 Conclusion

Since the 1970s, cannabis potency has continued to rise internationally. Increases in cannabis potency have been two-fold greater for cannabis resin than for herbal cannabis. During this time cannabis has potentially become a more harmful product, given accumulating evidence for associations of cannabis potency with cannabis use disorders and psychotic disorders. Current evidence from commercially-driven legal cannabis markets such as Washington State show that cannabis potency has risen particularly rapidly in these conditions. As the risk of psychosis (and other health harms) with cannabis appear to be dose-related, the increasing potency of cannabis and the proliferation of more potent cannabis products poses a public health and policy challenge internationally. While it is possible that alternative approaches to legalization could result in safer forms of cannabis on the market (e.g., through limits and/or taxes on potency) there is a lack of evidence to support the effectiveness of this strategy at present. Therefore, as major shifts in cannabis policy continue to be enacted, it is more important than ever to generate robust monitoring processes to evaluate the impact of these policies on the safety of cannabis products.

References

Arterberry, B. J., Padovano, H. T., Foster, K. T., et al. (2019). Higher average potency across the United States is associated with progression to first cannabis use disorder symptom. *Drug Alcohol Depend*, **195**, 186–192.

Barrus, D. G., Capogrossi, K. L., Cates, S. C., et al. (2016). Tasty THC: Promises and challenges of cannabis edibles. *Methods Rep RTI Press*, 10.3768.

Bergamaschi, M. M., Queiroz, R. H. C., Chagas, M. H. N., et al. (2011). Cannabidiol reduces the anxiety induced by simulated public speaking in treatment-naive social phobia patients. *Neuropsychopharmacology*, **36**, 1219–1226.

Budney, A. J., Sargent, J. D., and Lee, D. C. (2015). Vaping cannabis (marijuana): Parallel concerns to e-cigs? *Addiction*, **110**, 1699–1704.

Burgdorf, J. R., Kilmer, B., and Pacula, R. L. (2011). Heterogeneity in the composition of marijuana seized in California. *Drug Alcohol Depend*, **117**, 59–61.

Chandra, S., Radwan, M. M., Majumdar, C. G., et al. (2019). New trends in cannabis potency in USA and Europe during the last decade (2008–2017). *Eur Arch Psychiatry Clin Neurosci*, **269**, 5–15.

Chouvy, P.-A., and Afsahi, K. (2014). Hashish revival in Morocco. *Int J Drug Policy*, **25**, 416–423.

Craft, S., Winstock, A., Ferris, J., et al. (2020). Characterising heterogeneity in the use of different cannabis products: Latent class analysis with 55 000 people who use cannabis and associations with severity of cannabis dependence. *Psychol Med*, **50**, 2364–2373.

Curran, V. H., Brignell, C., Fletcher, S., et al. (2002). Cognitive and subjective dose–response effects of acute oral Δ9-tetrahydrocannabinol (THC) in infrequent cannabis users. *Psychopharmacology*, **164**, 61–70.

D'Souza, D. C., Perry, E., MacDougall, L., et al. (2004). The psychotomimetic effects of intravenous delta-9-tetrahydrocannabinol in healthy individuals: Implications for psychosis. *Neuropsychopharmacology*, **29**, 1558–1572.

Davenport, S. (2021). Price and product variation in Washington's recreational cannabis market. *Int J Drug Policy*, **91**, 102547.

De Meijer, E. P., Bagatta, M., Carboni, A., et al. (2003). The inheritance of chemical phenotype in *Cannabis sativa* L. *Genetics*, **163**, 335–346.

Di Forti, M., Marconi, A., Carra, E., et al. (2015). Proportion of patients in south London with first-episode psychosis attributable to use of high potency cannabis: A case-control study. *Lancet Psychiatry*, **2**, 233–238.

Di Forti, M., Quattrone, D., Freeman, T. P., et al. (2019). The contribution of cannabis use to variation in the incidence of psychotic disorder across Europe (EU-GEI): A multicentre case-control study. *Lancet Psychiatry*, **6**, 427–436.

Di Forti, M., Sallis, H., Allegri, F., et al. (2014). Daily use, especially of high-potency cannabis, drives the earlier onset of psychosis in cannabis users. *Schizophr Bull*, **40**, 1509–1517.

Dujourdy, L., and Besacier, F. (2017). A study of cannabis potency in France over a 25 years period (1992–2016). *Forensic Sci Int*, **272**, 72–80.

ElSohly, M. A., Chandra, S., Radwan, M., et al. (2021). A comprehensive review of cannabis potency in the United States in the last decade. *Biol Psychiatry: Cogn Neurosci Neuroimag*, **6**, 603–606.

ElSohly, M. A., Mehmedic, Z., Foster, S., et al. (2016). Changes in cannabis potency over the last 2 decades (1995–2014): Analysis of current data in the United States. *Biol Psychiatry*, **79**, 613–619.

EMCDDA. (2019). *European Monitoring Centre for Drugs and Drug Addiction. Developments in the European Cannabis Market.* Lisbon: EMCDDA Papers, Issue.

Freeman, A. M., Petrilli, K., Lees, R., et al. (2019). How does cannabidiol (CBD) influence the acute effects of delta-9-tetrahydrocannabinol (THC) in humans? A systematic review. *Neurosci Biobehav Rev*, **107**, 696–712.

Freeman, T., and Winstock, A. (2015). Examining the profile of high-potency cannabis and its association with severity of cannabis dependence. *Psychol Med*, **45**, 3181–3189.

Freeman, T. P., Craft, S., Wilson, J., et al. (2021). Changes in delta-9-tetrahydrocannabinol (THC) and cannabidiol (CBD) concentrations in cannabis over time: Systematic review and meta-analysis. *Addiction*, **116**, 1000–1010.

Freeman, T. P., Groshkova, T., Cunningham, A., et al. (2019). Increasing potency and price of cannabis in Europe, 2006–16. *Addiction*, **114**, 1015–1023.

Freeman, T. P., Hindocha, C., Baio, G., et al. (2020). Cannabidiol for the treatment of cannabis use disorder: A phase 2a, double-blind, placebo-controlled, randomised, adaptive Bayesian trial. *Lancet Psychiatry*, **7**, 865–874.

Freeman, T. P., and Lorenzetti, V. (2020). 'Standard THC units': A proposal to standardize dose across all cannabis products and methods of administration. *Addiction*, **115**, 1207–1216.

Freeman, T. P., Morgan, C. J., Hindocha, C., et al. (2014). Just say 'know': How do cannabinoid concentrations influence users' estimates of cannabis potency and the amount they roll in joints? *Addiction*, **109**, 1686–1694.

Freeman, T. P., van der Pol, P., Kuijpers, W., et al. (2018). Changes in cannabis potency and first-time admissions to drug treatment: A 16-year study in the Netherlands. *Psychol Med*, **48**, 2346–2352.

Hines, L. A., Freeman, T. P., Gage, S. H., et al. (2020). Association of high-potency cannabis use with mental health and substance use in adolescence. *JAMA Psychiatry*, **77**, 1044–1051.

Hurd, Y. L., Spriggs, S., Alishayev, J., et al. (2019). Cannabidiol for the reduction of cue-induced craving and anxiety in drug-abstinent individuals with heroin use disorder: A double-blind randomized placebo-controlled trial. *Am J Psychiatry*, **176**, 911–922.

Jikomes, N., and Zoorob, M. (2018). The cannabinoid content of legal cannabis in Washington State varies systematically across testing facilities and popular consumer products. *Sci Rep*, **8**, 4519.

Leung, J., Stjepanović, D., Dawson, D., et al. (2021). Do cannabis users reduce their THC dosages when using more potent cannabis products? A review. *Front Psychiatry*, **12**, 163.

Leweke, F., Piomelli, D., Pahlisch, F., et al. (2012). Cannabidiol enhances anandamide signaling and alleviates psychotic symptoms of schizophrenia. *Translat Psychiatry*, **2**, e94.

Loflin, M., and Earleywine, M. (2014). A new method of cannabis ingestion: The dangers of dabs? *Addict Behav*, **39**, 1430–1433.

Mahamad, S., Wadsworth, E., Rynard, V., et al. (2020). Availability, retail price and potency of legal and illegal cannabis in Canada after recreational cannabis legalisation. *Drug Alcohol Rev*, **39**, 337–346.

McGuire, P., Robson, P., Cubala, W. J., et al. (2018). Cannabidiol (CBD) as an adjunctive therapy in schizophrenia: A multicenter randomized controlled trial. *Am J Psychiatry*, **175**, 225–231.

Meacher, M., Nutt, D., Liebling, J., et al. (2019). Should the supply of cannabis be legalised now? *BMJ*, **366**, l4473.

Mehmedic, Z., Chandra, S., Slade, D., et al. (2010). Potency trends of Δ9-THC and other cannabinoids in confiscated cannabis preparations from 1993 to 2008. *J Forensic Sci*, **55**, 1209–1217.

Meier, M. H. (2017). Associations between butane hash oil use and cannabis-related problems. *Drug Alcohol Depend*, **179**, 25–31.

NIDA. (2021). *Establishing 5 mg of THC as the Standard Unit for Research*. Available at: https://nida.nih.gov/about-nida/noras-blog/2021/05/establishing-5mg-thc-standard-unit-research. Last accessed 18 March 2022.

Niesink, R. J., Rigter, S., Koeter, M. W., et al. (2015). Potency trends of Δ9-tetrahydrocannabinol, cannabidiol and cannabinol in cannabis in the Netherlands: 2005–15. *Addiction*, **110**, 1941–1950.

Pijlman, F., Rigter, S., Hoek, J., et al. (2005). Strong increase in total delta-THC in cannabis preparations sold in Dutch coffee shops. *Addict Biol*, **10**, 171–180.

Pitts, J., O'Neil, P., and Leggo, K. (1990). Survey variation in the THC content of illicitly imported cannabis* products: 1984–1989. *J Pharm Pharmacol*, **42**, 817–820.

van der Pol, P., Liebregts, N., Brunt, T., et al. (2014). Cross-sectional and prospective relation of cannabis potency, dosing and smoking behaviour with cannabis dependence: An ecological study. *Addiction*, **109**, 1101–1109.

Potter, D. J., Clark, P., and Brown, M. B. (2008). Potency of Δ9-THC and other cannabinoids in cannabis in England in 2005: Implications for psychoactivity and pharmacology. *J Forensic Sci*, **53**, 90–94.

Potter, D. J., Hammond, K., Tuffnell, S., et al. (2018). Potency of Δ9–tetrahydrocannabinol and other cannabinoids in cannabis in England in 2016: Implications for public health and pharmacology. *Drug Test Anal*, **10**, 628–635.

Poulsen, H., and Sutherland, G. (2000). The potency of cannabis in New Zealand from 1976 to 1996. *Sci Justice*, **40**, 171–176.

Rømer Thomsen, K., Lindholst, C., Thylstrup, B., et al. (2019). Changes in the composition of cannabis from 2000–2017 in Denmark: Analysis of confiscated samples of cannabis resin. *Exp Clin Psychopharmacol*, **27**, 402.

Schoeler, T., Petros, N., Di Forti, M., et al. (2016). Effects of continuation, frequency, and type of cannabis use on relapse in the first 2 years after onset of psychosis: An observational study. *Lancet Psychiatry*, **3**, 947–953.

Sevigny, E. L. (2013). Is today's marijuana more potent simply because it's fresher? *Drug Test Anal*, **5**, 62–67.

Smart, R., Caulkins, J. P., Kilmer, B., et al. (2017). Variation in cannabis potency and prices in a newly legal market: Evidence from 30 million cannabis sales in Washington state. *Addiction*, **112**, 2167–2177.

Taura, F., Sirikantaramas, S., Shoyama, Y., et al. (2007). Cannabidiolic-acid synthase, the chemotype-determining enzyme in the fiber-type Cannabis sativa. *FEBS Lett*, **581**, 2929–2934.

United Nations Office on Drugs and Crime. (2009). *Recommended Methods for the Identification and Analysis of Cannabis and Cannabis Products (revised and updated): Manual for Use By National Drug Analysis Laboratories*. New York: United Nations Publications.

Vandrey, R., Raber, J. C., Raber, M. E., et al. (2015). Cannabinoid dose and label accuracy in edible medical cannabis products. *JAMA*, **313**, 2491–2493.

Zamengo, L., Frison, G., Bettin, C., et al. (2014). Cannabis potency in the Venice area (Italy): Update 2013. *Drug Test Anal*, 7, 255–258.

Zuardi, A. W., Rodrigues, N. P., Silva, A. L., et al. (2017). Inverted U-shaped dose-response curve of the anxiolytic effect of cannabidiol during public speaking in real life. *Front Pharmacol*, **8**, 259.

6

Policy Implications of the Evidence on Cannabis Use and Psychosis

Wayne Hall and Louisa Degenhardt

The evidence on cannabis use and psychosis and other serious mental illnesses has often been evaluated through appraisers' pre-existing views on whether they think cannabis use by adults should or should not be legalized. Those who support the continuation of criminal penalties for cannabis use often cite evidence that cannabis use plays a causal role in psychosis to justify this policy (e.g., de Irala et al., 2005). Those who favour more liberal policies towards recreational cannabis use argue that there is insufficient evidence for a causal relationship (e.g., Ksir and Hart, 2016).

We first briefly assess whether the evidence is sufficient to warrant the conclusion that cannabis is a contributory cause of psychosis in young adults. We argue that even those who are sceptical that the relationship is causal should support a policy that informs young people who use cannabis about the possibility of their developing psychoses if they have a personal or family history of the disorder. We then discuss policies that could minimize the adverse effects that cannabis use has on psychosis risk in young people. These include discouraging cannabis use among to young people who have developed psychoses and currently use cannabis and informing young people about the mental health risks of cannabis use in ways that will dissuade those at higher risk of psychosis from using cannabis. We conclude with a discussion on policy implications of the link between cannabis use and psychosis, notably in those jurisdictions that have legalized cannabis use by adults.

6.1 Making Causal Inferences from Observational Data

There is consistent longitudinal evidence that young adults who are regular cannabis users have an increased risk of developing psychosis (Gage et al., 2016; Gilman et al., 2018; Hasan et al., 2020; Marconi et al., 2016; and see Chapter 17). In these studies, daily or near daily cannabis users report more psychotic symptoms and are much more likely to be diagnosed with a psychotic disorder than individuals who have not used cannabis. The risk of psychotic symptoms is higher in people who begin using cannabis in their mid-teens and who use regularly in young adulthood, and in young people who have a personal or family history of psychosis. Persons who develop psychosis when using cannabis, and who then cease using cannabis, have better clinical outcomes than those who continue to use cannabis. These relationships usually persist after controlling for confounding variables, such as personal characteristics, other types of drug use, and a family history of psychiatric disorder (Gilman et al., 2018; Hasan et al., 2020; Marconi et al., 2016).

The major reason for the continuing debate about whether the relationship is causal is that we cannot be sure that the baseline risk of psychosis is the same in young people who do and do not regularly use cannabis (Gage et al., 2016). One possibility, therefore, is that the association between cannabis use and psychosis arises from uncontrolled confounding, for example, regular cannabis users also use other drugs, such as psychostimulants and alcohol (both of which can produce psychotic symptoms). There could also be differences in environmental exposures (e.g., to childhood abuse) or shared genetic risk factors that increase the likelihood of first using cannabis and later developing a psychosis (Gage et al., 2016).

Longitudinal epidemiological studies have assessed the role of confounding by measuring and statistically adjusting for plausible confounding variables, such as other drug use, personal characteristics that predict psychosis, and a personal history of psychotic symptoms (e.g., Fergusson et al., 2003, 2005; Henquet et al., 2005; van Os et al., 2002; Zammit et al., 2002). The number and type of confounding variables that have been assessed and controlled for has varied between studies. Fixed effects regression has also been used to control for the effects of *unmeasured* confounders (Fergusson et al., 2005).

One type of confounding that presents special challenges is that between cannabis and tobacco smoking, both of which are very common among persons who develop schizophrenia. A systematic review of the epidemiological studies of tobacco use in schizophrenia (Hunter et al., 2020) argued that there was a compelling case that cigarette smoking played a causal role in the onset of schizophrenia. Disentangling the separate roles of tobacco and cannabis using statistical methods is a challenge because they are strongly correlated and the findings from individual studies are conflicted. One early study of the Avon cohort found that the association between cannabis use and psychosis was greatly attenuated after controlling for cigarette smoking (Gage et al., 2014). Later studies suggest that tobacco smoking does not explain the association between cannabis use and psychosis (e.g., Fergusson et al., 2015; Jones et al., 2018), including a subsequent follow-up of the Avon cohort (Jones et al., 2018).

Genetic epidemiological studies have assessed the degree to which the association between cannabis use and psychosis is explained by shared genetic factors that increase the risk of using cannabis and of developing a psychotic disorder. The main weakness of many of these studies is that they use lifetime or past year cannabis use rather than the much less prevalent but more causally relevant daily use. Another weakness is the difficulty in identifying genetic factors that accurately predict the risks of either cannabis use or psychosis. Gillespie and Kendler (2021) reviewed studies that used a variety of different genetically informed study designs to assessing genetic contributions to associations between cannabis use and schizophrenia. These included: studies of the association in cohorts of decreasing genetic relationships (e.g., twins, parents, siblings, cousins, and unrelated), Mendelian randomization studies, and studies that used polygenic risk scores to adjust the association between cannabis use and psychosis. Gillespie and Kendler argued that that there are shared genetic risks for cannabis use and psychosis and that an emerging psychosis increases the risks of cannabis use. They concluded, however, that there was also consistent evidence that cannabis use plays a small contributory causal role in the development of psychosis.

6.2 The Self-Medication Hypothesis

Another possible explanation of the association between cannabis use and psychosis is that cannabis use is a form of self-medication, that is, young people use cannabis to treat the emerging symptoms of a psychosis, such as social withdrawal, anhedonia, blunted affect, and depressed mood. The prevalence of cannabis use among first episode cases of psychosis is substantial (Hasan et al., 2020) so this possibility should be excluded (Moore et al., 2007).

Epidemiological studies have tested the self-medication hypothesis by only conducting analyses on data from those participants who reported no symptoms before the use of cannabis (e.g. Zammit et al., 2002). Other studies have specifically recruited participants who reported no history of psychotic symptoms (e.g. van Os et al., 2002) and others have statistically controlled for prior history of symptoms of mental disorders (Arseneault et al., 2002; Fergusson et al., 2003). These studies generally report that cannabis use preceded the onset of schizophrenia symptoms, suggesting that cannabis use increases the risk of psychosis rather than psychosis increasing cannabis use. Other evidence that is inconsistent with the self-medication hypothesis comes from prospective studies of the clinical outcomes in persons with psychoses who used cannabis before their diagnosis and who discontinued their cannabis use afterward. In systematic reviews of these studies, persons with psychoses who discontinue cannabis use have much better clinical outcomes than those who continue to use cannabis (e.g., lower rates of relapse and fewer positive symptoms) (Schoeler et al., 2016; Zammit et al., 2008).

6.3 Biological Plausibility

A causal relationship between regular cannabis use and psychosis is biologically plausible. The principal psychoactive ingredient in cannabis – tetrahydrocannabinol (THC) – acts upon CB_1 cannabinoid receptors in the brain (Atkinson and Abbott, 2018; Gilman et al., 2018; Iversen, 2012; and see Chapters 1 and 2). The cannabinoid system, in turn, interacts with dopaminergic and other neurotransmitters systems that have been implicated in the production of psychotic symptoms (Atkinson and Abbott, 2018). In double-blind provocation studies, intravenous THC increases positive and negative psychotic symptoms in a dose-dependent way in both persons with schizophrenia and in healthy volunteers (Cahill et al., 2018; Hindley et al., 2020; and see Chapter 16).

6.4 How Does the Evidence for Cannabis Compare with That for Alcohol- and Amphetamine-Related Psychoses?

The quality of the evidence that heavy alcohol use is a cause of psychosis is much weaker than that for cannabis. It largely consists of a case series of *delirium tremens* in severely alcohol dependent people undergoing alcohol withdrawal (Greenberg and Lee, 2001). There is one ethically questionable experimental study that deliberately induced *delirium tremens* in drinkers by abruptly stopping access to alcohol after several weeks of sustained heavy drinking in a hospital ward (Isbell et al., 1955). There are also case series of 'alcoholic hallucinosis' in heavy consumers of alcohol, but the status of this diagnostic entity, and the role of alcohol in producing these disorders, is uncertain (Greenberg and Lee, 2001; Lishman, 1987; Narasimha et al., 2019).

The evidence that heavy amphetamine use can induce a psychotic episode is stronger than is the case for alcohol (for a recent review of amphetamines and psychosis, see Voce et al., 2019). Connell (1958) published 200 case reports of persons who were heavy methamphetamine users who developed acute paranoid psychoses that remitted after they abstained from using methamphetamine for several days to a week. These psychoses were provoked by injections of large doses of methamphetamine given to problem amphetamine users (Bell, 1973), normal volunteers (Angrist et al., 1974), and medical students (Curran et al., 2004). Epidemiological studies have found a dose–response relationship between the frequency of amphetamine injection and the severity of psychotic symptoms (Hall and Hando, 1993; McKetin et al., 2013). A causal relationship is also biologically plausible because animal studies show that amphetamines inhibit monoamine (dopamine, norepinephrine, epinephrine, serotonin) reuptake, increasing monoamine concentrations in the neuronal synapse. The increased dopaminergic activity produces excess glutamate in the cerebral cortex, a pre-cursor to psychosis (Arunogiri et al., 2018; Lappin and Sara, 2019; Mullen et al., 2020).

In summary, the evidence that cannabis use is a contributory cause of psychosis is arguably stronger than the observational evidence that alcohol can produce psychoses. The epidemiological evidence is more extensive for cannabis than it is for methamphetamine but the magnitude of the risk of a psychosis is smaller for cannabis (2–3-fold) than for amphetamine (11-fold) (Degenhardt and Hall, 2001).

6.5 A Public Health Case for Prudence

If there was similar evidence of an association between a pharmaceutical drug and psychosis, regulators would withdraw the drug from the market (if the risk was large), or only allow it be prescribed if accompanied by warnings to patients and prescribers about these risks (Klein, 2006). There are important differences between the way that high income countries regulate pharmaceuticals and recreational drugs. We appropriately err in the direction of prudence when responding to evidence of harms caused by therapeutic drugs. We allow adults to voluntarily assume the risks of using alcohol and tobacco, only prohibiting their use by minors and prisoners. Until 2013, when Uruguay legalized adult use, cannabis was an exception to this policy (Hall et al., 2019) in all high-income countries that prohibited adults from using cannabis in accordance with the 1961 Single Convention on Narcotic Drugs (Room et al., 2010).

In deciding how to respond to this evidence, policymakers need to consider the costs and benefits of different potential policies. If the costs of a response are minimal, then we would be wise to implement it. For example, advising parents not to put infants to sleep in the prone position was advocated to reduce deaths from sudden infant death syndrome (SIDS) because: (1) this sleeping position was a strong risk factor for SIDS; (2) the change in behaviour carried few, if any, risks; and (3) if the relationship was *not* causal, parents and infants would not be greatly inconvenienced. The substantial reduction in SIDS deaths in countries that implemented this policy strengthened the evidence for a causal relationship between sleeping position and SIDS, even in the absence of an understanding of the underlying causal mechanisms (Dwyer et al., 1995).

The same prudential reasoning would support efforts to discourage young people from using cannabis or at least delaying their use until early adulthood (de Irala et al., 2005). The public health gain, if the relationship is causal, would be a possible reduction in schizophrenia incidence and prevalence. This gain would offset the pleasure foregone by young people who followed health advice not to use cannabis, or who delayed its use into adulthood. In principle, a reduction in cannabis use among incident cases of psychosis would provide evidence for the effectiveness of this policy but it may prove to be difficult to detect a reduction in psychosis incidence or prevalence (Degenhardt et al., 2003).

The case for preventing adolescent cannabis use is strengthened by other epidemiological evidence that young people who regularly use cannabis have a higher risk of other adverse psychosocial outcomes in young adulthood (Hall et al., 2008, 2020). These include: cannabis dependence (Connor et al., 2021); cognitive impairment (Lorenzetti et al., 2020); poor educational outcomes (Hall et al., 2020); the use of other illicit drugs (Fergusson et al., 2006; Hall and Lynskey, 2005); depression (Patton et al., 2002; and see Chapter 12); and lower quality-of-life and poorer social relationships in early adulthood (Fergusson and Boden, 2008; Patton et al., 2007). These adverse outcomes are all much more common among daily cannabis users than psychosis, but they have often been overshadowed in cannabis policy debates by psychosis. There are similar debates about whether cannabis dependence is a contributory cause of these outcomes (Macleod et al., 2004) but it is unlikely that cannabis plays no role in precipitating or worsening any of these outcomes. It is more likely that regular cannabis use is also a contributory cause of some of these adverse psychosocial outcomes in young adulthood (e.g., educational under-achievement and poorer quality-of-life) (Hall et al., 2020), thereby strengthening the case for discouraging adolescent cannabis use.

6.6 Responding to Young People with Psychoses Who Use Cannabis

Young people who develop psychotic symptoms and who use cannabis should be encouraged to stop using or reduce their frequency of use. There are major challenges in doing so. The first is finding effective ways to persuade young people with a psychotic predisposition to stop doing something that they enjoy when pleasures may be few and far between and their everyday lives may be very challenging. The second is providing effective help to those who want to stop using cannabis but find it difficult to do so. Recent evaluations (see Connor et al., 2021) of psychological interventions for cannabis dependence in persons *without* psychoses report only modest rates of abstinence at the end of treatment (20–40%) and substantial rates of relapse in the first year after treatment. Nonetheless, treatment substantially reduces cannabis

use and problems in those who do not quit, much like the outcomes of the treatment of alcohol dependence (Connor et al., 2021; Gates et al., 2016; Winters et al., 2020).

People with schizophrenia who use cannabis may have less chance of achieving abstinence because they often lack social support, are cognitively impaired, more likely to be unemployed, and may not adhere to antipsychotic treatment (Patel et al., 2020). A recent Cochrane review of 25 RCTs of treatments in persons with mental disorders found 'no compelling evidence to support any one psychosocial treatment over another to reduce substance use (or improve mental state) by people with serious mental illnesses' (Hunt et al., 2019). We accordingly need to develop more effective psychological and pharmacological treatments for cannabis dependence in persons with psychoses and other serious mental illnesses (see Chapter 24).

6.7 Informing Young People about the Mental Health Risks of Cannabis Use

We need more effective and persuasive ways of informing young people about the mental health risks of cannabis use, including the risks of cannabis dependence, impaired cognitive performance and reduced educational attainment, and depression (Hall et al., 2020). Providing credible advice on these risks is complicated by the polarized views on the health risks of cannabis in the community.

Well-conducted school-based universal drug prevention programmes for adolescents produce small reductions in illicit drug use (Faggiano et al., 2014; Norberg et al., 2013; Porath-Waller et al., 2010). There is some evidence from a small number of studies that these programmes can reduce cannabis use (Norberg et al., 2013; Porath-Waller et al., 2010).

Mass media campaigns are of uncertain effectiveness in reducing adolescent drug use because of weak study designs and heterogenous findings in evaluations of these approaches (Ferri et al., 2013). These campaigns are more often designed to meet the imperative that politicians demonstrate to parents that they are concerned about adolescent cannabis use. Their content is more likely to satisfy parents than provide credible and persuasive information to young people. Mass media and school-based campaigns must also address scepticism among *youth* about health advice given by *adults*. Adolescents are often sensitive to what they see as parental double standards in disapproving of cannabis use while drinking alcohol. They are also alert to what they see as dishonest information about cannabis because of a history of scare campaigns about cannabis.

Educating adolescents about the risks of cannabis use should ideally be part of broader health education about alcohol and other drug use and mental health (McBride, 2003). These programmes should: explain the mental health risks of intoxication using alcohol and cannabis and identify young people who are at high-risk of adverse effects, such as those with a family history of psychosis, and those who have had bad experiences with cannabis and alcohol (see also Chapter 16). Adolescents should also be encouraged to intervene with any peers who engage in risky cannabis and alcohol use, encouraging them to cease their use or seek help earlier than may otherwise be the case.

6.8 Policies towards Recreational Cannabis Use

A mistaken assumption is that if cannabis is a contributory cause of psychotic disorders then it follows that we should prohibit cannabis use (e.g., Cresswell, 2005). For example, de Irala et al. (2005, p. 358) pose the question that 'in light of all we know, should we recommend cannabis use to our youth and just wait and see until more evidence arises? Or is it wise to prohibit its use?'

This type of inference follows from a common media simplification of cannabis policy debates: that we should legalize cannabis if its use is harmless, and we should continue to prohibit it if its use can harm users (Hall, 1997; Hall and Pacula, 2010). Given this framing, it is understandable why those who defend cannabis prohibition often cite the evidence on psychosis and why advocates of legalization attempt to discredit this evidence for fear that it will undermine their most compelling argument for legalization, namely, that cannabis use causes no harm.

It does not follow, however, that cannabis use should be prohibited simply because it harms some users (Hall and Pacula, 2010). If it did, our society would be morally obliged to ban alcohol and tobacco use, as well as automobiles and motorbikes. The evidence that cannabis is a contributory cause of psychotic disorders is relevant to policy because they are serious disorders that adversely affect the life chances of the young people affected by them (Hall et al., 2001). Nonetheless, this health effect should not be the sole basis for cannabis policy. In making cannabis policy, we need to consider other evidence in addition to that on the harms arising from cannabis use. This other evidence bears on whether criminal penalties are the best way to discourage cannabis use and reduce cannabis-related harm, and whether the social and economic costs arising from criminal penalties are socially acceptable (Hall and Pacula, 2010; Pollack and Reuter, 2007; Room et al., 2010).

There are reasons for doubting that criminal penalties are very effective in deterring cannabis use. First, substituting civil for criminal penalties for cannabis use has not greatly increased rates of cannabis use in those jurisdictions that have made this change (MacCoun and Reuter, 2001; Room et al., 2010; Single, 1989). Second, imposing criminal penalties on an offence that is committed annually by around 10% of adults in many developed countries in any year means that the law is either not enforced or it is selectively enforced against social minorities and disadvantaged groups in the community (Hall and Pacula, 2010; Room et al., 2010). The latter practice has proven to be one of the most persuasive arguments used for cannabis legalization in the United States (Hall et al., 2019).

6.9 Minimizing Adverse Mental Health Effects of Cannabis Legalization

The legalization of adult cannabis use has been advocated in the United States and Canada as a better policy than cannabis prohibition because it eliminates criminal penalties for adult use and allows cannabis to be regulated in ways that protect users and minimize cannabis use by youth (McGinty et al., 2017). Experience to date with cannabis legalization in the United States has not lived up to these promises (Hall et al., 2019; Subritzky et al., 2016). Instead, legalization has increased cannabis users' access to more potent forms of cannabis (with THC content of 70% or more) than were available under prohibition (Smart et al., 2017). It has also greatly reduced cannabis prices (Dills et al., 2021), increased the availability of cannabis, and reduced the perceived risks of using cannabis (Carliner et al., 2017; Hall et al., 2019). And it has created a legal cannabis industry that has an interest in promoting daily cannabis use because daily users account for 80% of total cannabis consumption

(Chan and Hall, 2020) and, hence, generate the greatest profits for cannabis retailers (Hall et al., 2019).

In referendum campaigns to legalize cannabis in the United States, legalization has also been promoted as a way to save on the costs of law enforcement, generate new tax revenue for state governments, and provide a new source of legal employment (McGinty et al., 2017). In US states that have legalized cannabis, the industry has lobbied governments to reduce 'red tape' and cannabis taxes and regulation so that retailers can compete with the residual illicit cannabis market (Hall et al., 2019).

Policymakers could reduce cannabis-related harm in legal markets by looking to successful policy experiences with alcohol and tobacco (Pacula et al., 2014). For example, they could, in addition to setting age limits, place a cap on the THC content of cannabis products; base taxes on the THC content of cannabis products (much like we do with alcohol); and ban all advertising of cannabis products (Pacula et al., 2014; Shover and Humphreys, 2019).

Governments in Canada (Cox, 2018) and Uruguay (Hudak et al., 2018) have adopted some of these public health oriented policies (Hall et al., 2019; Pacula et al., 2014). Canada, for example, has set age limits on legal cannabis purchases; restricted the number and location of sales outlets; banned cannabis advertising; and required plain packaging of cannabis products. Uruguay has attempted to restrict the number of cannabis retail outlets, set limits on the THC content of cannabis products, and required all adult cannabis users to register with the state to legally access cannabis (Hudak et al., 2018). It remains to be seen whether these public health-oriented policies will continue in the face of concerted lobbying by the legal cannabis industry to reduce 'red tape and taxes'. In the longer term, if other high income countries adopt the same model of commercialized cannabis production and sales as in most of Canada and in US states that have legalized, we will see the creation of a large multinational cannabis industry that will look to expand its international markets.

6.10 Conclusion

The epidemiological evidence for a causal relationship between cannabis use and psychosis is consistent and arguably stronger than that for heavy alcohol use and similar to that for amphetamine use and psychotic symptoms. A causal relationship is biologically plausible because the cannabinoids interact with dopaminergic neurotransmission and high doses of THC can produce psychotic symptoms in people without psychosis.

Given the evidence, policymakers should discourage cannabis use among the clients of mental health services by screening all patients with psychotic symptoms and advising those who use cannabis to stop or to reduce their use. More research is needed on better ways to assist those who would like to stop but find it difficult to do so.

There is arguably an ethical imperative to inform young people of the probable mental health risks of cannabis use. It is also prudent to discourage young people from the early initiation of and frequent use of cannabis in adolescence and young adulthood. The challenge is to find credible and persuasive ways of doing so given the polarized debate about cannabis policy. Political imperatives to express community concern via mass media campaigns may work against effective education if they unwittingly foster sceptical views of the evidence. The tobacco industry's success in undermining tobacco control policies suggests that raising doubts about the quality of the evidence for harmful effects of cannabis will be an effective way of reassuring users that it is safe to continue using cannabis (Glantz et al., 1996).

Policymakers should not assume that, if the relationship between cannabis use and psychosis is causal, we should prohibit cannabis use by adults. Accepting a causal relationship removes the strongest case for liberalization – the absence of any harmful effects of cannabis on users. Given how seriously psychotic disorders can affect the life chances of young people, there is a need for caution in liberalizing cannabis regulations in ways that increase young people's access to highly potent cannabis, decrease their age of first use, and increase the frequency of their cannabis use. A considered decision about social policies towards adult cannabis requires an analysis of the harms caused by current policy, as well as the harms caused by cannabis use.

Acknowledgements

We would like to thank Sarah Yeates for her assistance in preparing this chapter for publication.

References

Angrist, B., Sathananthan, G., Wilk, S., et al. (1974). Amphetamine psychosis: Behavioral and biochemical aspects. *J Psychiatric Res*, **11**, 13–23.

Arseneault, L., Cannon, M., Poulton, R., et al. (2002). Cannabis use in adolescence and risk for adult psychosis: Longitudinal prospective study. *BMJ*, **325**, 1212–1213.

Arunogiri, S., Foulds, J. A., McKetin, R., et al. (2018). A systematic review of risk factors for methamphetamine-associated psychosis. *Aust NZ J Psychiatry*, **52**, 514–529.

Atkinson, D. L., and Abbott, J. K. (2018). Cannabinoids and the brain: The effects of endogenous and exogenous cannabinoids on brain systems and function. In: Compton, M. T., and Manseau, M. W. (eds.) *The Complex Connection between Cannabis and Schizophrenia* (pp. 37–74). San Diego: Academic Press.

Bell, D. S. (1973). The experimental reproduction of amphetamine psychosis. *Arch Gen Psychiatry*, **29**, 35–40.

Cahill, J. D., Gupta, S., Cortes-Briones, J., et al. (2018). Psychotomimetic and cognitive effects of Δ9-Tetrahydrocannabinol in laboratory settings. In: Compton, M. T., and Manseau, M. W. (eds.) *The Complex Connection between Cannabis and Schizophrenia* (pp. 75–128). San Diego: Academic Press.

Carliner, H., Brown, Q. L., Sarvet, A. L., et al. (2017). Cannabis use, attitudes, and legal status in the U.S.: A review. *Prevent Med*, **104**, 13–23.

Chan, G. C. K., and Hall, W. D. (2020). Estimation of the proportion of population cannabis consumption in Australia that is accounted for by daily users using Monte Carlo simulation. *Addiction*, **115**, 1182–1186.

Connell, P. H. (1958). *Amphetamine Psychosis*. (Maudsley Monograph). London: Published for the Institute of Psychiatry by Chapman and Hall.

Connor, J. P., Stjepanović, D., Le Foll, B., et al. (2021). Cannabis use and cannabis use disorder. *Nature Rev Dis Primers*, **7**, 16.

Cox, C. (2018). The Canadian Cannabis Act legalizes and regulates recreational cannabis use in 2018. *Health Policy*, **122**, 205–209.

Cresswell, A. (2005). Weak drug laws linked to madness. *The Australian*, 29 October.

Curran, C., Byrappa, N., and McBride, A. (2004). Stimulant psychosis: Systematic review. *Br J Psychiatry*, **185**, 196–204.

Degenhardt, L., and Hall, W. D. (2001). The association between psychosis and problematical drug use among Australian adults: Findings from the National Survey of Mental Health and Well-being. *Psychol Med*, **31**, 659–668.

Degenhardt, L., Hall, W. D., and Lynskey, M. (2003). Testing hypotheses about the relationship between cannabis use and psychosis. *Drug Alcohol Depend*, **71**, 37–48.

Dills, A., Goffard, S., Miron, J., et al. (2021). *The Effect of State Marijuana Legalizations: 2021 Update*. Washington, DC: Cato Institute.

Dwyer, T., Ponsonby, A. L., Blizzard, L., et al. (1995). The contribution of changes in the prevalence of prone sleeping position to the decline in sudden infant death syndrome in Tasmania. *JAMA*, **273**, 783–789.

Faggiano, F., Minozzi, S., Versino, E., et al. (2014). Universal school-based prevention for illicit drug use. *Cochrane Database Syst Rev*, CD003020.

Fergusson, D., and Boden, J. (2008). Cannabis use and later life outcomes. *Addiction*, **103**, 969–976; discussion 977–978.

Fergusson, D., Boden, J., and Horwood, L. (2006). Cannabis use and other illicit drug use: Testing the cannabis gateway hypothesis. *Addiction*, **101**, 556–569.

Fergusson, D., Hall, W. D., Boden, J., et al. (2015). Rethinking cigarette smoking, cannabis use, and psychosis. *Lancet Psychiatry*, **2**, 581–582.

Fergusson, D., Horwood, L., and Ridder, E. (2005). Tests of causal linkages between cannabis use and psychotic symptoms. *Addiction*, **100**, 354–366.

Fergusson, D., Horwood, L., and Swain-Campbell, N. (2003). Cannabis dependence and psychotic symptoms in young people. *Psychol Med*, **33**, 15–21.

Ferri, M., Allara, E., Bo, A., et al. (2013). Media campaigns for the prevention of illicit drug use in young people. *Cochrane Database Syst Rev*, CD009287.

Gage, S. H., Hickman, M., Heron, J., et al. (2014). Associations of cannabis and cigarette use with psychotic experiences at age 18: Findings from the Avon Longitudinal Study of Parents and Children. *Psychol Med*, **44**, 3435–3444.

Gage, S. H., Hickman, M., and Zammit, S. (2016). Association between cannabis and psychosis: Epidemiologic evidence. *Biol Psychiatry*, **79**, 549–556.

Gates, P. J., Sabioni, P., Copeland, J., et al. (2016). Psychosocial interventions for cannabis use disorder. *Cochrane Database Syst Rev*, **5**, CD005336.

Gillespie, N. A., and Kendler, K. S. (2021). Use of genetically informed methods to clarify the nature of the association between cannabis use and risk for schizophrenia. *JAMA Psychiatry*, **78**, 467–468.

Gilman, J. M., Sobolewski, S. M., and Eden Evins, A. (2018). Cannabis use as an independent risk factor for, or component cause of, schizophrenia and related psychotic disorders. In: Compton, M. T., and Manseau, M. W. (eds.) *The Complex Connection between Cannabis and Schizophrenia* (pp. 221–246). San Diego: Academic Press.

Glantz, S. A., Slade, J., Bero, L. A., et al. (eds.) (1996). *The Cigarette Papers*. Berkeley: University of California Press.

Greenberg, D. M., and Lee, J. W. (2001). Psychotic manifestations of alcoholism. *Curr Psychiatry Rep*, **3**, 314–318.

Hall, W. D. (1997). The recent Australian debate about the prohibition on cannabis use. *Addiction*, **92**, 1109–1115.

Hall, W. D., Degenhardt, L. D., and Lynskey, M. (2001). *The Health and Psychological Effects of Cannabis Use*. Canberra: Commonwealth Department of Health and Aged Care.

Hall, W. D., Degenhardt, L., and Patton, G. (2008). Cannabis abuse and dependence. In: Essau, C. A. (ed.) *Adolescent Addiction: Epidemiology, Treatment and Assessment* (pp. 117–148). London: Academic Press.

Hall, W. D., and Hando, J. (1993). Patterns of illicit psychostimulant use in Australia. In: Burrows, D., Flaherty, B. A., and MacAvoy, M. (eds.) *Psychostimulant Use in Australia*. Canberra: AGPS.

Hall, W. D., Leung, J., and Lynskey, M. (2020). The effects of cannabis use on the development of adolescents and young adults. *Ann Rev Develop Psychol*, **2**, 461–483.

Hall, W. D., and Lynskey, M. (2005). Is cannabis a gateway drug? Testing hypotheses about the relationship between cannabis use and the use of other illicit drugs. *Drug Alcohol Rev*, **24**, 39–48.

Hall, W. D., and Pacula, R. (2010). *Cannabis Use and Dependence: Public Health and Public Policy*. Cambridge: Cambridge University Press.

Hall, W. D., Stjepanović, D., Caulkins, J., et al. (2019). Public health implications of legalising the production and sale of cannabis for medicinal and recreational use. *Lancet*, **394**, 1580–1590.

Hasan, A., von Keller, R., Friemel, C. M., et al. (2020). Cannabis use and psychosis: A review of reviews. *Eur Arch Psychiatry Clin Neurosci*, **270**, 403–412.

Henquet, C., Krabbendam, L., Spauwen, J., et al. (2005). Prospective cohort study of cannabis use, predisposition for psychosis, and psychotic symptoms in young people. *BMJ*, **330**, 11.

Hindley, G., Beck, K., Borgan, F., et al. (2020). Psychiatric symptoms caused by cannabis constituents: A systematic review and meta-analysis. *Lancet Psychiatry*, **7**, 344–353.

Hudak, J., Ramsey, G., and Walsh, J. (2018). *Uruguay's Cannabis Law: Pioneering a New Paradigm*. Washington, DC: Center for Effective Public Management at Brookings.

Hunt, G. E., Siegfried, N., Morley, K., et al. (2019). Psychosocial interventions for people with both severe mental illness and substance misuse. *Cochrane Database Syst Rev*, **12**, CD001088.

Hunter, A., Murray, R., Asher, L., et al. (2020). The effects of tobacco smoking, and prenatal tobacco smoke exposure, on risk of schizophrenia: A systematic review and meta-analysis. *Nicotine Tobacco Res*, **22**, 3–10.

de Irala, J., Ruiz-Canela, M., and Martinez-Gonzalez, M. (2005). Causal relationship between cannabis use and psychotic symptoms or depression. Should we wait and see? A public health perspective. *Med Sci Monitor*, **11**, RA355–358.

Isbell, H., Fraser, H. F., Wikler, A., et al. (1955). An experimental study of the etiology of rum fits and delirium tremens. *Q J Stud Alcohol*, **16**, 1–33.

Iversen, L. (2012). How cannabis works in the human brain. In: Castle, D., Murray, R., and D'Souza, D. C. (eds.) *Marijuana and Madness* (pp. 1–11). Cambridge: Cambridge University Press.

Jones, H. J., Gage, S. H., Heron, J., et al. (2018). Association of combined patterns of tobacco and cannabis use in adolescence with psychotic experiences. *JAMA Psychiatry*, **75**, 240–246.

Klein, D. F. (2006). The flawed basis for FDA post-marketing safety decisions: The example of anti-depressants and children. *Neuropsychopharmacology*, **31**, 689–699.

Ksir, C., and Hart, C. L. (2016). Cannabis and psychosis: A critical overview of the relationship. *Curr Psychiatry Rep*, **18**, 12.

Lappin, J. M., and Sara, G. E. (2019). Psychostimulant use and the brain. *Addiction*, **114**, 2065–2077.

Lishman, W. A. (1987). *Organic Psychiatry: The Psychological Consequences of Cerebral Disorder*. Oxford: Blackwell Scientific.

Lorenzetti, V., Hoch, E., and Hall, W. (2020). Adolescent cannabis use, cognition, brain health and educational outcomes: A review of the evidence. *Eur Neuropsychopharmacol*, **36**, 169–180.

MacCoun, R. J., and Reuter, P. (2001). *Drug War Heresies: Learning from Other Vices, Times and Places*.

Cambridge: Cambridge University Press.

Macleod, J., Oakes, R., Copello, A., et al. (2004). Psychological and social sequelae of cannabis and other illicit drug use by young people: A systematic review of longitudinal, general population studies. *Lancet*, **363**, 1579–1588.

Marconi, A., Di Forti, M., Lewis, C. M., et al. (2016). Meta-analysis of the association between the level of cannabis use and risk of psychosis. *Schizophr Bull*, **42**, 1262–1269.

McBride, N. (2003). A systematic review of school drug education. *Health Educ Res*, **18**, 729–742.

McGinty, E. E., Niederdeppe, J., Heley, K., et al. (2017). Public perceptions of arguments supporting and opposing recreational marijuana legalization. *Prevent Med*, **99**, 80–86.

McKetin, R., Lubman, D. I., Baker, A. L., et al. (2013). Dose-related psychotic symptoms in chronic methamphetamine users: Evidence from a prospective longitudinal study. *JAMA Psychiatry*, **70**, 319–324.

Moore, T. H. M., Zammit, S., Lingford-Hughes, A., et al. (2007). Cannabis use and risk of psychotic or affective mental health outcomes: A systematic review. *Lancet*, **370**, 319–328.

Mullen, J. M., Richards, J. R., and Crawford, A. T. (2020). *Amphetamine Related Psychiatric Disorders*. Treasure Island, FL: StatPearls Publishing.

Narasimha, V. L., Patley, R., Shukla, L., et al. (2019). Phenomenology and course of alcoholic hallucinosis. *J Dual Diagn*, **15**, 172–176.

Norberg, M. M., Kezelman, S., and Lim-Howe, N. (2013). Primary prevention of cannabis use:

A systematic review of randomized controlled trials. *PLoS ONE*, **8**, e53187.

van Os, J., Bak, M., Hanssen, M., et al. (2002). Cannabis use and psychosis: A longitudinal population-based study. *Am J Epidemiol*, **156**, 319–327.

Pacula, R. L., Kilmer, B., Wagenaar, A. C., et al. (2014). Developing public health regulations for marijuana: Lessons from alcohol and tobacco. *Am J Public Health*, **104**, 1021–1028.

Patel, R. S., Sreeram, V., Vadukapuram, R., et al. (2020). Do cannabis use disorders increase medication non-compliance in schizophrenia?: United States nationwide inpatient cross-sectional study. *Schizophr Res*, **224**, 40–44.

Patton, G. C., Coffey, C., Carlin, J. B., et al. (2002). Cannabis use and mental health in young people: Cohort study. *BMJ*, **325**, 1195–1198.

Patton, G. C., Coffey, C., Lynskey, M. T., et al. (2007). Trajectories of adolescent alcohol and cannabis use into young adulthood. *Addiction*, **102**, 607–615.

Pollack, H. A., and Reuter, P. (2007). The implications of recent findings on the link between cannabis and psychosis. *Addiction*, **102**, 173–176.

Porath-Waller, A. J., Beasley, E., and Beirness, D. J. (2010). A meta-analytic review of school-based prevention for cannabis use. *Health Educ Behav*, **37**, 709–723.

Room, R., Fischer, B., Hall, W. D., et al. (2010). *Cannabis Policy: Moving beyond Stalemate*. Oxford: Oxford University Press.

Schoeler, T., Monk, A., Sami, M. B., et al. (2016). Continued versus discontinued cannabis use in

patients with psychosis: A systematic review and meta-analysis. *Lancet Psychiatry*, **3**, 215–225.

Shover, C. L., and Humphreys, K. (2019). Six policy lessons relevant to cannabis legalization. *Am J Drug Alcohol Abuse*, **45**, 698–706.

Single, E. W. (1989). The impact of marijuana decriminalization: An update. *J Public Health Policy*, **9**, 456–466.

Smart, R., Caulkins, J. P., Kilmer, B., et al. (2017). Variation in cannabis potency and prices in a newly legal market: Evidence from 30 million cannabis sales in Washington state. *Addiction*, **112**, 2167–2177.

Subritzky, T., Pettigrew, S., and Lenton, S. (2016). Issues in the implementation and evolution of the commercial recreational cannabis market in Colorado. *Int J Drug Policy*, **27**, 1–12.

Voce, A., McKetin, R., Burns, R., et al. (2019). A systematic review of the symptom profile and course of methamphetamine use and psychotic symptoms profiles associated psychosis. *Subst Use Misuse*, **54**, 549–559.

Winters, K. C., Mader, J., Budney, A. J., et al. (2020). Interventions for cannabis use disorder. *Curr Opin Psychology*, **38**, 67–74.

Zammit, S., Allebeck, P., Andréasson, S., et al. (2002). Self reported cannabis use as a risk factor for schizophrenia in Swedish conscripts of 1969: Historical cohort study. *BMJ*, **325**, 1199–1201.

Zammit, S., Moore, T. H., Lingford-Hughes, A., et al. (2008). Effects of cannabis use on outcomes of psychotic disorders: Systematic review. *Br J Psychiatry*, **193**, 357–363.

The Impact of Adolescent Exposure to Cannabis on the Brain
A Focus on Animal Studies

Erica Zamberletti and Tiziana Rubino

Cannabis is the most used drug globally (see Chapter 4), and adolescents and young adults account for the largest share of those using it (UNODC, 2020). In Europe, around 15% (18.0 million) of young adults (aged 15–34) report using cannabis in the last year, with males being typically twice as likely to report use than females (EMCDDA, 2020). When only 15–24-year-olds are considered, the prevalence of cannabis use is higher, with 19% having used the drug in the last year and 10% in the last month. Given this high prevalence of cannabis use among adolescents and the fact that cannabis is increasingly viewed as harmless by both adolescents and adults (Hammond et al., 2020; Hasin, 2018), there is an urgent need for a greater understanding of cannabis effects on the still developing adolescent brain.

7.1 Adolescence as a Critical Developmental Window

Adolescence represents a critical window of development which spans from childhood to adulthood. It is a period characterized by important processes of brain maturation devoted to a remodelling of its structure through a reduction in the grey matter volume and an increase in white matter, to make the brain more efficient (Gogtay et al., 2004). These processes encompass the refinement of specific neural circuits, characterized by a relatively early maturation of sub-cortical regions and a relatively delayed maturation of prefrontal control areas, with the result that the limbic and reward systems take control over the still immature prefrontal control system (Konrad et al., 2013). This period of transition is common to all mammals, with similar biological changes, including the brain remodelling processes (Hiller-Sturmhöfel and Spear, 2018). These similarities are very useful in the context of research, since the investigation of in-depth neurobiological mechanisms in humans still suffers substantial limitations. Moreover,

confounding factors, such as lifestyle, are difficult to control in humans and may result in divergent observations. Animal models, instead, enable us to establish a causal relationship and, thus, to better elucidate the neurobiological mechanisms underlying the process under study. Remarkably, all the main steps characterizing human adolescent brain maturation have also been described in rodents, thus providing researchers with the possibility to complement studies in human adolescents and address questions that are ethically or technically not amenable to study in humans (Hiller-Sturmhöfel and Spear, 2018).

In rodent models, too, the adolescent brain is highly plastic and undergoes developmental and biological changes that are required for proper behavioural and cognitive maturation. However, this dynamic nature of the adolescent brain places it in a state of higher vulnerability to harmful environmental manipulations, such as exposure to drugs.

In this chapter we will review studies that, through the use of animal models, have shed light on functional and structural alterations associated with adolescent cannabis use and the persistence of these phenotypes in adulthood.

7.2 Behavioural Consequences of Adolescent Cannabinoid Exposure

The majority of the studies performed in animal models suggest that an intense exposure to cannabinoids during adolescence exert long-term detrimental effects on emotional and cognitive functions, possibly contributing to the development of psychiatric disorders (Higuera Matas et al., 2015; Rubino and Parolaro, 2016).

7.3 Cannabinoids and Cognition

Cognitive deficits are among the best-described effects occurring after cannabinoid exposure and long-lasting alterations in cognitive functions have been observed in rodents repeatedly exposed to cannabinoids during adolescence (Prini et al., 2020). Impairments in working memory processes have been reported using object recognition and T-maze tasks in male and female rodent models following adolescent but not adult treatment (see, for review, Cuccurazzu et al., 2018; Kasten et al., 2017; Murphy et al., 2017; Prini et al., 2018; Renard et al., 2016; Rubino and Parolaro, 2016; Zamberletti et al., 2016). Additionally, enduring deficits on cognitive processes related to flexibility and decision-making have been described using attentional set-shifting tasks and probabilistic reward choice tasks (Gomes et al., 2014; Jacobs-Brichford et al., 2019). Long-term deficits in associative learning memory have also been reported, with rats exposed to THC during adolescence taking longer to learn a paired-associates learning task when tested in adulthood (Abela et al., 2019). Interestingly, this cognitive impairment appeared to be transient. Studies using pure spatial memory tasks such as water maze paradigms and Barnes maze test showed no deficits in learning and memory following chronic THC exposure during adolescence (Cha et al., 2006; Nelson et al., 2019), suggesting that THC effects only specific memory domains. In contrast, working memory performance was unaltered or slightly improved after adolescent self-administration of THC (Stringfield and Torregrossa, 2021b), as also reported after cannabis or THC smoke exposure (Bruijnzeel et al., 2019).

Overall, deficits in cognitive processing have been consistently demonstrated in both male and female animal models using experimenter-administration protocols. However, cannabinoid exposure under conditions of intravenous and smoke self-administration seems to have less detrimental effects on cognition, likely because, when adolescent rodents are given the opportunity to control the dose to which they are exposed to, they likely do not reach the high concentrations observed in experimenter administered exposure models and in human heavy abusers. Accordingly, the plasma concentration of cannabinoid metabolites obtained using smoke inhalation in these rats was comparable to a low-to-moderate dose exposure in humans (Stringfield and Torregrossa, 2021a).

7.4 Cannabinoids and Psychosis

One animal model to assess psychotic-like states in rodents is the pre-pulse inhibition (PPI) paradigm, whose impairment has been linked to a dysfunction in the sensorimotor gating mechanism, a cognitive abnormality also seen in schizophrenia. Alternatively, psychotic-like signs in animal models have been assessed through the investigation of hyperlocomotion, either at baseline or following stimulation by dopaminergic and glutamatergic agents. The majority of findings indicate that chronic exposure to THC during adolescence, but not during adulthood, induced long-lasting impairment of PPI in rats, although discrepant findings can be found depending on the rodent species used (De Felice et al., 2021; Levine et al., 2017; Rubino and Parolaro, 2016). Recently, it has been shown that PPI deficits triggered by adolescent cannabinoid exposure decreased after six months of abstinence (Abela et al., 2019). With respect to locomotor activity abnormalities, investigations of the spontaneous locomotor activity of rodents following adolescent cannabinoid treatments have generally been inconsistent. However, results seem to be more consistent when examining hyperlocomotion induced by dopaminergic and glutamatergic agents, indicating that adolescent THC exposure increased the locomotor response to both classes of compounds (Renard et al., 2016). Further suggestive of an inter-play between adolescent cannabinoid exposure and psychosis, especially when other risk factors are already present, is a recent study demonstrating that administration of THC during late adolescence can potentiate the development of schizophrenia-related behavioural phenotypes induced by neonatal exposure to phencyclidine in mice (Rodríguez et al., 2017).

7.5 Cannabinoids and Emotional Behaviour

In animal models, the link between cannabis use and anxiety is not as consistent as in humans. For instance, either anxiogenic, anxiolytic, or no effect have been described in the long-term following chronic administration of natural cannabinoid agonists in the elevated plus maze and in the open field tests (Renard et al., 2016). More recent findings also failed to provide a clear conclusion. An anxiolytic effect of adolescent THC exposure has been described preferentially in males when treated at a very early stage of adolescence and the main changes in baseline anxiety, either increases or decreases, have generally been demonstrated in the elevated plus maze test with respect to the open field test (Pushkin et al., 2019; Saravia et al., 2019; Silva et al., 2016). No effects on measures of anxiety have been reported after cannabis or THC exposure during adolescence (Bruijnzeel et al., 2019). Based on current literature data, it is therefore not possible to draw any conclusion on the long-lasting effects of adolescent cannabinoid exposure on measures of anxiety.

In contrast, available data clearly suggest that adolescent exposure to THC has detrimental effects on measures of depressive-like behaviours in adulthood. A depressive-like phenotype in adulthood has been described after adolescent exposure to cannabinoids in the sucrose preference test, in the forced swim test, and in the social interaction test (Levine et al., 2017). Long-term abnormalities related to aspects of depressive reactivity have also been observed after exposure to low THC doses in rats at the beginning of the adolescent period (1 mg/kg with exposure starting at post-natal day (PND) 30; De Gregorio et al., 2020). Of note, sexually dimorphic outcomes dominate the data for this domain of function. Indeed, female rats treated with cannabinoids during adolescence displayed more intense depressive behaviours compared to their male counterparts (Rubino and Parolaro, 2016). These findings support the theory that exposure to cannabinoids during adolescence may affect the susceptibility to developing mood disorders later in life, suggesting that female rats may be more susceptible to the affective consequences of adolescent cannabis exposure.

7.6 Gateway Effect

Epidemiological studies suggest an association between early cannabis use and a higher risk of progressing toward addiction to other drugs. This is known as the 'gateway hypothesis', that posits that the relationship between early cannabis use and the subsequent abuse of other addictive substances is causal in nature (Kandel and Kandel, 2015). Animal studies examining a causal link between adolescent cannabinoid exposure and subsequent abuse of illicit drugs at adulthood have mainly focused on opioids and cocaine. Adolescent THC exposure increased heroin intake (Ellgren et al., 2007) but did not facilitate the acquisition of heroin self-administration in adult rats (Ellgren et al., 2007; Stopponi et al., 2014). Furthermore, exposure to THC during adolescence was shown to increase the vulnerability to heroin relapse in adulthood (Stopponi et al., 2014), suggesting that a previous history of cannabinoid use during adolescence might be a risk factor for relapse following opioid use later in life. Also, inhaled THC

vapor during adolescence did not alter oxycodone self-administration in adult male and female rats (Nguyen et al., 2020). However, THC pre-exposure during adolescence increased fentanyl self-administration in female rats only (Nguyen et al., 2020). Overall, available data suggest that the association between adolescent THC exposure and adult vulnerability to opioids might be dependent on the sex of the animals and the potency of opioid tested. Recently, the influence of adolescent cannabis exposure on adult heroin reinforcement has been demonstrated in a model of genetic vulnerability to drug addiction. THC pre-exposure increased responding for heroin, heroin intake, and reinstatement in vulnerable male rats (Lecca et al., 2020), suggesting that genetic factors might play a pivotal role in determining the outcome of adolescent cannabinoid exposure on opioid vulnerability later in life.

There is pre-clinical evidence supporting the relationship between prior THC treatment and alterations in the rewarding or activating effects of cocaine (Aldhafiri et al., 2019; Dow-Edwards and Izenwasser, 2012; Friedman et al., 2019).

With regard to a possible association between adolescent cannabinoid exposure and subsequent use of legal drugs of abuse, such as nicotine, adolescent THC exposure did not alter the performance of intravenous nicotine self-administration in adulthood (Flores et al., 2020).

7.7 Molecular Underpinnings

Among the different maturational processes occurring in the adolescent brain, evidence from rodent – but also human – studies indicates that the different components of the endocannabinoid system undergo major changes during this specific developmental window, emphasizing the dynamic nature of this system in the adolescent brain (Bara et al., 2021; Rubino and Parolaro, 2016). Adolescent animals have lower amounts of CB1 receptors than adults, but they appear to be more efficiently coupled to G proteins, suggesting a stronger activation of the CB1-related intracellular pathways by endocannabinoid signalling (and also by exogenous cannabinoids) at this age. The levels of the two main endocannabinoids – AEA and 2-AG – undergo significant fluctuations during this period, and almost always display opposite alterations, that is, when AEA increases 2-AG decreases and vice-versa. This picture of intense changes points toward an active role of the endocannabinoid system in the developmental processes occurring in the adolescent brain, whose alteration could affect the proper shaping and functionality of the adult brain.

A growing body of evidence seems to suggest that this is exactly what THC does. Indeed, THC exposure during adolescence, activating indiscriminately all CB1 receptors present in the brain, disrupts the space- and time-specific action of the endocannabinoids, eventually impacting on the connectivity of neuronal networks and the specific neural refinement occurring in this developmental window (Molla and Tseng, 2020; Renard et al., 2018; Zamberletti and Rubino, 2021). Accordingly, some evidence suggests that THC may impact the ongoing remodelling of GABAergic and glutamatergic synapses in the PFC, thus disturbing the normative maturation of associated prefrontal networks. Blockade of the endocannabinoid tone from early to late adolescence significantly prevented the physiological decrease in some glutamatergic markers (i.e., PSD-95, gluN2A, and gluA2), suggesting a role for this system in the elimination of excitatory synapses (Rubino et al., 2015), a phenomenon also known as synaptic pruning, claimed to be responsible for the decrease in grey matter occurring in the adolescent brain. Therefore, it is not surprising that THC-overstimulation of CB1 receptors may lead to excessive pruning and disrupted glutamatergic receptor remodelling (Miller et al., 2019; Rubino et al., 2015). Again, blockade of the endocannabinoid tone from early- to mid-adolescence seems to promote the physiological increase in GAD67 expression (Simone et al., 2018), the main enzyme responsible for GABA production in the brain, suggesting an inhibitory role of the endocannabinoid tone in the maturational processes within the GABAergic system. On the contrary, adolescent THC exposure decreased GAD67 expression, thus preventing/delaying these processes (Renard et al., 2018; Zamberletti et al., 2014). This attenuation in GABAergic function seems to be related with a hyperactive neuronal state in PFC neurons and a reduced GABAergic control of prefrontal output, leading to disruptions in cortical gamma oscillatory activity and dysregulation of DAergic neurotransmission in sub-cortical areas (Molla and Tseng, 2020; Renard et al., 2018).

The long-term impact of adolescent THC exposure seems to suggest a contribution of epigenetic processes. Accordingly, adolescent THC exposure induced alterations in specific histone modifications in the PFC of both male and female rats, affecting mainly the transcription of genes related to synaptic plasticity (Miller et al., 2019; Prini et al., 2018). The effect of THC exposure on histone modifications displays an age-specific nature, being more intense and characterized by more complex kinetics in the adolescent brain when compared to the adult one (Prini et al., 2017, 2018). Remarkably, among the alterations, the increase in H3K9me3 appears to be causally linked with the cognitive impairment described in these animals, as the pharmacological blockade of H3K9me3 during adolescent exposure to THC prevented its development (Prini et al., 2018).

Neurons, however, are not the only cells impacted by THC in the brain. Glial cells, including microglia and astrocytes, are also influenced as they possess cannabinoid receptors (Melis et al., 2017). The few papers dealing with this topic suggest that adolescent THC exposure induced a significant increase of the percentage of reactive microglia in both male and female rats, suggesting the presence of neuroinflammation (Lopez Rodriguez et al., 2014; Zamberletti et al., 2015). Interestingly, in female rats, a causal link between this neuroinflammatory picture and THC-induced-cognitive deficits has been described, as co-treatment during adolescence with Ibudilast (an inhibitor of microglial activation) reduced both neuroinflammation and the long-lasting deficit in recognition memory (Zamberletti et al., 2015). Moreover, in males, adolescent THC exposure also induced alterations in astrocyte reactivity in the hippocampus (Jouroukhin et al., 2019; Zamberletti et al., 2016) and these changes too seem to play a role in THC-induced cognitive deficit. Interestingly, astrocyte genetic risk factors can exacerbate the impairment in cognition (Jouroukhin et al., 2019), suggesting that alterations in astrocyte functionality can enhance individual sensitivity toward the development of cognitive deficits after adolescent cannabis use.

7.8 Conclusion

The public debate on cannabis is frequently limited to very rigid and conflicting positions and is high in emotional content rather than being driven by science-based evidence. This often hinders an objective discussion of the potential specific risks associated with cannabis exposure. Available pre-clinical findings suggest that adolescents represent a vulnerable consumer group for cannabis preparations and seem to be at a higher risk of suffering from adverse consequences of cannabinoid exposure than the adult population. Indeed, animal research supports the hypothesis of the existence of long-term behavioural deficits in adulthood following adolescent cannabinoid exposure depending on three key factors: dosage, age of first exposure, and, maybe, THC/CBD ratio (we still need more experimental research to fully support this last assumption). Indeed, heavy THC exposure during adolescence triggers abnormal neurodevelopmental processes leading to an adult brain characterized by altered functionality. However, if the exposure starts in early adolescence, even moderate THC doses can lead to brain impairments. Finally, preliminary observations seem to suggest that the presence of CBD may mitigate THC detrimental effects, pointing to the existence of higher risks when exposed to cannabis strains rich in THC and/or poor in CBD.

Some issues still need further clarification, such as the existence of a sex-specificity in THC effect, the transient nature of the changes, the actual modulatory role of CBD, which THC doses may be really safe when administered chronically during this developmental window, and the genetic and/or environmental risk factors that can magnify THC effects. All these points need to be addressed by future research.

References

Abela, A. R., Rahbarnia, A., Wood, S., et al. (2019). Adolescent exposure to Δ9-tetrahydrocannabinol delays acquisition of paired-associates learning in adulthood. *Psychopharmacology*, **236**, 1875–1886.

Aldhafiri, A., Dodu, J. C., Alalawi, A., et al. (2019). Delta-9-THC exposure during zebra finch sensorimotor vocal learning increases cocaine reinforcement in adulthood. *Pharmacol Biochem Behav*, **185**, 172764.

Bara, A., Ferland, J. N., Rompala, G., et al. (2021). Cannabis and synaptic reprogramming of the developing brain. *Nat Rev Neurosci*, **22**, 423–438.

Bruijnzeel, A. W., Knight, P., Panunzio, S., et al. (2019). Effects in rats of adolescent exposure to cannabis smoke or THC on emotional behavior and cognitive function in adulthood. *Psychopharmacology*, **236**, 2773–2784.

Cha, Y. M., White, A. M., Kuhn, C. M., et al. (2006). Differential effects of delta9-THC on learning in adolescent and adult rats. *Pharmacol Biochem Behav*, **83**, 448–455.

Cuccurazzu, B., Zamberletti, E., Nazzaro, C., et al. (2018). Adult cellular neuroadaptations induced by adolescent THC exposure in female rats are rescued by enhancing anandamide signaling. *Int J Neuropsychopharmacol*, **21**, 1014–1024.

De Felice, M., Renard, J., Hudson, R., et al. (2021). l-Theanine prevents long-term affective and cognitive side effects of adolescent Δ-9-tetrahydrocannabinol exposure and blocks associated molecular and neuronal abnormalities in the mesocorticolimbic circuitry. *J Neurosci*, **41**, 739–750.

De Gregorio, D., Dean Conway, J., Canul, M. L., et al. (2020). Effects of chronic exposure to low doses of Δ9-tetrahydrocannabinol in adolescence and adulthood on serotonin/norepinephrine neurotransmission and emotional behaviors. *Int J Neuropsychopharmacol*, **23**, 751–761.

Dow-Edwards, D., and Izenwasser, S. (2012). Pretreatment with Delta9-tetrahydrocannabinol (THC) increases cocaine-stimulated activity in adolescent but not adult male rats. *Pharmacol Biochem Behav*, **100**, 587–591.

Ellgren, M., Spano, S. M., and Hurd, Y. L. (2007). Adolescent cannabis exposure alters opiate intake and opioid limbic neuronal populations in adult rats. *Neuropsychopharmacology*, **32**, 607–615.

EMCDDA, European Monitoring Centre for Drugs and Drug Addiction (2020). *European Drug Report 2020: Trends and Developments*. Luxembourg: Publications Office of the European Union.

Flores, Á., Maldonado, R., and Berrendero, F. (2020). THC exposure during adolescence does not modify nicotine reinforcing effects and relapse in adult male mice. *Psychopharmacology*, **237**, 801–809.

Friedman, A. L., Meurice, C., and Jutkiewicz, E. M. (2019). Effects of adolescent Δ9-tetrahydrocannabinol exposure on the behavioral effects of cocaine in adult Sprague–Dawley rats. *Exp Clin Psychopharmacol*, **27**, 326–337.

Gogtay, N., Giedd, J. N., Lusk, L., et al. (2004). Dynamic mapping of human cortical development during childhood through early adulthood. *Proc Natl Acad Sci USA*, **101**, 8174–8179.

Gomes, F. V., Guimarães, F. S., and Grace, A. A. (2014). Effects of pubertal cannabinoid administration on attentional set-shifting and dopaminergic hyper-responsivity in a developmental disruption model of schizophrenia. *Int J Neuropsychopharmacol*, **18**, pyu018.

Hammond, C. J., Chaney, A., Hendrickson, B., et al. (2020). Cannabis use among U.S. adolescents in the era of marijuana legalization: A review of changing use patterns, comorbidity, and health correlates. *Int Rev Psychiatry*, **32**, 221–234.

Hasin, D. S. U. S. (2018). Epidemiology of cannabis use and associated problems. *Neuropsychopharmacology*, **43**, 195–212.

Higuera-Matas, A., Ucha, M., and Ambrosio, E. (2015). Long-term consequences of perinatal and adolescent cannabinoid exposure on neural and psychological processes. *Neurosci Biobehav Rev*, **55**, 119–146.

Hiller-Sturmhöfel, S., and Spear, L. P. (2018). Binge drinking's effects on the developing brain-animal models. *Alcohol Res*, **39**, 77–86.

Jacobs-Brichford, E., Manson, K. F., and Roitman, J. D. (2019). Effects of chronic cannabinoid exposure during adolescence on reward preference and mPFC activation in adulthood. *Physiol Behav*, **199**, 395–404.

Jouroukhin, Y., Zhu, X., Shevelkin, A. V., et al. (2019). Adolescent Δ9-tetrahydrocannabinol exposure and astrocyte-specific genetic vulnerability converge on nuclear factor-κB-cyclooxygenase-2 signaling to impair memory in adulthood. *Biol Psychiatry*, **85**, 891–903.

Kandel, D., and Kandel, E. (2015). The gateway hypothesis of substance abuse: Developmental, biological and societal perspectives. *Acta Paediatr*, **104**, 130–137.

Kasten, C. R., Zhang, Y., Boehm, S. L. II. (2017). Acute and long-term effects of Δ9-tetrahydrocannabinol on object recognition and anxiety-like

activity are age- and strain-dependent in mice. *Pharmacol Biochem Behav*, **163**, 9–19.

Konrad, K., Firk, C., and Uhlhaas, P. J. (2013). Brain development during adolescence: Neuroscientific insights into this developmental period. *Dtsch Arztebl Int*, **110**, 425–431.

Lecca, D., Scifo, A., Pisanu, A., et al. (2020). Adolescent cannabis exposure increases heroin reinforcement in rats genetically vulnerable to addiction. *Neuropharmacology*, **166**, 107974.

Levine, A., Clemenza, K., Rynn, M., et al. (2017). Evidence for the risks and consequences of adolescent cannabis exposure. *J Am Acad Child Adolesc Psychiatry*, **56**, 214–225.

Lopez-Rodriguez, A. B., Llorente-Berzal, A., Garcia-Segura, L. M., et al. (2014). Sex-dependent long-term effects of adolescent exposure to THC and/or MDMA on neuroinflammation and serotoninergic and cannabinoid systems in rats. *Br J Pharmacol*, **171**, 1435–1447.

Melis, M., Frau, R., Kalivas, P. W., et al. (2017). New vistas on cannabis use disorder. *Neuropharmacology*, **124**, 62–72.

Miller, M. L., Chadwick, B., Dickstein, D. L., et al. (2019). Adolescent exposure to Δ9-tetrahydrocannabinol alters the transcriptional trajectory and dendritic architecture of prefrontal pyramidal neurons. *Mol Psychiatry*, **24**, 588–600.

Molla, H. M., and Tseng, K. Y. (2020). Neural substrates underlying the negative impact of cannabinoid exposure during adolescence. *Pharmacol Biochem Behav*, **195**, 172965.

Murphy, M., Mills, S., Winstone, J., et al. (2017). Chronic adolescent Δ9-tetrahydrocannabinol treatment of male mice leads to long-term cognitive and behavioral dysfunction, which are

prevented by concurrent cannabidiol treatment. *Cannabis Cannabinoid Res*, **2**, 235–246.

Nelson, N. G., Law, W. X., Weingarten, M. J., et al. (2019). Combined Δ9-tetrahydrocannabinol and moderate alcohol administration: Effects on ingestive behaviors in adolescent male rats. *Psychopharmacology*, **236**, 671–684.

Nguyen, J. D., Creehan, K. M., Kerr, T. M., et al. (2020). Lasting effects of repeated Δ9-tetrahydrocannabinol vapour inhalation during adolescence in male and female rats. *Br J Pharmacol*, **177**, 188–203.

Prini, P., Penna, F., Sciuccati, E., et al. (2017). Chronic Δ8-THC exposure differently affects histone modifications in the adolescent and adult rat brain. *Int J Mol Sci*, **18**, 2094.

Prini, P., Rusconi, F., Zamberletti, E., et al. (2018). Adolescent THC exposure in female rats leads to cognitive deficits through a mechanism involving chromatin modifications in the prefrontal cortex. *J Psychiatry Neurosci*, **43**, 87–101.

Prini, P., Zamberletti, E., Manenti, C., et al. (2020). Neurobiological mechanisms underlying cannabis-induced memory impairment. *Eur Neuropsychopharmacol*, **36**, 181–190.

Pushkin, A. N., Eugene, A. J., Lallai, V., et al. (2019). Cannabinoid and nicotine exposure during adolescence induces sex-specific effects on anxiety- and reward-related behaviors during adulthood. *PLoS ONE*, **14**, e0211346.

Renard, J., Rushlow, W. J., Laviolette, S. R. (2016). What can rats tell us about adolescent cannabis exposure? Insights from preclinical research. *Can J Psychiatry*, **61**, 328–334.

(2018). Effects of adolescent THC exposure on the prefrontal

GABAergic system: Implications for schizophrenia-related psychopathology. *Front Psychiatry*, **9**, 281.

Rodríguez, G., Neugebauer, N. M., Yao, K. L., et al. (2017). Δ9-tetrahydrocannabinol (Δ9-THC) administration after neonatal exposure to phencyclidine potentiates schizophrenia-related behavioral phenotypes in mice. *Pharmacol Biochem Behav*, **159**, 6–11.

Rubino, T., and Parolaro, D. (2016). The impact of exposure to cannabinoids in adolescence: Insights from animal models. *Biol Psychiatry*, **79**, 578–585.

Rubino, T., Prini, P., Piscitelli, F., et al. (2015). Adolescent exposure to THC in female rats disrupts developmental changes in the prefrontal cortex. *Neurobiol Dis*, **73**, 60–69.

Saravia, R., Ten-Blanco, M., Julià-Hernández, M., et al. (2019). Concomitant THC and stress adolescent exposure induces impaired fear extinction and related neurobiological changes in adulthood. *Neuropharmacology*, **144**, 345–357.

Silva, L., Black, R., Michaelides, M., et al. (2016). Sex and age specific effects of delta-9-tetrahydrocannabinol during the periadolescent period in the rat: The unique susceptibility of the prepubescent animal. *Neurotoxicol Teratol*, **58**, 88–100.

Simone, J. J., Baumbach, J. L., and McCormick, C. M. (2018). Effects of CB1 receptor antagonism and stress exposures in adolescence on socioemotional behaviours, neuroendocrine stress responses, and expression of relevant proteins in the hippocampus and prefrontal cortex in rats. *Neuropharmacology*, **128**, 433–447.

Stopponi, S., Soverchia, L., Ubaldi, M., et al. (2014). Chronic THC during adolescence increases the vulnerability to stress-induced relapse to heroin seeking in adult rats. *Eur Neuropsychopharmacol*, **24**, 1037–1045.

Stringfield, S. J., and Torregrossa, M. M. (2021a). Disentangling the lasting effects of adolescent cannabinoid exposure. *Prog Neuropsychopharmacol Biol Psychiatry*, **104**, 110067.

(2021b). Intravenous self-administration of delta-9-THC in adolescent rats produces long-lasting alterations in behavior and receptor protein expression. *Psychopharmacology*, **238**, 305–319.

UNODC, United Nation Office on Drugs and Crime (2020) *World Drug Report* 2020 (United Nations publication, Sales No. E.20.XI.6).

Zamberletti, E., and Rubino, T. (2021). Impact of endocannabinoid system manipulation on neurodevelopmental processes relevant to schizophrenia. *Biol Psychiatry Cogn Neurosci Neuroimaging*, **6**, 616–626.

Zamberletti, E., Beggiato, S., Steardo, L. Jr., et al. (2014). Alterations of prefrontal cortex GABAergic transmission in the complex psychotic-like phenotype induced by adolescent delta-9-tetrahydrocannabinol exposure in rats. *Neurobiol Dis*, **63**, 35–47.

Zamberletti, E., Gabaglio, M., Grilli, M., et al. (2016). Long-term hippocampal glutamate synapse and astrocyte dysfunctions underlying the altered phenotype induced by adolescent THC treatment in male rats. *Pharmacol Res*, **111**, 459–470.

Zamberletti, E., Gabaglio, M., Prini, P., et al. (2015). Cortical neuroinflammation contributes to long-term cognitive dysfunctions following adolescent delta-9-tetrahydrocannabinol treatment in female rats. *Eur Neuropsychopharmacol*, **25**, 2404–2415.

The Impact of Cannabis Exposure on the Adolescent Brain
Human Studies and Translational Insights

Jacqueline-Marie Ferland, Alexandra Chisholm, and Yasmin L. Hurd

Adolescence is the gradual transitional period from childhood to adulthood characterized by marked social, mental, and physical changes. It is also the prodromal stage where behavioural and cognitive changes can progress to psychiatric illnesses in certain individuals as they reach adulthood. While genetic risks are implicated in such vulnerability, so too are environmental factors experienced during this period, including cannabis exposure. Debates have ensued for decades regarding the *causal* role of cannabis use by teens in developing psychiatric illness. Such concerns have again grown in recent years as the perception of regular cannabis use being of any risk has decreased due to socio-political changes globally legalizing cannabis/marijuana for medicinal and recreational purposes. The concern is also fuelled by the fact that the potency of delta-9-tetrahydrocannabinol (Δ^9-THC), the main psychoactive component in cannabis, has increased over the years, with epidemiological studies showing an association to increased psychiatric risk (Di Forti et al., 2014; Hines et al., 2020). Many of the neurodevelopmental changes during adolescence, including maturation of prefrontal cortical (PFC) and mesolimbic regions of the brain, neurotransmitter signaling, myelination, and synaptic pruning, are modulated by the endogenous cannabinoid (endocannabinoid; eCB) system (Berghuis et al., 2007; Maccarone et al., 2014). As such, cannabis exposure during this phase of neurodevelopment can shape long-term behavioral and neurobiological trajectories relevant to psychiatric risk. Here, we discuss issues related to the pattern of cannabis use during adolescence and what neurobiological insights have been obtained that can guide translational pre-clinical studies to obtain deeper mechanistic knowledge that could help to improve early intervention and the development of novel treatments to reduce psychiatric illnesses.

8.1 Adolescent Cannabis Use

Although the availability of cannabis has shifted from the illegal to legal market (Choo et al., 2014; Hasin et al., 2015), it remains illicit for adolescents. Despite this perceived barrier to drug access, cannabis continues to be one of the most widely used drugs among teens, and while past-year use remained stable at 35% in the United States, recent data shows that the number of *daily* cannabis users has increased in this age group (Johnston et al., 2021). Teen perceptions of risk associated with regular cannabis use has dramatically declined with the belief that certain routes of administration are 'healthier'. For example, vaping cannabis has significantly increased in recent years, with users citing experimentation and taste as the top two reasons to vape cannabis. Smoking is nevertheless the most frequent and consistent route of administration reported by adolescent cannabis users, followed by vaping and then edibles (Knapp et al., 2019; Peters et al., 2018). However, adolescent cannabis use initiation typically progresses from smoking to edibles to vaping, which may facilitate progression to cannabis use disorder (CUD). In addition to the varied routes of administration, cannabis has become more potent, as evidenced by an increase in Δ^9-THC content from roughly 3% in the early 1990s to 15–20% today (see Chapter 5). Moreover, some administration routes, such as dabbing, can provide Δ^9-THC concentrations even up to 80%. As Δ^9-THC concentration increases, so too is the risk for CUD (Freeman and Winstock, 2015) and psychosis (Di Forti et al., 2014; Hines et al., 2020).

The decline in perceived risk associated with regular cannabis use and the increased Δ^9-THC potency, along with a wide variety of delivery systems, presents a unique challenge than ever before in our history. Nevertheless, widespread individual differences exist for cannabis use among adolescents. Not all those who try cannabis will continue to use it or develop cannabis use-associated problems. However, by 21, teen users of cannabis, regardless of onset category – late-onset occasional users (14%), early-onset occasional users (2.3%), and regular users (3.4%) – exhibited higher odds of harmful substance use compared to non-users (Taylor et al., 2017).

8.2 Endocannabinoid Function in the Adolescent Brain

The main psychoactive effects of cannabis, primarily ascribed to Δ^9-THC, occur via interaction with the eCB system that plays a critical role in the maturation of the adolescent brain. This system comprises the cannabinoid receptors that mediate the direct actions of cannabinoids as well as the eCB lipid ligands (anandamide and 2-arachidonoylglycerol) and enzymes responsible for their synthesis and degradation (Mechoulam et al., 2014). During adolescence, the eCB system facilitates neurodevelopment, particularly through its intricate involvement in neuroplasticity and synaptic function linked to the final establishment of mature neural processes. While there are still significant knowledge gaps regarding the eCB system during adolescent development, there are known dynamic fluctuations during this period of the eCB receptors and ligands relevant to the maturation of brain areas such as the PFC and striatum that are highly implicated in psychiatric and substance use disorders. For instance, there is a rapid, sustained increase in the cannabinoid receptor sub-type 1 (CB1R) binding during adolescence, particularly in the striatum, followed by a marked decline in early adulthood (Rodriguez de Fonseca et al., 1993). This pattern is also reflected at the level of the CB_1R gene expression, which is highest during adolescence and gradually decreases by adulthood, with the greatest alterations evident in limbic-related PFC regions (Heng et al., 2011). Concomitant to developmental changes in the CB_1R, eCB ligands also fluctuate throughout adolescence in a region- and time-specific manner (Ellgren et al., 2008). Such dynamic perturbations in eCB signalling due to supraphysiological levels of Δ^9-THC during adolescent development may prime the individual to long-term negative behavioural consequences. Indeed, greater psychiatric vulnerability is evident in adolescents who start using cannabis during early adolescence and for those who

use cannabis at higher rates (Chadwick et al., 2013; Hosseini and Oremus, 2019). In this chapter, we discuss some potential neurobiological outcomes associated with cannabis use during adolescence which may confer psychiatric vulnerability.

8.3 Neuroimaging: Window into the Adolescent Brain

Most knowledge about the adolescent human brain has been gleaned from neuroimaging studies. The important medical and societal implications of expanding knowledge about the adolescent brain was the foundation for longitudinal efforts including the IMAGEN study (Europe) and the ABCD consortium (USA) to track the impact of adolescent drug use on behaviour. Results from these and cross-sectional neuroimaging findings suggest that cannabis use during adolescence is associated with both structural and functional brain alterations (Figure 8.1), however, results vary.

8.3.1 Structural Neuroimaging

No change, reduced, or increased brain volume have been reported in association with adolescent cannabis exposure. For example, data from some retrospective studies indicate that occasional (<1–2 times per week) and frequent (>3 times per week) cannabis use during adolescence does not impact global or regional brain volumes, cortical thickness, or grey matter density when compared to non-users (Scott et al., 2019; Weiland et al., 2015). However, in occasional and regular users, the IMAGEN consortium reported that greater cannabis exposure is associated with a reduction in hippocampal and parahippocampal expansion and that cortical thinning displays a dose-dependent relationship with cannabis exposure where greater cannabis use predicted enhanced thinning of the PFC (Albaugh et al., 2021; Yu et al., 2020). Reports also exist that grey matter volume is increased in association with cannabis experience where 14-year-olds with only minimal (1–2) lifetime use had increased grey matter volume in the medial temporal lobes, posterior cingulate, lingual gyri, and cerebellum (Orr et al., 2019) and a retrospective study of recreational young adult cannabis users (average age 20–21, at least one use per week), with approximately four years of prior use, reported greater grey matter density in the nucleus accumbens,

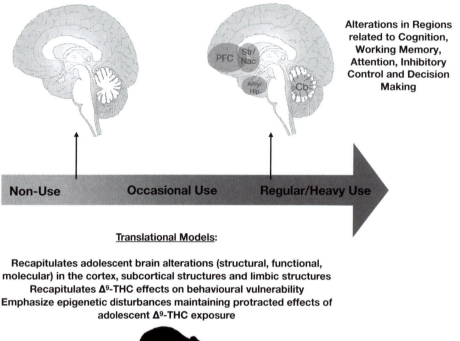

Alterations in Regions related to Cognition, Working Memory, Attention, Inhibitory Control and Decision Making

Non-Use   Occasional Use   Regular/Heavy Use

Translational Models:

Recapitulates adolescent brain alterations (structural, functional, molecular) in the cortex, subcortical structures and limbic structures
Recapitulates Δ⁹-THC effects on behavioural vulnerability
Emphasize epigenetic disturbances maintaining protracted effects of adolescent Δ⁹-THC exposure

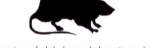

Figure 8.1 Schematic overview of global neural alterations observed in the brain associated with adolescent cannabis, which is most evident with regular/heavy use, and an overview of general findings in pre-clinical Δ⁹-THC adolescent exposure models. Amy/Hip, amygdala/hippocampus; Cb, cerebeullum; Str/Nac striatum/nucleus accumbens; PFC, prefrontal cortex. A black and white version of this figure will appear in some formats. For the colour version, please refer to the plate section.

hypothalamus, and amygdala relative to non-users (Gilman et al., 2014).

Despite inconsistencies, data from cross-sectional and longitudinal studies suggest that, relative to non-cannabis users, heavy adolescent cannabis users exhibit cortical alterations such as reduced volume in parietal, orbitofrontal, and frontal cortical regions (Churchwell et al., 2010; Epstein and Kumra, 2015; Kumra et al., 2012). Interestingly, these studies suggest that cortical alterations may be related to earlier initiation of cannabis use (Churchwell et al., 2010) and that cannabis use during this critical period of neurodevelopment may alter normal cortical thinning processes contributing to interactions in altered brain morphology associated with the development of psychiatric illness (Epstein and Kumra, 2015; Rais et al., 2010). Additionally, reduced cortical thickness in the PFC and insula was also documented in other cohorts of heavy adolescent cannabis users (Lopez-Larson et al., 2011). Evidence of reduced hippocampal

volumes, a brain region important for learning and memory, was also reported in abstinent heavy adolescent cannabis users (Ashtari et al., 2011); though not observed in all studies.

Although results are mixed, cross-sectional and longitudinal studies suggest cannabis use and its frequency of use may impact cortical and hippocampal development and alter normal thinning processes in structures relevant to cognition. Additionally, cannabis use during adolescence may increase volume in structures important for reward and emotional control.

8.3.2 Functional Neuroimaging

Resting State: Perturbations in cortical activation in baseline resting state neuroimaging conditions have been noted in adolescent cannabis users, with most suggesting increased activity. For example, high-risk adolescents with high cannabis use, but not low users, were reported to have enhanced activity of the middle frontal gyrus (Houck et al., 2013). Additionally, high-risk adolescents with cannabis dependence had greater activity in the right superior frontal gyrus and right superior parietal gyrus during resting state conditions where activation of the superior parietal and cerebellar regions positively related with the duration of cannabis use (Orr et al., 2013). Greater resting state activity within the parietal and cerebellar networks was also evident in association with greater cannabis use (Behan et al., 2014).

Working Memory: Altered activity with adolescent cannabis use is evident in brain regions mediating learning and working memory updating. For instance, during working memory tasks, regular, abstinent (5 days) adolescent users exhibited greater fMRI response throughout the PFC, insula, and left pre-central gyrus (Schweinsburg et al., 2010). Longitudinal assessment also suggests that functional differences in adolescence may predict cannabis initiation whereby enhanced frontoparietal activation and poor performance on a visual-spatial working memory task at age 13 is predictive of cannabis initiation by age 15 (Tervo-Clemmens et al., 2018). In addition to altered cortical activity, adolescent cannabis users also exhibit enhanced activity in the basal ganglia (Padula et al., 2007).

Attention, Inhibitory Control, and Decision-Making: During tasks designed to assess control of attention, chronic adolescent cannabis users have longer reaction times and make more errors, and their poor performance was associated with greater activation of the frontal cortex compared to controls (Abdullaev et al., 2010). During tasks used to assess inhibitory control, adolescent cannabis users appear to exhibit poorer inhibition compared to non-users with task-associated enhancement in activity across frontal, parietal, and cerebellar regions (Behan et al., 2014; Tapert et al., 2007). Data from the IMAGEN consortium also suggests that adolescent cannabis users may be hyper-responsive to emotional stimuli, whereby adolescents experimenting with cannabis have increased bilateral activation of the amygdala for negative (angry face) stimuli in contrast to controls (Spechler et al., 2015). Additionally, young adult (aged 20) cannabis users with an escalating trajectory of use from adolescence (from age 14 to 19) exhibit a negative functional connectivity between the nucleus accumbens and PFC (Lichenstein et al., 2017). These findings suggest that cannabis use alters the normal connectivity between the PFC and limbic regions of the brain and may prime neural processes critical for emotionality and reward.

Key Points:

1. Collectively, neuroimaging studies indicate that adolescent cannabis exposure can result in structural and functional brain alterations.

2. Overall, studies indicate that, relative to non-cannabis users, adolescent cannabis users exhibit cortical alterations in frontal and parietal brain regions and exhibit altered functional connectivity between frontal and limbic regions of the brain, which may facilitate behavioural vulnerability.

3. Functional neuroimaging studies indicate that cannabis exposure during adolescence is associated with alterations in brain regions relevant to higher order cognitive functioning, such as working memory, attention, inhibitory control, and decision-making (Figure 8.1).

4. Significant inconsistencies exist in the literature, with differences in the amount and frequency of use as well as psychiatric comorbidity and concomitant polysubstance use (often nicotine and/or alcohol), can be important contributing factors.

8.4 Translational Outcomes of Adolescent THC

Given the continued challenges of human studies with understandable caveats and confounds, pre-clinical animal models remain of significant value to understand the neurobiological consequences of adolescent cannabis exposure and its protracted effects that can be tracked over a shorter time course. Several reviews have been published regarding the long-term effects of adolescent exposure (Bara et al., 2021; Renard et al., 2016; Rubino and Parolaro, 2008). What is clear neurobiologically is that Δ^9-THC modulates mechanisms related to emotions, reward, and cognition to confer greater vulnerability to psychopathologies. For example, adolescent Δ^9-THC exposure has been found to recruit and modulate excitatory activity within the mesocorticolimbic circuit (Miladinovic et al., 2020; Renard et al., 2017), reduce PFC dendritic branching (De Felice et al., 2021; Miller et al., 2019), and influence amygdala morphology (Saravia et al., 2019), much of which is in line with global alterations observed in clinical populations. Recent data similarly suggests that dose plays an important role in the presentation of these phenotypes (Ruiz et al., 2021a, 2021b), where low dose has a strong influence on mechanisms relevant to reward and high dose on stress.

Animal models have also allowed the potential to identify fundamental biological mechanisms that have the potential to not only incorporate past cannabis experiences intracellularly, but also to alter current responses to the drug and to predict future brain and behavioural sensitivities. Such mechanisms are captured under the umbrella of 'epigenetics' that can also be influenced by individual genetics. The general definition of 'epigenetics' refers to the potentially heritable, and reversible, modulation of gene expression without altering the genetic code itself (Baedke, 2013; Van Speybroeck, 2002). While research has only touched the tip of the iceberg regarding epigenetic mechanisms related to the developmental effects of cannabis, significant evidence demonstrates that adolescent exposure does affect histone methylation that is maintained into adulthood and underlies dysregulation of gene expression and behaviour. For example, Δ^9-THC recruits methylation mechanisms that modulate the expression of transcripts that encode eCB genes and those related to synaptic plasticity, thus conferring greater behavioural vulnerability to addictive- and depressive-like phenotypes (Bara et al., 2021). Moreover, adolescent Δ^9-THC induces profound epigenetic dysregulation within the PFC along with a significant overlap between genes differentially altered across adolescent development in animals with Δ^9-THC exposure and gene networks dysregulated in the PFC of individuals diagnosed with schizophrenia (Miller et al., 2019). A great deal of research is needed to probe specific epigenetic alterations maintaining the molecular memory of adolescent cannabis exposure that can also help identify targets for future treatment interventions considering that epigenetics is reversible.

Although significant knowledge can be gained from animal studies (Figure 8.1), it is important to acknowledge that translating adolescent cannabis use in animal models usually does not capture all aspects of 'cannabis', since most pre-clinical studies have focused on the causal contribution of Δ^9-THC and not the plant. In addition, most studies have not used smoking or vaping models, but such efforts have recently been implemented. With the advent of vapor delivery systems and cannabis self-administration models (McLaughlin, 2018; Moore et al., 2021), research will be able to delve more deeply into the role of inhaled cannabis products on behaviour and neurobiological mechanisms underlying phenotypes associated with adolescent Δ^9-THC/cannabis experience.

8.5 Future Directions

As the field moves forward in attempts to expand knowledge regarding adolescent brain development and cannabis use, several factors should be considered. One critical factor is sex as a biological variable. Pre-clinical studies indicate sex-specific effects in the development of the eCB system, including cannabinoid receptor expression as well as physiological effects of cannabinoids and cannabinoid metabolism (Calakos et al., 2017). However, data is sparse regarding sex differences in the human literature though it is apparent that adolescent males and females use cannabis differently. Male adolescent users are also more likely to initiate cannabis use at a younger age (Pope et al., 2003), use cannabis more frequently (Leos-Toro et al., 2019; Schulenberg et al., 2005), use higher potency cannabis products (Baggio et al., 2014; Peters et al., 2018), and be at a greater risk of developing CUD (Hasin et al., 2015, 2019) compared to females. Another factor is the current cornucopia of cannabis/cannabinoid products. Converting information about such products to a common dosing system could improve insights about specific exposure conditions. Moreover, given the variability seen in longitudinal studies, it would be beneficial for the field to agree on common behavioural tasks across functional neuroimaging studies, even if the primary outcomes of the studies differ.

Overall, ongoing longitudinal efforts and improved translational pre-clinical models will significantly bridge the gap to improve neurobiological knowledge regarding adolescent cannabis exposure and to determine factors not only relevant to risk but also resilience to psychopathologies. Importantly, the significant contributions of epigenetic perturbation evident with adolescent cannabis exposure based on pre-clinical models suggest that early interventions have the potential to change the trajectory of cannabis effects and, thus, psychiatric risk.

References

Abdullaev, Y., Posner, M. I., Nunnally, R., et al. (2010). Functional MRI evidence for inefficient attentional control in adolescent chronic cannabis abuse. *Behav Brain Res*, **215**, 45–57.

Albaugh, M. D., Ottino-Gonzalez, J., Sidwell, A., et al. (2021). Association of cannabis use during adolescence with neurodevelopment. *JAMA Psychiatry*, **78**, 1–11.

Ashtari, M., Avants, B., Cyckowski, L., et al. (2011). Medial temporal structures and memory functions in adolescents with heavy cannabis use. *J Psychiatr Res*, **45**, 1055–1066.

Baedke, J. (2013). The epigenetic landscape in the course of time: Conrad Hal Waddington's methodological impact on the life sciences. *Stud Hist Philos Biol Biomed Sci*, **44**, 756–773.

Baggio, S., Deline, S., Studer, J., et al. (2014). Routes of administration of cannabis used for nonmedical purposes and associations with patterns of drug use. *J Adolesc Health*, **54**, 235–240.

Bara, A., Ferland, J. N., Rompala, G., et al. (2021). Cannabis and synaptic reprogramming of the developing brain. *Nat Rev Neurosci*, **22**, 423–438.

Behan, B., Connolly, C. G., Datwani, S., et al. (2014). Response inhibition and elevated parietal-cerebellar correlations in chronic adolescent cannabis users. *Neuropharmacology*, **84**, 131–137.

Berghuis, P., Rajnicek, A. M., Morozov, Y. M., et al. (2007). Hardwiring the brain: Endocannabinoids shape neuronal connectivity. *Science*, **316**, 1212–1216.

Calakos, K. C., Bhatt, S., Foster, D. W., et al. (2017). Mechanisms underlying sex differences in cannabis use. *Curr Addict Rep*, **4**, 439–453.

Chadwick, B., Miller, M. L., and Hurd, Y. L. (2013). Cannabis use during adolescent development: Susceptibility to psychiatric illness. *Front Psychiatry*, **4**, 129.

Choo, E. K., Benz, M., Zaller, N., et al. (2014). The impact of state medical marijuana legislation on adolescent marijuana use. *J Adolesc Health*, **55**, 160–166.

Churchwell, J. C., Lopez-Larson, M., and Yurgelun-Todd, D. A. (2010). Altered frontal cortical volume and decision making in adolescent cannabis users. *Front Psychol*, **1**, 225.

De Felice, M., Renard, J., Hudson, R., et al. (2021). L-Theanine prevents long-term affective and cognitive side effects of adolescent delta-9-tetrahydrocannabinol exposure and blocks associated molecular and neuronal abnormalities in the mesocorticolimbic circuitry. *J Neurosci*, **41**, 739–750.

Di Forti, M., Sallis, H., Allegri, F., et al. (2014). Daily use, especially of high-potency cannabis, drives the earlier onset of psychosis in cannabis users. *Schizophr Bull*, **40**, 1509–1517.

Ellgren, M., Artmann, A., Tkalych, O., et al. (2008). Dynamic changes of the endogenous cannabinoid and opioid mesocorticolimbic systems during adolescence: THC effects. *Eur Neuropsychopharmacol*, **18**, 826–834.

Epstein, K. A., and Kumra, S. (2015). Altered cortical maturation in adolescent cannabis users with and without schizophrenia. *Schizophr Res*, **162**, 143–152.

Freeman, T. P., and Winstock, A. R. (2015). Examining the profile of high-potency cannabis and its association with severity of cannabis dependence. *Psychol Med*, **45**, 3181–3189.

Gilman, J. M., Kuster, J. K., Lee, S., et al. (2014). Cannabis use is quantitatively associated with nucleus accumbens and amygdala abnormalities in young adult recreational users. *J Neurosci*, **34**, 5529–5538.

Hasin, D. S., Saha, T. D., Kerridge, B. T., et al. (2015). Prevalence of marijuana use disorders in the United States between 2001–2002 and 2012–2013. *JAMA Psychiatry*, **72**, 1235–1242.

Hasin, D. S., Shmulewitz, D., and Sarvet, A. L. (2019). Time trends in US cannabis use and cannabis use disorders overall and by sociodemographic subgroups: A narrative review and new findings. *Am J Drug Alcohol Abuse*, **45**, 623–643.

Heng, L., Beverley, J. A., Steiner, H., et al. (2011). Differential developmental trajectories for CB1 cannabinoid receptor expression in limbic/associative and sensorimotor cortical areas. *Synapse*, **65**, 278–286.

Hines, L. A., Freeman, T. P., Gage, S. H., et al. (2020). Association of high-potency cannabis use with mental health and substance use in adolescence. *JAMA Psychiatry*, **77**, 1044–1051.

Hosseini, S., and Oremus, M. (2019). The effect of age of initiation of cannabis use on psychosis, depression, and anxiety among youth under 25 years. *Can J Psychiatry*, **64**, 304–312.

Houck, J. M., Bryan, A. D., and Feldstein Ewing, S. W. (2013). Functional connectivity and cannabis use in high-risk adolescents. *Am J Drug Alcohol Abuse*, **39**, 414–423.

Johnston, L. D., Miech, R. A., O'Malley, P. M., et al. (2021). *Monitoring the Future National Survey Results on Drug Use 1975–2020: Overview, Key Findings on Adolescent Drug Use*. Ann Arbor: Institute for Social Research, University of Michigan.

Knapp, A. A., Lee, D. C., Borodovsky, J. T., et al. (2019). Emerging trends in cannabis administration among adolescent cannabis users. *J Adolesc Health*, **64**, 487–493.

Kumra, S., Robinson, P., Tambyraja, R., et al. (2012). Parietal lobe volume deficits in adolescents with schizophrenia and adolescents with cannabis use disorders. *J Am Acad Child Adolesc Psychiatry*, **51**, 171–180.

Leos-Toro, C., Rynard, V., Murnaghan, D., et al. (2019). Trends in cannabis use over time among Canadian youth: 2004–2014. *Prev Med*, **118**, 30–37.

Lichenstein, S. D., Musselman, S., Shaw, D. S., et al. (2017). Nucleus accumbens functional connectivity at age 20 is associated with trajectory of adolescent cannabis use and predicts psychosocial functioning in young adulthood. *Addiction*, **112**, 1961–1970.

Lopez-Larson, M. P., Bogorodzki, P., Rogowska, J., et al. (2011). Altered prefrontal and insular cortical thickness in adolescent marijuana users. *Behav Brain Res*, **220**, 164–72.

Maccarrone, M., Guzman, M., Mackie, K., et al. (2014). Programming of neural cells by (endo) cannabinoids: From physiological rules to emerging therapies. *Nat Rev Neurosci*, **15**, 786–801.

McLaughlin, R. J. (2018). Toward a translationally relevant preclinical model of cannabis use. *Neuropsychopharmacology*, **43**, 213.

Mechoulam, R., Hanus, L. O., Pertwee, R., et al. (2014). Early phytocannabinoid chemistry to endocannabinoids and beyond. *Nat Rev Neurosci*, **15**, 757–764.

Miladinovic, T., Manwell, L. A., Raaphorst, E., et al. (2020). Effects of chronic nicotine exposure on Delta(9)-tetrahydrocannabinol-induced locomotor activity and neural activation in male and female adolescent and adult rats. *Pharmacol Biochem Behav*, **194**, 172931.

Miller, M. L., Chadwick, B., Dickstein, D. L., et al. (2019). Adolescent exposure to Delta(9)-tetrahydrocannabinol alters the transcriptional trajectory and dendritic architecture of prefrontal pyramidal neurons. *Mol Psychiatry*, **24**, 588–600.

Moore, C. F., Davis, C. M., Harvey, E. L., et al. (2021). Appetitive, antinociceptive, and hypothermic effects of vaped and injected Delta-9-tetrahydrocannabinol (THC) in rats: Exposure and dose-effect comparisons by strain and sex. *Pharmacol Biochem Behav*, 202, 173116.

Orr, C., Morioka, R., Behan, B., et al. (2013). Altered resting-state connectivity in adolescent cannabis users. *Am J Drug Alcohol Abuse*, **39**, 372–381.

Orr, C., Spechler, P., Cao, Z., et al. (2019). Grey matter volume differences associated with extremely low levels of cannabis use in adolescence. *J Neurosci*, **39**, 1817–1827.

Padula, C. B., Schweinsburg, A. D., and Tapert, S. F. (2007). Spatial working memory performance and fMRI activation interaction in abstinent adolescent marijuana users. *Psychol Addict Behav*, **21**, 478–487.

Peters, E. N., Bae, D., Barrington-Trimis, J. L., et al. (2018). Prevalence and sociodemographic correlates of adolescent use and polyuse of combustible, vaporized, and edible cannabis products. *JAMA Netw Open*, **1**, e182765.

Pope, H. G., Gruber, A. J., Hudson, J. I., et al. (2003). Early-onset cannabis use and cognitive deficits: What is the nature of the association? *Drug Alcohol Depend*, **69**, 303–310.

Rais, M., Van Haren, N. E., Cahn, W., et al. (2010). Cannabis use and progressive cortical thickness loss in areas rich in CB1 receptors during the first five years of schizophrenia. *Eur*

Neuropsychopharmacol, 20, 855–865.

Renard, J., Rushlow, W. J., and Laviolette, S. R. (2016). What can rats tell us about adolescent cannabis exposure? Insights from preclinical research. *Can J Psychiatry*, **61**, 328–334.

Renard, J., Szkudlarek, H. J., Kramar, C. P., et al. (2017). Adolescent THC exposure causes enduring prefrontal cortical disruption of GABAergic inhibition and dysregulation of sub-cortical dopamine function. *Sci Rep*, 7, 11420.

Rodriguez de Fonseca, F., Ramos, J. A., Bonnin, A., et al. (1993). Presence of cannabinoid binding sites in the brain from early postnatal ages. *Neuroreport*, **4**, 135–138.

Rubino, T., and Parolaro, D. (2008). Long lasting consequences of cannabis exposure in adolescence. *Mol Cell Endocrinol*, **286**, S108–113.

Ruiz, C. M., Torrens, A., Castillo, E., et al. (2021a). Pharmacokinetic, behavioral, and brain activity effects of Delta(9)-tetrahydrocannabinol in adolescent male and female rats. *Neuropsychopharmacology*, **46**, 959–969.

Ruiz, C. M., Torrens, A., Lallai, V., et al. (2021b). Pharmacokinetic and pharmacodynamic properties of aerosolized ('vaped') THC in adolescent male and female rats. *Psychopharmacology (Berl)*, **238**, 3595–3605.

Saravia, R., Ten-Blanco, M., Julia-Hernandez, M., et al. (2019). Concomitant THC and stress adolescent exposure induces impaired fear extinction and related neurobiological changes in adulthood. *Neuropharmacology*, **144**, 345–357.

Schulenberg, J. E., Merline, A. C., Johnston, L. D., et al. (2005). Trajectories of marijuana use during the transition to adulthood: The big picture based on national panel data. *J Drug Issues*, **35**, 255–279.

Schweinsburg, A. D., Schweinsburg, B. C., Medina, K. L., et al. (2010). The influence of recency of use on fMRI response during spatial working memory in adolescent marijuana users. *J Psychoactive Drugs*, **42**, 401–412.

Scott, J. C., Rosen, A. F. G., Moore, T. M., et al. (2019). Cannabis use in youth is associated with limited alterations in brain structure. *Neuropsychopharmacology*, **44**, 1362–1369.

Spechler, P. A., Orr, C. A., Chaarani, B., et al. (2015). Cannabis use in early adolescence: Evidence of amygdala hypersensitivity to signals of threat. *Dev Cogn Neurosci*, **16**, 63–70.

Tapert, S. F., Schweinsburg, A. D., Drummond, S. P., et al. (2007) Functional MRI of inhibitory processing in abstinent adolescent marijuana users. *Psychopharmacology (Berl)*, **194**, 173–183.

Taylor, M., Collin, S. M., Munafo, M. R., et al. (2017). Patterns of cannabis use during adolescence and their association with harmful substance use behaviour: Findings from a UK birth cohort. *J Epidemiol Community Health*, **71**, 764–770.

Tervo-Clemmens, B., Simmonds, D., Calabro, F. J., et al. (2018). Early cannabis use and neurocognitive risk: A prospective functional neuroimaging study. *Biol Psychiatry Cogn Neurosci Neuroimaging*, **3**, 713–725.

Van Speybroeck, L. (2002). From epigenesis to epigenetics: The case of C. H. Waddington. *Ann NY Acad Sci*, **981**, 61–81.

Weiland, B. J., Thayer, R. E., Depue, B. E., et al. (2015). Daily marijuana use is not associated with brain morphometric measures in adolescents or adults. *J Neurosci*, **35**, 1505–1512.

Yu, T., Jia, T., Zhu, L., et al. (2020). Cannabis-associated psychotic-like experiences are mediated by developmental changes in the parahippocampal gyrus. *J Am Acad Child Adolesc Psychiatry*, **59**, 642–649.

Chapter

9

Cannabis and Cognition
An Update on Short- and Long-term Effects

Lisa-Marie Greenwood, Valentina Lorenzetti, and Nadia Solowij

9.1 Introduction

As detailed in Chapters 4 and 6, changes in the legal status of non-medicinal cannabis use have occurred in numerous international jurisdictions. In turn, there have been increases in the prevalence of recreational and daily use of cannabis (UNODC, 2020) and decreases in risk perception of cannabis use-related harms (Hughes et al., 2016). The commercialization of cannabis products has led to greater diversity of cannabis' phytochemical formulations and routes of delivery that appeal to its therapeutic (Bonn-Miller et al., 2018; T. P. Freeman et al., 2019) and mind-altering (Subbaraman and Kerr, 2021) properties. Research examining the effects of cannabis on cognition in humans has investigated specific neurotoxic and protective properties of cannabinoids. The two most researched cannabinoids from cannabis plant are delta-9-tetrahydrocannabinol (THC) and cannabidiol (CBD). As reviewed in Chapter 5, the concentration of THC, the primary psychoactive compound, has nearly doubled in recent years (Freeman et al., 2021). Cannabidiol has been effectively bred out of most recreationally used cannabis strains (Chandra et al., 2019; ElSohly et al., 2016; Potter et al., 2018) but has received renewed interest due to its therapeutic properties (Khan et al., 2020; and see Chapters 11 and 20) and potential to improve the safety profile of cannabis (Bonn-Miller et al., 2018).

With increasing legalization of cannabis, there is a need for greater public awareness of cannabis-related harms (Volkow et al., 2014). The clinical significance of cannabis' acute *short-term* effects on impaired cognition has important implications for emergency healthcare management of cannabis intoxication (Takakuwa and Schears, 2021) and for harm minimization policies, such as drug-driving (McCartney et al., 2021) and workplace safety (Hall et al., 2019). Of significant public health concern is increased prevalence of long-term recreational cannabis users seeking treatment for cannabis use disorder (CUD) (UNODC, 2016). Cannabis' *long-term* effects on

cognition have important clinical implications for discerning negative impacts on daily functioning, including increased risk of relapse following cannabis abstinence, poorer mental health (Hall et al., 2019; Murray et al., 2017), and lower educational attainment (Lorenzetti et al., 2020b).

In a previous version of this chapter (Solowij and Pesa, 2011), we reported a range of cognitive functions impaired during acute intoxication and in non-intoxicated regular cannabis users. Since that time, a considerable number of new studies have been published. This chapter summarizes the new findings in humans between 2011 and 2021, in order to clarify: the acute effects of cannabis intoxication on cognition, the residual effects of regular use on cognition, and the recovery of cognitive function following prolonged periods of abstinence. We then discuss factors that confer greater risk and resilience to cognitive impairment following cannabis use.

Box 9.1 Time-course of acute cannabis intoxication and residual non-acute effects of regular cannabis use

Acute Cannabis Intoxication: Acute cannabis intoxication manifests in transient symptoms with different onset and duration depending on the route of administration. Symptoms typically occur within minutes after inhalation and start to decline approximately two-to-four hours following use. Oral consumption, such as edibles, has a delayed onset (~30 minutes) and results in lower and delayed peak concentrations due to the pharmacokinetic profile of slower absorption rates and lower bioavailability compared to inhalation.

Residual Non-Acute Effects of Regular Cannabis Use: The continued effects of cannabis use on cognition have been assessed from 12 hours after last cannabis use through to prolonged periods of abstinence (e.g., several months or years). Biological measures, such as blood and urinary cannabinoid metabolites, are often measured to index the sub-acute residual effects of cannabis.

9.2 Learning and Memory

The most frequently studied domains with strongest evidence for the *acute* and dose-dependent effects of cannabis on cognition are verbal learning and memory (Broyd et al., 2016b; Curran et al., 2020; Kroon et al., 2021). Research studies typically use immediate recall trials of word lists to test encoding of novel information, and delayed recall and recognition trials to test consolidation and retrieval from episodic memory. A recent meta-analysis reported moderate-to-large effects of acute intoxication with CB1 receptor agonists on verbal learning and memory (Zhornitsky et al., 2021). This evidence is consistent with a previous systematic review reporting a large effect size of acute cannabinoid intoxication in humans (Broyd et al., 2016b). There is mixed evidence for whether a history of regular cannabis use increases tolerance to these effects.

The consumption of high THC cannabis products with no or insignificant amounts of CBD may impair the ability to reliably form new memories. THC administered prior to learning disrupts immediate (Ranganathan et al., 2017) and delayed (Curran et al., 2020; Ranganathan et al., 2017) verbal recall, but not spatial memory (Borgan et al., 2019). Conversely, THC administered prior to delayed trials did not affect verbal recall accuracy (Doss et al., 2018; Ranganathan et al., 2017). Therefore, THC intoxication may impair encoding of novel information and, thus, compromise memory retrieval, but does not seem to affect recall accuracy of previously established memories. Cannabis users consuming THC *and* CBD cannabis strains (but not THC-based) had intact verbal recall accuracy following cannabis use in a naturalistic setting (Curran et al., 2020). CBD may mitigate THC impairment on brain function in memory networks (Batalla et al., 2014). However, findings from controlled experiments on the behavioral effects of combined THC *and* CBD are mixed (Englund et al., 2013; Morgan et al., 2018). Differences in dose, timing, and route of administration may be further critical factors for inconsistent findings.

Recent systematic reviews and meta-analyses provide evidence for *residual* cannabis effects on learning and memory in regular users (Broyd et al., 2016b; Krzyzanowski and Purdon, 2020; Lovell et al., 2020; Nader and Sanchez, 2018; Schoeler et al., 2016; Scott et al., 2017). More prolonged and heavier use is associated with poorer learning and memory (Broyd et al.,

2016b; Cuttler et al., 2012; Kroon et al., 2021; Solowij et al., 2011; Thames et al., 2014), while greater cannabis use frequency during adolescence predicts poorer verbal memory (Duperrouzel et al., 2019). A recent review found longer durations of regular cannabis use were associated with shorter abstinence periods prior to neuropsychological assessment of verbal learning performance (Krzyzanowski and Purdon, 2020), which may confound interpretations. Age of onset of cannabis use, and cannabinoid composition and dosage, may also moderate these effects. There is inconclusive evidence on the long-term effects of cannabis on visuospatial learning and memory (Lorenzetti et al., 2021; Sneider et al., 2013).

There remains insufficient and mixed evidence for the recovery of verbal learning and memory deficits following one or more months of cannabis abstinence (Broyd et al., 2016b; Kroon et al., 2021), with findings of persistent deficits (Lorenzetti et al., 2021; Meier et al., 2012; Riba et al., 2015), partial recovery (Roten et al., 2015), and full recovery (Broyd et al., 2016a; Medina et al., 2007; Tait et al., 2011; Thames et al., 2014). Lorenzetti et al. (2021) report recovery in visuospatial but not verbal learning following 2.5 years of cannabis abstinence and suggest abstinence may affect different constructs of learning and memory in distinct ways. Recovery of memory function in adolescent cannabis users has been observed following 72 hours abstinence (Scott et al., 2017). Additional studies should determine whether early age of cannabis use onset contributes to residual and chronic effects on learning and memory. Cross-sectional studies face methodological challenges in mapping the effects of age on cognition. Some limitations include earlier onset cannabis use being associated with longer durations of exposure and the narrow age range in which cannabis initiation typically occurs during youth (EMCDDA, 2015; GOC, 2019).

Several mechanisms may underlie learning and memory impairments following acute and chronic cannabis use, respectively. THC decreases acetylcholine release in the hippocampus and prefrontal cortex (Gessa et al., 1998) and disrupts endocannabinoid-mediated synaptic plasticity via induction of long-term synaptic depression (Prini et al., 2020). Impaired verbal learning and memory in heavy and early onset cannabis users has been associated with aberrant brain structure and function implicated in memory and motivation, including reduced thickness of the entorhinal and left orbitofrontal cortices

(Wittemann et al., 2021) and altered function of the para-hippocampus and midbrain (Blest-Hopley et al., 2021). A finding of brain functional alterations without impaired behavioural performance on a recognition task (Smith et al., 2017) warrants further mechanistic studies to inform cannabis-related brain dysfunctions and their recovery with abstinence.

9.2.1 False Memories

Acutely administered THC may lead to suggestive bias and susceptibility to false memories when recalling details of an event (Ballard et al., 2012; Kloft et al., 2020). Oral THC (15 mg) administered during delayed recall trials did not affect recall accuracy, but did increase false recollection of neutral and emotion-related pictures and words in healthy controls (Doss et al., 2018). Vaporized THC (300 µg/kg) in occasional cannabis users lead to higher spontaneous false-recognition in a word-list association task and greater susceptibility to suggestion bias and false memories when recalling virtual reality scenarios (Kloft et al., 2020). These findings suggest cannabis weakens the association between presented and unrelated stimuli during encoding, which contributes to later response bias (Kloft et al., 2020). Ongoing susceptibility to false memories has also been demonstrated after one week (Kloft et al., 2020) and four weeks (Riba et al., 2015) abstinence in cannabis users. False memories increase the risk of human error and have important implications for social relationships, occupational performance, and eye-witness testimony.

9.3 Working Memory

Inconsistent results emerge on how *acute* cannabis intoxication affects working memory across verbal, visual, and spatial contents. Disruptions to working memory affect everyday actions that require mental workspace to achieve goal-directed behaviours, such as driving and problem-solving. Several recent reviews in cannabis users are inconsistent in reporting small-to-moderate (Bourque and Potvin, 2021; McCartney et al., 2021; Zhornitsky et al., 2021), mixed (Broyd et al., 2016b), or no (Oomen et al., 2018) deficits in working memory. Well-controlled studies are needed to determine the role of regular cannabis use history in mediating acute effects of THC on working memory as there is insufficient evidence for the development of tolerance.

Neurocognitive tasks indexing working memory tap into diverse cognitive constructs that may be more, or less, sensitive to the impairing effects of cannabis. The N-back task is one of the most frequently reported and impaired working memory tasks (Oomen et al., 2018). This task overlaps with attention and memory and there is evidence for use of different processing strategies across the lifespan to drive task performance (Gajewski et al., 2018). A latent factor analysis supports the division of working memory across visuo-spatial versus numerical–verbal contents rather than underlying sub-processes (Waris et al., 2017). In a well-controlled experimental design, Adam et al. (2020) found that oral THC (15 mg) impairs visual working memory. They also conducted a systematic review and used a down-sampling technique to demonstrate that insufficient sample size and shorter task durations (e.g., less than three minutes) led to many previous studies being underpowered. Variability in measurement and methodology may contribute to mixed reports on the acute effects of cannabis on working memory.

Impairments in working memory performance following cannabis use is subject to task complexity and required cognitive load. At lower memory loads THC increases brain activation in memory networks (Bossong et al., 2012). Intact behavioural performance at low cognitive loads may be sub-served by neural compensatory mechanisms to overcome cannabis' effects on brain function (Mizrahi et al., 2017). Evidence for neural compensation in CUD is found for connectivity differences in the dorsolateral prefrontal cortex compared to controls during an N-back task (Ma et al., 2018). Further neuroimaging and neurophysiological studies may inform neural compensation mechanisms through reorganization of the brain's neural resources. THC has also been shown to increase mind wandering and decrease metacognitive accuracy of visual working memory (Adam et al., 2020). Research has yet to break down the role of attention in task-unrelated thoughts that may mitigate behavioural impairment across cognitive domains.

There is mixed evidence that CBD mitigates the effects of THC-impairment on working memory. Oral CBD (600 mg) increased cerebral blood flow in the hippocampus in healthy controls but did not affect working memory (Bloomfield et al., 2020). This finding concurs with working memory performance following vaporized CBD (16 mg), which did not differ from placebo (Morgan et al., 2018). When CBD (16 mg) was combined with THC (8 mg) it did not attenuate THC impairment. This finding is contrary to that of a study using nabiximols (1:1 ratio THC to CBD) where performance was similar to placebo (Schoedel et al., 2011). Differences in the effects of combined CBD and THC across studies may be due to different ratios of cannabinoids, routes of administration, or the different working memory tasks used across studies.

There is some evidence for *residual* effects of cannabis on working memory, primarily for verbal domains in young adult cannabis users (Fried et al., 2005; Herzig et al., 2014; Wadsworth et al., 2006) and spatial domains in adolescent users (Day et al., 2013). A recent review suggests more severe cannabis-related impairment in adolescents than adults (Gorey et al., 2019). However, a separate systematic review and meta-analysis found no cognitive effects for studies requiring a minimum 72 hours abstinence (Scott et al., 2018). In the largest study to date, Owens et al. (2019) assessed working memory in 1,038 cannabis users. They found positive urinary THC predicted poorer performance on the N-back and reported altered brain activity in memory networks mediated this relationship. Cousijn et al. (2014) reported no differences in brain activation during the N-back between controls and cannabis users who remained abstinent for 1.8 days prior to assessment. Together, these findings suggest recovery in working memory function following short periods of abstinence.

9.4 Attentional Control

Impaired attention during *acute* cannabis intoxication is consistently reported in human trials measuring selective, divided, and sustained attention. Several systematic reviews support THC-mediated impairments in attention (Bourque and Potvin, 2021; Broyd et al., 2016b; Kroon et al., 2021), with evidence for an increasing dose-dependent effect (Broyd et al., 2016b; Kroon et al., 2021; Schlienz et al., 2020; Vandrey et al., 2017). THC has been shown to disrupt activation of brain networks needed to redirect behaviour during salience processing (Ramaekers et al., 2021). Impaired divided attention is also evident following acute administration of other cannabinoids in some studies (Bedi et al., 2013; Schoedel et al.,

2012; Wesnes et al., 2009) but not others (Schoedel et al., 2011; Vandrey et al., 2013). A recent meta-analysis of CB1 receptor agonists found only mild effects on attention (Zhornitsky et al., 2021). Whether CBD mitigates THC-related impairment in attention remains under investigation, with a recent study finding no effects of oral pre-treatment with CBD (800 mg) on THC (20 mg) impaired performance (Woelfl et al., 2020).

The ability to direct stimulus- and goal-directed attention is important for optimizing behaviours required for daily functioning. There is evidence for tolerance to the acute effects of cannabis on selected (Colizzi and Bhattacharyya, 2018; McCartney et al., 2021) and divided (McCartney et al., 2021) attention in regular users. One study reported THC effects on attention were associated with baseline THC levels but not with a history of regular cannabis use (Ramaekers et al., 2016). A separate study found that altered functional connectivity and increased striatal glutamate concentrations following THC (300 µg/kg) were associated with poorer attention in occasional, but not frequent users (Mason et al., 2021). Further studies are needed to determine whether tolerance is mediated by sub-acute effects of THC and whether it is consistent across different routes of administration, as well as to assess timeframes for recovery in less-frequent users.

There is evidence for small-to-moderate *residual* effects of cannabis on attention processing in cannabis users (Bourque and Potvin, 2021; Broyd et al., 2016b; Lorenzetti et al., 2020b; Paige and Colder, 2020; Scott et al., 2018), with sub-acute residual effects contributing to poorer attention (Broyd et al., 2016b; Kroon et al., 2021). A recent study supports neural compensatory mechanisms in regular cannabis users who had altered functional connectivity between prefrontal and occipital brain regions while performing within the normal range on a visual attention task (Rangel-Pacheco et al., 2021). Cannabis dependence may be related to poorer sustained and selective attention (Cengel et al., 2018; Ortega-Mora et al., 2021) and increased alertness (Ortega-Mora et al., 2021). Earlier cannabis use onset has shown to predict poorer attentional control in later adolescence (18–21 years) (Paige and Colder, 2020) and has been associated with impaired selective attention in current users (Ortega-Mora et al., 2021) and poorer attention after 23 days (Bosker et al., 2013) and 30 days

(Hooper et al., 2014) abstinence. Together, these findings suggest that critical periods of brain neurodevelopment during adolescence may be particularly vulnerable to the long-term effects of cannabis on attentional control.

9.4.1 Attentional Bias

Acute administration of THC increases dopamine release in the striatum (Bossong et al., 2015) and impairs attentional salience processing (Sami et al., 2015). Morgan et al. (2010) found that people who use cannabis with higher ratios of CBD to THC had reduced attentional bias to cannabis-related cues during intoxication. Oral THC (10 mg) has shown to disrupt attentional salience to a greater degree in controls than in cannabis users (Colizzi et al., 2018), suggesting the development of tolerance on stimulus salience processing. However, heavier cannabis use leads to greater attentional bias toward cannabis and related stimuli (Cousijn et al., 2013; O'Neill et al., 2020; Vujanovic et al., 2016; Zhang et al., 2020). These biases have been linked to the reinforcing properties of drug use (Koob and Volkow, 2016) that increase the risk of a dependence syndrome inclusive of craving (Zhang et al., 2020). THC acutely increases dopamine and glutamate (Bossong et al., 2015) in brain regions involved in reward and dependence (Scofield et al., 2016). Evidence suggests these effects are related to automatic orienting to cannabis-related stimuli (Alcorn et al., 2019; O'Neill et al., 2020) and this automatic bias may interfere with other attentional processes (Van Kampen et al., 2020).

9.5 Processing Speed

Evidence consistently shows that *acute* THC administration impairs processing speed (McCartney et al., 2021; Petker et al., 2019; Woelfl et al., 2020). A recent systematic review found the size of these effects were larger for inhalation of CB1 receptor agonists compared to oral administration (Bourque and Potvin, 2021). This finding is consistent with oral THC administration leading to lower peak THC plasma concentrations relative to inhalation (Dinis-Oliveira, 2016). Poorer processing speed may be driven by subacute effects of recent cannabis exposure measured by the presence of positive urinary THC in young adults (Petker et al., 2019). The role of chronicity of cannabis use on processing speed is unclear, with evidence for no effects (Petker et al., 2019) and also impairment in chronic users compared to non-users and occasional users (Frolli et al., 2021). Further studies are needed to examine how cannabis use history and prolonged abstinence affect processing speed.

9.6 Inhibition

Inhibitory control is a key component of executive function that suppresses learned or primed responses to a stimulus in support of goal-directed behaviour. Inhibitory control can be measured by tasks such as Go/No-Go, which measures response inhibition via the suppression of an action, and the Stroop task, which measures the ability to resist interference from task-irrelevant distractions. *Acute* administration of THC impairs performance on a number of tasks: the Stop-Signal (Jacobs et al., 2016; Metrik et al., 2012; Theunissen et al., 2012; van Wel et al., 2013), the Go/No-Go task (Moreno et al., 2012; Spronk et al., 2016), and the Stroop task (Metrik et al., 2012; Theunissen et al., 2015). These deficits may be underscored by increased regional cerebral blood flow and metabolism in brain inhibitory control pathways (Wrege et al., 2014), and altered brain function in inferior frontal regions in association with increased transient psychotic symptoms (Bhattacharyya et al., 2015; and see Chapter 16).

Findings for the *residual* effects of cannabis on inhibitory control in cannabis users are mixed, with evidence of impairment (Fontes et al., 2018; Lisdahl and Price, 2012; Solowij et al., 2012) and of no alterations (Gonzalez et al., 2012; Grant et al., 2012). There is preliminary evidence that risk motivation affects the degree of impaired inhibitory control (Griffith-Lendering et al., 2012). Evidence for an effect of sex is mixed, with reduced performance on the Go/No-Go task in young male compared to female cannabis users (Crane et al., 2013), and no effects of sex on verbal inhibition (Lisdahl and Price, 2012). The residual effects of inhibitory control may be ascribed to altered brain function in the frontal cortex during response inhibition (Moeller et al., 2016), and the left frontal cortex, cingulate cortex, and thalamus following two weeks of abstinence (Wallace et al., 2020). Overall, regular and dependent cannabis use may have residual effects on inhibitory control and underlying brain dysfunction may persist following periods of abstinence.

9.7 Discussion

Significant evidence has emerged in recent years to support that *acute* exposure to cannabis impairs cognitive function in humans, particularly in the domains of learning, episodic memory, attention, and processing speed. Mixed-findings across other areas of cognition, such as working memory, are likely due to methodological heterogeneity in examining distinct cognitive constructs. Emerging evidence supports dose-dependent effects of cannabis on cognition. Yet, research is still to determine whether there is a 'safe' dose range related to daily cognitive skills. The evidence for non-intoxicating *residual* effects of chronic cannabis use is less consistent, with small-to-moderate effect sizes on learning and memory, and small effects on attention. Evidence for the persistence of cognitive deficits following longer periods of abstinence are insufficient to ascertain recovery timelines. There is a need for further research to investigate risk factors that may slow or prevent recovery of cognitive impairment in some regular users.

The effects of cannabis on cognition appear to be mediated by a complex interaction of cannabis use metrics (history, frequency, age and duration of use), route of administration (oral, vaporized, smoked), and the ratio of different cannabinoids (particularly CBD:THC). There are field-wide challenges in systematically controlling for periods of abstinence, sub-acute cannabis effects, types of cannabis strains, and in quantifying cannabis use history. The role of neurodevelopment and cannabis dependence in the onset and maintenance of cannabis' cognitive effects remain under-investigated. It is reasonable to assume that the medical conditions of different patient groups will influence the effects of cannabis. However, there is a lack of mechanistic understanding on how cannabis may mitigate harmful versus therapeutic benefits across varying cognitive domains. Despite growing evidence for the protective effects of CBD on neural functioning, there is no dose-dependent profile for CBD in mitigating THC impairment on cognition.

9.7.1 History of Heavy Cannabis Use and Tolerance

Cross-sectional studies in chronic cannabis users rely on self-report retrospective measures and lack measurement consistency in quantifying cannabis use history. Some further limitations include residual sub-acute effects of cumulative cannabis exposure and controlling for abstinence. Heavy and prolonged cannabis use has been associated with blunted effects of cannabis on verbal memory and attention (Broyd et al., 2016b; Colizzi and Bhattacharyya, 2018; McCartney et al., 2021), and more recently with attentional salience (Gunasekera et al., 2022) and reward processing (Gunasekera et al., 2022; Mason et al., 2021), suggesting the development of tolerance. Sub-acute effects (Desrosiers et al., 2014) and pharmaco-dynamic changes (Ramaekers et al., 2020) following cumulative cannabis exposure may further mediate observed tolerance to impaired cognition (Krzyzanowski and Purdon, 2020). Longer durations of cannabis use may lead to more persistent cognitive impairments and the development of cannabis dependence (van de Giessen et al., 2017; Volkow et al., 2014). However, most studies to date have not sufficiently addressed the role of cannabis dependence, independent from regular and heavy use, in contributing to the effects of cannabis on cognition.

9.7.2 Neurobiology of Tolerance and Chronic Use

A neurobiological model of tolerance proposes pharmacodynamic changes in chronic cannabis users that may dampen the effects of cannabis on select cognitive domains. This model also accounts for residual cognitive impairment following short periods of abstinence in regular and heavy cannabis users (Oomen et al., 2018; Ramaekers et al., 2021). Downregulation of CB1 receptors and endocannabinoids is observed following repeated THC exposure (Bhattacharyya et al., 2017; Ceccarini et al., 2015; D'Souza et al., 2016; Hirvonen, 2015; Hirvonen et al., 2012; Spindle et al., 2021), with greater effects in heavier cannabis users (Ceccarini et al., 2015; Hirvonen et al., 2012). Reduced receptor density and activity may mediate THC's receptor binding properties (Colizzi et al., 2015) and lead to normalization of dopaminergic neurotransmission in mesocorticolimbic pathways to mitigate cannabis' effects on reward (Mason et al., 2021) and other cognitive processes.

There is insufficient and inconclusive neuroanatomical evidence to suggest altered brain morphology following persistent cannabis use and whether they contribute to cannabis-related effects on cognition. Chronic cannabis use may disrupt neuronal dynamics that lead to altered synaptic plasticity and perturbed brain structural alterations (Battistella et al., 2014; Chye et al., 2021; Filbey et al., 2014; Hill et al., 2016). Regular and heavy use of cannabis also leads to N-methyl-D-aspartate receptor (NMDAR) hypofunction (Fan et al., 2010), a decrease in glutamate-derived metabolites (Colizzi et al., 2020; Muetzel et al., 2013; Prescot et al., 2013), and excitotoxicity due to excessive increases in Ca2+ concentrations at post-synaptic ion channels (Plitman et al., 2014). These neural changes may lead to long-lasting effects on brain plasticity (Fishbein et al., 2012; Zamberletti et al., 2016) and atrophy (Barfi et al., 2021) in regions important for cognition. Recent meta-analyses support cannabis dependence as an important metric for ascertaining the impact of cannabis on regional brain structure and function (Chye et al., 2019; Lorenzetti et al., 2020a). Research has yet to establish the role of dependence-related brain alterations in slowing or preventing cognitive recovery following chronic cannabis use.

9.7.3 Neurobiology of Abstinence and Cognition

Abstinence from cannabis following regular use is associated with reduced tolerance to cannabis' intoxicating effects and upregulation of CB1 receptors (D'Souza et al., 2016; Hirvonen et al., 2012). CB1 receptor upregulation has shown to begin after as little as two days' abstinence (D'Souza et al., 2016). Following four weeks of abstinence, these receptor changes have been associated with improved cognition (Hirvonen et al., 2012), suggesting recovery from the cumulative effects of cannabis exposure. These latter findings are consistent with broader evidence of cognitive recovery after six-weeks in regular cannabis users (Broyd et al., 2016b). Studies investigating CB1 receptor density in humans primarily include dependent cannabis users. In humans, there is a need to confirm whether cannabis dependence mediates the recovery of CB1 receptor hypofunction following chronic cannabis use. Neurobiological models of tolerance may interact with learned behavioural strategies to compensate for the acute effects of cannabis on cognitive performance; however, evidence for these behavioural strategies is limited (Ramaekers et al., 2020).

9.7.4 Age of Cannabis Use and Sex

Adolescence is a critical period of neurodevelopment and brain maturation that may increase the risk and resilience to cannabis' effects on cognition (Hurd et al., 2019; Larsen and Luna, 2018; Lubman et al., 2015). Younger cannabis users show similar patterns of impairment to adults, particularly for learning and memory, but show poorer inhibitory control that is more likely to persist following abstinence (Gorey et al., 2019; Morin et al., 2018). Interpretation of research supporting recovery of function during adolescence (Castellanos-Ryan et al., 2017; Lorenzetti et al., 2019) requires caution due to the small number of studies. Cognitive impairment during adolescence may be less related to age of cannabis use initiation (Lovell et al., 2020; Scott et al., 2018) and more strongly with heavier cannabis use (Ganzer et al., 2016; Lovell et al., 2020; Sagar and Gruber, 2018). Brain anatomy develops differently across discrete neurodevelopmental periods (Tamnes et al., 2017). Therefore, there is a need to track the cognitive effects of cannabis across brain pubertal and developmental markers rather than age (Matheson and Le Foll, 2020). There are well known sex differences in neurodevelopmental trajectories (Kaczkurkin et al., 2019). Mounting evidence for an effect of sex on dopamine release (Zachry et al., 2021), CB1 receptor density (Spindle et al., 2021), and response to THC metabolism and intoxication (Sholler et al., 2021) warrant further investigation of sex as an individual risk factor contributing to the effects of cannabis on cognition.

9.7.5 Cannabinoids

The dose and ratios of different cannabinoids vary across cannabis products (Freeman et al., 2014; T. P. Freeman et al., 2019). The deleterious effects of acute and chronic cannabis use on cognition are primarily attributed to action of THC on the endocannabinoid system. Although CBD is thought to be non-intoxicating (Colizzi and Bhattacharyya, 2017; Englund et al., 2017), one study found vaporized CBD (400 mg) produced subjectively intoxicating symptoms (Solowij et al., 2019). Research has not sufficiently identified mechanisms by which acutely administered CBD, or other cannabinoids such as Δ-9-tetrahydrocannabivarin (Englund et al., 2015), may protect against THC-mediated impairment in cognition. There is no clear dose-dependent profile for acute CBD on cognitive performance and results are generally mixed (A. M. Freeman et al., 2019). Empirical studies typically administer CBD doses that are higher than available in the cannabis plant (Niesink and van Laar, 2013) and may not represent the phytochemical formulations consumed by recreational users. Studies of cannabinoid potencies and ratios representative of cannabis use in the community are needed to guide harm minimization policies and guidelines.

9.8 Conclusion

Recent research has focused on increasing the safety profile of cannabis to reduce potential harms. There is accumulating evidence that furthers our understanding of factors that increase risk and resilience to the effects of cannabis on cognition: history and frequency of cannabis use, routes of administration, ratio of different cannabinoids, cannabis potency, sub-acute cannabis effects, cannabis dependence, and neurodevelopment. However, methodological challenges need to be tackled to delineate the cognitive domains that are most vulnerable to cannabis exposure. We need consistent metrics for quantifying cannabis use in recreational and medical settings, and repeated measures assessing cognitive constructs in samples before and after cannabis use onset, as well as over time, including with prolonged abstinence. Increasing trends toward the legalization and medicalization of cannabis means that new findings are necessary to inform targets for preventative interventions and public health policies to mitigate the harms that people can experience when using cannabis.

References

Adam, K. C. S., Doss, M. K., Pabon, E., et al. (2020). Δ9-tetrahydrocannabinol (THC) impairs visual working memory performance: A randomized crossover trial. *Neuropsychopharmacology*, **45**, 1807–1816.

Alcorn, J. L. 3rd, Marks, K. R., Stoops, W. W., et al. (2019). Attentional bias to cannabis cues in cannabis users but not cocaine users. *Addict Behav*, **88**, 129–136.

Ballard, M. E., Gallo, D. A., and De Wit, H. (2012). Psychoactive drugs and false memory: Comparison of dextroamphetamine and δ-9-tetrahydrocannabinol on false recognition. *Psychopharmacology (Berl)*, **219**, 15–24.

Barfi, E., Tehrani, A. M., Mohammadpanah, M., et al. (2021). The role of tetrahydrocannabinol in inducing disrupted signaling cascades, hippocampal atrophy and memory defects. *J Chem Neuroanat*, **113**, 101943.

Batalla, A., Crippa, J. A., Busatto, G. F., et al. (2014). Neuroimaging studies of acute effects of THC and CBD in humans and animals: A systematic review. *Curr Pharm Des*, **20**, 2168–2185.

Battistella, G., Fornari, E., Annoni, J.-M., et al. (2014). Long-term effects of cannabis on brain structure. *Neuropsychopharmacology*, **39**, 2041–2048.

Bedi, G., Cooper, Z. D., & Haney, M. (2013). Subjective, cognitive and cardiovascular dose–effect profile of nabilone and dronabinol in marijuana smokers. *Addict Biol*, **18**, 872–881.

Bhattacharyya, S., Atakan, Z., Martin-Santos, R., et al. (2015). Impairment of inhibitory control processing related to acute psychotomimetic effects of cannabis. *Eur Neuropsychopharmacol*, **25**, 26–37.

Bhattacharyya, S., Egerton, A., Kim, E., et al. (2017). Acute induction of anxiety in humans by delta-9-tetrahydrocannabinol related to amygdalar cannabinoid-1 (CB1) receptors. *Sci Rep*, 7, 15025.

Blest-Hopley, G., O'Neill, A., Wilson, R., et al. (2021). Disrupted parahippocampal and midbrain function underlie slower verbal learning in adolescent-onset regular cannabis use. *Psychopharmacology (Berl)*, **238**, 1315–1331.

Bloomfield, M. A. P., Green, S. F., Hindocha, C., et al. (2020). The effects of acute cannabidiol on cerebral blood flow and its relationship to memory: An arterial spin labelling magnetic resonance imaging study. *J Psychopharmacol*, **34**, 981–989.

Bonn-Miller, M. O., Elsohly, M. A., Loflin, M. J. E., et al. (2018). Cannabis and cannabinoid drug development: Evaluating botanical versus single molecule approaches. *Int Rev Psychiatry*, **30**, 277–284.

Borgan, F., Beck, K., Butler, E., et al. (2019). The effects of cannabinoid 1 receptor compounds on memory: A meta-analysis and systematic review across species. *Psychopharmacology (Berl)*, **236**, 3257–3270.

Bosker, W. M., Karschner, E. L., Lee, D., et al. (2013). Psychomotor function in chronic daily cannabis smokers during sustained abstinence. *PLoS ONE*, **8**, e53127.

Bossong, M. G., Jansma, J. M., Van Hell, H. H., et al. (2012). Effects of δ9-tetrahydrocannabinol on human working memory function. *Biol Psychiatry*, **71**, 693–699.

Bossong, M. G., Mehta, M. A., Van Berckel, B. N., et al. (2015). Further human evidence for striatal dopamine release induced by administration of Δ9-tetrahydrocannabinol (THC): Selectivity to limbic striatum. *Psychopharmacology (Berl)*, **232**, 2723–2729.

Bourque, J., and Potvin, S. (2021). Cannabis and cognitive functioning: From acute to residual effects, from randomized controlled trials to prospective designs. *Front Psychiatry*, **12**, 919.

Broyd, S.J., Greenwood, L.-M., Van Hell, H. H., et al. (2016a). Mismatch negativity and P50 sensory gating in abstinent former cannabis users. *Neural Plast*, **2016**, 6526437.

Broyd, S.J., Van Hell, H. H., Yucel, M., et al. (2016b). Acute and chronic effects of cannabinoids on human cognition: A systematic review. *Biol Psychiatry*, **79**, 557–567.

Castellanos-Ryan, N., Pingault, J.-B., Parent, S., et al. (2017). Adolescent cannabis use, change in neurocognitive function, and high-school graduation: A longitudinal study from early adolescence to young adulthood. *Dev Psychopathol*, **29**, 1253–1266.

Ceccarini, J., Kuepper, R., Kemels, D., et al. (2015). [18f]mk-9470 pet measurement of cannabinoid CB1 receptor availability in chronic cannabis users. *Addict Biol*, **20**, 357–367.

Cengel, H. Y., Bozkurt, M., Evren, C., et al. (2018). Evaluation of cognitive functions in individuals with synthetic cannabinoid use disorder and comparison to individuals with cannabis use disorder. *Psychiatry Res*, **262**, 46–54.

Chandra, S., Radwan, M. M., Majumdar, C. G., et al. (2019). New trends in cannabis potency in USA and Europe during the last decade (2008–2017). *Eur Arch Psychiatry Clin Neurosci*, **269**, 5–15.

Chye, Y., Kirkham, R., Lorenzetti, V., et al. (2021). Cannabis, cannabinoids, and brain morphology: A review of the evidence. *Biol Psychiatry Cogn Neurosci Neuroimaging*, **6**, 627–635.

Chye, Y., Lorenzetti, V., Suo, C., et al. (2019). Alteration to hippocampal volume and shape confined to cannabis dependence: A multi-site study. *Addict Biol*, **24**, 822–834.

Colizzi, M., and Bhattacharyya, S. (2017). Does cannabis composition matter? Differential effects of delta-9-tetrahydrocannabinol and cannabidiol on human cognition. *Curr Addic Rep*, **4**, 62–74.

(2018). Cannabis use and the development of tolerance: A systematic review of human evidence. *Neurosci Biobehav Rev*, **93**, 1–25.

Colizzi, M., Fazio, L., Ferranti, L., et al. (2015). Functional genetic variation of the cannabinoid receptor 1 and cannabis use interact on prefrontal connectivity and related working memory behavior. *Neuropsychopharmacology*, **40**, 640–649.

Colizzi, M., McGuire, P., Giampietro, V., et al. (2018). Previous cannabis exposure modulates the acute effects of delta-9-tetrahydrocannabinol on attentional salience and fear processing. *Exp Clin Psychopharmacol*, **26**, 582–598.

Colizzi, M., Weltens, N., Mcguire, P., et al. (2020). Delta-9-tetrahydrocannabinol increases striatal glutamate levels in healthy individuals: Implications for psychosis. *Mol Psychiatry*, **25**, 3231–3240.

Cousijn, J., Goudriaan, A. E., Ridderinkhof, K. R., et al. (2013). Neural responses associated with cue-reactivity in frequent cannabis users. *Addict Biol*, **18**, 570–580.

Cousijn, J., Wiers, R. W., Ridderinkhof, K. R., et al. (2014). Effect of baseline cannabis use and working-memory network function on changes in cannabis use in heavy cannabis users: A prospective FMRI study. *Hum Brain Mapp*, **35**, 2470–2482.

Crane, N. A., Schuster, R. M., and Gonzalez, R. (2013). Preliminary evidence for a sex-specific relationship between amount of cannabis use and neurocognitive performance in young adult cannabis users. *J Int Neuropsychol Soc*, **19**, 1009–1015.

Curran, T., Devillez, H., Yorkwilliams, S. L., et al. (2020). Acute effects of naturalistic THC vs. CBD use on recognition memory: A preliminary study. *J Cannabis Res*, **2**, 28.

Cuttler, C., Mclaughlin, R. J., and Graf, P. (2012). Mechanisms underlying the link between cannabis use and prospective memory. *PLoS ONE*, **7**, e36820.

D'Souza, D. C., Cortes-Briones, J. A., Ranganathan, M., et al. (2016). Rapid changes in CB1 receptor availability in cannabis dependent males after abstinence from cannabis. *Biol Psychiatry Cogn Neurosci Neuroimaging*, **1**, 60–67.

Day, A. M., Metrik, J., Spillane, N. S., et al. (2013). Working memory and impulsivity predict marijuana-related problems among frequent users. *Drug Alcohol Depend*, **131**, 171–174.

Desrosiers, N. A., Himes, S. K., Scheidweiler, K. B., et al. (2014). Phase I and II cannabinoid disposition in blood and plasma of occasional and frequent smokers following controlled smoked cannabis. *Clin Chem*, **60**, 631–643.

Dinis-Oliveira, R. J. (2016). Metabolomics of δ9-tetrahydrocannabinol:

Implications in toxicity. *Drug Metab Rev*, **48**, 80–87.

Doss, M. K., Weafer, J., Gallo, D. A., et al. (2018). Δ9-tetrahydrocannabinol at retrieval drives false recollection of neutral and emotional memories. *Biol Psychiatry*, **84**, 743–750.

Duperrouzel, J. C., Hawes, S. W., Lopez-Quintero, C., et al. (2019). Adolescent cannabis use and its associations with decision-making and episodic memory: Preliminary results from a longitudinal study. *Neuropsychology*, **33**, 701–710.

ElSohly, M. A., Mehmedic, Z., Foster, S., et al. (2016). Changes in cannabis potency over the last 2 decades (1995–2014): Analysis of current data in the united states. *Biol Psychiatry*, **79**, 613–619.

Englund, A., Atakan, Z., Kralj, A., et al. (2015). The effect of five day dosing with THCV on THC-induced cognitive, psychological and physiological effects in healthy male human volunteers: A placebo-controlled, double-blind, crossover pilot trial. *J Psychopharmacol*, **30**, 140–151.

Englund, A., Freeman, T. P., Murray, R. M., et al. (2017). Can we make cannabis safer? *Lancet Psychiatry*, **4**, 643–648.

Englund, A., Morrison, P. D., Nottage, J., et al. (2013). Cannabidiol inhibits THC-elicited paranoid symptoms and hippocampal-dependent memory impairment. *J Psychopharmacol (Oxford)*, **27**, 19–27.

European Monitoring Centre for Drugs and Drug Addiction (EMCDDA). (2015). *European Drug Report 2015: Trends and Developments*. Luxembourg: Publications Office of the European Union.

Fan, N., Yang, H., Zhang, J., et al. (2010). Reduced expression of glutamate receptors and phosphorylation of creb are responsible for in vivo δ9-THC exposure-impaired hippocampal synaptic plasticity. *J Neurochem*, **112**, 691–702.

Filbey, F. M., Aslan, S., Calhoun, V. D., et al. (2014). Long-term effects of marijuana use on the brain. *PNAS*, **111**, 16913.

Fishbein, M., Gov, S., Assaf, F., et al. (2012). Long-term behavioral and biochemical effects of an ultra-low dose of δ9-tetrahydrocannabinol (THC): Neuroprotection and erk signaling. *Exp Brain Res*, **221**, 437–448.

Fontes, M. A., Bolla, K. I., Cunha, P. J., et al. (2018). Cannabis use before age 15 and subsequent executive functioning. *Br J Psychiatry*, **198**, 442–447.

Freeman, A. M., Petrilli, K., Lees, R., et al. (2019). How does cannabidiol (CBD) influence the acute effects of delta-9-tetrahydrocannabinol (THC) in humans? A systematic review. *Neurosci Biobehav Rev*, **107**, 696–712.

Freeman, T. P., Craft, S., Wilson, J., et al. (2021). Changes in delta-9-tetrahydrocannabinol (THC) and cannabidiol (CBD) concentrations in cannabis over time: Systematic review and meta-analysis. *Addiction*, **116**, 1000–1010.

Freeman, T. P., Hindocha, C., Green, S. F., et al. (2019). Medicinal use of cannabis based products and cannabinoids. *BMJ*, **365**, l1141.

Freeman, T. P., Morgan, C. J., Hindocha, C., et al. (2014). Just say 'know': How do cannabinoid concentrations influence users' estimates of cannabis potency and the amount they roll in joints? *Addiction*, **109**, 1686–1694.

Fried, P. A., Watkinson, B., and Gray, R. (2005). Neurocognitive consequences of marihuana: A comparison with pre-drug performance. *Neurotoxicol Teratol*, **27**, 231–239.

Frolli, A., Ricci, M. C., Cavallaro, A., et al. (2021). Cognitive development and cannabis use in adolescents. *Behav Sci (Basel)*, **11**, 37.

Gajewski, P. D., Hanisch, E., Falkenstein, M., et al. (2018). What does the N-back task measure as we get older? Relations between working-memory measures and other cognitive functions across the lifespan. *Front Psychol*, **9**, 2208.

Ganzer, F., Bröning, S., Kraft, S., et al. (2016). Weighing the evidence: A systematic review on long-term neurocognitive effects of cannabis use in abstinent adolescents and adults. *Neuropsychol Rev*, **26**, 186–222.

Gessa, G. L., Casu, M. A., Carta, G., et al. (1998). Cannabinoids decrease acetylcholine release in the medial-prefrontal cortex and hippocampus, reversal by sr 141716a. *Eur J Pharmacol*, **355**, 119–124.

van de Giessen, E., Weinstein, J. J., Cassidy, C. M., et al. (2017). Deficits in striatal dopamine release in cannabis dependence. *Mol Psychiatry*, **22**, 68–75.

Gonzalez, R., Schuster, R. M., Mermelstein, R. J., et al. (2012). Performance of young adult cannabis users on neurocognitive measures of impulsive behavior and their relationship to symptoms of cannabis use disorders. *J Clin Exp Neuropsychol*, **34**, 962–976.

Gorey, C., Kuhns, L., Smaragdi, E., et al. (2019). Age-related differences in the impact of cannabis use on the brain and cognition: A systematic review. *Eur Arch Psychiatry Clin Neurosci*, **269**, 37–58.

Government of Canada (GOC). (2019). *Canadian tobacco, alcohol and drugs survey (CTADS): Summary of results for 2017*. Available at: www.canada.ca/en/health-canada/services/canadian-tobacco-alcohol-drugs-survey/2017-summary.html (Last accessed 9 April 2021).

Grant, J. E., Chamberlain, S. R., Schreiber, L., et al. (2012). Neuropsychological deficits associated with cannabis use in young adults. *Drug Alcohol Depend*, **121**, 159–162.

Griffith-Lendering, M. F. H., Huijbregts, S. C. J., Vollebergh, W. A. M., et al. (2012). Motivational and cognitive inhibitory control in recreational cannabis users. *J Clin Exp Neuropsychol*, **34**, 688–697.

Gunasekera, B., Diederen, K., and Bhattacharyya, S. (2022). Cannabinoids, reward processing, and psychosis. *Psychopharmacology (Berl)*, **239**, 1157–1177.

Hall, W., Hoch, E., and Lorenzetti, V. (2019). Cannabis use and mental health: Risks and benefits. *Eur Arch Psychiatry Clin Neurosci*, **269**, 1–3.

Herzig, D. A., Nutt, D. J., and Mohr, C. (2014). Alcohol and relatively pure cannabis use, but not schizotypy, are associated with cognitive attenuations. *Front Psychiatry*, **5**, 133.

Hill, S. Y., Sharma, V., and Jones, B. L. (2016). Lifetime use of cannabis from longitudinal assessments, cannabinoid receptor (CNR1) variation, and reduced volume of the right anterior cingulate. *Psychiatry Res Neuroimaging*, **255**, 24–34.

Hirvonen, J. (2015). In vivo imaging of the cannabinoid CB1 receptor with positron emission tomography. *Clin Pharmacol Ther*, **97**, 565–567.

Hirvonen, J., Goodwin, R. S., Li, C. T., et al. (2012). Reversible and regionally selective downregulation of brain cannabinoid CB1 receptors in chronic daily cannabis smokers. *Mol Psychiatry*, **17**, 642–649.

Hooper, S. R., Woolley, D., and De Bellis, M. D. (2014). Intellectual, neurocognitive, and academic achievement in abstinent adolescents with cannabis use disorder. *Psychopharmacology (Berl)*, **231**, 1467–1477.

Hughes, A., Lipari, R. N., and Williams, M. R. (2016). Marijuana use and perceived risk of harm from marijuana use varies within and across states. In: *The CBHSQ Report*. Rockville, MD: Substance Abuse and Mental Health Services Administration (US). Available at: www.ncbi.nlm.nih.gov/books/NBK396156/. Last accessed 30 October 2022.

Hurd, Y. L., Manzoni, O. J., Pletnikov, M. V., et al. (2019). Cannabis and the developing brain: Insights into its long-lasting effects. *J Neurosci*, **39**, 8250.

Jacobs, D. S., Kohut, S. J., Jiang, S., et al. (2016). Acute and chronic effects of cannabidiol on δ^9-tetrahydrocannabinol (δ^9-THC)-induced disruption in stop signal task performance. *Exp Clin Psychopharmacol*, **24**, 320–330.

Kaczkurkin, A. N., Raznahan, A., and Satterthwaite, T. D. (2019). Sex differences in the developing brain: Insights from multimodal neuroimaging. *Neuropsychopharmacology*, **44**, 71–85.

Khan, R., Naveed, S., Mian, N., et al. (2020). The therapeutic role of cannabidiol in mental health: A systematic review. *J Cannabis Res*, **2**, 2.

Kloft, L., Otgaar, H., Blokland, A., et al. (2020). Cannabis increases susceptibility to false memory. *PNAS*, **117**, 4585.

Koob, G. F. D., and Volkow, N. D. M. D. (2016). Neurobiology of addiction: A neurocircuitry analysis. *Lancet Psychiatry*, **3**, 760–773.

Kroon, E., Kuhns, L., and Cousijn, J. (2021). The short-term and long-term effects of cannabis on

cognition: Recent advances in the field. *Curr Opin Psychol*, **38**, 49–55.

Krzyzanowski, D. J., and Purdon, S. E. (2020). Duration of abstinence from cannabis is positively associated with verbal learning performance: A systematic review and meta-analysis. *Neuropsychology*, **34**, 359–372.

Larsen, B., and Luna, B. (2018). Adolescence as a neurobiological critical period for the development of higher-order cognition. *Neurosci Biobehav Rev*, **94**, 179–195.

Lisdahl, K. M., and Price, J. S. (2012). Increased marijuana use and gender predict poorer cognitive functioning in adolescents and emerging adults. *J Int Neuropsychol Soc*, **18**, 678–688.

Lorenzetti, V., Chye, Y., Silva, P., et al. (2019). Does regular cannabis use affect neuroanatomy? An updated systematic review and meta-analysis of structural neuroimaging studies. *Eur Arch Psychiatry Clin Neurosci*, **269**, 59–71.

Lorenzetti, V., Chye, Y., Suo, C., et al. (2020a). Neuroanatomical alterations in people with high and low cannabis dependence. *Aust NZ J Psychiatry*, **54**, 68–75.

Lorenzetti, V., Hoch, E., and Hall, W. (2020b). Adolescent cannabis use, cognition, brain health and educational outcomes: A review of the evidence. *Eur Neuropsychopharmacol*, **36**, 169–180.

Lorenzetti, V., Takagi, M., Van Dalen, Y., et al. (2021). Investigating the residual effects of chronic cannabis use and abstinence on verbal and visuospatial learning. *Front Psychiatry*, **12**, 663701.

Lovell, M. E., Akhurst, J., Padgett, C., et al. (2020). Cognitive outcomes associated with long-term, regular, recreational cannabis use in adults: A meta-analysis. *Exp*

Clin Psychopharmacol, **28**, 471–494.

Lubman, D. I., Cheetham, A., and Yücel, M. (2015). Cannabis and adolescent brain development. *Pharmacol Ther*, **148**, 1–16.

Ma, L., Steinberg, J. L., Bjork, J. M., et al. (2018). Fronto-striatal effective connectivity of working memory in adults with cannabis use disorder. *Psychiatry Res Neuroimaging*, **278**, 21–34.

Mason, N. L., Theunissen, E. L., Hutten, N. R. P. W., et al. (2021). Reduced responsiveness of the reward system is associated with tolerance to cannabis impairment in chronic users. *Addict Biol*, **26**, e12870.

Matheson, J., and Le Foll, B. (2020). Cannabis legalization and acute harm from high potency cannabis products: A narrative review and recommendations for public health. *Front Psychiatry*, **11**, 1017.

McCartney, D., Arkell, T. R., Irwin, C., et al. (2021). Determining the magnitude and duration of acute δ(9)-tetrahydrocannabinol (δ(9)-THC)-induced driving and cognitive impairment: A systematic and meta-analytic review. *Neurosci Biobehav Rev*, **126**, 175–193.

Medina, K. L., Hanson, K. L., Schweinsburg, A. D., et al. (2007). Neuropsychological functioning in adolescent marijuana users: Subtle deficits detectable after a month of abstinence. *J Int Neuropsychol Soc*, **13**, 807–820.

Meier, M. H., Caspi, A., Ambler, A., et al. (2012). Persistent cannabis users show neuropsychological decline from childhood to midlife. *PNAS*, **109**, E2657–E2664.

Metrik, J., Kahler, C. W., Reynolds, B., et al. (2012). Balanced placebo design with marijuana: Pharmacological and expectancy effects on impulsivity and risk taking. *Psychopharmacology (Berl)*, **223**, 489–499.

Mizrahi, R., Watts, J. J., and Tseng, K. Y. (2017). Mechanisms contributing to cognitive deficits in cannabis users. *Neuropharmacology*, **124**, 84–88.

Moeller, S. J., Bederson, L., Alia-Klein, N., et al. (2016). Neuroscience of inhibition for addiction medicine: From prediction of initiation to prediction of relapse. *Prog Brain Res*, **223**, 165–188.

Moreno, M., Estevez, A. F., Zaldivar, F., et al. (2012). Impulsivity differences in recreational cannabis users and binge drinkers in a university population. *Drug Alcohol Depend*, **124**, 355–362.

Morgan, C. J. A., Freeman, T. P., Hindocha, C., et al. (2018). Individual and combined effects of acute delta-9-tetrahydrocannabinol and cannabidiol on psychotomimetic symptoms and memory function. *Transl Psychiatry*, **8**, 181.

Morgan, C. J. A., Freeman, T. P., Schafer, G. L., et al. (2010). Cannabidiol attenuates the appetitive effects of δ9-tetrahydrocannabinol in humans smoking their chosen cannabis. *Neuropsychopharmacology*, **35**, 1879–1885.

Morin, J.-F. G., Afzali, M. H., Bourque, J., et al. (2018). A population-based analysis of the relationship between substance use and adolescent cognitive development. *Am J Psychiatry*, **176**, 98–106.

Muetzel, R. L., Marjańska, M., Collins, P. F., et al. (2013). In vivo 1h magnetic resonance spectroscopy in young-adult daily marijuana users. *Neuroimage Clin*, **2**, 581–589.

Murray, R. M., Englund, A., Abi-Dargham, A., et al. (2017). Cannabis-associated psychosis: Neural substrate and clinical impact. *Neuropharmacology*, **124**, 89–104.

Nader, D. A., and Sanchez, Z. M. (2018). Effects of regular cannabis use on neurocognition, brain structure, and function: A systematic review of findings in adults. *Am J Drug Alcohol Abuse*, **44**, 4–18.

Niesink, R. J., and van Laar, M. W. (2013). Does cannabidiol protect against adverse psychological effects of THC? *Front Psychiatry*, **4**, 130.

O'Neill, A., Bachi, B., and Bhattacharyya, S. (2020). Attentional bias towards cannabis cues in cannabis users: A systematic review and meta-analysis. *Drug Alcohol Depend*, **206**, 107719.

Oomen, P. P., Van Hell, H. H., and Bossong, M. G. (2018). The acute effects of cannabis on human executive function. *Behav Pharmacol*, **29**, 605–616.

Ortega-Mora, I. E., Caballero-Sánchez, U., Román-López, T. V., et al. (2021). The alerting and orienting systems of attention are modified by cannabis dependence. *J Int Neuropsychol Soc*, **27**, 520–532.

Owens, M. M., Mcnally, S., Petker, T., et al. (2019). Urinary tetrahydrocannabinol is associated with poorer working memory performance and alterations in associated brain activity. *Neuropsychopharmacology*, **44**, 613–619.

Paige, K. J., and Colder, C. R. (2020). Long-term effects of early adolescent marijuana use on attentional and inhibitory control. *J Stud Alcohol Drugs*, **81**, 164–172.

Petker, T., Owens, M. M., Amlung, M. T., et al. (2019). Cannabis involvement and neuropsychological performance: Findings from the human connectome project. *J Psychiatry Neurosci*, **44**, 414–422.

Plitman, E., Nakajima, S., De La Fuente-Sandoval, C., et al. (2014). Glutamate-mediated excitotoxicity in schizophrenia: A review. *Eur*

Neuropsychopharmacol, 24, 1591–1605.

Potter, D. J., Hammond, K., Tuffnell, S., et al. (2018). Potency of δ(9)-tetrahydrocannabinol and other cannabinoids in cannabis in England in 2016: Implications for public health and pharmacology. *Drug Testing Anal*, 10, 628–635.

Prescot, A. P., Renshaw, P. F., and Yurgelun-Todd, D. A. (2013). γ-amino butyric acid and glutamate abnormalities in adolescent chronic marijuana smokers. *Drug Alcohol Depend*, 129, 232–239.

Prini, P., Zamberletti, E., Manenti, C., et al. (2020). Neurobiological mechanisms underlying cannabis-induced memory impairment. *Eur Neuropsychopharmacol*, 36, 181–190.

Ramaekers, J. G., Mason, N. L., Kloft, L., et al. (2021). The why behind the high: Determinants of neurocognition during acute cannabis exposure. *Nat Rev Neurosci*, 22, 439–454.

Ramaekers, J. G., Mason, N. L., and Theunissen, E. L. (2020). Blunted highs: Pharmacodynamic and behavioral models of cannabis tolerance. *Eur Neuropsychopharmacol*, 36, 191–205.

Ramaekers, J. G., Van Wel, J. H., Spronk, D. B., et al. (2016). Cannabis and tolerance: Acute drug impairment as a function of cannabis use history. *Sci Rep*, 6, 26843–26843.

Ranganathan, M., Radhakrishnan, R., Addy, P. H., et al. (2017). Tetrahydrocannabinol (THC) impairs encoding but not retrieval of verbal information. *Prog Neuropsychopharmacol Biol Psychiatry*, 79, 176–183.

Rangel-Pacheco, A., Lew, B. J., Schantell, M. D., et al. (2021). Altered fronto-occipital connectivity during visual selective attention in regular cannabis users.

Psychopharmacology (Berl), 238, 1351–1361.

Riba, J., Valle, M., Sampedro, F., et al. (2015). Telling true from false: Cannabis users show increased susceptibility to false memories. *Mol Psychiatry*, 20, 772–777.

Roten, A., Baker, N. L., and Gray, K. M. (2015). Cognitive performance in a placebo-controlled pharmacotherapy trial for youth with marijuana dependence. *Addict Behav*, 45, 119–123.

Sagar, K. A., and Gruber, S. A. (2018). Marijuana matters: Reviewing the impact of marijuana on cognition, brain structure and function, & exploring policy implications and barriers to research. *Int Rev Psychiatry*, 30, 251–267.

Sami, M. B., Rabiner, E. A., and Bhattacharyya, S. (2015). Does cannabis affect dopaminergic signaling in the human brain? A systematic review of evidence to date. *Eur Neuropsychopharmacol*, 25, 1201–1224.

Schlienz, N. J., Spindle, T. R., Cone, E. J., et al. (2020). Pharmacodynamic dose effects of oral cannabis ingestion in healthy adults who infrequently use cannabis. *Drug Alcohol Depend*, 211, 107969.

Schoedel, K. A., Addy, C., Chakraborty, B., et al. (2012). Human abuse potential and cognitive effects of taranabant, a cannabinoid 1 receptor inverse agonist: A randomized, double-blind, placebo- and active-controlled, crossover study in recreational polydrug users. *J Clin Psychopharmacol*, 32, 492–502.

Schoedel, K. A., Chen, N., Hilliard, A., et al. (2011). A randomized, double-blind, placebo-controlled, crossover study to evaluate the subjective abuse potential and cognitive effects of nabiximols oromucosal spray in subjects with a history of recreational cannabis use. *Hum Psychopharmacol Clin Exp*, 26, 224–236.

Schoeler, T., Kambeitz, J., Behlke, I., et al. (2016). The effects of cannabis on memory function in users with and without a psychotic disorder: Findings from a combined meta-analysis. *Psychol Med*, 46, 177–188.

Scofield, M. D., Heinsbroek, J. A., Gipson, C. D., et al. (2016). The nucleus accumbens: Mechanisms of addiction across drug classes reflect the importance of glutamate homeostasis. *Pharmacol Rev*, 68, 816.

Scott, J. C., Slomiak, S. T., Jones, J. D., et al. (2018). Association of cannabis with cognitive functioning in adolescents and young adults: A systematic review and meta-analysis. *JAMA Psychiatry*, 75, 585–595.

Scott, J. C., Wolf, D. H., Calkins, M. E., et al. (2017). Cognitive functioning of adolescent and young adult cannabis users in the Philadelphia neurodevelopmental cohort. *Psychol Addict Behav*, 31, 423–434.

Sholler, D. J., Strickland, J. C., Spindle, T. R., et al. (2021). Sex differences in the acute effects of oral and vaporized cannabis among healthy adults. *Addict Biol*, 26, e12968.

Smith, J. L., De Blasio, F. M., Iredale, J. M., et al. (2017). Verbal learning and memory in cannabis and alcohol users: An event-related potential investigation. *Front Psychol*, 8, 2129.

Sneider, J. T., Gruber, S. A., Rogowska, J., et al. (2013). A preliminary study of functional brain activation among marijuana users during performance of a virtual water maze task. *J Addict*, 2013, 461029.

Solowij, N., Broyd, S., Greenwood, L.-M., et al. (2019). A randomised controlled trial of vaporised δ9-tetrahydrocannabinol and cannabidiol alone and in combination in frequent and infrequent cannabis users: Acute intoxication effects. *Eur Arch Psychiatry Clin Neurosci*, **269**, 17–35.

Solowij, N., Jones, K. A., Rozman, M. E., et al. (2011). Verbal learning and memory in adolescent cannabis users, alcohol users and non-users. *Psychopharmacology (Berl)*, **216**, 131–144.

et al. (2012). Reflection impulsivity in adolescent cannabis users: A comparison with alcohol-using and non-substance-using adolescents. *Psychopharmacology (Berl)*, **219**, 575–586.

Solowij, N., and Pesa, N. (2011). Cannabis and cognition: Short- and long-term effects. In Castle, D., Murray, R., and D'Souza, D. (eds.) *Marijuana and Madness* (pp. 91–102). Cambridge: Cambridge University Press.

Spindle, T. R., Kuwabara, H., Eversole, A., et al. (2021). Brain imaging of cannabinoid type I (CB1) receptors in women with cannabis use disorder and male and female healthy controls. *Addict Biol*, **26**, e13061.

Spronk, D. B., De Bruijn, E. R. A., Van Wel, J. H. P., et al. (2016). Acute effects of cocaine and cannabis on response inhibition in humans: An erp investigation. *Addict Biol*, **21**, 1186–1198.

Subbaraman, M. S., and Kerr, W. C. (2021). Cannabis use frequency, route of administration, and co-use with alcohol among older adults in Washington State. *J Cannabis Res*, **3**, 17.

Tait, R. J., Mackinnon, A., and Christensen, H. (2011). Cannabis use and cognitive function: 8-year trajectory in a young adult cohort. *Addiction*, **106**, 2195–2203.

Takakuwa, K. M., and Schears, R. M. (2021). The emergency department care of the cannabis and synthetic cannabinoid patient: A narrative review. *Int J Emerg Med*, **14**, 10.

Tamnes, C. K., Herting, M. M., Goddings, A. L., et al. (2017). Development of the cerebral cortex across adolescence: A multisample study of inter-related longitudinal changes in cortical volume, surface area, and thickness. *J Neurosci*, **37**, 3402–3412.

Thames, A. D., Arbid, N., and Sayegh, P. (2014). Cannabis use and neurocognitive functioning in a non-clinical sample of users. *Addict Behav*, **39**, 994–999.

Theunissen, E. L., Heckman, P., de Sousa Fernandes Perna, E. B., et al. (2015). Rivastigmine but not vardenafil reverses cannabis-induced impairment of verbal memory in healthy humans. *Psychopharmacology (Berl)*, **232**, 343–353.

Theunissen, E. L., Kauert, G. F., Toennes, S. W., et al. (2012). Neurophysiological functioning of occasional and heavy cannabis users during THC intoxication. *Psychopharmacology (Berl)*, **220**, 341–350.

United Nations Office on Drugs and Crime. (2016). *World Drug Report 2016 (United Nations publication, Sales No. E.16.XI.7)*. New York: United Nations.

(2020). *World Drug Report 2020 (United Nations publication, Sales No. E.20.XI.6)*. New York: United Nations.

Van Kampen, A.D., Cousijn, J., Engel, C., et al. (2020). Attentional bias, craving and cannabis use in an inpatient sample of adolescents and young adults diagnosed with cannabis use disorder: The moderating role of cognitive control. *Addict Behav*, **100**, 106126.

Van Wel, J. H. P., Kuypers, K. P. C., Theunissen, E. L., et al. (2013). Single doses of THC and cocaine decrease proficiency of impulse control in heavy cannabis users. *Br J Pharmacol*, **170**, 1410–1420.

Vandrey, R., Herrmann, E. S., Mitchell, J. M., et al. (2017). Pharmacokinetic profile of oral cannabis in humans: Blood and oral fluid disposition and relation to pharmacodynamic outcomes. *J Anal Toxicol*, **41**, 83–99.

Vandrey, R., Stitzer, M. L., Mintzer, M. Z., et al. (2013). The dose effects of short-term dronabinol (oral THC) maintenance in daily cannabis users. *Drug Alcohol Depend*, **128**, 64–70.

Volkow, N. D., Baler, R. D., Compton, W. M., et al. (2014). Adverse health effects of marijuana use. *N Engl J Med*, **370**, 2219–2227.

Vujanovic, A. A., Wardle, M. C., Liu, S., et al. (2016). Attentional bias in adults with cannabis use disorders. *J Addict Dis*, **35**, 144–153.

Wadsworth, E. J., Moss, S. C., Simpson, S. A., et al. (2006). Cannabis use, cognitive performance and mood in a sample of workers. *J Psychopharmacol*, **20**, 14–23.

Wallace, A. L., Maple, K. E., Barr, A. T., et al. (2020). Bold responses to inhibition in cannabis-using adolescents and emerging adults after 2 weeks of monitored cannabis abstinence. *Psychopharmacology (Berl)*, **237**, 3259–3268.

Waris, O., Soveri, A., Ahti, M., et al. (2017). A latent factor analysis of working memory measures using large-scale data. *Front Psychol*, **8**, 1062.

Wesnes, K. A., Annas, P., Edgar, C. J., et al. (2009). Nabilone produces marked impairments to cognitive function and changes in subjective state in healthy volunteers. *J Psychopharmacol*, **24**, 1659–1669.

Wittemann, M., Brielmaier, J., Rubly, M., et al. (2021). Cognition and cortical thickness in heavy cannabis users. *Eur Addict Res*, **27**, 115–122.

Woelfl, T., Rohleder, C., Mueller, J. K., et al. (2020). Effects of cannabidiol and delta-9-tetrahydrocannabinol on emotion, cognition, and attention: A double-blind, placebo-controlled, randomized experimental trial in healthy volunteers. *Front Psychiatry*, **11**, 576877.

Wrege, J., Schmidt, A., Walter, A., et al. (2014). Effects of cannabis on impulsivity: A systematic review of neuroimaging findings. *Curr Pharm Des*, **20**, 2126–2137.

Zachry, J. E., Nolan, S. O., Brady, L. J., et al. (2021). Sex differences in dopamine release regulation in the striatum. *Neuropsychopharmacology*, **46**, 491–499.

Zamberletti, E., Gabaglio, M., Grilli, M., et al. (2016). Long-term hippocampal glutamate synapse and astrocyte dysfunctions underlying the altered phenotype induced by adolescent THC treatment in male rats. *Pharmacol Res*, **111**, 459–470.

Zhang, M., Fung, D. S. S., and Smith, H. (2020). A literature review of attentional biases amongst individuals with substance dependency: Individual differences and modulating factors. *Psychiatry Intl*, **1**, 125–134.

Zhornitsky, S., Pelletier, J., Assaf, R., et al. (2021). Acute effects of partial CB(1) receptor agonists on cognition: A meta-analysis of human studies. *Prog Neuropsychopharmacol Biol Psychiatry*, **104**, 110063.

Is There a Cannabis-Associated Psychosis Sub-type?

Lessons from Biological Typing in the B-SNIP Project and Implications for Treatment

Godfrey D. Pearlson and Matcheri S. Keshavan

10.1 Introduction: Overarching Questions

There is increasing evidence for cannabis use being a significant risk factor for first episode psychosis, particularly schizophrenia, as summarized by Di Forti et al. (2019), who, in a multi-site, multi-country study, were able to demonstrate a clear-cut dose–response relationship with frequent users of high-THC cannabis possessing at least double the risk of developing the illness. In any psychiatric disorder, whenever a risk factor of large effect size is identified, be it genetic or environmental, an obvious question is whether the associated clinical picture, underlying biology, illness course, or treatment response is distinct in any regard. If so, this can provide a window into the illness with potential practical import for clinicians.

Because of the evidence that cannabis may precipitate psychotic disorders in addition to schizophrenia (e.g., see Chapter 13, on bipolar illness), we prefer the term 'cannabis-associated psychosis' (CAP) for chronic psychotic illnesses that arise in the context of significant current or past cannabis use. Setting aside acute psychotic states occurring in the context of cannabis use that may spontaneously remit or that resolve rapidly following antipsychotic treatment, and focusing only on these chronic persistent illnesses, one question to examine is whether there is a characteristic symptomatic profile or distinct longer-term clinical picture or clinical course that distinguishes cases of CAP compared to similar diagnoses where cannabis does not seem to be etiologically involved.

A related issue, covered in Chapters 14, 15, and 22, is what is known currently regarding the aetiopathological mechanism whereby cannabis use translates for some individuals into manifestations of CAP.

In other words, is there evidence that such cases have an identifiable biological underpinning or risk profile that is distinct from individuals with psychosis whose aetiology is not related to cannabis use? Or is cannabis merely a non-specific precipitant of the illness in individuals harbouring pre-existing vulnerabilities, for example higher polygenic risk scores for psychotic or affective illness?

One approach taken by the current authors to address these questions is to look for clues within a large-scale, multi-centre cross-sectional study of individuals with an established psychotic illness, the Bipolar–Schizophrenia Network on Intermediate Phenotypes (B-SNIP). B-SNIP used biological characteristics to sub-divide individuals with psychotic illnesses (schizophrenia, schizoaffective disorder, and psychotic bipolar disorder) into distinct subgroups known as 'Biotypes', that cut across DSM diagnoses. Observations from that study identified a sub-type (Biotype-3) associated with adolescent cannabis exposure, that manifests distinct biological characteristics. As detailed in Section 10.5, while biologically unremarkable in many respects, this cannabis exposure-associated sub-type is associated with hippocampal abnormalities. This leads to speculation that the hippocampus may be a key hub in the aetiology of CAP, both because of its broader role in the pathophysiology of psychosis and because of the high concentrations of cannabinoid type-1 receptors (CB_1R) in this brain region. Thus, if the underlying biology of CAP is provoked by THC and involves the endocannabinoid system (see Chapters 2, 16, and 18), then might the 'anti-THC' phytocannabinoid cannabidiol (CBD) provide a more targeted treatment for biologically-defined individuals from the B-SNIP study (a theme touched on in Chapter 21)?

10.2 Is There a Specific Clinical Picture for Cannabis-Associated Psychosis?: Chronic Symptoms and Course

It is important in framing the discussion here to point out that schizophrenia is currently conceptualized not as a disease, but a syndrome defined by symptoms (none of which is unique to schizophrenia) and illness course. Its underlying biology is unclear. Schizophrenia is heterogeneous and shares boundaries with other psychotic illnesses in multiple domains, including symptoms, candidate risk genes, pharmaceutical treatments, and familial expression. Attempts to distinguish schizophrenia using a unique biological 'fingerprint' from other psychotic illnesses have been notably unsuccessful (Keshavan et al., 2011; Tamminga et al., 2014), the authors proceeding from a broader perspective that uses the term 'psychosis' to delineate chronic illnesses characterized by hallucinations delusions, thought disorder, and negative symptoms.

What is the evidence for a distinct schizophrenia-like psychosis caused by cannabis? Boydell et al. (2007) examined a large population of individuals with schizophrenia with and without histories of cannabis abuse, enumerating detailed symptom measures and family histories of schizophrenia, and finding few distinct differences on these measures between the two groups. However, multiple studies provide evidence that cannabis use in patients with schizophrenia is unexpectedly associated with a greater likelihood of preserved cognition, compared to the multi-domain 1–1.5 standard deviation decrements typical of the disorder compared to the general population (Green, 1996; Mallet et al., 2017; Stip, 2006). Such relative preservation is surprising (Yucel et al., 2012), given the acute impairment of cognition produced by THC exposure and possible more persistent cognitive effects of chronic cannabis use (Crane et al., 2013; Grant et al., 2003; Ranganathan and D'Souza, 2006) (Chapters 9 and 17). Ferraro et al. (2013, 2020) carefully examined questions related to better cognition in cannabis users with first onset psychotic illness. They both confirmed the phenomenon and suggested that, in part, it is attributable to the better pre-morbid IQ of cannabis users. In addition, the better pre-morbid social functioning of the latter may have contributed to their likelihood of initiating cannabis use.

Also for psychosis patients currently using cannabis, there is some evidence for a greater degree of cognitive recovery after abstinence, also suggesting less underlying irreversible cognitive impairment (Helle et al., 2013, 2014; Houston et al., 2011). Alongside this cognitively-based presumptive evidence of less developmental damage is convergent evidence that CAP is associated with significantly fewer neurologic soft signs (Mallet et al., 2017).

One way to explore the issue of CAP is to assess psychosis endophenotypes, that represent a familial biological liability trait to develop psychosis, and sort with genetic risk, in psychotic individuals with and without histories of cannabis abuse. Consistent with the cognitive studies (Crane et al., 2013; Ranganathan and D'Souza, 2006), one hypothesis is that non-cannabis using psychosis patients have a greater biological pre-disposition to the disorder identified through a greater degree of abnormalities in additional psychosis endophenotype measures. Conversely, individuals whose psychosis was provoked in the context of heavy cannabis use (hypothetically an environmental precipitant of the illness) hypothetically have a lesser biological pre-disposition to the disorder, as indexed by their more normal psychosis endophenotype scores. Loberg et al. (2014) speculate that the better cognition in cannabis-using patients with schizophrenia may be a consequence of psychosis having being triggered by the drug in individuals with a lower inherent vulnerability for the disorder, and who thereby have more intact brains from a developmental perspective. As well as data from neurocognitive performance (Rabin et al., 2011; Schoeler et al., 2015; Stirling et al., 2005; Yucel et al., 2012), patients with cannabis-associated schizophrenia evidence fewer neurological abnormalities (i.e., soft signs) (Mallet et al., 2017) and fewer structural MRI abnormalities, including more normal hippocampal volumes (Cunha et al., 2013; Koenders et al., 2015; Malchow et al., 2013) and fewer negative symptoms (Mallet et al., 2017). Greater degrees of childhood trauma and maltreatment (Alemany, 2014; Carr et al., 2013) have also been noted in several studies to be significant co-precipitants or moderators of the drug's risk for psychotic illness.

A recent meta-analysis (Sami and Bhattacharyya, 2018) examined endophenotype measures, including structural and functional MRI, electrophysiology and eye movements, as well as biochemical markers of the endocannabinoid, GABA, glutamate, and dopamine systems. Electrophysiologically, while some reports indicated that CAP patients had more abnormal P50 paired auditory stimulus and auditory oddball P300 responses, other studies did not replicate P300 differences (van Tricht et al., 2013). Unclear differences pertain to evoked potentials; for example auditory oddball P300 amplitude has been reported as both increased (Rentzsch et al., 2016) and decreased (van Tricht et al., 2013) compared to non-cannabis using schizophrenia patients.

In structural MRI studies overall grey and white matter findings are difficult to interpret as group sizes are generally small, effect sizes unimpressive, and findings inconsistent, with findings of no differences (Dekker et al., 2010), increases (Schnell et al., 2012), and smaller volumes. Overall, these papers do not report consistent agreement on the type and location of differences between psychosis with and without cannabis involvement, although three papers noted hippocampal sparing in association with CAP.

In more recent work on eye movements, Sami et al. (2021) quantified smooth pursuit eye movements and anti-saccade responses in early-phase psychosis patients with and without histories of cannabis use, plus matched healthy controls with and without histories of cannabis use. Cannabis-using and non-using psychosis patients were not different in diagnosis, symptom severity, or level of functioning. They found a significant (with large effect size) cannabis effect, patient effect, and patient × cannabis interaction for smooth pursuit velocity gain, identifying more severely impaired smooth pursuit in psychosis patients without a history of cannabis use. The authors (in agreement with Loberg et al.'s (2014) earlier conjectures) interpreted their findings as consistent with the hypothesis that endophenotypic neurobiological alterations (such as oculomotor findings) in psychosis are less prominent in patients whose illness developed in the context of cannabis use, because such individuals had less neurobiological pre-disposition to develop the illness, requiring an environmental 'second hit', that is, cannabis use, in order to trigger their psychosis.

Other investigators have probed possible underlying biological vulnerabilities pre-disposing an individual to cannabis-triggered psychosis. Mallet et al.'s (2017) small study raised the idea of greater family liability for psychosis in cannabis-associated psychosis patients. This is supported by more recent epidemiologic studies (e.g., that of Kendler et al., 2019), that indicated that individuals who ultimately developed a persistent psychotic state in the context of cannabis use were both more likely to have had prior short-lived cannabis-provoked psychotic episodes followed by recovery and also had moderately more family histories of psychotic illnesses (and of alcohol and drug abuse). Kendler et al. (2019) concluded that schizophrenia following substance-induced psychosis is likely a drug-precipitated disorder in highly vulnerable individuals, not a syndrome predominantly caused by drug exposure. These conclusions are modified by a recent report of Quattrone et al. (2020) that concluded that schizophrenia risk variance and cannabis use mapped independently onto specific dimensions of positive symptoms, contributing to variation across the psychosis continuum. A complicating factor is that there is some evidence for a shared vulnerability for both psychotic disorders and cannabis use via genetic vulnerability and/or stress (Haney and Evins, 2016; Ksir and Hart, 2016).

On the environmental side, cannabis interacts with other environmental risk factors, including developmental trauma and child maltreatment, minority group position, and growing up in an urban environment, cumulatively with increasing number of risk factors.

In summary, more comprehensive models have attempted to integrate genetic vulnerability alongside cannabis use and childhood maltreatment in a complex gene-by-environment interactive model (Van Gastel et al., 2013). Thus, CAP may be associated alongside cannabis, with a greater number of environmental risk factors and possibly greater genetic vulnerability for the disorder.

10.3 Glutamate Abnormalities in CAP

Focusing on how the syndrome might be mediated, Sami and Bhattacharyya's (2018) earlier comprehensive review examines evidence for dopaminergic, glutamatergic and GABA-ergic abnormalities in CAP. The first (cross-sectional) paper that used magnetic resonance spectroscopy to assess glutamate reported prefrontal reductions in psychosis patients who use cannabis compared to those who did not, in association with impaired working memory (Rigucci et al., 2017). The neurocognitive impairment in that publication, measured using the MATRICS battery, was in contradistinction to the multiple papers cited in showing greater cognitive disturbances rather than cognitive sparing in cannabis-using psychosis patients. Elsewhere, a recent paper (Colizzi et al.,

2019) summarizes the evidence for the hypothesis that cannabis might induce psychosis by disrupting glutamate signalling in the striatum. Sami et al. (2020) assessed MR spectroscopic measures of glutamate in the associative striatum (hippocampus, caudate head, anterior cingulate, and other cortical regions) that are known to express high levels of CB_1R, and to be sites of significant glutamatergic projections. They assessed these areas spectroscopically, alongside MR structural measures, in early psychosis patients and matched controls with and without histories of cannabis use. The authors detected no significant group differences in spectroscopic glutamate measures in any region. However, in psychosis patients with heavy cannabis use compared to those with minimal use, grey matter volume explained a significant proportion of the variance in caudate glutamate measures (in fact there was no such relationship in the light cannabis-using patients). The authors speculated that a history of cannabis use could lead to morphologic changes in associative stratum that then influence striatal glutamatergic levels in the context of psychosis.

10.4 The Hippocampus Plays an Important Role in Psychosis in General, and in THC-Provoked Psychosis Specifically

As already mentioned, the hippocampus has constituted a focus of interest for CAP researchers because of its role in psychosis and its high concentration of CB_1 receptors. As reviewed by Lieberman, there is considerable evidence that the hippocampus is consistently deviant in psychotic disorders, particularly schizophrenia. Studies consistently show reductions in hippocampal volumes in schizophrenia and schizoaffective disorders, as well as increased basal perfusion/activation deficits during declarative memory and reductions in neurogenesis in the dentate gyrus (Winterburn et al., 2013). Such findings are also found in patients with bipolar disorder (Treadway et al., 2015), but particularly in individuals with bipolar disorder with psychosis (Lieberman et al., 2018). Furthermore, among the many cortical and subcortical regions implicated in psychosis, abnormal resting state connectivity between the hippocampus, parahippocampal gyrus, and other brain areas has been described in schizophrenia (Wannan et al.,

2019) and in subjects at increased risk for the disorder (Antoniades et al., 2018; Makowski et al., 2017). Hippocampal dysfunction is likely related to memory deficits found in psychosis (Tamminga et al., 2021). Again, this structure contains one of the highest brain concentrations of CB_1 receptors (Hibar et al., 2016; Strasser et al., 2005; Zhou et al., 2008).

There is some evidence that hippocampal and parahippocampal (Koenders et al., 2015) volumes are larger in schizophrenia patients with a history of cannabis use (Cunha et al., 2013; Koenders et al., 2015), although not all studies show this effect (Malchow et al., 2013) and some have shown the opposite (Smith et al., 2015; Solowij et al., 2013) or, alternatively, hippocampal shape differences. In a recent abstract, Scheffler et al. (2021) explored the effects of cannabis use on hippocampal sub-field volumes in male cannabis-using versus non-using psychosis patients and matched healthy controls. They reported a significant diagnosis-by-cannabis use interaction in the subiculum, with smaller volumes in the cannabis-using compared to the non-cannabis-using patients and smaller volumes in the cannabis-using than the cannabis non-using controls.

For schizophrenia in general Lieberman et al. (2018) hypothesize a process where dysregulated glutamate neurotransmission begins in the CA1 region of the hippocampus. This excites local neuronal activity as assessed by measures of metabolism and blood flow and evokes attenuated psychotic symptoms, provoking prodromal symptoms. Lieberman et al. hypothesize that a continuation of this abnormal glutamatergic state then progresses to fully-evolved syndromal psychosis. As this process continues, it begins to involve regions connected to the hippocampus and its projections including the frontal cortex. Continued excitotoxicity ultimately leads to hippocampal cell death and loss of inter-neurons. Evidence for this includes previous neuroimaging research demonstrating structural (volume reduction, shape anomalies) and functional abnormalities (increased metabolism measured by blood flow and glucose metabolism) in the medial temporal lobe structures of patients with schizophrenia. Specifically the CA1 and subiculum sub-regions of the anterior hippocampus (Ho et al., 2017; Kraguljac et al., 2017) appear particularly affected. In addition, administration of the glutamatergic agent ketamine to healthy individuals produces a behavioural syndrome that mimics both positive and negative symptoms (Krystal et al.,

1994; Moghaddam and Javitt, 2012) of schizophrenia. Finally, clinical proton magnetic resonance spectroscopy studies report increased hippocampal glutamate levels in prodromal schizophrenia patients compared to healthy control subjects that are associated with hyper-metabolism in different brain regions of such patients (Shakory et al., 2018). In summary, the literature is somewhat inconsistent, with increases as well as decreases being observed in hippocampal glutamate in this context.

Regarding hippocampal involvement more specifically in THC-provoked psychosis, Atakan et al. (2013) reported on results of a double-blind, placebo-controlled, pseudo-randomized design experiment, where healthy men with minimal cannabis experience were given oral THC or placebo. Behavioural and functional magnetic resonance imaging measures were then recorded while participants performed a cognitive task. During the THC condition, temporarily psychotic subjects (~50% of sample) made more frequent inhibition errors and showed differential activation in the left parahippocampal gyrus, bilateral middle temporal gyri, and right cerebellum. THC produced opposite effects on regional activation relative to placebo in the two groups. Because manifesting acute psychotic symptoms was associated with a differential effect of THC on activation in the medial and ventral temporal cortex and cerebellum, the authors concluded that these regions mediate THC's effects on psychotic symptoms (O'Neill et al., 2021; Paul and Bhattacharyya, 2021).

To summarize, the hippocampus, along with other regions, seems central to the pathophysiology of both schizophrenia and THC-provoked acute psychotic symptoms.

Examining THC more closely, the substance and its metabolites affect the human brain primarily as partial but persistent CB_1 (and weak CB_2) receptor agonists. This mechanism is not only responsible for most of cannabis' psychoactive effects (e.g., intoxication), rewarding effects and dependence, but many studies also have shown THC is pro-psychotic. Intravenous THC acutely provokes both positive and negative psychotic symptoms, both in healthy non-psychotic individuals (D'Souza et al., 2004) and can lead to temporary relapse/exacerbations of positive symptoms in those with pre-existing psychosis (Morrison et al., 2009). Also, schizophrenia patients have higher CSF levels of the endogenous CB receptor-linked anandamide neurotransmitter, which

normalize with both antipsychotic treatment and clinical remission (Huang et al., 2007; Leweke et al., 2012). Other evidence linking THC's effects on the brain to psychosis comes from studies of chronic cannabis abusers. Used chronically, THC raises the risk for short-lived psychotic episodes and for schizophrenia, with a longer duration of dose, higher THC concentrations, and adolescent use being major contributors to subsequent increased risk (Colizzi et al., 2015; Morrison et al., 2009).

Links between the endocannabinoid system (ECS) and psychosis via CB-receptor mediated neurotransmission are supported by two persuasive indirect arguments as well. First and possibly most salient is that THC persistently alters ECS function during a highly sensitive neurodevelopmental period of adolescence when (a) cannabis use/abuse dramatically increases, (b) psychosis typically emerges, and (c) the brain is vulnerable to persisting THC-related disruptions (Danijua et al., 2020; Di Forti et al., 2019; Gage et al., 2016; Koethe et al., 2009; Leweke et al., 2012; Meyer et al., 2018; Raver et al., 2013; Renard et al., 2014). The ECS' crucial roles in foetal axonal growth, guidance, migration, maturation, and synaptic development peak in adolescence, where it is vital to pruning, brain development, and plasticity (Leweke et al., 2012). This period is, thus, a particularly sensitive window to ECS perturbation (Lee et al., 2016; Realini et al., 2009). In adolescent rodents, THC specifically disrupts neural pruning, with subsequent permanent effects on adult behaviour, for example, altered spatial working memory (Dow-Edwards and Silva, 2017; Meyer et al., 2018; Renard et al., 2014; Rubino and Parolaro, 2016). Other THC-driven alterations in adolescent rodents include hippocampal cell loss, changes in brain energetics, impaired LTD, and disruption of endogenous cannabinoid neurotransmitters AEA (anandamide) and 2-AG – many of which are prolonged effects that are non-physiological and, thus, potentially disruptive to any processes (e.g., neurodevelopmental) that are under the influence of the ECS. Such ECS alterations can profoundly dysregulate developmental processes in cortical GABA and glutamate (Lee et al., 2016), resulting in a change that 'resembles the ones present in schizophrenic patients' (Meyer et al., 2018). Collectively, this confluence of epidemiological, clinical, and biochemical findings suggest teenage cannabis use might be promoting disadvantageous changes to the ECS system that contribute to the

95

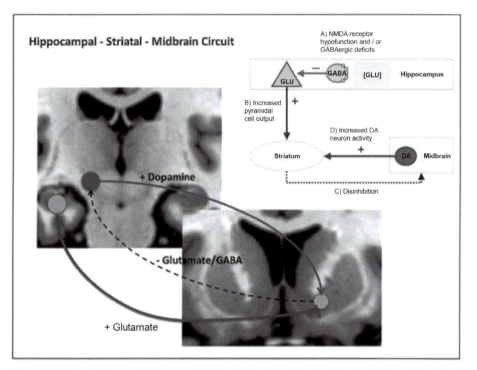

Figure 10.1 Cannabis-impacted hippocampal/midbrain/striatal circuit involved in striatal DA regulation (from Danijua et al., 2020). In psychosis, dysregulation of glutamate (due to GLU/GABA imbalance) elevates hippocampal neural activity, hyper-perfusion (A) and output (B, blue line), altering hippocampal function. Hippocampal hyperactivity leads to increased striatal/DA function (C and D, dashed & red lines).

neurobiological impairments that underlie psychosis symptom expression in some patients with psychotic illness. Second, the ECS modulates DA neurotransmission both acutely and chronically in both animals and humans (albeit less convincingly so), suggesting its role in psychosis symptom expression might be neuromodulatory (Lubman et al., 2015; Rubino and Parolaro, 2008; Schneider, 2008; Sullivan, 2000). Human studies reveal DA effects of THC that are more complex than are seen in animals (Bloomfield et al., 2016; Bossong et al., 2015; Cheer et al., 2004; French, 1997; Rubino et al., 2015; Schneider, 2008; Tanda and Goldberg, 2003). These complex findings suggest models of THC-induced psychosis based solely on DA are likely inadequate. These ideas have led to recently-proposed theoretical models (Figure 10.1) that summarize what is known about the likely biochemical/neurotransmitter pathways that underlie ECS modulation over glutamate/GABA/dopamine dysfunction in psychosis. These models again incorporate the hippocampus as a key node and recognize THC as a possible trigger (Abush et al., 2018).

10.5 What Is B-SNIP?

Currently, psychiatric diagnoses are determined, for the most part, on the basis of clinical phenomenology and illness course. This is problematic in that it fails to address underlying causes, and also because such candidate defining features as deficit states clearly cut across major psychiatric diagnoses and are not specific to schizophrenia (Keshavan et al., 2020). In an effort to better understand psychotic illness to gain new insights into intervention development, over the past approximately 10 years, the NIMH-funded multi-site Bipolar-Schizophrenia Network on Intermediate Phenotypes (B-SNIP) has collected deep phenotyping data in over 3,000 individuals across the psychosis spectrum with conventional DSM diagnostic, clinical, and demographic data (clinically stable, mainly mid-course psychosis patients with either schizophrenia, schizoaffective disorder, or bipolar disorder with psychosis) (Tamminga et al., 2021). It should be emphasized that the B-SNIP project collected information from psychotic individuals defined as meeting DSM criteria for these three disorders, rather than only focusing on persons with schizophrenia. The initial purpose of the study was to collect a wide variety of clinical and biomarker information from individuals with psychosis (and in B-SNIP-1 from their first-degree relatives), as well as from matched non-psychotic individuals. The candidate biomarkers were selected from a variety of domains, including cognitive, oculomotor (smooth pursuit and saccades), electrophysiological (both resting EEG and ERP's), imaging (structural, functional, diffusion tensor imaging, and, in a sub-sample, spectroscopy), and genetic. The initial purpose was to determine whether or not, individually or in combination, the measures from this biomarker panel might identify a distinctive biological 'fingerprint' that characterized each of the three major psychiatric disorders. That enterprise failed; what quickly became apparent is that each of the three DSM disorders showed abnormality on each of the biomarkers that differed only in degree, with substantial overlap such that no single biomarker or combination thereof distinguished one syndromal diagnosis from another (Keshavan et al., 2011; Tamminga et al., 2021). Neither were patients with separate DSM diagnoses separable, employing commonly-used symptomatic scales (Tamminga et al., 2013). The obvious next step was to put aside conventional diagnoses, merge individuals from all three psychotic disorders into a single pool, and to then attempt to separate them statistically into distinct sub-groups, using an unsupervised machine-learning approach applied to a selection of all variables from among the overall biomarker data. Healthy controls were not part of the Biotype classification. This approach was much more successful and yielded three, non-overlapping, biologically-defined presumptive disease entities (termed Biotypes B1, B2, B3) each with a distinctive neurobiological profile (Clementz et al., 2016). Variables used in defining the Biotypes were a sub-set of the overall biomarkers derived from the cognitive, oculomotor, and electrophysiological domains. Using external biological validators, that is, biological markers not used in defining the Biotypes themselves, such as MRI, MR spectroscopic, and genetic information, confirms the distinctiveness of the Biotypes (e.g., Ivleva et al., 2017). The Biotype structure has now been decisively replicated in an N > 900 independent sample (Clementz et al., 2022). The B-SNIP Biotypes are highly stable over time, as determined using repeated biomarker measurements in the same individuals at 6- and 12-month retest.

The three distinct proband Biotypes comprise Biotype-1 (B1), which is characterized by severely deficient neural response to salient stimuli combined with very low levels of intrinsic brain activity, and significant cognitive impairment. Biotype-2 (B2) displays normal sensory responses to salient stimuli, but prominently accentuated intrinsic electrophysiological neural activity and generally similar cognitive impairment to B1. Biotype 3 (B3) is defined by minimal deviation from normal function, with near-normal cognitive and electrophysiological responses. Importantly, conventional DSM diagnoses are spread across Biotypes, with the implication that what clinicians broadly see as 'psychotic illness' arises from demonstrably different neurobiological routes, and that each of the three DSM psychosis diagnoses is heterogeneous and contains and admixture of all three Biotypes. Notably, within each diagnosis the different Biotypes may display values on measures such as intrinsic electrophysiological neural activity that can be opposite in direction.

Patients who fall into the Biotype 3 category have less genetic risk for schizophrenia in the form of lower psychosis polygenic risk scores (PRS) (Tamminga et al., 2021) and fewer first-degree relatives with psychosis, and are also the least socially and cognitively impaired (Clementz et al., 2016). However, while B3 patients are the 'least abnormal' with regard to many biological measures, they still have frank, debilitating psychotic illness.

Our recently published and pilot data indicate B3 patients stand out from other Biotypes because they have specific hippocampal structural abnormalities (Guimond et al., 2021), normal cognition on the BACS (Keefe et al., 2004), and significantly greater histories of adolescent cannabis use (Hanna et al., 2016). This is consistent with a premise that B3 patients' pathophysiology might be specifically related to dysfunction of the brain's endocannabinoid system (ECS). This dysfunction might be more malleable using novel targeted pharmacological manipulation of the ECS compared to other psychosis Biotypes.

In general, the overarching hope of B-SNIP's current programme of research is that the Biotypes represent footholds for targeted treatments via understanding their underlying biology. The B-SNIP context gives us an opportunity to match novel intervention to Biotype-specific pathophysiology in targeted ways that are likely to be more productive than prior attempts to find effective new treatments

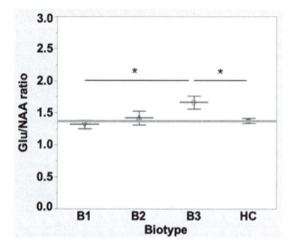

Figure 10.2 MR spectroscopy results showing abnormal glutamate:NAA ratios only in B3

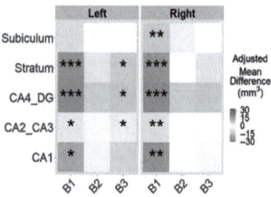

Figure 10.3 Hippocampal morphometry results that show Biotype-specific abnormality profiles

regardless of psychosis patients' different neurobiological impairments. Within B-SNIP, B3 is the only Biotype so far in which we have the evidence that cannabis-linked abnormalities seem to drive the Biotype's neurobiological abnormalities. To emphasize, despite gathering numerous biomarkers across several domains, B3's *only* discernible neurobiological abnormalities in our extensive research so far are hippocampal-related, manifesting against a background of adolescent cannabis use. This alone suggests that an intervention that specifically targets ECS could be more effective for B3 patients than for Biotype 1 and 2 patients who have more complex, multi-system pathophysiology. For instance, B3 manifests unique hippocampal spectroscopic abnormalities. In a B-SNIP pilot proton spectroscopy study (Bolo et al., 2021) we assessed 103 total subjects comprising 60 healthy controls, 13 B1, 13 B2, and 17 B3 subjects, imaged at 3T in a single $1.5 \times 1.5 \times 1.5$ cm^3 hippocampal voxel, located in the anterior pole of the left hippocampus, to measure glutamate and N-acetyl aspartate (NAA) concentrations. As shown in Figure 10.2, B3 patients uniquely showed tissue-corrected, elevated glutamate:NAA ratios. This B3 finding was due to elevated glutamate and reduced NAA in the face of normal grey matter concentrations. This may imply that these neurons in B3 are less viable, or perhaps more subject to excitotoxicity. The significantly abnormal glutamate and glutamate/NAA ratios in B3 also suggest abnormal functional activity of the structure. One possible explanation is

that activation in anterior hippocampal input regions is high and in output regions low in B3 versus controls, consistent with increased glutamatergic activity (high glutamate) in input regions (dentate gyrus, entorhinal cortex) and increased (compensating) GABAergic activity in output regions (e.g., CA3). It is also consistent with reports of high resting state GABA being associated with decreased task-related activation. This could also have therapeutic implications, as CBD is neuroprotective and anti-excitotoxic (Stokes et al., 2012). Second, despite normal-appearing global grey matter density in the medial temporal lobe (Bloomfield et al., 2014), the hippocampal morphometry reveals the profile of volume reduction in B3 is distinct from HCs and the other Biotypes. We assessed differences in the volume and shape of the amygdala and hippocampus contrasting traditional clinical diagnoses and with Biotype classification. The study used MAGeT (van de Giessen et al., 2017; Volkow et al., 2014) in 481 B-SNIP-1 subjects (Figure 10.3). B3 had significantly smaller volumes (N = 199) for the left hippocampus compared to healthy controls, as well as significantly smaller (again left-sided) stratum, CA4/DG and CA2/CA3. In contrast, hippocampal morphometry in B1 (N = 121) showed a different overall profile. In B1, volume diminution was bilateral and more severe, while in B2 (N = 161) the hippocampi were near-normal (Guimond et al., 2021). Together, this suggests B3 hippocampal function and structure are selectively abnormal compared to other psychosis patients. It is important that the two brain measures where B3 shows significant abnormalities are both hippocampal because the wealth of empirical evidence for hippocampal abnormalities lies at the heart of many current psychosis models (Wiers et al., 2016).

Finally, compared to other Biotypes, B3 contains a significant excess of individuals who used cannabis during adolescence prior to psychosis onset (pilot data derived from the Dallas site in BSNIP-1 and from all sites in BSNIP-2). Lifetime cannabis use disorders were more frequent in B3 (78/278: 28.1%) compared to B1 (36/198: 18.2%) and B2 (51/ 235: 21.7%) ($\chi^2(2) = 6.67$, $p = 0.036$). This overall effect was driven by significantly higher rates of lifetime cannabis use disorders in B3 versus B1 ($p = 0.017$) and B3 versus B1 and B2 (combined) ($p = 0.018$).

Furthermore, in B-SNIP, psychosis patients overall who used cannabis as adolescents tend to have relatively preserved structural MRI grey matter patterns and cognitive profile characteristics, features typical of B3. As such, we re-examined whole brain and regional grey matter density (GMD) estimated from a Voxel-Based Morphometry approach in B-SNIP1 psychosis probands (N = 109) stratified by history of adolescent cannabis use (Benetti et al., 2009). Probands with adolescent use had whole brain and regional GMDs not different from controls, whereas those without such use showed typical GMD reductions, especially in SZ.

We also compared BACS cognitive composite scores in 97 B-SNIP1 individuals with SZ, SAD, and psychotic BP versus healthy controls (Rasetti et al., 2011). Cognitive performance was significantly higher in psychosis individuals with adolescent cannabis use compared to those without. Essentially, the relative profile of preserved cognitive and overall grey matter profiles in our psychosis patients stratified by history of adolescent cannabis use before they were formally Biotyped is consistent with the profile of B3 (Benetti et al., 2009; Rasetti et al., 2011). Also, as reviewed at the beginning of this chapter, many historical reports of cannabis-associated psychosis stress the relatively intact cognition of such patients (Aguiar et al., 2014; Szallasi et al., 2007).

Finally, structural hippocampal deficits have been observed in individuals with a history of childhood trauma, with or without psychopathology, suggesting that early life stress exposure affects hippocampal development. del Re et al. (2022) investigated the effects of childhood trauma and cannabis use, together with their interactions, on hippocampal volume within the B-SNIP sample. These investigators explored the risk factors together with age of psychosis onset in relation to anterior and posterior hippocampal volumes using path analysis, in a large trans-diagnostic sample of B-SNIP psychotic probands (N = 1,138) and controls (N = 535). 3T MRI structural T1 images showed significant inverse correlations between trauma score and volumes of both anterior and posterior hippocampus in psychosis probands but not healthy controls, as well as correlations with age of onset of psychotic illness (the higher the CTQ score, the lower the onset age). Probands with a history of cannabis use had higher trauma scores and an earlier age of psychosis onset, consistent with studies cited at the beginning of this chapter.

Together, these B-SNIP findings raise the possibility that early cannabis use may precipitate psychosis in individuals with less prominent cognitive or neuroanatomic risk factors, displaying for the most part normal anatomy (except for the hippocampus) and cognition that characterize B3, and/or that adolescent cannabis use could be a feature of a unique psychosis sub-group.

While these data do not demonstrate conclusively that a disturbed ECS is the main underlying etiopathology for B3, given the extensive background data on THC's ECS-mediated impact on the adolescent brain and particularly on downstream hippocampal-mediated mechanisms, available evidence suggests that this may be one reasonable conclusion.

10.6 Synthesis, Conceptual Model

Figure 10.4 illustrates the overall conceptual model and premise underlying the proposed research. Briefly, we propose that B3 psychosis stems from more environmentally driven factors (including more adolescent cannabis use and greater childhood trauma) in the context of a lower genetic risk, at least as assessed by schizophrenia polygenic risk scores. We hypothesize that B3 psychopathology is more specifically driven by ECS dysfunction than that of B1 or B2. A recent model (Hu and Mackie, 2015) (Figure 10.1) suggests these hypothetical ECS alterations may be provoked by a mechanism whereby THC alters glutamatergic and GABA-ergic neurotransmission within the ECS and by disrupting the system's neuromodulatory control over DA, resulting in clinical expression of psychosis. The hippocampus, by virtue of its prominence in the

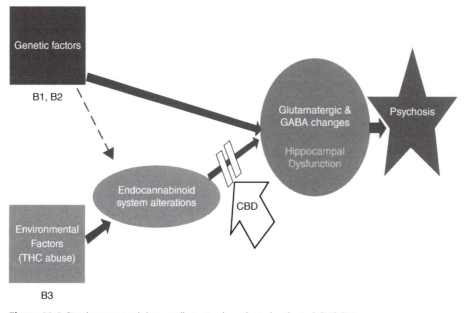

Figure 10.4 Simple conceptual diagram illustrating hypothetical paths to B-SNIP Biotypes

ECS and its central role in some psychosis models (and influence by CBD in fMRI tasks), is an important structure in which to measure this dysfunction. Part of our argument arises from the recognition that environmental influences (e.g., cannabis abuse) seem implicated both in psychosis and B3 in particular. Importantly, we are not advancing an argument that there is a sub-group of psychosis that is *exclusively* 'caused' by cannabis use. More realistically, the substantial evidence for ECS dysfunction in psychosis suggests there could be a proportion of psychosis patients, perhaps those with specific pre-existing ECS abnormalities, whose psychotic symptom expression arises following ECS dysregulation of dopaminergic function through complex biochemical pathways that are still a focus of active empirical study. One prominent source of such ECS disruption among others could be adolescent cannabis use. Regardless of how future studies ultimately characterize any ECS-specific pathway to psychosis, as a corollary we hypothesize here that B3 in particular may be more pre-disposed to respond therapeutically to a drug known to act on the ECS, that blocks THC's deleterious psychosis-promoting effects on hippocampal function, and that has several documented potential mechanistic pathways of action within the ECS, that is, cannabidiol (CBD), and should thus be considered as a targeted intervention for B3 patients.

Figure 10.4 suggests that B-SNIP Biotypes 1 and 2 have relatively greater genetic loadings for psychosis, associated with more neurodevelopmental abnormalities, which ultimately lead to primary GABA and glutamate neurotransmitter changes that in turn precipitate psychosis. In the case of Biotype 3, there is less genetic loading and a greater environmental component, primarily consisting of adolescent cannabis use, but additional factors, such as childhood abuse, that impinge primarily on the endocannabinoid system (ECS), with secondary effects on glutamate and GABA, leading to psychosis. The implication is that, because of ECS involvement, Biotype 3 patients may be more responsive to treatment with cannabidiol (CBD).

10.7 Conclusion

Our knowledge of CAP is still growing. Issues of what sort of psychosis is provoked in some individuals from a clinical and biological point of view, in the context of the cannabis use, is increasingly coming into focus. However, many questions still remain unanswered, in part because of problems with existing studies. Many relevant publications to date have examined patients with psychotic illnesses, predominantly schizophrenia, who at the time of assessment were regular cannabis smokers, compared to similar patients who were not (and sometimes to healthy control subjects). While such assessments are undoubtedly informative, any observations are influenced by both acute and chronic effects of cannabis on biological and symptomatic measures. Because cannabis itself can have effects on electrophysiology and cognition, evaluating individuals were still regularly using the drug requires disambiguation of these effects through experimental designs that probably account for their presence.

By and large, studies have not addressed issues of whether individuals with CAP associated with substantial past rather than current cannabis use differ from those without such histories. Publications have also been restricted for the most part to schizophrenia, whereas B-SNIP data argue for a broader examination of patients across the psychotic illness spectrum. Finally, many relevant publications are based on relatively small samples, making effect sizes difficult to estimate and restricting generalizability. Thus, there is a strong need for efforts to pool data from multiple centres in order to construct a more informative, generalizable, and broad-based analysis of CAP.

Despite some limitations with the literature described, several broad themes emerge from existing data on which seems to be general agreement. In general, compared to matched non-cannabis associated same-diagnosis patients, individuals with CAP seem to manifest less impaired cognition, with this being a well-replicated finding.

In addition, there is some (but less) support CAP for earlier onset of illness, greater likelihood of childhood abuse, the presence of fewer negative symptoms and neurological soft signs, more normal resting state and evoked EEG patterns, more normal smooth pursuit and saccadic eye movements, and fewer structural MRI abnormalities. There may be relative hippocampal sparing on MRI measures, but other suggestions that the hippocampus is functionally or biochemically implicated in the illness. Some studies have brought forward evidence for striatal and perhaps hippocampal glutamatergic mechanisms in the context of CAP. There is also some evidence for greater familial liability to schizophrenia by history.

In what way does our knowledge of B-SNIP Biotype 3 help illuminate the above facts, or help with them in context? Biotype 3 is characterized by the following: a significant excess of adolescent cannabis use histories preceding the onset of psychosis, histories of childhood abuse, distinctly preserved cognition, characteristic abnormalities of hippocampal morphology and some evidence for a characteristic pattern of hippocampal glutamate elevations. In addition, Biotype 3 has more normal MRI grey matter patterns, the lowest schizophrenia polygenic risk scores, normal evoked and resting electrophysiology, near-normal saccades and smooth pursuit eye movements. Supporting observations across the entire B-SNIP population show that individuals with histories of cannabis use manifest more normal cognition and more normal MRI grey matter distributions. In general, then, there is a collection of similar or shared features across observations made in cases of CAP across the existing literature and the documented features of B-SNIP Biotype 3.

One conclusion is that Biotype 3 is a psychosis sub-type that could be studied further as a novel window into CAP. Such studies may prove important – for example, as implied in Figure 10.4, cannabidiol or glutamatergic antipsychotic agents might be especially effective in treating individuals with CAP. Speculating further, the pathophysiological mechanisms hypothesized to underlie Biotype 3 may also provide one possible explanation as to why only some schizophrenia patients have responded to CBD in clinical trials of the drug, and why one third of patients with schizophrenia fail to respond to dopaminergic agents.

If we can define the biology of a particular sub-set of cases of psychosis spectrum disorders, that might bring us closer to finding a specific treatment or treatments for those individuals.

References

Abush, H., Ghose, S., van Enkevort, E. A., et al. (2018). Associations between adolescent cannabis use and brain structure in psychosis. *Psychiatry Res Neuroimaging*, **276**, 53–64.

Aguiar, D. C., Moreira, F. A., Terzian, A. L., et al. (2014). Modulation of defensive behavior by Transient Receptor Potential Vanilloid Type-1 (TRPV1) channels. *Neurosci Biobehav Rev*, **46**, 418–428.

Alemany, S. (2014). Psychosis-inducing effects of cannabis are related to both childhood abuse and COMT genotypes. *Acta Psychiatr Scand*, **129**, 54–62.

Antoniades, M., Schoeler, T., Radua, J., et al. (2018). Verbal learning and hippocampal dysfunction in schizophrenia: A meta-analysis. *Neurosci Biobehav Rev*, **86**, 166–175.

Atakan, Z., Bhattacharyya, S., Allen, P., et al. (2013). Cannabis affects people differently: Inter-subject variation in the psychotogenic effects of D9-tetrahydrocannabinol: A functional magnetic resonance imaging study with healthy volunteers. *Psychol Med*, **43**, 1255–1267.

Benetti, S., Mechelli, A., Picchioni, M., et al. (2009). Functional integration between the posterior hippocampus and prefrontal cortex is impaired in both first episode schizophrenia and the at risk mental state. *Brain*, **132**, 2426–2436.

Bloomfield, M. A., Ashok, A. H., Volkow, N. D., et al. (2016). The effects of Delta(9)-tetrahydrocannabinol on the dopamine system. *Nature*, **539**, 369–377.

Bloomfield, M. A., Morgan, C. J., Egerton, A., et al. (2014). Dopaminergic function in cannabis users and its relationship to cannabis-induced psychotic symptoms. *Biol Psychiatry*, **75**, 470–478.

Bolo, N., Zeng, V., Clementz, B. A., et al. (2021). Hippocampal glutamate, verbal episodic memory and intrinsic neural activity in the psychosis spectrum *Soc Biol Psychiatry*, **89**, S345.

Bossong, M. G., Mehta, M. A., van Berckel, B. N., et al. (2015). Further human evidence for striatal dopamine release induced by administration of 9-tetrahydrocannabinol (THC): Selectivity to limbic striatum. *Psychopharmacology (Berl)*, **232**, 2723–2729.

Boydell, J., Dean, K., Dutta, R., et al. (2007). A comparison of symptoms and family history in schizophrenia with and without

prior cannabis use: Implications for the concept of cannabis psychosis. *Schizophr Res*, **93**, 203–210.

Carr, C. P., Martins, C. M., Stingel, A. M., et al. (2013). The role of early life stress in adult psychiatric disorders: A systematic review according to childhood trauma subtypes. *J Nerv Ment Dis*, **201**, 1007–1020.

Cheer, J. F., Wassum, K. M., Heien, M. L., et al. (2004). Cannabinoids enhance subsecond dopamine release in the nucleus accumbens of awake rats. *J Neurosci*, **24**, 4393–4400.

Clementz, B. A., Parker, D. A., Trotti, R. L., et al. (2022). Psychosis biotypes: Replication and validation from the B-SNIP Consortium. *Schizophr Bull*, **48**, 56–68.

Clementz, B. A., Sweeney, J. A., Hamm, J. P., et al. (2016). Identification of distinct psychosis biotypes using brain-based biomarkers. *Am J Psychiatry*, **173**, 373–383.

Colizzi, M., Iyegbe, C., and Powell, J., et al. (2015). Interaction between DRD2 and AKT1 genetic variations on risk of psychosis in cannabis users: A case control study. *NPJ Schizophren*, **1**, 15049.

Colizzi, M., Weltens, N., McGuire, P., et al. (2019). Does cannabis induce psychosis by altering glutamate signaling in the striatum? *Schizophr Bull*, **45**, S166–S167.

Crane, N. A., Schuster, R. M., Fusar-Poli, P., et al. (2013). Effects of cannabis on neurocognitive functioning: Recent advances, neurodevelopmental influences, and sex differences. *Neuropsychol Rev*, **23**, 117–137.

Cunha, P. J., Rosa, P. G. P., and Ayres Ade, M. (2013). Cannabis use, cognition and brain structure in first-episode psychosis. *Schizophr Res*, **147**, 209–215.

D'Souza, D. C., Perry, E., MacDougall, L., et al. (2004). The psychotomimetic effects of intravenous delta-9-tetrahydrocannabinol in healthy individuals: Implications for psychosis. *Neuropsychopharmacology*, **29**, 1558–1572.

Danijua, Y., Bossong, M. G., Brandt, K., et al. (2020). Do the effects of cannabis on the hippocampus and striatum increase risk for psychosis? *Neurosci Biobehav Rev*, **112**, 324–335.

Dekker, N., Schmitz, N., and Peters, B. D. (2010). Cannabis use and callosal white matter structure and integrity in recent-onset schizophrenia. *Psychiatry Res*, **181**, 51–56.

Di Forti, M., Quattrone, D., Freeman, T. P., et al. (2019). The contribution of cannabis use to variation in the incidence of psychotic disorder across Europe (EU-GEI): A multicentre case-control study. *Lancet Psychiatry*, **6**, 427–436.

Dow-Edwards, D., and Silva, L. (2017). Endocannabinoids in brain plasticity: Cortical maturation, HPA axis function and behavior. *Brain Res*, **1654**, 157–164.

Ferraro, L, La Cascia, C., Quattrone, D., et al. (2020). Premorbid adjustment and IQ in patients with first-episode psychosis: A multisite case-control study of their relationship with cannabis use. *Schizophr Bull*, **46**, 517–529.

Ferraro, L., Russo, M., O'Connor, J., et al. (2013). Cannabis users have higher premorbid IQ than other patients with first onset psychosis. *Schizophr Res*, **150**, 129–135.

French, E. D. (1997) delta9-Tetrahydrocannabinol excites rat VTA dopamine neurons through activation of cannabinoid CB1 but not opioid receptors. *Neurosci Lett*, **226**, 159–162.

Gage, S. H., Hickman, M., and Zammit, S. (2016). Association between cannabis and psychosis: Epidemiologic evidence. *Biol Psychiatry*, **79**, 549–556.

van de Giessen, E., Weinstein, J. J., Cassidy, C. M., et al. (2017). Deficits in striatal dopamine release in cannabis dependence. *Mol Psychiatry*, **22**, 68–75.

Grant, I., Gonzalez, R., Carey, C. L., et al. (2003). Non-acute (residual) neurocognitive effects of cannabis use: A meta-analytic study. *J Int Neuropsychol Soc*, **9**, 679–689.

Green, M. F. (1996). What are the functional consequences of neurocognitive deficits in schizophrenia? *Am J Psychiatry*, **153**, 321–330.

Guimond, S., Gu, F., Shannon, H., et al. (2021). A diagnosis and biotype comparison across the psychosis spectrum: Investigating volume and shape amygdala-hippocampal differences from the B-SNIP study. *Schizophr Bull*, **47**, 1706–1717.

Haney, M., and Evins, A. E. (2016). Does cannabis cause, exacerbate or ameliorate psychiatric disorders? An oversimplified debate discussed. *Neuropsychopharmacology*, **41**, 393–401.

Hanna, R. C., Shalvoy, A., Cullum, C. M., et al. (2016). Cognitive function in individuals with psychosis: Moderation by adolescent cannabis use. *Schizophr Bull*, **42**, 1496–1503.

Helle, S., Gjestad, R., Johnsen, E., et al. (2013). Cognitive changes in non-affective psychosis the first 4–6 weeks after admission to a psychiatric acute ward: Effects of substance use. *Schizophr Bull*, **39**, 262.

(2014). Cognitive changes in patients with acute phase psychosis: Effects of illicit drug use. *Psychiatry Res*, **220**, 818–824.

Hibar, D. P., Westlye, L. T., and van Erp, T. G. M. (2016). Subcortical volumetric abnormalities in bipolar disorder. *Mol Psychiatry*, **21**, 1710–1716.

Ho, N. F., Iglesias, J. E., Sum, M. Y., et al. (2017). Progression from selective to general involvement of hippocampal subfields in schizophrenia. *Mol Psychiatry*, **22**, 142–152.

Houston, J. E., Murphy, J., Shevlin, M., et al. (2011). Cannabis use and psychosis: Re-visiting the role of childhood trauma. *Psychol Med*, **41**, 2339–2348.

Hu, S. S., and Mackie, K. (2015). Distribution of the endocannabinoid system in the central nervous system. *Handb Exp Pharmacol*, **231**, 59–93.

Huang, J. T.-J., Leweke, F. M., Tsang, T. M., et al. (2007). CSF metabolic and proteomic profiles in patients prodromal for psychosis. *PLoS ONE*, **2**, e756.

Ivleva, E. I., Clementz, B. A., and Dutcher, A. M. (2017). Brain structure biomarkers in the psychosis biotypes: Findings from the bipolar-schizophrenia network for intermediate phenotypes. *Biol Psychiatry*, **82**, 26–39.

Keefe, R. S. E., Goldberg, T. E., Harvey, P. D., et al. (2004). The Brief Assessment of Cognition in Schizophrenia: Reliability, sensitivity, and comparison with a standard neurocognitive battery. *Schizophr Res*, **68**, 283–297.

Kendler, K. S., Ohlsson, H., Sundquist, J., et al. (2019). Prediction of onset of substance-induced psychotic disorder and its progression to schizophrenia in a Swedish national sample. *Am J Psychiatry*, **176**, 711–719.

Keshavan, M. S., Kelly, S., and Hall, M. H. (2020). The core deficit of 'classical' schizophrenia cuts across the psychosis spectrum. *Can J Psychiatry*, **65**, 231–234.

Keshavan, M. S., Morris, D. W., Sweeney, J. A., et al. (2011). A dimensional approach to the psychosis spectrum between bipolar disorder and schizophrenia: The Schizo-Bipolar Scale. *Schizophr Res*, **133**, 250–254.

Koenders, L., Machielsen, M. W. J., and van der Meer, F. J. (2015). Brain volume in male patients with recent onset schizophrenia with and without cannabis use disorders. *J Psychiatry Neurosci*, **40**, 197–206.

Koethe, D., Giuffrida, A., Schreiber, D., et al. (2009). Anandamide elevation in cerebrospinal fluid in initial prodromal states of psychosis. *Br J Psychiatry*, **194**, 371–372.

Kraguljac, N. V., Karper, L. P., Seibyl, J. P., et al. (2017). Ketamine modulates hippocampal neurochemistry and functional connectivity: A combined magnetic resonance spectroscopy and resting-state fMRI study in healthy volunteers. *Mol Psychiatry*, **22**, 562–569.

Krystal, J. H., Karper, L. P., Seibyl, J. P., et al. (1994). Subanesthetic effects of the noncompetitive NMDA antagonist, ketamine, in humans. Psychotomimetic, perceptual, cognitive, and neuroendocrine responses. *Arch Gen Psychiatry*, **51**, 199–214.

Ksir, C., and Hart, C. L. (2016). Correlation still does not imply causation. *Lancet Psychiatry*, **3**, 401.

Lee, T. T., Hill, M. N., and Lee, F. S. (2016). Developmental regulation of fear learning and anxiety behavior by endocannabinoids. *Genes Brain Behav*, **15**, 108–124.

Leweke, F. M., Piomelli, D., Pahlisch, F., et al. (2012). Cannabidiol enhances anandamide signaling and alleviates psychotic symptoms of schizophrenia. *Transl Psychiatry*, **2**, e94.

Lieberman, J. A., Girgis, R. R., Brucato, G., et al. (2018). Hippocampal dysfunction in the pathophysiology of schizophrenia: A selective review and hypothesis for early detection and intervention. *Mol Psychiatry*, **23**, 1764–1772.

Loberg, E.-M., Helle, S., Nygard, M., et al. (2014). The cannabis pathway to non-affective psychosis may reflect less neurobiological vulnerability. *Front Psychiatry*, **5**, 159.

Lubman, D. I., Cheetham, A., and Yucel, M. (2015). Cannabis and adolescent brain development. *Pharmacol Ther*, **148**, 1–16.

Makowski, C., Bodnar, M., Shenker, J. J., et al. (2017). Linking persistent negative symptoms to amygdala-hippocampus structure in first-episode psychosis. *Transl Psychiatry*, **7**, e1195.

Malchow, B., Hasan, A., Schneider-Axmann, T., et al. (2013). Effects of cannabis and familial loading on subcortical brain volumes in first-episode schizophrenia. *Eur Arch Psychiatry Clin Neurosci*, **263**, S155–S168.

Mallet, J., Ramoz, N., Le Strat, Y., et al. (2017). Heavy cannabis use prior psychosis in schizophrenia: Clinical, cognitive and neurological evidences for a new endophenotype? *Eur Arch Psychiatry Clin Neurosci*, **267**, 629–638.

Meyer, H. C., Lee, F. S., and Gee, D. G. (2018). The role of the endocannabinoid system and genetic variation in adolescent brain development. *Neuropsychopharmacology*, **43**, 21–33.

Moghaddam, B., and Javitt, D. (2012). From revolution to evolution: The glutamate hypothesis of schizophrenia and its implication for treatment. *Neuropsychopharmacology*, **37**, 4–15.

Morrison, P. D., Zois, V., McKeown, D. A., et al. (2009). The acute effects of synthetic intravenous Delta9-tetrahydrocannabinol on psychosis, mood and cognitive functioning. *Psychol Med*, **39**, 1607–1616.

O'Neill, A., Annibale, L., Blest-Hopley, G., et al. (2021). Cannabidiol modulation of hippocampal glutamate in early psychosis. *J Psychopharmacol*, **35**, 814–822.

Paul, S., and Bhattacharyya, S. (2021). Cannabis use-related working memory deficit mediated by lower left hippocampal volume. *Addict Biol*, **26**, e12984.

Quattrone, D., Ferraro, L., Tripoli, G., et al. (2020). *The Relation of the Psychosis Continuum with Schizophrenia Polygenic Risk Score and Cannabis Use*. Schizophrenia International Research Society.

Rabin, R. A., Zakzanis, K. K., and George, T. P. (2011). The effects of cannabis use on neurocognition in schizophrenia: A meta-analysis. *Schizophr Res*, **128**, 111–116.

Ranganathan, M., and D'Souza, D. C. (2006). The acute effects of cannabinoids on memory in humans: A review. *Psychopharmacologia*, **188**, 425–444.

Rasetti, R., Sambataro, F., Chen, Q., et al. (2011). Altered cortical network dynamics: A potential intermediate phenotype for schizophrenia and association with ZNF804A. *Arch Gen Psychiatry*, **68**, 1207–1217.

Raver, S. M., Haughwout, S. P., and Keller, A. (2013). Adolescent cannabinoid exposure permanently suppresses cortical oscillations in adult mice. *Neuropsychopharmacology*, **38**, 2338–2347.

del Re, E. C., Yassine, W., Zeng, V., et al. (2022). Childhood trauma and cannabis interactions in affecting psychosis onset: Role of the anterior–posterior axis of the hippocampus and differences in cannabis use before or after psychosis onset. *medRxiv*.

Realini, N., Rubino, T., and Parolaro, D. (2009). Neurobiological alterations at adult age triggered by adolescent exposure to cannabinoids. *Pharmacol Res*, **60**, 132–138.

Renard, J., Krebs, M. O., Le Pen, G., et al. (2014). Long-term consequences of adolescent cannabinoid exposure in adult psychopathology. *Front Neurosci*, **8**, 361.

Rentzsch, J., Stadtmann, A., Montag, C., et al. (2016). Attentional dysfunction in abstinent long-term cannabis users with and without schizophrenia. *Eur Arch Psychiatry Clin Neurosci*, **266**, 409–421.

Rigucci, S., Xin, L., Klauser, P., et al. (2017). Cannabis use in early psychosis is associated with reduced glutamate levels in the prefrontal cortex. *Psychopharmacologia*, **235**, 13–22.

Rubino, T., and Parolaro, D. (2008). Long lasting consequences of cannabis exposure in adolescence. *Mol Cell Endocrinol*, **286**, S108–S113.

(2016). The impact of exposure to cannabinoids in adolescence: Insights from animal models. *Biol Psychiatry*, **79**, 578–585.

Rubino, T., Prini, P., Piscitelli, F., et al. (2015). Adolescent exposure to THC in female rats disrupts developmental changes in the prefrontal cortex. *Neurobiol Dis*, **226**, 159–162.

Sami, M. B., Annibale, L., O'Neill, A., et al. (2021). Eye movements in patients in early psychosis with and without a history of cannabis use. *NPJ Schizophrenia*, **7**, 1–7.

Sami, M. B., and Bhattacharyya, S. (2018). Are cannabis-using and non-using patients different groups? Towards understanding the neurobiology of cannabis use in psychotic disorders. *J Psychopharmacol*, **32**, 825–849.

Sami, M. B., Worker, A., Colizzi, M., et al. (2020). Association of cannabis with glutamatergic levels in patients with early psychosis: Evidence for altered volume striatal glutamate relationships in patients with a history of cannabis use in early psychosis. *Transl Psychiatry*, **10**, 111.

Scheffler, F., Plessis, S. D., Asmal, L., et al. (2021). Cannabis use and hippocampal subfield volumes in males with a first episode of a schizophrenia spectrum disorder and healthy controls. *Schizophr Res*, **231**, 13–21.

Schneider, M. (2008). Puberty as a highly vulnerable developmental period for the consequences of cannabis exposure. *Addict Biol*, **13**, 253–263.

Schnell, T., Kleiman, A., Gouzoulis-Mayfrank, E., et al. (2012). Increased gray matter density in patients with schizophrenia and cannabis use: A voxel-based morphometric study using DARTEL. *Schizophr Res*, **138**, 183–187.

Schoeler, T., Kambeitz, J., and Bhattacharyya, S. (2015) The effect of cannabis on memory function in users with and without a psychotic disorder: A meta-analysis. *Psychol Med*, **10**, 1–12.

Shakory, S., Watts, J. J., Hafizi, S., et al. (2018). Hippocampal glutamate metabolites and glial activation in clinical high risk and first episode psychosis. *Neuropsychopharmacology*, **43**, 2249–2255.

Smith, M. J., Cobia, D. J., Reilly, J. L., et al. (2015). Cannabis-related episodic memory deficits and hippocampal morphological differences in healthy individuals and schizophrenia subjects. *Hippocampus*, **25**, 1042–1051.

Solowij, N., Malterfang, M., Lubman, D. I., et al. (2013). Alteration to hippocampal shape in cannabis users with and without schizophrenia. *Schizophr Res*, **143**, 179–184.

Stip, E. (2006). Cognition, schizophrenia and the effect of antipsychotics. *Encephale*, **32**, 341–350.

Stirling, J., Lewis, S., and Hopkins, R., et al. (2005). Cannabis use prior to first onset psychosis predicts spared neurocognition at 10-year follow-up. *Schizophr Res*, **75**, 135–137.

Stokes, P. R., Egerton, A., Watson, B., et al. (2012). History of cannabis use is not associated with alterations in striatal dopamine D2/D3 receptor availability. *J Psychopharmacol*, **26**, 144–149.

Strasser, H. C., Lilyestrom, J., Ashby, E. R., et al. (2005). Hippocampal and ventricular volumes in psychotic and nonpsychotic bipolar patients compared with schizophrenia patients and community control subjects: A pilot study. *Biol Psychiatry*, **57**, 633–639.

Sullivan, J. M. (2000). Cellular and molecular mechanisms underlying learning and memory impairments produced by cannabinoids. *Learn Mem*, **7**, 132–139.

Szallasi, A., Cortright, D. N., Blum, C. A., et al. (2007). The vanilloid receptor TRPV1: 10 years from channel cloning to antagonist proof-of-concept. *Nat Rev Drug Discov*, **6**, 357–372.

Tamminga, C. A., Clementz, B. A., Pearlson, G. D., et al. (2021). Biotyping in psychosis: Using multiple computational approaches with one data set. *Neuropsychopharmacology*, **46**, 143–155.

Tamminga, C. A., Ivleva, E. I., Keshavan, M. S., et al. (2013). Clinical phenotypes of psychosis in the Bipolar-Schizophrenia Network on Intermediate Phenotypes (B-SNIP). *Am J Psychiatry*, **170**, 1263–1274.

Tamminga, C. A., Pearlson, G. D., Keshavan, M., et al. (2014). Bipolar and schizophrenia network for intermediate phenotypes: Outcomes across the psychosis continuum. *Schizophr Bull*, **40**, S131–S137.

Tanda, G., and Goldberg, S. R. (2003). Cannabinoids: Reward, dependence, and underlying neurochemical mechanisms – A review of recent preclinical data. *Psychopharmacology (Berl)*, **232**, 2723–2729.

Treadway, M. T., Waskom, M. L., Dillon, D. G., et al. (2015). Illness progression, recent stress, and morphometry of hippocampal subfields and medial prefrontal cortex in major depression. *Biol Psychiatry*, **77**, 285–294.

van Tricht, M. J., Harmsen, E. C., Koelman, J. H. T. M., et al. (2013). Effects of cannabis use on event related potentials in subjects at ultra high risk for psychosis and healthy controls. *Int J Psychophysiol*, **88**, 149–156.

Van Gastel, W. A., Schubart, C. D., Van Eijk, K. R., et al. (2013). The effect of childhood maltreatment and cannabis use on adult psychotic symptoms is modified by the COMT Val158Met polymorphism. *Schizophr Res*, **150**, 303–311.

Volkow, N. D., Wang, G. J., Telang, F., et al. (2014). Decreased dopamine brain reactivity in marijuana abusers is associated with negative emotionality and addiction severity. *Proc Natl Acad Sci USA*, **111**, E3149–E3156.

Wannan, C. M. J., Cropley, V. L., Chakravarty, M. M., et al. (2019). Evidence for network-based cortical thickness reductions in schizophrenia. *Am J Psychiatry*, **176**, 552–563.

Wiers, C. E., Shokri-Kojori, E., Wong, C. T., et al. (2016). Cannabis abusers show hypofrontality and blunted brain responses to a stimulant challenge in females but not in males. *Neuropsychopharmacology*, **41**, 2596–2605.

Winterburn, J. L., Pruessner, J. C., Chavez, S., et al. (2013). A novel in vivo atlas of human hippocampal subfields using high-resolution 3 T magnetic resonance imaging. *Neuroimage*, **74**, 254–265.

Yucel, M., Bora, E., Lubman, D. I., et al. (2012). The impact of cannabis use on cognitive functioning in patients with schizophrenia: A meta-analysis of existing findings and new data in a first-episode sample. *Schizophr Bull*, **38**, 316–330.

Zhou, Y., Shu, N., Liu, Y., et al. (2008). Altered resting-state functional connectivity and anatomical connectivity of hippocampus in schizophrenia. *Schizophr Res*, **100**, 120–132.

Cannabis and Anxiety

Grace Lethbridge, Beth Patterson, and Michael Van Ameringen

11.1 Introduction

Anxiety disorders, such as panic disorder (PD), agoraphobia, social anxiety disorder (SAD), generalized anxiety disorder (GAD), and specific phobias, are among the most prevalent mental health disorders. They are chronic conditions with a lifetime prevalence of 29% (Kessler et al., 2005). Anxiety disorders are associated with significant burden for afflicted individuals, their families, and society. This burden is characterized by substantial functional impairment, as well as increased use of health services and decreased work productivity (Baxter et al., 2013; Katzman et al., 2014). Cognitive behavioural therapy is the first-line psychological treatment for anxiety disorders and yields response rates of 46–77%. Unfortunately, this treatment is not widely available and is often associated with significant costs to the patient (Katzman et al., 2014). First-line pharmacological treatments for anxiety disorders include antidepressants which target serotonin and/or noradrenalin reuptake. These include selective serotonin reuptake inhibitors (SSRIs) and serotonin noradrenalin reuptake inhibitors (SNRIs). Treatment response rates to these standard agents are less than optimal, with ~50% of patients continuing to have residual, impairing symptoms (Bystritsky, 2006). Pharmacological treatments are also associated with significant, often disabling side-effects leading to non-compliance and discontinuation (Olfson et al., 2006). As a result, there is a great need to identify new treatments targeting novel etiological pathways and the associated mechanisms of action.

Cannabis, a derivative of the *Cannabis Sativa* plant, is commonly used recreationally for its euphoric and relaxing effects. Although cannabis is considered an illicit substance in many parts of the world, regulatory bodies in the Netherlands, Canada, and a number of US States have legalized its use for either medicinal or recreational use or both (see Chapter 4). The primary components of cannabis include the phytocannabinoids, delta-9-tetrahydrocannabinol (THC), and cannabidiol (CBD). Cannabis exerts its effects primarily through the endocannabinoid system, which is involved in immune system regulation, pain perception, insulin sensitivity, fat and energy metabolism, and fear and anxiety responses.

Although the research on the mechanism of action, safety, and efficacy of cannabis continues to evolve, cannabis has been gaining popularity in the community as an alternative treatment for anxiety disorders. This chapter summarizes the current research evidence regarding cannabis as a treatment for anxiety.

> **Box 11.1   The endocannabinoid system as a target for anxiety treatment**
>
> First line interventions for anxiety disorders, such as antidepressants and cognitive behavioural therapies, yield moderate response rates. Therefore, investigating treatments which target alternative neuropathways may be of great importance. The endocannabinoid system presents a potential novel target for the treatment of anxiety disorders.

11.2 Surveys of Medicinal Cannabis Use

Medicinal cannabis for the treatment of a wide variety of health conditions has become increasingly common across the globe. Surveys of medicinal cannabis users indicate that many patients endorse using their prescribed cannabis to treat anxiety, regardless of the condition for which it was prescribed.

In 2016, a large-scale survey (n = 1,784) explored the patterns of medical cannabis use in Australia: 15% of the sample reported anxiety as the main medical condition they treated with cannabis and 51% reported using cannabis to treat any symptoms of anxiety. With regard to the subjective efficacy of cannabis, 84% of the sample reported their symptoms 'very much improved or much improved' and less than 1% reported their cannabis use exacerbated their symptoms or resulted in intolerable side-effects (Lintzeris et al., 2018). In another cross-sectional study of self-identified CBD users (n = 2,409), 62% of users reported using CBD to treat a medical condition, and 22.4% of the sample reported anxiety as their reason for using CBD (Corroon and Phillips, 2018). Although the authors did not differentiate between medical conditions, in terms of the subjective efficacy of CBD across these conditions, 36% of the participants reported that CBD worked very well by itself, 30% reported it worked moderately well by itself, 30% reported it worked well when combined with conventional medicine, and 4% reported it did not work very well.

In 2018, a survey using the Strainprint™ Cannabis Tracker examined the subjective effects of cannabis. The Strainprint™ Cannabis Tracker allows medical cannabis users to track their symptoms as a function of cannabis use and is available for free download on Google Play and the Apple App. Users can track their doses and the THC:CBD ratio of their cannabis. Within 5,085 tracking sessions of where users were treating anxiety with cannabis, significantly lower anxiety levels following cannabis use in 93.5% of the sessions was reported (Cuttler et al., 2018). Only 2.1% of the users experienced exacerbated symptoms, while 4.4% experienced no symptom change. Interestingly, most respondents reported the greatest stress reductions from products with a high CBD concentration.

The Tilray Observational Patient Survey collected data from 2,032 patients who had been prescribed medical cannabis. Although respondents reported using medicinal cannabis for many issues, 44% reported using cannabis for anxiety symptoms (Turna et al., 2019). Validated symptom severity scale cut-scores were used to estimate the rates of probable anxiety disorders, which were high: Generalized Anxiety Disorder (GAD), 46%; Social Anxiety Disorder (SAD), 42%; Panic Disorder (PD), 5%. Most (92%) of the sample reported that cannabis improved their anxiety symptoms. Around half (49%) reported substituting cannabis to some degree for a prescription drug and, within this group, 61% reported that cannabis had completely replaced a prescription drug. The majority of the anxiety group reported that cannabis improved their 'anxiety,

worry, fears' (92.0%), 'irritability' (76%), 'difficulty falling to sleep' (72%), 'anxiety attacks' (59%), and 'low mood' (57%). On a scale of 1 (not at all effective) to 5 (very effective), 65% of respondents scored the effectiveness of their cannabis use at alleviating anxiety symptoms greater than 4, indicating high perceived effectiveness. Interestingly, 99.5% of respondents reported using cannabis recreationally prior to using it medically. A substantial proportion (42%) of respondents reported using 1–2 g of cannabis per day, 35% used less than 1 g/day, and 23% used more than 3 g/day. Anxiety score severity (GAD-7, $p < 0.001$) was positively associated with the amount of cannabis used per day. Heavy users (>3 g/day) had significantly higher anxiety scores than moderate (1–2 g/day) or light users (<1 g/day) (GAD-7, $p < 0.01$). No differences were observed between light and moderate users.

A recent systematic review uncovered the persistent gaps in the literature regarding the association between cannabis use and the long-term outcomes on anxiety and mood disorders (Mammen et al., 2018). The authors suggested that clinical trials are needed to examine the long-term effects of cannabis with specific data on cannabinoid concentrations, route of administration (e.g., oral pill, inhalant), dosage, and interactions with medications (e.g., anti-anxiety drugs), as these factors may differentially affect the long-term outcomes associated with cannabis use. Furthermore, most of the current literature does not examine within-individual changes on anxiety severity scales between baseline and follow-up assessments, with most studies simply suggesting that cannabis use, compared to no cannabis, is associated with greater symptom severity over time (Mammen et al., 2018).

Box 11.2 Perceptions of users regarding anxiolytic effects of cannabis

Many survey studies indicate that individuals in the community are using cannabis to treat anxiety and perceive that it is efficacious. These results are limited, however, and important factors such as dose, frequency of use, age of cannabis use onset, routes of administration, symptom severity, and a priori beliefs about the anxiolytic role of cannabis are not adequately addressed. These factors may differentially affect the long-term prognosis of cannabis users.

11.3 Clinical Trials

The anxiolytic effects of the main active components of cannabis (THC and CBD) have both been evaluated scientifically. Studies in healthy adults have indicated that THC, putatively, has dose-dependent anxiolytic (low dose) or anxiogenic (high dose) effects, as well as antidepressant and hypnotic effects (Bossong et al., 2013; Fusar-Poli et al., 2009). The behavioural, cognitive, and endocrine effects of 0 mg, 2.5 mg, and 5 mg intravenous THC were also described in a 3-day, double-blind, randomized, and counterbalanced study in 22 healthy participants (D'Souza et al., 2004). Heightened levels of anxiety and lowered levels of calmness were reported, 3 hours following 2.5 mg or 5 mg of THC infusion (D'Souza et al., 2004). Alternatively, CBD has demonstrated analgesic, anticonvulsant, and anxiolytic properties in both human and animal models. In humans, 300 mg of CBD was shown to have the same post-stress anxiolytic effects as 5 mg of ipsapirone, a selective partial agonist of 5-HT1A (Bhattacharyya et al., 2010). Healthy volunteers have reported decreased levels of subjective anxiety 90-minutes following 400 mg of CBD administration (Fusar-Poli et al., 2009). The ratio of THC to CBD varies greatly between strains of cannabis plants, and these variations have been shown to induce a wide variety of psychological effects from relaxation (Bonn-Miller et al., 2007) to psychosis (National Academies of Sciences, Engineering, and Medicine, 2017). When THC and CBD are combined, CBD recurrently exhibits the ability to mitigate the anxiogenic effects of THC in both human and animal models (Bhattacharyya et al., 2010; Crippa et al., 2004; Fusar-Poli et al., 2009; Karniol et al., 1974; Zuardi et al., 1982); however, this effect depends on the ratio of CBD to THC administered (Zeyl et al., 2020; Zuardi et al., 2012). Further, the anxiolytic effects of CBD have been described as an inverted 'bell-shaped' dose–response curve (Crippa et al., 2018). The terminology used in the literature describing the dose–response relationship between CBD and anxiety depends on the outcome variable that is plotted on the y-axis. If a higher score on the outcome measure indicates an anxiolytic effect, the dose–response curve for CBD may be described as an inverted U-shape or bell-shape; both terms are synonymous. In contrast, if a lower score on the outcome measure indicates an anxiolytic effect (e.g., STAI), the curve may be described as U-shaped or as an inverted bell-shape. For CBD, moderate doses exhibit anxiolytic effects, whereas lower and higher doses elicit minimal effects (Fusar-Poli et al., 2009). It has been suggested that the activation of TRPV1 receptors, which occurs at high doses of CBD, contributes to this observed dose–response relationship (Campos and Guimarães, 2009). Activation of TRPV1 receptors can increase the release of glutamate, which is a neurotransmitter that can oppose the anxiolytic effects produced by CBD (Crippa et al., 2018).

There have been very few clinical trials examining the efficacy of cannabis as a treatment for anxiety disorders. The bulk of the literature is comprised of single-dose studies in healthy adults, where symptoms of anxiety have been measured. Only the effects of CBD and the synthetic cannabinoid, nabilone, have been examined in anxiety disorders using a clinical trial design.

11.3.1 CBD and Anxiety

In regard to individual anxiety disorders, CBD has been examined in two small SAD studies (Bergamashi et al., 2011; Crippa et al., 2011) and nabilone has been evaluated in GAD (Glass et al., 1981). In a study of drug-naïve SAD patients, the participants were administered either 600 mg of CBD (capsule) or placebo 1.5 hours prior to a stimulated public speaking task (SPST). The treatment group exhibited lower anxiety levels than the placebo group ($p = 0.012$), as per the speech phase of the Visual Analogue Mood Scales (VAMS) (Bergamashi et al., 2011). The placebo group also exhibited greater cognitive impairment, discomfort, and alertness. In a study of 10 socially anxious men, the pathogenesis of SAD was examined using neuroimaging (Crippa et al., 2011). The participants were administered either 400 mg of CBD (capsule) or placebo. The anxiety-evoking stimulus was the Single Photon-Emission Computed Tomography (SPECT) procedure itself, as it involves insertion of a cannula to administer a tracer intravenously, as well as exposure to an unfamiliar medical environment for the imaging. The study acquired subjective ratings on the VAMS at five different time points: 30 minutes before drug intake (CBD or placebo), at the time of drug intake, during intravenous injection of the tracer, pre-SPECT imaging (15 minutes post-tracer injection), and just after the SPECT imaging. In comparison to the placebo group, the CBD group demonstrated decreased VAMS anxiety scores during venous cannula insertion (60 minutes post-CBD intake; t = 2.74, p = 0.02), pre-SPECT imaging (75 minutes post-CBD intake; t = 3.61, p = 0.006), and post-SPECT imaging (140 minutes post-CBD intake; t = 3.94, p = 0.003).

Although not conducted in an anxiety-disordered sample, a double-blind study of 40 healthy volunteers compared the effects of 5 mg of ipsapirone, 300 mg of CBD, 10 mg of diazepam, and placebo on subjective anxiety prior to and following a SPST (Zuardi et al., 1993). Anxiety was evaluated through the VAMS and the State-Trait Anxiety Inventory (STAI), following the SPST. Results indicated that ipsapirone mitigated SPST-induced anxiety, while CBD decreased anxiety post-SPST. Conversely, diazepam was anxiolytic pre- and post-SPST, but it had no effect on the increase in anxiety induced by the SPST and was found to be sedating. The results provide evidence for the anxiolytic properties of ipsapirone and CBD in healthy volunteers exposed to a stressful performance-based stimulus. In a double-blind study of 57 healthy male subjects asked to do a SPST, the effects of CBD at different doses were compared (Linares et al., 2019). The subjects were administered either 150 mg of CBD (n = 15), 300 mg of CBD (n = 15), 600 mg of CBD (n = 12), or placebo (n = 15). During the SPST, subjective VAMS scores were obtained at six different time points. The 300 mg dose of CBD significantly reduced anxiety during the speech task, in comparison to the placebo. No significant differences in VAMS scores were observed between groups receiving 150 mg of CBD, 600 mg of CBD, or placebo, thereby illustrating the inverted U-shaped dose–response curve of CBD (Linares et al., 2019).

A crossover RCT in 43 healthy individuals aimed to determine whether CBD expectancy alone could influence stress, anxiety, and mood (Spinella et al., 2021). Subjective stress, anxiety, and mood were measured using a single-item Numerical Rating Scale (NRS), the six-item shortened version of the STAI (STAI-S-SF; Marteau and Bekker, 1992), and the 10-item International Positive and Negative Affect Schedule Short Form (I-PANAS-SF; Thompson, 2007), respectively. This study also evaluated the extent to which a priori beliefs regarding CBD's therapeutic effects predicted these responses. Overall, there were no changes in subjective stress or anxiety in the CBD expectancy condition; however, subjects with strong a priori beliefs of CBD as an anxiolytic agent reported significantly decreased anxiety scores in the CBD expectancy condition (NRS and STAI). The findings highlight the importance of controlling for the effects of CBD expectancy in clinical research.

> **Box 11.3 Anxiolytic effects of CBD**
>
> The anxiolytic effects of CBD can be conceptualized as having a bell-shaped dose–response curve – moderate doses exhibit anxiolytic effects, whereas lower and higher doses elicit minimal effects. Although several studies suggest the anxiolytic role of CBD following episodic anxiety-inducing stimuli, more research is needed to investigate the long-term outcomes of regular, repeated CBD administration for chronic anxiety treatment.

11.3.2 Nabilone and Anxiety

Nabilone is an oral synthetic analogue of Δ9-THC, which is the principal psychoactive component of the cannabis plant. Although it mimics the structure and function of Δ9-THC through weak partial agonism of the CB1 and CB2 receptors (Borgelt et al., 2013; Pertwee, 2009), nabilone is considered to be more potent than Δ9-THC (Bedi et al., 2013). Due to its antiemetic and appetite stimulating properties (Amar, 2006), it is typically used for treating anorexia and weight loss in patients with HIV, as well as nausea and vomiting in cancer patients undergoing chemotherapy. However, in both an open-label (n = 5) and a double blind (n = 20) study, the effects of nabilone on psychoneurotic anxiety were examined. The dosage was adjustable in the open-label trial (mean dose = 2.8 mg; range = 2–8 mg/day). The researchers found that nabilone significantly reduced anxiety as per the Hamilton Anxiety Scale (HAM-A) (p < 0.001) from day seven onward (Fabre and McLendon, 1981). In the RCT, 1 mg of nabilone administered three times per day (3 mg/day) was more effective in reducing anxiety than the placebo, as per the HAM-A (p < 0.001) and Physician's Global Impression scale (p = 0.002) by day seven (Fabre and McLendon, 1981).

In a single-blind balanced Latin-square study, the effects of single oral doses of nabilone were examined in eight anxious volunteers (Glass et al., 1981). Each subject was exposed to placebo twice and received three different doses of nabilone at one-week intervals. Subjective effects on anxiety were quantitatively measured using the Profile of Mood States (POMS). The study consisted of two phases. In Phase I, subjective anxiolytic effects were reported in 50% of patients at low doses (1–2 mg) of nabilone. Phase II used doses that were 58% less than those used in Phase I, due to the occurrence of adverse events: there was no difference in reported anxiety at these lower doses (Glass et al., 1981).

11.3.3 Clinical Trials Where Anxiety Was a Secondary Outcome

Evidence regarding the utility of medicinal cannabis for comorbid anxiety may be drawn from studies where it has been assessed as a secondary outcome. This includes studies which have examined the efficacy of cannabis in treating symptoms of multiple sclerosis, Huntington's disease, migraines, fibromyalgia, neuropathy, and Parkinson's disease. These studies are presented in Table 11.1. Many of these studies used nabiximols spray, which is a whole plant extract from the *Cannabis sativa* plant that contains a balanced ratio of CBD (2.5 mg/spray) and Δ9-THC (2.7 mg/spray). Overall, the findings suggest that nabiximols spray does not have significant anxiolytic effects, in comparison to placebo, for patients with multiple sclerosis (Aragona et al., 2009; Rog et al., 2005) or Huntington's disease (Moreno et al., 2016). However, nabilone has demonstrated significant anxiolytic effects, relative to placebo, at a dose of 1–4 mg/day in patients with fibromyalgia (Skrabek et al., 2008) and neuropathy (Toth et al., 2012). Conversely, nabilone has not yielded significant anxiolytic effects, relative to ibuprofen (400 mg/day) or dihydrocodeine (30–240 mg/day), in patients with medication use headache (Pini et al., 2012) or neuropathy (Frank et al., 2008). Dronabinol (10–20 mg/day), another

---

Box 11.4 Anxiolytic effects of cannabinoids in medical conditions

Anxiety is often measured as a secondary outcome to another medical condition. Various RCTs have examined the anxiolytic role of cannabis, CBD, nabiximols, and nabilone when measured as a secondary outcome. The results suggest these agents, adjunctive to standard treatments, have the potential to improve anxiety-related symptoms in patients with Huntington's disease, fibromyalgia, neuropathy, and burning mouth syndrome.

---

synthetic form of Δ9-THC, has not produced significant anxiolytic effects in patients with chronic pain, relative to placebo (Malik et al., 2017; Narang et al., 2008). Although CBD oil (5–25 mg/kg/day) has not demonstrated efficacy in relieving symptoms of anxiety in patients with Parkinson's disease (Leehey et al., 2020), *Cannabis sativa* oil (10–40 drops/day) has shown symptomatic improvement of anxiety in patients with primary burning mouth syndrome (Gambino et al., 2021).

11.4 Reviews and Meta-analyses

A systematic review of 31 studies investigated the association between anxiety and cannabis use/CUD in the general population (Kedzior and Laeber, 2014). Cannabis use at baseline was significantly associated with anxiety at follow-up in five studies (OR = 1.28; 95% CI = 1.06–1.54; $p = 0.01$) after adjusting for confounders (e.g., other substance use, psychiatric comorbidity, certain demographics). There was a small positive association between anxiety and either cannabis use (OR = 1.24; 95% CI = 1.06–1.45; $p = 0.006$; n = 15 studies) or CUD (OR = 1.68; 95% CI = 1.23–2.31; $p = 0.001$; n = 13 studies), and between comorbid anxiety and depression and cannabis use (OR = 1.68; 95% CI = 1.17–2.40; $p = 0.004$; n = 5 studies). In 2017, the National Academies of Sciences, Engineering, and Medicine (NASEM) reviewed the evidence regarding the health effects of cannabis and cannabinoids. The review employed five levels of evidence: conclusive, substantial, moderate, limited, and insufficient. There was insufficient evidence to support a statistical association between cannabis use and the development of any type of anxiety disorder, with the exception of SAD, which had moderate level evidence. There was also limited evidence to suggest increased anxiety symptom severity in daily cannabis users.

In a meta-analysis of 40 RCTs (n = 3,067), the role of cannabinoids in the treatment of various mental health disorders was examined (Black et al., 2019). In studies where anxiety was secondary to another medical condition, mainly chronic pain and multiple sclerosis (seven studies, n = 252), a small reduction in anxiety symptoms was found following THC (with or without CBD) (SMD = –0.25; 95% CI = –0.49 to –0.01); however, the quality of the evidence was rated as very low. Most studies were based on synthetic cannabinoids, rather than medicinal cannabis, further

Table 11.1 Clinical trials of cannabinoids where anxiety was a secondary outcome

Study	Primary Condition	Design	N	Methods	Drug Intervention	Results for Anxiety
Aragona et al. (2009)	Multiple Sclerosis	Crossover RCT	17	• 3 weeks for each intervention • 2-week washout period • Self-rating Anxiety Scale (SAS)	• 100 µL nabiximols spray (2.7 mg THC and 2.5 mg CBD per spray) (mean daily sprays = 8.20 ± 3.15) • Placebo (mean daily sprays = 15.16 ± 4.51)	No significant difference for post-treatment SAS scores between groups (Nabiximols = PBO, $p = 0.21$)
Rog et al. (2005)	Multiple Sclerosis	Parallel RCT	64	• 5 weeks • Hospital Anxiety and Depression Scale	• Adjunctive nabiximols spray (2.7 mg THC and 2.5 mg CBD per spray) (mean daily sprays in week 4 = 9.6, range = 2–25, SD = 6.1) • Placebo (adjunct to analgesics)	No significant between-group difference for change in HADS scores over time (cannabis = PBO) 1 dropout due to an adverse event with cannabis treatment (tachycardia and hypertension)
Moreno et al. (2016)	Huntington's Disease	Crossover RCT	26	• 12 weeks for each intervention • 4-week washout period • Hospital Anxiety and Depression Scale	• Nabiximols spray (2.7 mg THC and 2.5 mg CBD per spray, 12 sprays/day) • Placebo	No significant differences in HADS scores during treatment with Nabiximol Spray, relative to placebo (Nabiximols = PBO, $p = 0.405$)
Pini et al. (2012)	Medication Use Headache	Crossover RCT	30	• 8 weeks for each intervention • 1-week washout period • Zung Anxiety Scale (ZAS)	• Oral nabilone (0.5 mg/day) • Oral ibuprofen (400 mg/day)	No significant difference in anxiety scores between groups (nabilone = ibuprofen) 2 dropouts due to adverse events (gastric discomfort with ibuprofen and loss of concentration/memory with nabilone)
Skrabek et al. (2008)	Fibromyalgia	Parallel RCT	40	• 4 weeks • Fibromyalgia Impact Questionnaire 10-point anxiety scale	• Nabilone (0.5 mg PO titrated to 1 mg, BID) • Placebo	Significant improvement of anxiety scores from baseline in nabilone group (Nabilone > PBO, $p < 0.02$)
Abrams et al. (2007)	Neuropathy	Parallel RCT	50	• 5 days • Profile of Mood States	• Smoked cannabis (3.56% THC, TID) • Placebo (TID)	No significant difference between groups in the reduction of total mood disturbance (Cannabis = PBO, 33% vs. 29%, $p = 0.28$)

Study	Condition	Design	N	Duration / Measures	Intervention	Results
Frank et al. (2008)	Neuropathy	Crossover RCT	96	• 6 weeks for each intervention • 2-week washout period • Hospital Anxiety and Depression Scale	• Nabilone (250 μg–2 mg) • Dihydrocodeine (30–240 mg)	No significant treatment effect on HADS scores (Nabilone = dihydrocodeine)
Toth et al. (2012)	Neuropathy	Parallel RCT	26	• 5 weeks • Hospital Anxiety and Depression Scale	• Adjunctive nabilone (1–4 mg/day) • Placebo (adjuvant to current pain medications)	Significant improvement in HADS scores for nabilone group in comparison to placebo group (Nabilone > PBO, $F = 2.24$, $p < 0.05$)
Narang et al. (2008)	Chronic Pain	Crossover RCT	30	• 3, 8-hour visits • Minimum 3-day washout period • Anxiety (Sum of Pain Intensity Difference, SPID)	• Oral dronabinol (10 mg or 20 mg) • Placebo	No significant difference between treatment groups and placebo group (dronabinol = PBO)
Malik et al. (2017)	Chronic Pain	Parallel RCT	19	• 4 weeks • Beck Anxiety Inventory (BAI)	• Oral dronabinol (5 mg, BID) • Placebo	No significant differences in BAI scores from pre-treatment to post-treatment or between the two groups (dronabinol = PBO)
De Vries et al. (2017)	Chronic Pain	Parallel RCT	65	• 50–52 days • Pain Anxiety Symptom Scale, Hospital Anxiety and Depression Scale	• Oral THC tablet (Namisol; 3–8 mg, TID) • Placebo	No significant differences in post-treatment measures of anxiety between groups (THC = PBO)
Gambino et al. (2021)	Primary Burning Mouth Syndrome	Prospective, open-label single-arm pilot study	17	• 4 weeks • Hospital Anxiety and Depression Scale	• Cannabis sativa oil (Bediol, 6.3% THC, 8% CBD, 1 g of cannabis in 10 g of olive oil, 5–20 drops BID)	Decreased anxiety symptoms at 12 weeks ($p = 0.030$) and 24-weeks ($p = 0.031$) follow-up
Leehey et al. (2020)	Parkinson's Disease	Open label, dose escalation study	13	• Mean duration was 26.8 (8.0) days • Quality-of-Life in Neurological Disorders (Neurol-QoL) short form for anxiety	• CBD oil (Epidiolex with ≤0.15% THC twice daily) • Titrated from 5 to 20–25 mg/kg/day	No significant change in anxiety scores from baseline ($n = 10$, $p = 0.783$) 3 patients dropped out due to adverse effects: • Rash at 5 mg/kg/day • Abdominal pain and gas at 17.5 mg/kg/day • Fatigue, diarrhoea, and hepatitis at 25 mg/kg/day

suggesting the need for high-quality studies directly examining the effect of cannabis on treating mental disorders. Finally, a large retrospective chart review investigated whether adjunctive CBD improved sleep and/or anxiety in out-patients whose primary complaints were either anxiety (n = 47) or poor sleep (n = 25) (Shannon et al., 2019). Most patients received 25 mg of CBD per day for at least one month. Their sleep and anxiety scores were measured at baseline and post-CBD treatment. Hamilton Anxiety Rating Scale (HAM-A) scores decreased within the first month in 57 patients (79.2%) and this effect was maintained for the study's duration. Although Pittsburgh Sleep Quality Index (PSQI) scores improved within the first month in 48 patients (66.7%), they seemed to fluctuate over time. Three patients who did not tolerate CBD well discontinued treatment. Two patients discontinued CBD treatment within the first week due to fatigue. One patient with a developmental disorder was taken off CBD due to increased sexually inappropriate behaviour. The psychiatrist in the study suggested this behaviour was related to disinhibition, resulting from substantial improvements in the patient's anxiety (Shannon et al., 2019).

11.5 Longitudinal Studies

A three-year longitudinal survey of cannabis use in 3,723 patients with a primary anxiety disorder compared the outcomes between cannabis users, patients with CUD, and non-users (Feingold et al., 2018). Remission rates of 66%, 53%, and 47% in non-users, cannabis users, and individuals with CUD, respectively, were found but were not significantly different from each other, after adjusting for confounders (Feingold et al., 2018). These results suggest that long-term cannabis use neither harms nor improves the trajectory of anxiety disorders, but it may increase the risk of disordered use. In contrast, a systematic review of 12 prospective cohort studies examined the longitudinal effects of cannabis use on anxiety and mood disorder (AMD) symptoms (n = 11,959). In 11 studies, recent cannabis use (past 6 months) was associated with elevated symptoms of anxiety relative to comparison groups. Ten studies further proposed that cannabis use was associated with less symptomatic improvement from adjunctive treatments (e.g., medication and psychotherapy) (Mammen et al., 2018). Although these results oppose other studies suggesting that cannabis may improve AMD-related

symptoms, it was proposed this can be attributed to differences in study period lengths. The effects of long-term exogenous administration of cannabinoids, such as THC, on the endocannabinoid system to improve anxiety symptoms is understudied. The researchers speculated that cannabis may be suitable for acute symptomatic improvement; however, with long-term exposure, the drug may lead to persistent symptoms and the prevention of symptomatic recovery (Mammen et al., 2018).

11.6 Cannabis: Anxiolytic or Anxiogenic?

Although cannabis is often used in the community to reduce stress and anxiety (Korem et al., 2016), many individuals report that it may also exacerbate these problems. At this point, the direction of the association between cannabis and anxiety is unclear: Is it that anxious people are more likely to use cannabis as a form of self-medication or is cannabis use related to anxiety onset?

11.6.1 Cannabis Use as a Predictor of Anxiety Symptoms

Two meta-analyses suggest that cannabis use at baseline is associated with anxiety symptoms at follow-up, after adjusting for confounders (OR = 1.28, 95% CI = 1.06–1.54, n = 5 studies; OR = 1.15, 95% CI = 1.03–1.29, n = 10 studies) (Kedzior and Laeber, 2014; Twomey, 2017). Cohorts with anxiety were more likely to use cannabis or have CUD (Kedzior and Laeber, 2014). More recently, a systematic review (n = 24 studies) and meta-analysis (n = 7 studies) investigated the prospective long-term association between cannabis use and anxiety (Xue et al., 2020). Cannabis use was found to be significantly associated with increased odds of developing anxiety at follow-up (OR = 1.25; 95% CI = 1.01–1.54; I^2 = 39%). When the analysis was restricted to studies using a structured diagnostic interview rather than self-report, the strength of the association decreased (OR = 1.15; 95% CI = 1.01–1.30). When the analysis was restricted to high-quality studies, the association was statistically insignificant (OR = 1.10; 95% CI = 0.82–1.47). When specific anxiety disorders were considered individually, cannabis use was not associated with increased odds of developing GAD (OR = 1.44; 95% CI = 0.94–2.22, I^2 = 35%), SAD (OR = 1.12; 95%

CI = 0.61–2.05; I^2 = 38%), or PD (OR = 1.52; 95% CI = 0.96–2.40, I^2 = 0%).

Many studies have used data collected over a three-year period from the National Epidemiologic Survey on Alcohol and Related Conditions (NESARC). One such study found that cannabis use in the 12 months preceding the survey was not associated with an increased prevalence of anxiety disorders (OR = 1.0; 95% CI = 0.8–1.2) after adjusting for confounders (Blanco et al., 2016). At the 3-year follow-up, although no significant relationship between cannabis use and the prevalence of PD, SAD, specific phobia, or GAD was found, increased frequency of cannabis use was associated with significantly increased odds of incident SAD (OR = 1.8; 95% CI = 1.1–2.8). In another three-year prospective study, the association between cannabis use, CUD, and anxiety disorders was explored. The study concluded that cannabis use was not associated with increased incidence of any anxiety disorder at follow-up (AOR = 1.12; 95% CI = 0.63–0.98) (Feingold et al., 2016). Heavy cannabis use was associated with incident SAD, but the association was not fully retained in the final adjusted model, except among adults (OR = 2.83; 95% CI = 1.26–6.35). There was a significant association between baseline CUD and incident SAD among young adults (AOR = 2.45; 95% CI = 1.19–5.06).

11.6.2 Anxiety as a Predictor of Cannabis Use

Fewer studies have investigated the reverse association: anxiety as a predictor of cannabis use. In a 14-year prospective longitudinal study, after adjusting for confounding variables, such as mood disorders, conduct disorder, gender, and other anxiety disorders, the presence of SAD at the first interview was not significantly associated with greater odds of cannabis abuse in men (OR = 0.99; 95% CI = 0.38–2.59; p = 0.98) or women (OR = 2.40; 99% CI = 0.77–7.52; p = 0.048) (Buckner et al., 2008). Similarly, a three-year prospective study concluded that a baseline anxiety disorder was not associated with future initiation of cannabis (AOR = 0.93; 95% CI = 0.58–1.51) or onset of CUD (AOR = 0.68; 95% CI = 0.41–1.14). When the data were stratified, having PD at baseline increased the risk of cannabis use at follow-up among older adults (AOR = 2.83; 95% CI = 1.44–5.55), but not young adults (AOR = 1.04; 95% CI = 0.21–5.18) (Feingold et al., 2016).

> **Box 11.5 Cannabis as a predictor of anxiety**
>
> The data is equivocal across studies investigating cannabis use as a predictor of anxiety. This may be attributed to differences in sample location, sample sizes, and time between baseline and follow-up assessments of cannabis use and anxiety disorders/symptoms.

11.7 Cannabis Use Disorder and Anxiety

The United Nations estimated that there were 192 million past-year cannabis users worldwide in 2018 (United Nations, 2020). Prevalence rates of past-year cannabis use vary across countries and continents, with higher estimates reported in North America (12.4%), West and Central Africa (12.4%), and Oceania (10.3%) than across Asia (1.8%), North Africa (4.3%), and Eastern and Southern Europe (2.4%) (Peacock et al., 2018). CUD is defined as a problematic pattern of cannabis use leading to clinically significant impairment or distress. Globally, it is estimated that 22.1 million people met CUD diagnostic criteria in 2016 (289.7 cases per 100,000 people) (Degenhardt et al., 2018). Unfortunately, very few countries have collected longitudinal data on cannabis use disorders. Nevertheless, data from the United States suggests that approximately 30% of those who use cannabis will develop CUD (Hasin et al., 2015). Hasin et al. reported the past-year prevalence of DSM-IV CUD was 1.5% (0.08) in 2001–2002 compared to 2.9% (0.13) in 2012–2013 ($p < 0.05$). Consistent with data from the United States, Health Canada suggests that one in three cannabis users will develop problems with their usage, and 9% will develop an addiction (Health Canada, 2019). If an individual uses cannabis daily, there is a 25–50% risk of developing an addiction (Health Canada, 2019). Changes to the potency, legal status, and social acceptance of cannabis are speculated to contribute to the observed changes in cannabis use and CUD prevalence rates over time (Connor et al., 2021). For further discussion of these issues, the reader is referred to Chapters 4–6.

Meta-analytic evidence has indicated positive associations between both anxiety and CUD (OR = 1.68, 95% CI = 1.23–2.31, p = 0.004) (Kedzior and Laeber, 2014), and between CUD and GAD (OR = 2.99; 95% CI = 2.14–4.16) (Onaemo et al., 2020). However, the current evidence appears to be strongest for an association between CUD and SAD. Approximately 25–33% of people with cannabis dependence have comorbid SAD, which is a higher rate than for comorbid PD (6–10%), GAD (12–21%), or PTSD (18–20%) (Agosti et al., 2002; Stinson et al., 2006). In non-clinical samples, heightened social anxiety symptoms have been correlated with greater problems associated with cannabis consumption, such as using cannabis to cope in social situations. Conversely, individuals with heightened social anxiety symptoms may avoid social situations altogether where cannabis is unavailable or where they fear judgment for either their use of an illicit substance or their behaviour while intoxicated (Buckner et al., 2006, 2007, 2008, 2011, 2012a). In a sample of past-month cannabis users, aged 18–36, elevated social anxiety was associated with greater cannabis-related impairment in social, occupational, physical, and personal life facets (Foster et al., 2016). Finally, a cross-sectional study from the Wave 1 NESARC data examined individuals with SAD, CUD, or SAD-CUD comorbidity. The study found that SAD onset precedes CUD onset in most individuals with SAD-CUD comorbidity. SAD-CUD comorbidity led to greater psychiatric comorbidity and impairment than either disorder alone (Buckner et al., 2012b).

11.8 Conclusion

Many large-scale survey studies suggest that cannabis is being used in the community for the treatment of anxiety symptoms. Unfortunately, the evidence examining cannabis as a psychopharmacological treatment for anxiety consists of a few, primarily single-dose studies with small sample sizes. Although there is a signal for efficacy, the limitations of the study designs limit the clinical application of these findings. Further RCT investigations using repeated administration in clinical populations are urgently required to adequately address this important issue. Additionally, the current literature mainly focuses on cannabinoid compounds rather than plant-based cannabis. No recommendations can be made regarding the clinical utility of cannabis as a treatment for anxiety disorders without evaluating the effects of the plant as a whole. Plant-based studies are needed to identify the specific effects of different cannabis strains, frequencies, dosages, times of intake, and routes of administration (D'Souza and Ranganathan, 2015). Additionally, cannabis is rarely used independently, as it is often used concurrently with alcohol (Downey et al., 2013). Therefore, it is important for future studies to investigate the interactions between cannabis, other medications, and recreational substances. Further studies should also investigate whether the therapeutic benefits of cannabis are comparable to conventional psychopharmacological treatments in order to better understand the potential role of cannabis in the compendium of psychopharmacological treatment of anxiety disorders.

References

Abrams, D. I., Jay, C. A., Shade, S. B., et al. (2007). Cannabis in painful HIV-associated sensory neuropathy: A randomized placebo-controlled trial. *Neurology*, **68**, 515–521.

Agosti, V., Nunes, E., and Levin, F. (2002). Rates of psychiatric comorbidity among US residents with lifetime cannabis dependence. *Am J Drug Alcohol Abuse*, **28**, 643–652.

Amar, M. B. (2006). Cannabinoids in medicine: A review of their therapeutic potential. *J Ethnopharmacol*, **105**, 1–25.

Aragona, M., Onesti, E., Tomassini, V., et al. (2009). Psychopathological and cognitive effects of therapeutic cannabinoids in multiple sclerosis: A double-blind, placebo controlled, crossover study. *Clin Neuropharmacol*, **32**, 41–47.

Baxter, A. J., Scott, K. M., Vos, T., et al. (2013). Global prevalence of anxiety disorders: A systematic review and meta-regression. *Psychol Med*, **43**, 897–910.

Bedi, G., Cooper, Z. D., and Haney, M. (2013). Subjective, cognitive and cardiovascular dose-effect progile of nabilone and dronabinol in marijuana smokers. *Addict Biol*, **18**, 872–881.

Bergamaschi, M. M., Queiroz, R. H. C., Chagas, M. H. N., et al. (2011). Cannabidiol reduces the anxiety induced by simulated public speaking in treatment-naive social phobia patients. *Neuropsychopharmacology*, **36**, 1219–1226.

Bhattacharyya, S., Morrison, P. D., Fusar-Poli, P., et al. (2010). Opposite effects of Δ-9-tetrahydrocannabinol and cannabidiol on human brain function and psychopathology. *Neuropsychopharmacology*, **35**, 764–774.

Black, N., Stockings, E., Campbell, G., et al. (2019). Cannabinoids for the treatment of mental disorders and symptoms of mental disorders: A systematic review and meta-analysis. *Lancet Psychiatry*, **6**, 995–1010.

Blanco, C., Hasin, D. S., Wall, M. M., et al. (2016). Cannabis use and risk of psychiatric disorders: Prospective evidence from a US national longitudinal study. *JAMA Psychiatry*, **73**, 388–395.

Bonn-Miller, M. O., Zvolensky, M. J., and Bernstein, A. (2007). Marijuana use motives: Concurrent relations to frequency of past 30-day use and anxiety sensitivity among young adult marijuana smokers. *Addict Behav*, **32**, 49–62.

Borgelt, L., Franson, K., Nussbaum, A., et al. (2013). The pharmacologic and clinical effects of medical cannabis. *Pharmacotherapy*, **33**, 195–209.

Bossong, M. G., Van Hell, H. H., Jager, G., et al. (2013). The endocannabinoid system and emotional processing: A pharmacological fMRI study with Δ9-tetrahydrocannabinol. *Eur Neuropsychopharmacol*, **23**, 1687–1697.

Buckner, J. D., Bonn-Miller, M. O., Zvolensky, M. J., et al. (2007). Marijuana use motives and social anxiety among marijuana-using young adults. *Addict Behav*, **32**, 2238–2252.

Buckner, J. D., Heimberg, R. G., Matthews, R. A., et al. (2012a). Marijuana-related problems and social anxiety: The role of marijuana behaviors in social situations. *Psychol Addict Behav*, **26**, 151.

Buckner, J. D., Heimberg, R. G., and Schmidt, N. B. (2011). Social anxiety and marijuana-related problems: The role of social avoidance. *Addict Behav*, **36**, 129–132.

Buckner, J. D., Heimberg, R. G., Schneier, F. R., et al. (2012b). The relationship between cannabis use disorders and social anxiety

disorder in the National Epidemiological Study of Alcohol and Related Conditions (NESARC). *Drug Alcohol Depend*, **124**, 128–134.

Buckner, J. D., Schmidt, N. B., Bobadilla, L., et al. (2006). Social anxiety and problematic cannabis use: Evaluating the moderating role of stress reactivity and perceived coping. *Behav Res Ther*, **44**, 1007–1015.

Buckner, J. D., Schmidt, N. B., Lang, A. R., et al. (2008). Specificity of social anxiety disorder as a risk factor for alcohol and cannabis dependence. *J Psychiatr Res*, **42**, 230–239.

Bystritsky, A. (2006). Treatment-resistant anxiety disorders. *Mol Psychiatry*, **11**, 805–814.

Campos, A. C., and Guimarães, F. S. (2009). Evidence for a potential role for TRPV1 receptors in the dorsolateral periaqueductal gray in the attenuation of the anxiolytic effects of cannabinoids. *Prog Neuro-Psychopharmacol Biol Psychiatry*, **33**, 1517–1521.

Connor, J. P., Stjepanović, D., Le Foll, B., et al. (2021). Cannabis use and cannabis use disorders. *Nat Rev Dis Primers*, **7**, 1–24.

Corroon, J., and Phillips, J. A. (2018). A cross-sectional study of cannabidiol users. *Cannabis Cannabinoid Res*, **3**, 152–161.

Crippa, J. A., Derenusson, G. N., Ferrari, T. B., et al. (2011). Neural basis of anxiolytic effects of cannabidiol (CBD) in generalized social anxiety disorder: A preliminary report. *J Psychopharmacol*, **25**, 121–130.

Crippa, J. A., Guimaraes, F. S., Campos, A. C., et al. (2018). Translational investigation of the therapeutic potential of cannabidiol (CBD): Toward a new age. *Front Immunol*, **9**, 2009.

Crippa, J. A., Zuardi, A. W., Garrido, G. E., et al. (2004). Effects of cannabidiol (CBD) on regional

cerebral blood flow. *Neuropsychopharmacology*, **29**, 417–426.

Cuttler, C., Spradlin, A., and McLaughlin, R. J. (2018). A naturalistic examination of the perceived effects of cannabis on negative affect. *J Affect Disord*, **235**, 198–205.

D'Souza, D. C., Perry, E., MacDougall, L., et al. (2004). The psychotomimetic effects of intravenous delta-9-tetrahydrocannabinol in healthy individuals: Implications for psychosis. *Neuropsychopharmacology*, **29**, 1558–1572.

D'Souza, D. C., and Ranganathan, M. (2015). Medical marijuana: Is the cart before the horse? *JAMA*, **313**, 2431–2432.

De Vries, M., Van Rijckevorsel, D. C., Vissers, K. C., et al. (2017). Tetrahydrocannabinol does not reduce pain in patients with chronic abdominal pain in a phase 2 placebo-controlled study. *Clin Gastroenterol Hepatol*, **15**, 1079–1086.

Degenhardt, L., Charlson, F., Ferrari, A., et al. (2018). The global burden of disease attributable to alcohol and drug use in 195 countries and territories, 1990–2016: A systematic analysis for the Global Burden of Disease Study 2016. *Lancet Psychiatry*, **5**, 987–1012.

Downey, L. A., King, R., Papafotiou, K., et al. (2013). The effects of cannabis and alcohol on simulated driving: Influences of dose and experience. *Accid Anal Prev*, **50**, 879–886.

Fabre, L. F., and McLendon, D. (1981). The efficacy and safety of nabilone (a synthetic cannabinoid) in the treatment of anxiety. *J Clin Pharmacol*, **21**, 377S–382S.

Feingold, D., Rehm, J., Factor, H., et al. (2018). Clinical and functional outcomes of cannabis use among individuals with anxiety disorders:

A 3-year population-based longitudinal study. *Depress Anxiety*, **35**, 490–501.

Feingold, D., Weiser, M., Rehm, J., et al. (2016). The association between cannabis use and anxiety disorders: Results from a population-based representative sample. *Eur Neuropsychopharmacology*, **26**, 493–505.

Foster, D. W., Buckner, J. D., Schmidt, N. B., et al. (2016). Multisubstance use among treatment-seeking smokers: Synergistic effects of coping motives for cannabis and alcohol use and social anxiety/depressive symptoms. *Subst Use Misuse*, **51**, 165–178.

Frank, B., Serpell, M. G., Hughes, J., et al. (2008). Comparison of analgesic effects and patient tolerability of nabilone and dihydrocodeine for chronic neuropathic pain: Randomised, crossover, double blind study. *BMJ*, **336**, 199–201.

Fusar-Poli, P., Crippa, J. A., Bhattacharyya, S., et al. (2009). Distinct effects of Δ9-tetrahydrocannabinol and cannabidiol on neural activation during emotional processing. *Arch Gen Psychiatry*, **66**, 95–105.

Gambino, A., Cabras, M., Panagiotakos, E., et al. (2021). Evaluating the suitability and potential efficiency of cannabis sativa oil for patients with primary burning mouth syndrome: A prospective, open-label, single-arm pilot study. *Pain Med*, **22**, 142–151.

Glass, R. M., Uhlenhuth, E. H., Hartel, F. W., et al. (1981). Single-dose study of nabilone in anxious volunteers. *J Clin Pharmacol*, **21**, 383S–396S.

Hasin, D. S., Saha, T. D., Kerridge, B. T., et al. (2015). Prevalence of marijuana use disorders in the United States between 2001–2002 and 2012–2013. *JAMA Psychiatry*, **72**, 1235–1242.

Health Canada. (2019). *Addiction to Cannabis*. Available at: www.canada.ca/en/health-canada/services/drugs-medication/cannabis/health-effects/addiction.html. Last accessed 30 October 2022.

Karniol, I. G., Shirakawa, I., Kasinski, N., et al. (1974). Cannabidiol interferes with the effects of Δ9-tetrahydrocannabinol in man. *Eur J Pharmacol*, **28**, 172–177.

Katzman, M. A., Bleau, P., Blier, P., et al. (2014). Canadian clinical practice guidelines for the management of anxiety, posttraumatic stress and obsessive-compulsive disorders. *BMC Psychiatry*, **14**, 1.

Kedzior, K. K., and Laeber, L. T. (2014). A positive association between anxiety disorders and cannabis use or cannabis use disorders in the general population: A meta-analysis of 31 studies. *BMC Psychiatry*, **14**, 1–22.

Kessler, R. C., Chiu, W. T., Demler, O., et al. (2005). Prevalence, severity, and comorbidity of 12-month DSM-IV disorders in the National Comorbidity Survey Replication. *Arch Gen Psychiatry*, **62**, 617–627.

Korem, N., Zer-Aviv, T. M., Ganon-Elazar, E., et al. (2016). Targeting the endocannabinoid system to treat anxiety-related disorders. *J Basic Clinical Physiol Pharmacol*, **27**, 193–202.

Leehey, M. A., Liu, Y., Hart, F., et al. (2020). Safety and tolerability of cannabidiol in Parkinson disease: An open label, dose-escalation study. *Cannabis Cannabinoid Res*, **5**, 326–336.

Linares, I. M., Zuardi, A. W., Pereira, L. C., et al. (2019). Cannabidiol presents an inverted U-shaped dose–response curve in a simulated public speaking test. *Braz J Psychiatry*, **41**, 9–14.

Lintzeris, N., Driels, J., Elias, N., et al. (2018). Medicinal cannabis in Australia, 2016: The cannabis as medicine survey (CAMS-16). *Med J Aust*, **209**, 211–216.

Malik, Z., Bayman, L., Valestin, J., et al. (2017). Dronabinol increases pain threshold in patients with functional chest pain: A pilot double-blind placebo-controlled trial. *Dis Esophagus*, **30**, 1–8.

Mammen, G., Rueda, S., Roerecke, M., et al. (2018). Association of cannabis with long-term clinical symptoms in anxiety and mood disorders: A systematic review of prospective studies. *J Clin Psychiatry*, **79**, 2248.

Marteau, T. M., and Bekker, H. (1992). The development of a six-item short-form of the state scale of the Spielberger State – Trait Anxiety Inventory (STAI). *Br J Clin Psychol*, **31**, 301–306.

Moreno, J. L. L. S., Caldentey, J. G., Cubillo, P. T., et al. (2016). A double-blind, randomized, cross-over, placebo-controlled, pilot trial with Sativex in Huntington's disease. *J Neurol*, **263**, 1390–1400.

Narang, S., Gibson, D., Wasan, A. D., et al. (2008). Efficacy of dronabinol as an adjuvant treatment for chronic pain patients on opioid therapy. *J Pain*, **9**, 254–264.

National Academies of Sciences, Engineering, and Medicine. (2017). *The Health Effects of Cannabis and Cannabinoids: The Current State of Evidence and Recommendations for Research*. Washington, DC: National Academies Press, pp. 289–327.

Olfson, M., Marcus, S. C., Tedeschi, M., et al. (2006). Continuity of antidepressant treatment for adults with depression in the United States. *Am J Psychiatry*, **163**, 101–108.

Onaemo, V. N., Fawehinmi, T. O., and D'Arcy, C. (2020). Comorbid cannabis use disorder with major depression and generalized anxiety disorder: A systematic review and meta-analyses of nationally representative epidemiological surveys. *J Affect Disord*, **281**, 467–475.

Peacock, A., Leung, J., Larney, S., et al. (2018). Global statistics on alcohol, tobacco and illicit drug use: 2017 status report. *Addiction*, **113**, 1905–1926.

Pertwee, R. (2009). Emerging strategies for exploiting cannabinoid receptor agonists as medicines. *Br J Pharmacol*, **156**, 397–411.

Pini, L. A., Guerzoni, S., Cainazzo, M. M., et al. (2012). Nabilone for the treatment of medication overuse headache: Results of a preliminary double-blind, active-controlled, randomized trial. *J Headache Pain*, **13**, 677–684.

Rog, D. J., Nurmikko, T. J., Friede, T., et al. (2005). Randomized, controlled trial of cannabis-based medicine in central pain in multiple sclerosis. *Neurology*, **65**, 812–819.

Shannon, S., Lewis, N., Lee, H., et al. (2019). Cannabidiol in anxiety and sleep: A large case series. *Perm J*, **23**, 18-041.

Skrabek, R. Q., Galimova, L., Ethans, K., et al. (2008). Nabilone for the treatment of pain in fibromyalgia. *J Pain*, **9**, 164–173.

Spinella, T. C., Stewart, S. H., Naugler, J., et al. (2021). Evaluating cannabidiol (CBD) expectancy effects on acute stress and anxiety in healthy adults: A randomized crossover study. *Psychopharmacology*, **238**, 1965–1977.

Stinson, F. S., Ruan, W. J., Pickering, R., et al. (2006). Cannabis use disorders in the USA: Prevalence, correlates and co-morbidity. *Psychol Med*, **36**, 1447.

Thompson, E. R. (2007). Development and validation of an internationally reliable short-form of the Positive and Negative Affect Schedule (PANAS). *J Cross-Cult Psychol*, **38**, 227–242.

Toth, C., Mawani, S., Brady, S., et al. (2012). An enriched-enrolment, randomized withdrawal, flexible-dose, double-blind, placebo-controlled, parallel assignment efficacy study of nabilone as adjuvant in the treatment of diabetic peripheral neuropathic pain. *Pain*, **153**, 2073–2082.

Turna, J., Simpson, W., Patterson, B., et al. (2019). Cannabis use behaviors and prevalence of anxiety and depressive symptoms in a cohort of Canadian medicinal cannabis users. *J Psychiatr Res*, **111**, 134–139.

Twomey, C.D. (2017). Association of cannabis use with the development of elevated anxiety symptoms in the general population: A meta-analysis. *J Epidemiol Community Health*, **71**, 811–816.

United Nations (2020). *World Drug Report 2020*. Vienna: UNODC.

Xue, S., Husain, M. I., Zhao, H., et al. (2020). Cannabis use and prospective long-term association with anxiety: A systematic review and meta-analysis of longitudinal studies. *Can J Psychiatry*, **66**, 126–138.

Zeyl, V., Sawyer, K., and Wightman R. S. (2020). What do you know about maryjane? A systematic review of the current data on the THC:CBD ratio. *Subst Use Misuse*, **55**, 1223–1227.

Zuardi, A. W., Cosme, R. A., Graeff, F. G., et al. (1993). Effects of ipsapirone and cannabidiol on human experimental anxiety. *J Psychopharmacol*, **7**(1_suppl), 82–88.

Zuardi, A. W., Hallak, J. E., and Crippa, J. A. (2012). Interaction between cannabidiol (CBD) and Δ(9)-tetrahydrocannabinol (THC): Influence of administration interval and dose ratio between the cannabinoids. *Psychopharmacology*, **219**, 247–249.

Zuardi, A. W., Shirakawa, I., Finkelfarb, E., et al. (1982). Action of cannabidiol on the anxiety and other effects produced by Δ9-THC in normal subjects. *Psychopharmacology*, **76**, 245–250.

Cannabis Consumption and Risk of Depression and Suicidal Behaviour

Gabriella Gobbi

Depression affects about 5% of the population and represents the leading cause of absenteeism from work. Depression (also known as major depressive disorder) is characterized by a persistent depressed mood and/or anhedonia (i.e., lack of interest or pleasure in all or most activities). In addition to these primary symptoms, individuals may present with additional symptoms, including difficulties in concentration and indecisiveness, reduced energy, slowed thought and physical movement, changes in weight and sleep, feelings of worthlessness and guilt, as well as recurrent thoughts of death and recurrent suicidal ideation (American Psychiatric Association, 2013).

The causes of depression are not fully elucidated, and it is probably caused by multiple factors. In recent years, a plethora of animal studies and epidemiological studies, including meta-analyses, have affirmed a neurobiological link between cannabis use and the risk of developing mood disorders.

12.1 The Link between Cannabis and Depression: Evidence from Animal Studies

The link between CB1 agonists and the development of depression has been evaluated in several animal studies. The potent CB1 agonist WIN55,212-2, at low doses, increases serotonin 5-HT firing activity (5-HT being the main neurotransmitter implicated in depression), paralleled by increased swimming in the forced swimming tests (a measure of anti-depressant effect) but, at higher doses, it decreases 5-HT electrical activity (Bambico et al., 2007). Chronic administration of WIN55,212-2 in adolescent rats, but not adult rats, produces a depressive-like phenotype and anxiety-like phenotype, with a decrease in 5-HT activity and low norepinephrine (NE) activity, which is a hallmark of increased anxiety-like behaviour. Similarly, adolescent delta-9-tetrahydrocannabinol (THC) exposure results

in depressive behaviours and increased anxiety. Interestingly, increased anxiety, as well as a significant reduction in 5-HT neural activity, was also detected after THC adult exposure, suggesting that long-term exposure to cannabis may also affect the mature adult brain (De Gregorio et al., 2020). Studies have also demonstrated that, following chronic adolescent cannabinoid exposure, dopamine neurons become less responsive to the stimulating action of cannabinoids and a long-lasting cross-tolerance for morphine, cocaine, and amphetamine occur (Pistis et al., 2004). Rats administered THC during adolescence also have fewer synaptic contacts during adulthood and reduced efficiency of hippocampal networks (Rubino et al., 2009); these differences may constitute the neurobiological underpinning of the cognitive and behavioural deficits that are observed in humans. Some of the detrimental effects of cannabis on social behaviour, anhedonia, and depressive-like behaviour seem more pronounced in females, in both animals and humans (Rubino and Parolaro, 2016). The behavioural changes are paralleled by a decrease in anandamide (the naturally occurring substrate for the CB1 receptor) and increase in CB1 receptor density (Rubino et al., 2015), suggesting that long-term cannabis exposure changes the endogenous endocannabinoid system.

12.2 The Link between Cannabis and Depression: Evidence from Human Studies

It is well known that cannabis is frequently used by people who suffer from depression, especially adolescents, since, in the short-term, it produces an elevation of mood (called 'high') as well as a decrease in anxiety and irritability; however, after long-term use, the depressive symptomatology worsens.

People with depressive symptoms use cannabis to cope with negative emotions (Moitra et al., 2015). For example, it was reported that 50% of medical cannabis users observed a reduction in depression and 58% reduction in anxiety and stress following cannabis smoking (Cuttler et al., 2018). The link between depression and frequent cannabis use (or cannabis use disorder) might, thus, be a symptom of maladaptive coping efforts (Ketcherside and Filbey, 2015).

On the other hand, some research indicates that even adolescents without pre-morbid depressive symptoms, who start using cannabis only for recreational purposes, are more likely to develop depression later in life after long-term use (Gobbi et al., 2019).

Here we present the studies in subjects who (i) use cannabis to self-medicate depressive mood and (ii) started recreational cannabis use for social/personal reasons and then developed depression.

12.2.1 Cannabis Use as Self-Medication for Depression

The relationship may be bidirectional, meaning that individuals with a cannabis use disorder are at increased risk of a depressive episode (Smolkina et al., 2017), and individuals who initiate cannabis use while experiencing considerable depressive symptoms are more likely to develop a cannabis use disorder (Rhew et al., 2017).

Cannabis is a commonly used substance among individuals experiencing symptoms of depression (Leadbeater et al., 2019), and especially those seeking treatment for major depression (Bahorik et al., 2017). Several studies have reported that depression is related to more frequent cannabis use among males (Assari et al., 2018; Crane et al., 2015).

Depression can trigger cannabis use (Bahorik et al., 2017; Wilkinson et al., 2016), although not all individuals who experience depression use cannabis regularly. For example, in adolescents, the rate of cannabis use is higher in depressed individuals compared to non-depressed: 41% of depressed adolescents consume cannabis versus 27% of non-depressed adolescents consume cannabis (Degenhardt et al., 2010). However, it must be noted that, in this study, 59% of adolescents with depression never consumed cannabis, suggesting that other factors must be present to increase the risk of cannabis consumption in the presence of depressive symptomatology.

Indeed, depression per se is *not a risk factor* for cannabis consumption (Womack et al., 2016) and there is limited evidence for a self-medication

hypothesis. It was reported that depression eventually becomes a risk factor for cannabis/alcohol use in grade 10, only when it is associated with other factors in grade 7–8, such as low school grades, alcohol intoxication, delinquency, poor communication with parents, lack of parental rules, conflict with parents, separated parents, and drug use by closest friends (Briere et al., 2011). Other studies have found that the peer pressure as well as a poor school bonding are also significant contributing factors for recreational cannabis use (Gobbi et al., 2019; Marmorstein and Iacono, 2011).

Cannabis use may worsen depression and contribute to poorer overall mental health (Bahorik et al., 2017; Mammen et al., 2018); on the other hand, abstinence from cannabis leads to reductions in symptom severity (Jacobus et al., 2017). For these reasons, the cannabis use disorder should be always addressed in the treatment of patients with major depression.

12.2.2 Cannabis Use (Non-Self-Medication) and Risk of Depression

Gobbi et al. (2019) investigated the question of whether cannabis consumption can increase the risk of depression even in adolescents who did not have any symptoms of depression *before* starting their recreational cannabis use. A systematic review and meta-analysis of international studies comprising 23,317 individuals revealed that cannabis use in adolescence could harmfully alter mental health, even in adolescents who did not report any depressive symptoms before starting cannabis use. Indeed, these individuals reported an increase of 40% in the risk of depression (see Figure 12.1), a 50% increase in suicidal ideation, and a 300% elevation in suicide attempts.

It is important to emphasize that, in studies that have controlled for pre-existing depression (depression before starting recreational cannabis), there was minimal heterogeneity, meaning a good concordance in the association between cannabis consumption and increased risk of depression (D. W. Brook et al., 2002; J. S. Brook et al., 2001; Degenhardt et al., 2013; Georgiades and Boyle, 2007; Marmorstein and Iacono, 2011; Silins et al., 2014).

Interestingly, a few studies that also adjusted for childhood depression (Brook et al., 2002) and maternal/paternal depression (Marmorstein and Iacono, 2011) found that the risk for depression after recreational cannabis consumption is still high: OR = 1.44,

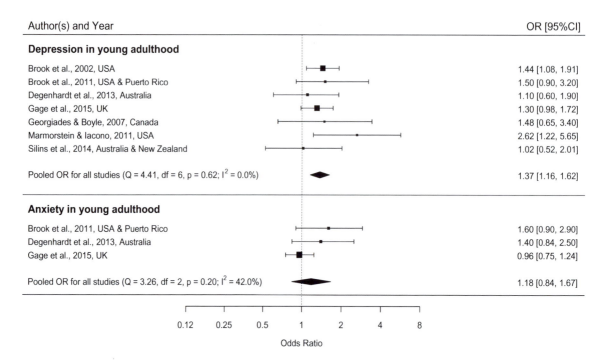

Forest plot showing adjusted ORs and 95% CIs for depression and anxiety in young adulthood according to cannabis use in individual studies

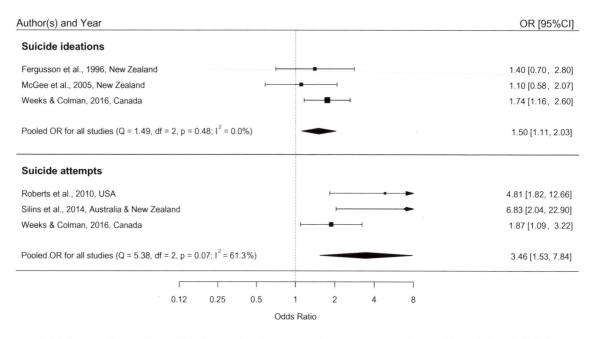

Forest plot showing adjusted ORs and 95% CIs for suicidal ideations and attempts according to cannabis use in individual studies.

Figure 12.1 Random effects meta-analysis of whether cannabis use during adolescence increases the odds of developing depression and anxiety in young adulthood

95% CI = 1.08–1.91 and OR = 2.62, 95% CI = 1.22–5.65, respectively. When the risk of depression is not adjusted for other factors, the OR is 15 or more (Patton et al., 2002).

Several meta-analyses have tested whether cannabis use leads to the development of depression within several months or many years following the initiation of cannabis use. Results from these analyses indicate that cannabis use is associated with increased risk of developing depression. In the general population, the risk is relatively low, especially after accounting for confounding variables, including the absence of premorbid depression, alcohol and substance use, age, sex, ethnicity, and education (Lev-Ran et al., 2014; Mammen et al., 2018; Moore et al., 2007). However, given the high prevalence of cannabis consumption among adolescents and young adults (about 20–30% in industrialized countries), the moderate risk of depression translates into a high number of depressions caused by cannabis (Gobbi et al., 2019).

Harder et al. (2008), in a mixed longitudinal-retrospective study, applied the high-dimensional propensity score (PS) adjustment to control for baseline depression in adolescent cannabis consumers and found that young adult depression was still elevated, with an OR of 1.33 (95% CI = 0.76–2.33).

Other studies have confirmed this evidence. Schoeler et al. (2018) studied a cohort from the Cambridge Study in Delinquent Development (CSDD) (N = 285) from age 8 to 48 years to prospectively investigate the association between cannabis use and risk of major depressive disorder (MDD). Early-onset cannabis use (before age 18), but not late-onset cannabis use (after age 27), was associated with a higher risk and shorter time until a subsequent MDD diagnosis. Conversely, MDD in adulthood (age 18–32) was linked to a reduction in subsequent cannabis use (age 32–48), suggesting the evidence that frequent cannabis use especially during neurodevelopment is a risk factor for later life depression.

More than 35 epidemiological studies have reported an association between cannabis and depression. Interestingly, most of these studies reported a positive correlation between adolescent cannabis use and later depression (Baggio et al., 2014; Fergusson and Horwood, 1997; Fleming et al., 2008; Wilkinson et al., 2016; Womack et al., 2016). A few studies analysed the different trajectories of cannabis use patterns from adolescence through to young adulthood. For example, one study of 1,232 first-year college students delineated six cannabis use trajectories encompassing non-use, late-increase use, college-peak use, and chronic use (Caldeira et al., 2012). The six trajectory groups were not significantly different in terms of year 1 health-related variables but differed on all 10-year mental health outcomes tested, including depression and anxiety. Non-users fared significantly better than most of the cannabis-using trajectory groups on every outcome tested. Chronic and late-increase users of cannabis fared the worst for the depression score of all groups, after controlling for gender, ethnicity, socioeconomic status, and tobacco and alcohol use.

In a different study, there was evidence that younger users of cannabis (aged 14–15) were at significantly higher risk for suicidal behaviours, although, overall, the association between cannabis use and depression did not vary with age (Fergusson et al., 2002). Another study (Otten and Engels, 2013) found an increased risk of depression among adolescents who possessed the short allele of the 5-HTTLPR genotype (s/s), evincing an interaction between genetics and an environmental exposure (Silins et al., 2014). Other trajectory studies likewise found positive associations between cannabis use during adolescence and later anxiety and depression ($p = 0.002$) paralleled by academic unpreparedness, delinquency ($p < 0.001$), and poorer academic performance ($p = 0.032$) (D'Amico et al., 2016).

In contrast, a few studies failed to find a statistical correlation between cannabis and depressive symptoms (Meier et al., 2015; Scholes-Balog et al., 2016; Van Gastel et al., 2014; Wilkinson et al., 2016; Windle and Wiesner, 2004). One study found no evidence of increased depression among non-users versus other groups, though the chronic group of users reported significantly more anxiety symptoms at age 33 than the other groups, after controlling for baseline anxiety (Epstein et al., 2015). Another study supported a self-medication hypothesis in males, in which adolescents with higher depressive symptoms at baseline used more cannabis (Wilkinson et al., 2016). This study failed to support a link between using cannabis as an adolescent and later depression in males or females, but found a positive association between tobacco and depression. A study of Swedish conscripts did not support an association between the use of cannabis and depression, but only with schizoaffective disorder (Manrique-Garcia et al., 2012); remarkably, in this study, subjects consuming cannabis were aged 18–20 at baseline, supporting the hypothesis that the late consumption of cannabis has less impact on subsequent risk of depression.

123

In synthesis, a plethora of evidence suggests that the use of cannabis is high in people with depressive symptoms, in a low social-economic environment, with poor school bonding, and use of other drugs and alcohol. In these 'vulnerable' people, the association between cannabis and depression is thus quite high. However, in studies that have controlled for pre-morbid condition, socio-economic status, and use of other drugs, the risk of developing depression after (recreational) cannabis exposure still remains moderate. The risk is low–medium but, given the high numbers of adolescents exposed to cannabis (20–30%), the increase in cases of depression remains high at a population level. Indeed, a rough estimation from our studies suggests that approximately 7% of cases of depression in Canadians and Americans between the ages of 18–30 is attributable to cannabis.

12.3 Cannabis and Suicidality

The risk of suicidality (i.e., suicide death, suicidal ideation, and suicide attempts) increases with the presence of psychiatric disorders, with depression, psychosis, and substance use disorders being the most relevant risk factors (Bradvik, 2018). Bagge and Borges (2017) showed that acute alcohol consumption, more than acute ingestion of cannabis, is responsible for suicidal attempts. However, a meta-analysis suggests that chronic cannabis use is associated with suicidal behaviour, albeit there is a high degree of heterogeneity among studies (Borges et al., 2016). The pooled ORs estimate for any cannabis use and suicide attempts was 2.23 (95% CI = 1.24–4), and for any heavy use, 3.2 (95% CI = 1.72–5.94).

A 14-year prospective study among adolescents and young adults (i.e., ages 11–21 years) found that drug use (cannabis and other drugs) was not associated with suicidal ideation, but that suicidal ideation increases the use of illicit drugs, suggesting a pattern of 'self-medication' for suicidal youth (Zhang and Wu, 2014). However, a 30-year follow-up of a population based cohort (van Ours et al., 2013) reported a large dose–response relation of cannabis with onset of suicidal ideation; this finding is consistent with other work that showed heavy cannabis use (in terms of high usage frequency) in adolescence to be associated with suicide attempts in young adulthood (Silins et al., 2014). A study of male Swedish conscripts

followed for 33 years reported that death by suicide was more common among those who had used cannabis more than 50 times, although this association disappeared after controlling for confounders (e.g., alcohol, tobacco, other drugs, psychiatric disorders) (Price et al., 2009).

Gobbi et al. (2019) pooled data from three studies examining the association of cannabis use during adolescence and subsequent suicidal ideation within adolescence and young adulthood and found an OR of 1.50 (95% CI = 1.11–2.03; $I^2 = 0\%$) (see Figure 12.1). For the number of suicide attempt outcomes within adolescence during young adulthood, the results were pooled with a consequential OR of 3.46 (95% CI = 1.53–7.84; $I^2 = 61.3\%$). However, the results for suicidal attempts showed a high degree of heterogeneity ($I^2 = 61.3\%$), meaning that these results are not conclusive. On the other hand, the results for suicidal ideation are quite consistent since the heterogeneity among studies was low ($I^2 = 0\%$). This latter finding is consonant with other primary studies (Delforterie et al., 2015; Kung et al., 2003, 2005; Moore et al., 2007; Shalit et al., 2016) as well as with the systematic review of Borges et al. (2016) reporting an increased risk of suicidal behaviours among both adolescents and young adults who have used cannabis.

Overall, chronic cannabis use is a risk factor for suicidal ideation as well as suicidal behaviours. There appear to be sex differences in this association. For example, there is evidence that the association between cannabis use and the incidence of suicidal ideation is significant only in males, while an association between baseline suicidality and new cannabis use is significantly only in females (van Ours et al., 2013; Shalit et al., 2016). On the other hand, a recent study by Han et al. (2021) found an association between cannabis use and suicidal ideation and attempts in all adult men and women, higher in women. Therefore, one must keep in mind that the relationship between cannabis use and suicidal behaviours is complex since it is influenced by factors beyond frequency of lifetime cannabis use, age at onset, and genetic pre-disposition.

The association between cannabis consumption and suicidality have recently been validated by using two-sample Mendelian randomization, which is a method using measured variation in genes of known function to examine the causal effect of a modifiable exposure on disease outcomes. Orri et al. (2021) found evidence supporting a possible causal role of cannabis (OR = 1.18; 95% CI = 1.01–1.37, $p = 0.032$), alcohol (OR = 1.95; 95% CI = 1.15–3.32, $p = 0.013$), and cigarette smoking (initiation, OR = 1.90; 95% CI = 1.54–2.34, $p < 0.001$) on suicide attempts. Interestingly, multivariate modelling showed that only cannabis showed a direct pathway to suicide attempt ($p = 0.001$). These results, using this sophisticated genetic analysis, suggest that cannabis plays a causal role in suicidality.

12.4 Conclusion

In summary, clinical studies suggest that cannabis is consumed by young people with depression largely for self-medication; however, its use, even in the absence of pre-morbid conditions, may also increase the risk of developing a mood disorder, and can drive impulsive and suicidal behaviours. Further studies are needed to understand why young people are more vulnerable than adults to the effects of cannabis on the brain.

References

American Psychiatric Association. (2013). *Diagnostic and Statistical Manual of Mental Disorders*, 5th ed. Washington, DC: American Psychiatric Association.

Assari, S., Lankarani, M. M., and Caldwell, C. H. (2018). Does discrimination explain high risk of depression among high-income African American men? *Behav Sci*, **8**, 40.

Bagge, C. L., and Borges, G. (2017). Acute substance use as a warning sign for suicide attempts: A case-crossover examination of the 48 hours prior to a recent suicide attempt. *J Clin Psychiatry*, **78**, 20169.

Baggio, S, N'Goran, A. A., Deline, S, et al. (2014). Patterns of cannabis use and prospective associations with health issues among young males. *Addiction*, **109**, 937–945.

Bahorik, A. L., Leibowitz, A., Sterling, S. A., et al. (2017). Patterns of marijuana use among psychiatry patients with depression and its impact on recovery. *J Affect Disord*, **213**, 168–171.

Bambico, F. R., Katz, N., Debonnel, G., et al. (2007). Cannabinoids elicit antidepressant-like behavior and activate serotonergic neurons through the medial prefrontal cortex. *J Neurosci*, **27**, 11700–11711.

Borges, G., Bagge, C. L., and Orozco, R. (2016). A literature review and meta-analyses of cannabis use and suicidality. *J Affect Disord*, **195**, 63–74.

Bradvik, L. (2018). Suicide risk and mental disorders. *Int J Environ Res Public Health*, **15**, 2028.

Briere, F. N., Fallu, J. S., Descheneaux, A., et al. (2011). Predictors and consequences of simultaneous alcohol and cannabis use in adolescents. *Addict Behav*, **36**, 785–788.

Brook, D. W., Brook, J. S., Zhang, C., et al. (2002). Drug use and the risk of major depressive disorder, alcohol dependence, and substance use disorders. *Arch Gen Psychiatry*, **59**, 1039–1044.

Brook, J. S., Brook, D. W., Arencibia-Mireles, O., et al. (2001). Risk factors for adolescent marijuana use across cultures and across time. *J Genet Psychol*, **162**, 357–374.

Caldeira, K. M., O'Grady, K. E., Vincent, K. B., et al. (2012). Marijuana use trajectories during the post-college transition: Health outcomes in young adulthood. *Drug Alcohol Depend*, **125**, 267–275.

Crane, N. A., Langenecker, S. A., and Mermelstein, R. J. (2015). Gender differences in the associations among marijuana use, cigarette use, and symptoms of depression during adolescence and young adulthood. *Addict Behav*, **49**, 33–39.

Cuttler, C., Spradlin, A., and McLaughlin, R. J. (2018). A naturalistic examination of the perceived effects of cannabis on negative affect. *J Affect Disord*, **235**, 198–205.

D'Amico, E. J., Tucker, J. S., Miles, J. N., et al. (2016). Alcohol and marijuana use trajectories in a diverse longitudinal sample of adolescents: Examining use patterns from age 11 to 17 years. *Addiction*, **111**, 1825–1835.

De Gregorio, D., Dean Conway, J., Canul, M. L., et al. (2020). Effects of chronic exposure to low doses of Delta9-tetrahydrocannabinol in adolescence and adulthood on serotonin/norepinephrine neurotransmission and emotional behaviors. *Int J Neuropsychopharmacol*, **23**, 751–761.

Degenhardt, L., Coffey, C., Carlin, J. B., et al. (2010). Outcomes of occasional cannabis use in adolescence: 10-year follow-up study in Victoria, Australia. *Br J Psychiatry*, **196**, 290–295.

Degenhardt, L., Coffey, C., Romaniuk, H., et al. (2013). The persistence of the association between adolescent cannabis use and common mental disorders into young adulthood. *Addiction*, **108**, 124–133.

Delforterie, M. J., Lynskey, M. T., Huizink, A. C., et al. (2015). The relationship between cannabis involvement and suicidal thoughts and behaviors. *Drug Alcohol Depend*, **150**, 98–104.

Epstein, M., Hill, K. G., Nevell, A. M., et al. (2015). Trajectories of marijuana use from adolescence into adulthood: Environmental and individual correlates. *Dev Psychol*, **51**, 1650–1663.

Fergusson, D. M., and Horwood, L. (1997). Early onset cannabis use and psychosocial adjustment in young adults. *Addiction*, **92**, 279–296.

Fergusson, D. M., Horwood, L. J., and Swain-Campbell, N. (2002). Cannabis use and psychosocial adjustment in adolescence and young adulthood. *Addiction*, **97**, 1123–1135.

Fleming, C. B., Mason, W. A., Mazza, J. J., et al. (2008). Latent growth modeling of the relationship between depressive symptoms and substance use during adolescence. *Psychol Addict Behav*, **22**, 186–197.

Georgiades, K., and Boyle, M. H. (2007). Adolescent tobacco and cannabis use: Young adult outcomes from the Ontario Child Health Study. *J Child Psychol Psychiatry*, **48**, 724–731.

Gobbi, G., Atkin, T., Zytynski, T., et al. (2019). Association of cannabis use in adolescence and risk of depression, anxiety, and suicidality in young adulthood: A systematic review and meta-analysis. *JAMA Psychiatry*, **76**, 426–434.

Han, B., Compton, W. M., Einstein, E. B., et al. (2021). Associations of suicidality trends with cannabis use as a function of sex and depression status. *JAMA Netw Open*, **4**, e2113025.

Harder, V. S., Stuart, E. A., and Anthony, J. C. (2008). Adolescent cannabis problems and young adult depression: Male–female stratified propensity score analyses. *Am J Epidemiol*, **168**, 592–601.

Jacobus, J., Squeglia, L., Escobar, S., et al. (2017). Changes in marijuana use symptoms and emotional functioning over 28-days of monitored abstinence in adolescent marijuana users. *Psychopharmacology*, **234**, 3431–3442.

Ketcherside, A., and Filbey, F. M. (2015). Mediating processes between stress and problematic marijuana use. *Addict Behav*, **45**, 113–118.

Kung, H. C., Pearson, J. L., and Liu, X. (2003). Risk factors for male and female suicide decedents ages 15–64 in the United States. Results from the 1993 National Mortality Followback Survey. *Soc Psychiatry Psychiatr Epidemiol*, **38**, 419–426.

Kung, H. C., Pearson, J. L., and Wei, R. (2005). Substance use, firearm availability, depressive symptoms, and mental health service utilization among white and African American suicide decedents aged 15 to 64 years. *Ann Epidemiol*, **15**, 614–621.

Leadbeater, B. J., Ames, M. E., and Linden-Carmichael, A. N. (2019). Age-varying effects of cannabis use frequency and disorder on symptoms of psychosis, depression and anxiety in adolescents and adults. *Addiction*, **114**, 278–293.

Lev-Ran, S., Roerecke, M., Le Foll, B., et al. (2014). The association between cannabis use and depression: A systematic review and meta-analysis of longitudinal studies. *Psychol Med*, **44**, 797–810.

Mammen, G., Rueda, S., Roerecke, M., et al. (2018). Association of cannabis with long-term clinical symptoms in anxiety and mood disorders: A systematic review of prospective studies. *J Clin Psychiatry*, **79**, 2248.

Manrique-Garcia, E., Zammit, S., Dalman, C., et al. (2012). Cannabis use and depression: A longitudinal study of a national cohort of Swedish conscripts. *BMC Psychiatry*, **12**, 112.

Marmorstein, N. R., and Iacono, W. G. (2011). Explaining associations between cannabis use disorders in adolescence and later major depression: A test of the psychosocial failure model. *Addict Behav*, **36**, 773–776.

Meier, M. H., Hill, M. L., Small, P. J., et al. (2015). Associations of adolescent cannabis use with academic performance and mental health: A longitudinal study of upper middle class youth. *Drug Alcohol Depend*, **156**, 207–212.

Moitra, E., Christopher, P. P., Anderson, B. J., et al. (2015). Coping-motivated marijuana use correlates with DSM-5 cannabis use disorder and psychological distress among emerging adults. *Psychol Addict Behav*, **29**, 627–632.

Moore, T. H., Zammit, S., Lingford-Hughes, A., et al. (2007). Cannabis use and risk of psychotic or affective mental health outcomes: A systematic review. *Lancet*, **370**, 319–328.

Orri, M., Seguin, J. R., Castellanos-Ryan, N., et al. (2021). A genetically informed study on the association of cannabis, alcohol, and tobacco smoking with suicide attempt. *Mol Psychiatry*, **26**, 5061–5070.

Otten, R., and Engels, R. C. (2013). Testing bidirectional effects between cannabis use and depressive symptoms: Moderation by the serotonin transporter gene. *Addict Biol*, **18**, 826–835.

van Ours, J. C., Williams, J., Fergusson, D., et al. (2013). Cannabis use and suicidal ideation. *J Health Econ*, **32**, 524–537.

Patton, G. C., Coffey, C., Carlin, J. B., et al. (2002). Cannabis use and mental health in young people: Cohort study. *BMJ*, **325**, 1195–1198.

Pistis, M., Perra, S., Pillolla, G., et al. (2004). Adolescent exposure to cannabinoids induces long-lasting changes in the response to drugs of abuse of rat midbrain dopamine neurons. *Biol Psychiatry*, **56**, 86–94.

Price, C., Hemmingsson, T., Lewis, G., et al. (2009). Cannabis and suicide: Longitudinal study. *Br J Psychiatry*, **195**, 492–497.

Rhew, I. C., Fleming, C. B., Vander Stoep, A., et al. (2017). Examination of cumulative effects of early adolescent depression on cannabis and alcohol use disorder in late adolescence in a community-based cohort. *Addiction*, **112**, 1952–1960.

Rubino, T., and Parolaro, D. (2016). The impact of exposure to cannabinoids in adolescence: Insights from animal models. *Biol Psychiatry*, **79**, 578–585.

Rubino, T., Prini, P., Piscitelli, F., et al. (2015). Adolescent exposure to THC in female rats disrupts developmental changes in the prefrontal cortex. *Neurobiol Dis*, **73**, 60–69.

Rubino, T., Realini, N., Braida, D., et al. (2009). Changes in hippocampal morphology and neuroplasticity induced by adolescent THC treatment are associated with cognitive impairment in adulthood. *Hippocampus*, **19**, 763–772.

Schoeler, T., Theobald, D., Pingault, J. B., et al. (2018). Developmental sensitivity to cannabis use patterns and risk for major depressive disorder in mid-life: Findings from 40 years of follow-up. *Psychol Med*, **48**, 2169–2176.

Scholes-Balog, K. E., Hemphill, S. A., Evans-Whipp, T. J., et al. (2016). Developmental trajectories of adolescent cannabis use and their relationship to young adult social and behavioural adjustment: A longitudinal study of Australian youth. *Addict Behav*, **53**, 11–18.

Shalit, N., Shoval, G., Shlosberg, D., et al. (2016). The association between cannabis use and suicidality among men and women: A population-based longitudinal study. *J Affect Disord*, **205**, 216–224.

Silins, E., Horwood, L. J., Patton, G. C., et al. (2014). Young adult sequelae of adolescent cannabis use: An integrative analysis. *Lancet Psychiatry*, **1**, 286–293.

Smolkina, M., Morley, K. I., Rijsdijk, F., et al. (2017). Cannabis and depression: A twin model approach to co-morbidity. *Behav Genet*, **47**, 394–404.

Van Gastel, W. A., Vreeker, A., Schubart, C. D., et al. (2014). Change in cannabis use in the general population: A longitudinal study on the impact on psychotic experiences. *Schizophr Res*, **157**, 266–270.

Wilkinson, A. L., Halpern, C. T., and Herring, A. H. (2016). Directions of the relationship between substance use and depressive symptoms from adolescence to young adulthood. *Addict Behav*, **60**, 64–70.

Windle, M., and Wiesner, M. (2004). Trajectories of marijuana use from adolescence to young adulthood: Predictors and outcomes. *Devel Psychopathol*, **16**, 1007–1027.

Womack, S. R., Shaw, D. S., Weaver, C. M., et al. (2016). Bidirectional associations between cannabis use and depressive symptoms from adolescence through early adulthood among at-risk young men. *J Stud Alcohol Drugs*, **77**, 287-297.

Zhang, X., and Wu, L. T. (2014). Suicidal ideation and substance use among adolescents and young adults: A bidirectional relation? *Drug Alcohol Depend*, **142**, 63–73.

Cannabis and Bipolar Disorder

Jairo Vinícius Pinto and Mauren Letícia Ziak

13.1 Introduction

Bipolar disorder (BD) is a common psychiatric disorder that has a global prevalence of 1–2% and whose onset usually occurs in early adulthood (Merikangas et al., 2012). BD is also one of the leading causes of disability and suicide worldwide (Gore et al., 2011). However, the course of BD can vary widely: Some patients have few mood episodes and mild psychosocial or neurocognitive functioning over time; conversely, others have a chronic, relapsing-remitting course with poor outcomes, psychosis, and suicide attempts, thereby resulting in progressive functional decline (Pinto et al., 2021). These differences in symptoms over time are partially due to comorbidities, particularly substance use disorders (SUD) (Berk et al., 2017).

BD has the highest prevalence of SUD among the major psychiatric conditions: SUDs affect over 30% of this population (Gibbs et al., 2015; Hunt et al., 2016a). Convergent evidence indicates that persons with co-occurring BD and SUD experience poorer treatment outcomes, such as more suicide attempts, higher rates of refractoriness to lithium, as well as more frequent and longer mood episodes (Hunt et al., 2016b; Pinto et al., 2019). It is noteworthy that cannabis has a complex association with bipolar disorder, being one of the most used substances in this population, with a growing number of studies addressing this association in recent years. However, the causality is yet to be clarified since the relationship between both disorders is complex and not unidirectional. For instance, lifetime SUD do not predict time to recovery from a depressive episode in persons with BD, but those with current or a past history of SUD are more likely to switch from depression to a manic, hypomanic, or mixed episode (Ostacher et al., 2010).

In this chapter we will summarize and appraise the evidence associating BD and cannabis use. First, we discuss the prevalence of cannabis use and the prevalence of co-occurring BD and cannabis use disorder (CUD). Second, we discuss the clinical characteristics and longitudinal outcomes associated with this co-occurrence. Third, we outline the findings on neurobiology and the current evidence on therapeutics. Finally, we highlight gaps in the current knowledge and suggest future directions for research.

13.2 Characteristics and Outcomes Associated with Cannabis Use in Bipolar Disorder

Although cannabis use is widespread in the general population, with approximately 192 million users worldwide (UNDOC, 2018), it is even more common in persons with BD. This population is 6.8 times more likely to report a lifetime history of cannabis use (Agrawal et al., 2011), reaching a point prevalence of up to 70% (Bally et al., 2014). Moreover, CUD is more common in persons with BD than in the general population, with meta-analyses estimating a pooled point prevalence of 17–24% (Hunt et al., 2016b; Pinto et al., 2019). Understanding the characteristics of persons with BD who use cannabis may shed light on the impact of co-occurring BD and CUD.

Several studies have described the sociodemographic and clinical characteristics of persons with co-occurring BD and CUD (Pinto et al., 2019). A meta-analysis of observational studies indicates that persons with co-occurring BD and CUD tend to be younger, male, single, and have fewer years of education, compared to persons with BD and without CUD (Pinto et al., 2019). Further, persons with co-occurring BD and CUD tend to experience an earlier onset of mood symptoms, are more likely to have psychotic symptoms and suicide attempts and have higher prevalence of other SUDs in comparison to persons with BD without CUD. Although this meta-analysis provides clinically relevant insights on the association between cannabis use and negative outcomes in BD, it was based on cross-sectional data, thereby hindering conclusions regarding causality (Pinto et al., 2019).

The onset of BD and cannabis use is essential for the investigation of clinical outcomes. For example, does cannabis use trigger the early onset of BD? Or, conversely, does the early onset of mood symptoms lead adolescents and young adults to use cannabis? Similarly, does cannabis use increase the chance of suicide attempts among persons with BD, or do persons with severe BD use cannabis to deal with suicide-related affect, cognitions, and behaviours?

Cross-sectional studies have the potential to characterize the sociodemographic and clinical features of persons with BD who use cannabis, whereas prospective longitudinal studies enable the researchers to investigate the temporal relationship between substance use and mood symptoms. Therefore, it is essential to gather data from longitudinal studies to better understand this relationship since this type of study may allow the comprehension of the temporal sequence of events.

A longitudinal study demonstrated in a five-year follow-up that cannabis use was associated with more time in affective episodes, as well as with rapid cycling bipolar disorder, which is defined as having at least four mood episodes in the previous year. Although most patients with CUD presented remission after hospitalization, they also experienced shorter time to recurrence of mood episodes (Strakowski et al., 2007). Likewise, other longitudinal studies showed lower remission rates in persons with BD who use cannabis, as well as more frequent recurrence and longer duration of mood episodes (Kim et al., 2015; Zorrilla et al., 2015).

Similar results regarding the outcomes were found in another study that investigated the course of BD according to individual patterns of cannabis use after a manic or mixed mood episode. During the 2-year follow-up, persons with BD who use cannabis had lower rates of recovery (defined as absent or nearly absent symptoms without relapse) and remission (defined as achieving functional remission and reporting adequate social functioning). They also presented a higher recurrence rate, defined as a new episode after remission, as well as poorer psychosocial functioning in comparison to cannabis-naïve persons with BD. Conversely, persons with BD and past but not current cannabis use had similar outcomes to

cannabis-naïve persons with BD, suggesting that persons with BD who stop using cannabis may be able to avoid some negative effects associated with the use of this substance (Zorrilla et al., 2015).

Besides discussing recurrence, remission, and psychosocial functioning, it is also crucial to investigate the impact of cannabis use on mortality, especially death by suicide. For instance, a population study showed that, despite the fact that SUD are predictors of all-cause mortality in persons with BD, cannabis use alone was not a significant predictor of all-cause deaths in this population (Hjorthøj et al., 2015). Although cannabis use alone did not predict deaths by suicide or by accidents in persons with BD, alcohol and other substances were significantly associated with such causes of death (Hjorthøj et al., 2015). However, another registry-based study involving persons with BD found an association between current – but not prior – cannabis use and a higher risk of completed suicide (Østergaard et al., 2017).

The studies described thus far showed that the use of cannabis has an impact on the longitudinal course of BD. However, they also showed that stopping the use of cannabis may avoid negative outcomes that are related to the use of this substance.

It is noteworthy that psychoactive substances, such as cannabis, can worsen mood or psychotic symptoms not only by their direct neurobiological effects, but also by decreasing the patient's adherence to treatment. This fact is demonstrated in a cohort in which persons with co-occurring BD and CUD were less likely to adhere to the pharmacotherapies than persons with BD and without CUD (González-Pinto et al., 2010). Thus, interventions for reducing substance use among persons with BD may improve clinical outcomes, which is especially critical during early adulthood, given growing evidence highlighting the effectiveness of early intervention (Pinto et al., 2021).

In Section 13.3, we will address the impact of CUD on the course of the illness throughout the life cycle, discussing the chronological aspects of this comorbidity.

13.3 Cannabis Use Disorder throughout the Course of Bipolar Disorder

The literature has shown that people at risk of developing BD can be identified before the emergence of manic or hypomanic episodes, even though the definitive diagnosis of BD requires the presence of full-blown symptoms. One of the most common approaches is to assess people that may have a genetic liability for developing BD, which consists of having at least one biological parent diagnosed with BD or with others serious mental illnesses, such as major depressive disorder or schizophrenia (Pinto et al., 2021). In longitudinal studies, cannabis use is associated with negative outcomes in persons with BD; therefore, it is crucial to study at-risk populations to understand the temporal relationship between cannabis use and the development of BD, as well as its impact on outcomes.

As an example, a longitudinal study investigated the relationship of substance use in high-risk offspring of parents with BD, showing that 23.7% of this at-risk population had comorbid SUD and cannabis was the most commonly used substance (16.6%). It is noteworthy that some of the clinical characteristics associated with the co-occurrence of BD and CUD were already seen in this at-risk population: males had an increased risk of SUD and the presence of a SUD increased the risk of subsequent psychotic symptoms (Duffy et al., 2012). Still, the relationship between cannabis use and the development of mood disorders is multidirectional and complex. While a prior history of mood disorders increased the risk of SUD by approximately 2.5-fold, a previous diagnosis of SUD also increased the risk of the subsequent development of BD by 3.4-fold, as well as of other mood disorders by 3-fold. Moreover, it is noteworthy that a history of SUD in parents with BD increased the risk of SUD in the offspring by 3-fold (Duffy et al., 2012).

Early-onset and delay in starting treatment are related to more severe symptoms and more frequent mood episodes in persons with BD. Thus, an early diagnosis with subsequent evidence-based treatment is necessary to improve outcomes (Post et al., 2010). Furthermore, early interventions should also include the correct identification and treatment of the co-occurring SUDs. In this sense, a cross-sectional study sought to investigate the prevalence and the characteristics of adolescents aged between 13 and 19 years old with BD who also had a SUD, comparing them to adolescents with BD and without SUD. Among the 33% of the adolescents with BD who had a co-occurring SUD, 25% had CUD. In 61% of the sample, the onset of SUD preceded that of BD, whereas in 18% the BD onset was before that of SUD. Further, diagnoses of panic disorder and oppositional defiant disorder were significantly associated with BD and SUD (Scavone et al., 2018).

Another longitudinal study assessed the temporal association between the onset of BD and the onset of CUD. Of all 144 patients evaluated, 47.9% had co-occurring BD and CUD. Approximately 25% were first diagnosed with BD and subsequently with CUD and 22.9% received the diagnosis of CUD first and were then diagnosed with BD. Notably, those who were diagnosed first with BD experienced an earlier onset of the illness, with a mean age at onset of seven years less than those diagnosed with CUD first (Strakowski et al., 2007). Similarly, another study showed that earlier onset of BD is associated with lifetime cannabis use, regardless of which disorder was recognized first (Lagerberg et al., 2011). The authors also showed, in another study, that persons with co-occurring BD and CUD had significantly earlier ages at onset of hypomanic/manic or depressive episodes (Lagerberg et al., 2014). Together, these studies demonstrate an association between cannabis use and earlier onset of BD; however, despite their longitudinal designs, these studies entailed retrospective data collection, and are thereby susceptible to recall and other types of biases.

The risk of developing BD among persons who use cannabis is a matter of ongoing controversy and requires longitudinal data to provide meaningful insights. An example is a populational study of 45,057 men in Sweden that had a 35-year follow-up period and aimed to assess whether cannabis use at ages of 18–20 years-old increases the risk of developing mood disorders. The authors found no impact of previous cannabis use on the development of BD, even among persons classified as engaging in 'high use' (defined as using cannabis more than 50 times during their lifetime) (Manrique-Garcia et al., 2012). Likewise, the populational study of the National Epidemiological Survey on Alcohol and Related Conditions (NESARC) sought to investigate the impact and the chronological relationship of cannabis use and mood disorders. The NESARC showed that, even though a previous diagnosis of major depressive disorder was significantly associated with starting cannabis use, an initial diagnosis of BD was not significantly associated with an incidence of cannabis use, after adjusting for covariates. Although weekly to almost daily cannabis use was associated with an increased incidence of BD after adjustment, daily use was not, a finding that requires further investigation (Feingold et al., 2015).

Although the studies investigating the relationship between cannabis use and mood disorders usually assess patients with a well-established diagnosis of BD, the clinical features of BD often change throughout life and the course of illness. Therefore, it is essential to investigate these characteristics, assessing longitudinal outcomes from the early stages of the illness, including not only patients at the first episode of mania, but also persons at high risk of developing BD. It is also important to carry out further studies that investigate the use of cannabis across different phases of the illness or along the life course.

13.4 Neurobiological Basis of Cannabis Use and Bipolar Disorder

Considering that cannabis use may have multi-pronged effects on the course of BD, it is important to understand the effects of cannabis and its constituent cannabinoids on the pathophysiology of BD. The components of the endocannabinoid system are present in neuronal and immune cell lines, which are critical for the neurobiological mechanisms of BD. In addition, endocannabinoids have neuromodulatory effects in the central and peripheral nervous system, modulating many biological functions that are important for BD, such as mood, anxiety, appetite, sleep, and memory processing (Pinto et al., 2020). More information regarding the endocannabinoid system and its components can be found in Chapters 1 and 2.

Cannabis is known to induce and exacerbate psychotic symptoms, probably by partial activation of the cannabinoid receptor 1 (CB1R) by delta-9-tetrahydrocannabinol (THC), which is its main cannabinoid constituent (D'Souza et al., 2004, 2005). Further, cannabis may be involved in the pathophysiological processes that underlie mania, since cannabis use can exacerbate manic symptoms among persons with BD (Gibbs et al., 2015) and is associated with worse manic symptoms among persons with first-episode psychosis (Stone et al., 2014). Cannabis is also associated with an increased risk of new-onset manic-like symptoms in the general population and, especially during adolescence, may be an independent risk factor for the development of hypomania in young adulthood (Gibbs et al., 2015; Marwaha et al., 2018). These findings suggest that cannabinoid CB1R agonists may precipitate mania among those who have a genetic predisposition. Conversely, CB1R antagonists, such as rimonabant, are known to induce depression-like

syndrome in pre-clinical models and humans (Christensen et al., 2007). This evidence indicates a role of brain cannabinoid receptors in the pathophysiology of BD: CB1R agonism may tilt the mood polarity toward mania, whereas CB1R antagonism might be favouring the expression of depressive symptoms.

Furthermore, cannabis use may have a lasting impact by disrupting endocannabinoid system signalling, especially in adolescence and early adulthood. In a longitudinal observational study conducted in Scandinavia, cannabis-induced psychosis showed a high conversion rate to BD, suggesting that cannabis may increase the risk of developing a primary psychotic disorder (Starzer et al., 2018). However, there is still a lack of studies investigating peripheral biomarkers of the endocannabinoid system in BD. The few studies in this field mainly assessed the polymorphism of CB1R, CB2R, and fatty acid amide hydrolase (FAAG) genes, finding conflicting results (Arjmand et al., 2019). Thus, more studies are required to draw conclusions. Moreover, no published studies up to date have investigated the peripheral endocannabinoids, such as anandamide and 2-arachidonoylglycerol in persons with BD (Arjmand et al., 2019; Navarrete et al., 2020)

Due to this lack of evidence of direct measurements of endocannabinoids, neuroimaging studies may provide a viable way to investigate the biological effects of cannabis in the pathophysiology of BD. As an example, a cross-sectional study investigated functional magnetic resonance imaging (MRI) brain activation in adolescents and young adults with co-occurring BD and CUD. Persons with BD without CUD had significantly greater brain activation in the right amygdala, left nucleus accumbens, and both thalami in comparison to those with co-occurring BD and CUD. On the other hand, persons with BD and without CUD exhibited significantly greater activation in the left nucleus accumbens, right thalamus, and left striatum than healthy controls. These results show that the brain regions involved in emotional processing of young persons with co-occurring BD and CUD are different from the regions activated in those with BD without CUD. These findings would suggest that cannabis use can alter the activation of areas related to emotional processing among persons with BD or persons with co-occurring BD and CUD present a unique neurobiological endophenotype (Bitter et al., 2014).

Another study aimed to investigate the association of regional grey matter volumes (GMV) with the future development of substance use adolescents and young adults with BD, through the assessment of high-resolution structural MRI scans of persons with minimal or no prior substance use at the baseline assessment, but who had also reported substance use at follow-up of six years. The authors found that lower GMV in the dorsolateral prefrontal cortex was observed at baseline in both males and females who reported subsequent alcohol and cannabis use compared to those who did not report it. In female participants, lower GMV in regions related to emotional regulation, such as orbitofrontal and insula, were associated with future substance use. On the other hand, lower GMV in regions related to attention and executive process, such as the rostral prefrontal cortex, were associated with future use in male participants. These results suggest that GMV is associated with future risk of substance use in young persons with CBD, with some preliminary findings indicating neurobiological differences between males and females (Lippard et al., 2017).

To investigate the relationship between cannabis use and brain structures in adolescents with BD, volume, thickness, and surface area in MRI scans of this clinical population were assessed in a cross-sectional study. Participants with co-occurring BD and CUD had larger volume and surface area in parietal regions, as well as smaller thickness in frontal regions, while patients with BD without CUD had smaller volume, surface area, and thickness both in the parietal and frontal regions. Although a cross-sectional study – thus not establishing causal relations – a larger volume and larger surface area in the parietal region may represent effects of cannabis on the brain, while the reduction in the prefrontal cortex may reflect a genetic predisposition to the use of cannabis (Sultan et al., 2021).

Hartberg et al. (2018) studied whether there were differences in brain morphology of persons with schizophrenia and BD who use cannabis using MRI. They found that persons who use cannabis had reduced cortical thickness in the right caudal middle frontal gyrus when starting the cannabis use before illness onset, but otherwise the study did not find evidence of specific morphological brain associations of cannabis use in BD or schizophrenia.

To investigate the impact of cannabis use in adolescence as a neurobiological risk for psychosis, Abush et al. (2018) evaluated total and regional grey matter density (GMD) through a voxel-based morphometry analysis in persons with psychotic disorders (schizophrenia, schizoaffective disorder, and BD with psychotic features) and healthy controls. In general, persons with BD had lower GMD in comparison to healthy controls. However, when stratifying history of cannabis use, persons with BD and cannabis use in adolescence did not differ from healthy persons without cannabis use. Moreover, the comparisons revealed no significant GMD differences when contrasting BD with adolescent cannabis use versus those without cannabis use. These intriguing findings require cautious interpretation, since the data was collected through a cross-sectional design, using retrospective information. Thus, further prospective, transdiagnostic and longitudinal investigations are necessary to clarify the effects of cannabis on the neurobiology of psychotic disorders (Abush et al., 2018).

Similar intriguing findings were observed in another study with a retrospective analysis of a cohort that aimed to compare clinical features and neurocognitive performance in patients with BD with a history of CUD compared to those without a history of CUD. The neurocognitive analyses indicated an overall pattern of superior performance in attention, working memory, and processing speed in patients with a history of CUD (Braga et al., 2012). Curiously, another study from the same research group showed that schizophrenia has the opposite pattern, possibly suggesting different underlying neurobiological mechanisms in both psychotic disorders (Ringen et al., 2010).

Regarding neurocognitive characteristics, a systematic review aimed to investigate the literature on cannabis use and neurocognition in persons with BD and found a small number of studies (Jordan Walter et al., 2021). Among the six studies included in the review, three showed no differences between persons with BD who use cannabis and those who do not. Two of the studies found better neurocognitive performances in domains such as attention, processing speed, working memory, and semantic verbal fluency in those participants who use cannabis. Only one of the included studies found a worse performance associated with cannabis use; however, this study used cannabis dependence as an inclusion criterion, in contrast to the other studies that included cannabis use, CUD, cannabis abuse, etc. Although most studies included in this systematic review suggested that cannabis use is not associated with neurocognitive impairment in BD, this evidence is limited not only by the lack of studies but also by the heterogeneity found among them and by their cross-sectional designs (Jordan Walter et al., 2021).

Although important, these are initial findings from cross-sectional data. Thus, not only is further longitudinal neuroimaging investigation necessary, but also further investigations on peripheral biomarkers related to the endocannabinoid system are fundamental to better understand how cannabis can influence the neurobiology of BD.

13.5 Treatment of Co-occurring Bipolar Disorder and Cannabis Use Disorder, and Cannabinoids as Therapeutic Options

Although the impact of CUD on the course of BD is known, there are no published randomized controlled trials so far that have explicitly focused on this important clinical issue (Yatham et al., 2018). This limitation is not a specificity of CUD, since the quality of the evidence for the treatment of BD co-occurring with other SUD is, in general, also low (Beaulieu et al., 2012; Ostacher et al., 2010). This phenomenon is due to several reasons, including not only the complexity of the study designs, since many patients use more than one substance, but also the inconsistency of the variables used as outcomes, not allowing the direct comparison of the results. For example, when assessing alcohol use disorder, the clinical interview can include the number of drinks per drinking day as an outcome, while the assessment of other substances use can include urine test results, thus showing the heterogeneity of measurements.

Despite these limitations, the main clinical guidelines provide treatment recommendations for co-occurring BD and SUD, such as avoiding medications like antidepressants that may increase the risk of mood destabilization, as well as choosing parsimonious pharmacotherapies that treat both conditions (Yatham et al., 2018). More specifically, lithium and valproate present some preliminary evidence of efficacy in the concomitant treatment of BD mood symptoms and substance use disorder (Albanese et al., 2000; Brady et al., 1995; Geller et al., 1998), even though valproate is preferably recommended over lithium to treat acute manic episodes in patients with co-occurring SUD (Yatham et al., 2018). Thus, the combination of valproate and lithium is suggested as a first-choice treatment for co-occurring BD and SUD, while monotherapy with lithium or valproate, or the combination of valproate with other medications, are second-choice options (Beaulieu et al.,

2012). Furthermore, a small trial provided preliminary evidence that lithium can effectively reduce substance use and treat mood symptoms in adolescents with co-occurring BD and SUD (Geller et al., 1998). In terms of psychosocial interventions, a randomized controlled trial showed that a cognitive-behavioural based therapy called integrated group psychotherapy has the potential to reduce substance use in people with BD and SUD (Weiss et al., 2007). Moreover, family-focused therapy can also be considered, especially in adolescents (Yatham et al., 2018).

It is known that SUD may negatively impact the course of BD; however, data from qualitative interviews suggest that cannabis use may have a positive impact on mood symptoms and has often been viewed as a self-treatment for BD (Arjmand et al., 2019; Healey et al., 2009). In addition, anecdotal evidence also demonstrates that many people claim to use cannabis in order to cope with mood symptoms (Grinspoon and Bakalar, 1998; Gruber et al., 1996). A naturalistic study found significant reductions in depressive symptoms after using medical cannabis with relatively low THC levels and high levels of cannabidiol (CBD); even though continued use of cannabis worsened the depressive symptoms over time (Cuttler et al., 2018). A longitudinal study asked participants to rate their mood symptoms three times a day and after using cannabis over a four-week period in order to investigate whether cannabis use may impact on the psychopathology in persons with BD. The result of this approach, called ecological momentary assessment, showed improvements in self-reported mood symptoms, especially depressive, among people with BD after using cannabis (Sagar et al., 2016). In spite of this self-reported evidence, a better comprehension on the pharmacology of cannabis constituents, and their impact on BD, is necessary to draw conclusions. However, relying on retrospective studies of self-report is fraught with challenges, especially in substance use disorders, which are often characterized by lack of insight regarding the amount of substance use and the consequent functional impairment. Furthermore, given that cannabis impairs memory, retrospective recall of subjective effects may not be accurate. Therefore, it may be necessary to conduct prospective experimental studies carefully characterizing the effects of cannabis on symptoms of BD in real-time, so that the acute effects of cannabis in BD can be fully understood, akin to studies conducted in schizophrenia (D'Souza et al., 2005; Henquet et al., 2010).

Understanding the relationship between cannabis use and mood disorders is complex due to the existence of more than 100 phytocannabinoids in cannabis (Pinto et al., 2020). THC and CBD are the most studied natural cannabinoids and some evidence indicates that they have antagonistic effects: while THC induces anxiety and psychotic symptoms, cannabidiol does not induce psychotomimetic effects and has been reported to counteract anxiety symptoms due to its action on CB1R and 5-hydroxytryptamine receptors (Szkudlarek et al., 2019). CBD has already been studied for anxiety disorder (Wright et al., 2020), schizophrenia (McGuire et al., 2018), and substance use disorders (Freeman et al., 2020; Hurd et al., 2019; Mongeau-Pérusse et al., 2021), showing promising results for some of these conditions. Given that CBD also has antiepileptic and neuroprotective properties, its use in mood disorders, especially in bipolar disorder, seems plausible (Pinto et al., 2020).

In spite of the potential antidepressant actions in pre-clinical studies, a systematic review did not find any published trial investigating the use of CBD among persons with BD (Pinto et al., 2020). After a comprehensive review, this study assessed several trials and observational studies that evaluated depressive symptoms as secondary outcomes; however, none of the trials focused on persons with mood disorders (Pinto et al., 2020). Only one report included persons with BD: it was a case series with two persons whose manic episodes were treated with CBD 600–1,200 mg. Although the patients tolerated CBD well and did not report side-effects, monotherapy with CBD did not improve the manic symptoms (Zuardi et al., 2010). To this date, there is one ongoing double-blind placebo-controlled trial investigating CBD as a treatment for BD (https://clinicaltrials.gov/ct2/show/NCT03310593), whose results have yet to be published.

13.6 Conclusion

Persons with BD commonly use cannabis and have a high prevalence of co-occurring CUD. In addition, persons with BD and co-occurring CUD tend to have earlier onset of symptoms and are more likely to have psychosis, suicide attempts, and other SUDs in comparison to those without CUD. Moreover, convergent evidence indicates that CUD is associated with longitudinal impacts on the course of BD, demonstrating an association with longer and more frequent mood episodes, lower recovery, and remission rates, as well as poorer psychosocial functioning; however, abstinence from cannabis may improve clinical outcomes, partly by increasing treatment adherence.

There are still gaps in the knowledge regarding the relationship between BD and cannabis use, and there is no evidence yet to guide the treatment of co-occurring BD and CUD. As society's attitudes toward cannabis and its constituents have been rapidly shifting, studying the impact of this substance in persons with BD, as well as the use of cannabinoids for therapeutic purposes, is increasingly important. Therefore, further clinical trials investigating pharmacotherapies and psychosocial interventions for persons with co-occurring BD and CUD are needed, as well as further studies investigating the neurobiological impact of cannabinoids among persons with BD, especially focusing on exogenous cannabinoid actions on the eCB system during adolescence and early adulthood. Finally, preliminary evidence indicates that some cannabinoids, such as CBD, hold promise to treat BD and SUD. Rigorously studying the effects of cannabinoids, with placebo-controlled experimental designs, especially in combination with well-established treatments for BD, is crucial to guide clinical decision-making.

References

Abush, H., Ghose, S., Van Enkevort, E. A., et al. (2018). Associations between adolescent cannabis use and brain structure in psychosis. *Psychiatry Res Neuroimaging*, **276**, 53–64.

Agrawal, A., Nurnberger, J. I. J., and Lynskey, M. T. (2011). Cannabis involvement in individuals with bipolar disorder. *Psychiatry Res*, **185**, 459–461.

Albanese, M. J., Clodfelter, R. C. J., and Khantzian, E. J. (2000). Divalproex sodium in substance abusers with mood disorder. *J Clin Psychiatry*, **61**, 916–921.

Arjmand, S., Behzadi, M., Kohlmeier, K. A., et al. (2019). Bipolar disorder and the endocannabinoid system. *Acta Nuropsychiatr*, **31**, 193–201.

Bally, N., Zullino, D., and Aubry, J.-M. (2014). Cannabis use and first manic episode. *J Affect Disord*, **165**, 103–108.

Beaulieu, S., Saury, S., Sareen, J., et al. (2012). The Canadian Network for Mood and Anxiety Treatments (CANMAT) task force recommendations for the management of patients with mood disorders and comorbid substance use disorders. *Ann Clin Psychiatry*, **24**, 38–55.

Berk, M., Post, R., Ratheesh, A., et al. (2017). Staging in bipolar disorder: From theoretical framework to clinical utility. *World Psychiatry*, **16**, 236–244.

Bitter, S. M., Adler, C. M., Eliassen, J. C., et al. (2014). Neurofunctional changes in adolescent cannabis users with and without bipolar disorder. *Addiction*, **109**, 1901–1909.

Brady, K. T., Sonne, S. C., Anton, R., et al. (1995). Valproate in the treatment of acute bipolar affective episodes complicated by substance abuse: A pilot study. *J Clin Psychiatry*, **56**, 118–121.

Braga, R. J., Burdick, K. E., Derosse, P., et al. (2012). Cognitive and clinical outcomes associated with cannabis use in patients with bipolar I disorder. *Psychiatry Res*, **200**, 242–245.

Christensen, R., Kristensen, P. K., Bartels, E. M., et al. (2007). Efficacy and safety of the weight-loss drug rimonabant: A meta-analysis of randomised trials. *Lancet*, **370**, 1706–1713.

Cuttler, C., Spradlin, A., and McLaughlin, R. J. (2018). A naturalistic examination of the perceived effects of cannabis on negative affect. *J Affect Disord*, **235**, 198–205.

D'Souza, D. C., Abi-Saab, W. M., Madonick, S., et al. (2005). Delta-9-tetrahydrocannabinol effects in schizophrenia: Implications for cognition, psychosis, and addiction. *Biol Psychiatry*, **15**, 594–608.

D'Souza, D. C., Perry, E., MacDougall, L., et al. (2004). The psychotomimetic effects of intravenous delta-9-tetrahydrocannabinol in healthy individuals: Implications for psychosis. *Neuropsychopharmacology*, **29**, 1558–1572.

Duffy, A., Horrocks, J., Milin, R., et al. (2012). Adolescent substance use disorder during the early stages of bipolar disorder: A prospective high-risk study. *J Affect Disord*, **142**, 57–64.

Feingold, D., Weiser, M., Rehm, J., et al. (2015). The association between cannabis use and mood disorders: A longitudinal study. *J Affect Disord*, **172**, 211–218.

Freeman, T. P., Hindocha, C., Baio, G., et al. (2020). Cannabidiol for the treatment of cannabis use disorder: A phase 2a, double-blind, placebo-controlled, randomised, adaptive Bayesian trial. *Lancet Psychiatry*, **7**, 865–874.

Geller, B., Cooper, T. B., Sun, K., et al. (1998). Double-blind and placebo-controlled study of lithium for adolescent bipolar disorders with secondary substance dependency. *J Am Acad Child Adolesc Psychiatry*, **37**, 171–178.

Gibbs, M., Winsper, C., Marwaha, S., et al. (2015). Cannabis use and mania symptoms: A systematic review and meta-analysis. *J Affect Disord*, **171**, 39–47.

González-Pinto, A., Reed, C., Novick, D., et al. (2010). Assessment of medication adherence in a cohort of patients with bipolar disorder. *Pharmacopsychiatry*, **43**, 263–270.

Gore, F. M., Bloem, P. J., Patton, G. C., et al. (2011). Global burden of disease in young people aged 10–24 years: A systematic analysis. *Lancet*, **377**, 2093–2102.

Grinspoon, L., and Bakalar, J. B. (1998). The use of cannabis as a mood stabilizer in bipolar disorder: Anecdotal evidence and the need for clinical research. *J Psychoactive Drugs*, **30**, 171–177.

Gruber, A. J., Pope, H. G. J., and Brown, M. E. (1996). Do patients use marijuana as an antidepressant? *Depression*, **4**, 77–80.

Hartberg, C. B., Lange, E. H., Lagerberg, T. V., et al. (2018). Cortical thickness, cortical surface area and subcortical volumes in schizophrenia and bipolar disorder patients with cannabis use. *Eur Neuropsychopharmacol*, **28**, 37–47.

Healey, C., Peters, S., Kinderman, P., et al. (2009). Reasons for substance use in dual diagnosis bipolar disorder and substance use disorders: A qualitative study. *J Affect Disord*, **113**, 118–126.

Henquet, C., van Os, J., Kuepper, R., et al. (2010). Psychosis reactivity to cannabis use in daily life: An experience sampling study. *Br J Psychiatry*, **196**, 447–453.

Hjorthøj, C., Østergaard, M. L. D., Benros, M. E., et al. (2015). Association between alcohol and substance use disorders and all-cause and cause-specific mortality in schizophrenia, bipolar disorder, and unipolar depression: A nationwide, prospective, register-based study. *Lancet Psychiatry*, **2**, 801–808.

Hunt, G. E., Malhi, G. S., Cleary, M., et al. (2016a). Comorbidity of bipolar and substance use disorders in national surveys of general populations, 1990–2015: Systematic review and meta-analysis. *J Affect Disord*, **206**, 321–330.

(2016b). Prevalence of comorbid bipolar and substance use disorders in clinical settings, 1990–2015: Systematic review and meta-analysis. *J Affect Disord*, **206**, 331–349.

Hurd, Y. L., Spriggs, S., Alishayev, J., et al. (2019). Cannabidiol for the reduction of cue-induced craving and anxiety in drug-abstinent individuals with heroin use disorder: A couble-blind randomized placebo-controlled trial. *Am J Psychiatry*, **176**, 911–922.

Jordan Walter, T., Pocuca, N., Young, J. W., et al. (2021). The relationship between cannabis use and cognition in people with bipolar disorder: A systematic scoping review. *Psychiatry Res*, **297**, 113695.

Kim, S.-W., Dodd, S., Berk, L., et al. (2015). Impact of cannabis use on long-term remission in bipolar I and schizoaffective disorder. *Psychiatry Invest*, **12**, 349–355.

Lagerberg, T. V., Kvitland, L. R., Aminoff, S. R., et al. (2014). Indications of a dose–response relationship between cannabis use and age at onset in bipolar disorder. *Psychiatry Res*, **215**, 101–104.

Lagerberg, T. V., Sundet, K., Aminoff, S. R., et al. (2011). Excessive cannabis use is associated with earlier age at onset in bipolar disorder. *Eur Arch Psychiatry Clin Neurosci*, **261**, 397–405.

Lippard, E. T. C., Mazure, C. M., Johnston, J. A. Y., et al. (2017). Brain circuitry associated with the development of substance use in bipolar disorder and preliminary evidence for sexual dimorphism in adolescents. *J Neurosci Res*, **95**, 777–791.

Manrique-Garcia, E., Zammit, S., Dalman, C., et al. (2012). Cannabis use and depression: A longitudinal study of a national cohort of Swedish conscripts. *BMC Psychiatry*, **12**, 112.

Marwaha, S., Winsper, C., Bebbington, P., et al. (2018). Cannabis use and hypomania in young people: A prospective analysis. *Schizophr Bull*, **44**, 1267–1274.

McGuire, P., Robson, P., Cubala, W. J., et al. (2018). Cannabidiol (CBD) as an adjunctive therapy in schizophrenia: A multicenter randomized controlled trial. *Am J Psychiatry*, **175**, 225–231.

Merikangas, K. R., Jin, R., He, J.-P., et al. (2012). Prevalence and correlates for bipolar spectrum disorder in the World Mental Health Survey Initiative. *Arch Gen Psychiatry*, **68**, 241–251.

Mongeau-Pérusse, V., Brissette, S., Bruneau, J., et al. (2021). Cannabidiol as a treatment for craving and relapse in individuals with cocaine use disorder: A randomized placebo-controlled trial. *Addiction*, **116**, 2431–2442.

Navarrete, F., García-Gutiérrez, M. S., Jurado-Barba, R., et al. (2020). Endocannabinoid system components as potential biomarkers in psychiatry. *Front Psychiatry*, **11**, 315.

Ostacher, M. J., Perlis, R. H., Nierenberg, A. A., et al. (2010). Impact of substance use disorders on recovery from episodes of depression in bipolar disorder patients: Prospective data from the Systematic Treatment Enhancement Program for Bipolar Disorder (STEP-BD). *Am J Psychiatry*, **167**, 289–297.

Østergaard, M. L. D., Nordentoft, M., and Hjorthøj, C. (2017). Associations between substance use disorders and suicide or suicide attempts in people with mental illness: A Danish nation-wide, prospective, register-based study of patients diagnosed with schizophrenia, bipolar disorder, unipolar depression or personality disorder. *Addiction*, **112**, 1250–1259.

Pinto, J. V., Kauer-Sant'Anna, M., and Yatham, L. N. (2021). What impact does bipolar disorder staging have on the use of pharmacotherapy? *Expert Opin Pharmacother*, **22**, 1513–1516.

Pinto, J. V., Medeiros, L. S., da Rosa, G. S., et al. (2019). The prevalence and clinical correlates of cannabis use and cannabis use disorder among patients with bipolar disorder: A systematic review with meta-analysis and meta-regression. *Neurosci Biobehav Rev*, **101**, 78–84.

Pinto, J. V., Saraf, G., Frysch, C., et al. (2020). Cannabidiol as a treatment for mood disorders: A systematic review. *Can J Psychiatry*, **65**, 213–227.

Post, R. M., Leverich, G. S., Kupka, R. W., et al. (2010). Early-onset bipolar disorder and treatment delay are risk factors for poor outcome in adulthood. *J Clin Psychiatry*, **71**, 864–872.

Ringen, P. A., Vaskinn, A., Sundet, K., et al. (2010). Opposite relationships between cannabis use and neurocognitive functioning in bipolar disorder and schizophrenia. *Psychol Med*, **40**, 1337–1347.

Sagar, K. A., Dahlgren, M. K., Racine, M. T., et al. (2016). Joint effects: A pilot investigation of the impact of bipolar disorder and marijuana use on cognitive function and mood. *PLoS ONE*, **11**(6), e0157060.

Scavone, A., Timmins, V., Collins, J., et al. (2018). Dimensional and categorical correlates of substance use disorders among Canadian adolescents with bipolar disorder. *J Can Acad Child Adolesc Psychiatry*, **27**, 159–166.

Starzer, M. S. K., Nordentoft, M., and Hjorthøj, C. (2018). Rates and predictors of conversion to schizophrenia or bipolar disorder following substance-induced psychosis. *Am J Psychiatry*, **175**, 343–350.

Stone, J. M., Fisher, H. L., Major, B., et al. (2014). Cannabis use and first-episode psychosis: Relationship with manic and psychotic symptoms, and with age at presentation. *Psychol Med*, **44**, 499–506.

Strakowski, S. M., DelBello, M. P., Fleck, D. E., et al. (2007). Effects of co-occurring cannabis use disorders on the course of bipolar disorder after a first hospitalization for mania. *Arch Gen Psychiatry*, **64**, 57–64.

Sultan, A. A., Kennedy, K. G., Fiksenbaum, L., et al. (2021). Neurostructural correlates of cannabis use in adolescent bipolar disorder. *Int J Neuropsychopharmacol*, **24**, 181–190.

Szkudlarek, H. J., Desai, S. J., Renard, J., et al. (2019). Delta-9-tetrahydrocannabinol and cannabidiol produce dissociable effects on prefrontal cortical executive function and regulation of affective behaviors. *Neuropsychopharmacology*, **44**, 817–825.

UNDOC. (2018). *World Drug Report 2018. Global Overview of Drug Demand and Supply.* Available at: www.unodc.org/wdr2018 (Last accessed 12 November 2022).

Weiss, R. D., Griffin, M. L., Kolodziej, M. E., et al. (2007). A randomized trial of integrated group therapy versus group drug counseling for patients with bipolar disorder and substance dependence. *Am J Psychiatry*, **164**, 100–107.

Wright, M., Di Ciano, P., and Brands, B. (2020). Use of cannabidiol for the treatment of anxiety: A short synthesis of pre-clinical and clinical evidence. *Cannabis Cannabinoid Res*, **5**, 191–196.

Yatham, L. N., Kennedy, S. H., Parikh, S. V., et al. (2018). Canadian Network for Mood and Anxiety Treatments (CANMAT) and International Society for Bipolar Disorders (ISBD) 2018 guidelines for the management of patients with bipolar disorder. *Bipolar Disord*, **20**, 97–170.

Zorrilla, I., Aguado, J., Haro, J. M., et al. (2015). Cannabis and bipolar disorder: Does quitting cannabis use during manic/mixed episode improve clinical/functional outcomes? *Acta Psychiat Scand*, **131**, 100–110.

Zuardi, A., Crippa, J., Dursun, S., et al. (2010). Cannabidiol was ineffective for manic episode of bipolar affective disorder. *J Psychopharmacol*, **24**, 135–137.

Cannabis and Psychosis Proneness

Rajiv Radhakrishnan, Shubham Kamal, Sinan Guloksuz, and Jim van Os

14.1 Introduction

Cannabis is one of the most commonly used drugs worldwide (2021 World Drug report). With the increase in legalization of medical and recreational use of cannabis, and decrease in the perception of harm, adolescents and young adults are more likely to use cannabis. Converging lines of evidence from epidemiological studies (Di Forti et al., 2019; Linscott and van Os, 2013; Marconi et al., 2016), human laboratory studies (Ganesh et al., 2020; Hindley et al., 2020), and genetic studies (Johnson et al., 2021; Quattrone et al., 2021) suggest that cannabis use is a risk factor for the later development of psychosis (Radhakrishnan et al., 2014a, 2014b). Hence, there is a pressing need to identify individuals who are at risk of developing psychosis following cannabis use.

The concept of psychosis proneness has undergone many transformations since its initial conceptualization in the early twentieth century. These include early taxonomic concepts such as schizotypy (Rado), schizotaxia (Meehl), and dimensional constructs such as psychoticism (Eysenck) and the fully dimensional model of Claridge. These made way for the concepts of endophenotype, familial high-risk for schizophrenia, prodromal states, basic symptoms, clinical high-risk for psychosis (CHR)/ultra-high-risk for psychosis (UHR), and attenuated psychosis syndrome. These conceptualizations of psychosis proneness are based on the idea that psychotic disorders such as schizophrenia emerge on the backdrop of less intense symptoms resembling psychosis. The presence of less intense symptoms resembling psychosis may, hence, identify a group that is at increased risk (i.e., psychosis proneness). Of note, these conceptualizations have focused largely on the positive symptoms of psychosis. With the advent of large, genome-wide association studies (GWAS) in schizophrenia, psychosis proneness has been defined in terms of genetic risk independent of the presence of less intense symptoms resembling psychosis, that is, highest tertile of polygenic risk score for schizophrenia. More recent epidemiological studies have also identified symptom clusters that increase the risk for psychotic experiences in the general population.

While there are conceptual differences in how psychosis proneness has been defined over the years, research on the effects of cannabis on different constructs of psychosis proneness point to some consistent threads of evidence. In this chapter, we focus primarily on the effects of cannabis on symptom-based conceptualizations of psychosis-proneness such as schizotypy, CHR/UHR, and sub-clinical psychotic symptoms in the general population. The reader is also directed to Chapters 10, 15, and 16 of this book.

14.2 Psychosis Proneness: Historical Perspective

The concept of psychosis proneness has its roots in early efforts to identify individuals who are at risk of developing schizophrenia. The initial observation that psychiatric disorders ran in families resulted in a longitudinal follow-up of children of people diagnosed with schizophrenia to identify those who are at increased risk of developing the disorder (Pearson and Kley, 1957). Concurrently, cross-sectional studies also noted the presence of schizophrenia-like traits (e.g., social isolation, suspiciousness, irritability, eccentricity) among their family members, as observed by Bleuler, Kraepelin and others (see Castle and Buckley, 2015). These cross-sectional studies were referred to as investigations of psychosis-proneness (Claridge, 1994)

Enshrined in a psychodynamic framework, Rado (1953) introduced the term 'schizotype' (schizophrenic phenotype) to denote an ensemble of psychodynamic traits (i.e., anhedonia, emotional imbalance, and inter-personal impairment) that are present throughout life and undergo 'a sequence of schizotypal changes' with time; this became known as schizotypal personality organization. Meehl (1962) expanded on this concept to define four core features (thought disorder; associative dyscontrol or 'cognitive slippage'; inter-personal aversiveness; anhedonia; and ambivalence). He hypothesized that this was the result of a genetically determined neurophysiological 'neural integrative defect', called schizotaxia. It was noted that only a small proportion of people with schizotypy develop schizophrenia and this allowed for interaction with environmental risk factors.

This concept, that is, that there was a continuity of traits even in non-clinical populations in the absence of symptoms of schizophrenia, was further refined by Eysenck (1992) and Claridge (1994). During a period when the Kraepelin–Bleuler dichotomy of schizophrenia and bipolar disorder was challenged and the existence of a single unitary psychosis was proposed, Eysenck suggested that if schizotypy existed as a dimension that resulted in schizophrenia at one extreme, there ought to be another entity that resulted in bipolar disorder since '. . . we cannot have a single dimension with "psychosis" at both ends' (Eysenck, 1992). In order to resolve this, he proposed the existence of three personality dimensions: Psychoticism, Extraversion, and Neuroticism. According to Eysenck's model, psychotic disorders were considered as extreme points along quantitative dimensions (i.e., extreme values of Psychoticism combined with individual expressions of varying values of Extraversion and Neuroticism) resulting in different clinical syndromes, for example, schizoid personality, schizotypy, and schizophrenia (Eysenck, 1992). 'Psychoticism' was, hence, conceptualized as the underlying dimensional liability for all psychotic disorders, in keeping with the concept of *Einheitspsychose* (unitary psychosis).

Several scales were developed to measure schizotypy in non-clinical populations, including the Chapman scales, Schizotypal Personality Questionnaire (SPQ) (Raine, 1991), Schizotypal Trait Questionnaire (STQ) (Claridge and Broks, 1984), Oxford–Liverpool Inventory of Feelings and Experiences (O-LIFE) (Mason and Claridge, 2006), Structured Interview for Schizotypy (SIS) (Kendler et al., 1989), for specific schizotypal dimensions: positive (e.g., Magical Ideation (Eckblad and Chapman, 1983), Perceptual Aberration Scale (scale by Chapman and Chapman, unpublished)) and negative (e.g., Scales for Physical Anhedonia and Social Anhedonia (Chapman et al., 1976)). Claridge proposed a fully dimensional model of schizotypy and

schizophrenia based on factor analysis of the different scales developed to measure schizotypy. They identified a three-factor model, comprising (i) cognitive–perceptual or positive schizotypy dimension, (ii) inter-personal deficit or negative schizotypy dimension, and (iii) disorganization dimension; this appeared to recapitulate the factor structure of schizophrenia (Raine, 2006; Wuthrich and Bates, 2006). Eysenck's psychoticism scale appears to map onto a personality dimension more closely related to non-conformity and antisocial traits. The Community Assessment of Psychic Experiences (CAPE) (Stefanis et al., 2002) provides measures of positive and negative dimensions (as well as an affective–depressive dimension) in the general population.

14.3 Effect of Cannabis Use on Schizotypy

14.3.1 Does Schizotypy Increase Sensitivity to the Psychotomimetic Effects of Cannabis?

Schizotypy did not moderate the psychotomimetic effects of delta-9-tetrahydrocannabinol (THC) in a pooled analysis of 128 cannabis users who received THC in double-blind, randomized, placebo-controlled, crossover design, laboratory challenge studies (Freeman et al., 2021). An online survey (n = 129, 64% women, predominantly students) who had used cannabis at least once in their lifetime, however, found that schizotypy (measured using O-LIFE scale) was the only significant predictor of unusual experiences and this did not correlate with frequency of cannabis use. Schizotypy was positively correlated with cognitive impairment and negatively correlated with age (Airey et al., 2020). A meta-analysis of 29 cross-sectional studies found that 'ever' using cannabis was associated with higher schizotypy scores with moderate effect-sizes (0.3–0.4 range) on domains of positive schizotypy and disorganization; and small effect-sizes (0.15–0.2 range) on the domain of negative schizotypy (Szoke et al., 2014).

Among those with high schizotypy, cannabis use was not associated with divergent thinking, a measure of creativity. However, cannabis use was associated with divergent thinking in the non-schizotypy group (Minor et al., 2014). In another study, cannabis use increased verbal fluency in those with low divergent thinking to levels similar to those with high divergent thinking. Although the group with higher divergent thinking had significantly higher trait schizotypy, they did not show a change in verbal fluency with cannabis use (Schafer et al., 2012).

An interesting study from the Netherlands and Flanders employed sibling-control and cross-sibling comparison among patients with a psychotic disorder (n = 1,120), their siblings (n = 1,057), and community controls (n = 590). Compared to controls, siblings displayed greater sensitivity to the effects of current cannabis use on positive schizotypy and negative schizotypy. The analyses suggested that familial risk increased sensitivity to cannabis (i.e., moderation) rather than familial risk increasing use of cannabis (mediation) (Genetic Risk and Outcome in Psychosis Investigators, 2011).

14.3.2 Does Cannabis Use Increase Rates of Schizotypy?

In a study on a non-clinical population comprising university students (n = 910), higher frequency of cannabis use was associated with higher schizotypy as measured by the positive- and disorganization subscales of the SPQ. The SPQ sub-scales 'odd beliefs', 'ideas of reference', 'unusual perceptual experiences', 'odd speech', and total SPQ scores were found to be mediated by measures of aberrant salience (measured using the aberrant salience inventory (ASI)) (O'Tuathaigh et al., 2020).

The effect of age on the relationship between cannabis use and schizotypy has been examined in a number of studies. In a study of 155 cannabis users, aged 15–24 years, who were assessed at six-month intervals, younger age was associated with increased negative schizotypy over time among frequent cannabis users. Contrarily, younger age was associated with decreasing negative schizotypy over time among occasional cannabis users (Albertella et al., 2018).

14.3.3 Does Cannabis Impact the Rate of Conversion from Schizotypy to Schizophrenia?

Rates of transition from schizotypal disorder to schizophrenia has been estimated to be approximately 25–50% (Albert et al., 2017; Hjorthoj et al., 2018; Nordentoft et al., 2006; Parnas et al., 2011). In the Danish OPUS trial, the rate of conversion to a psychotic disorder at 2-year follow-up was 25% for those

randomized to integrated treatment versus 48.3% for those who received standard treatment (Nordentoft et al., 2006). In the OPUS-II study, at 3.5-year follow-up, the rate of conversion from schizotypal disorder to schizophrenia was 32% (Albert et al., 2017). The Copenhagen Prodromal Study found that the rate of conversion from schizotypal personality disorder to schizophrenia was 25% at 5-year follow-up (Parnas et al., 2011). In a large Danish nationwide prospective cohort study including all individuals born between 1 January 1981 through 10 August 2014, with an incident diagnosis of schizotypal disorder and without a previous diagnosis of schizophrenia, 2,539 participants with schizotypal disorder were identified (57.0% male) (Hjorthoj et al., 2018). The rate of conversion to schizophrenia was 16.3% (95% CI = 14.8–17.8%) after 2 years, and 33.1% (95% CI = 29.3–37.3%) after 20 years. Among those with cannabis use disorder, the rate of conversion at 20 years was 58.2% (95% CI = 44.8–72.2%). Adjusting for covariates, cannabis use disorder, in addition to amphetamine-, and opioid-use disorder, the greater risk of conversion to schizophrenia remained significant (HR = 1.34; 95% CI = 1.11–1.63).

14.4 Effect of Cannabis Use on Clinical-High Risk for Psychosis (CHR)/Ultra-High Risk for Psychosis (UHR)

14.4.1 Does CHR/UHR Increase Sensitivity to the Psychosis-like Effects of Cannabis?

The question of whether CHR/UHR individuals show increased sensitivity to the psychosis-like effects of cannabis has not been well studied in experimental paradigms. CHR/UHR individuals who use cannabis were found to experience a transient increase in paranoia and anxiety, and a decrease in neurocognitive performance following cannabis intoxication in a small laboratory study (Vadhan et al., 2017). This is consistent with the clinical finding that CHR/UHR individuals who use cannabis have higher rates of unusual thought content and suspiciousness than non-users (Carney et al., 2017).

14.4.2 Does Cannabis Use Increase Rates of CHR/UHR?

CHR/UHR has been shown to be associated with higher rates of current and lifetime cannabis use, for example, 36.5% versus 11.1% in healthy controls in one study (Auther et al., 2012). In a meta-analysis of

30 studies, UHR individuals (n = 4,205 versus n = 667 controls) were found to have high rates of current (26.7%) and lifetime (52.8%) cannabis use, and cannabis-use disorder (CUD) (12.8%); and increased odds of lifetime cannabis use (OR = 2.09) and CUD (OR = 5.49) compared to controls (Carney et al., 2017). UHR cannabis users were observed to have had higher rates of unusual thought content and suspiciousness than non-users. Intriguingly, CHR with a lifetime history of cannabis use has been found to have less social anhedonia and better social functioning compared to CHR who did not use cannabis (Auther et al., 2012).

14.4.3 Does Cannabis Impact the Rate of Conversion from CHR/UHR to Schizophrenia?

Studies suggest that current cannabis abuse/dependence, but not lifetime cannabis use, is associated with higher risk of transition to psychosis. For example, in a study of 182 CHR individuals, risk factors for transition to psychosis included cannabis use before age 15 years and frequent use of cannabis. However, within the whole sample, current cannabis users were not more likely to develop psychosis than those who had never used cannabis. Of note, in this study although lifetime prevalence of cannabis use 73.6%, the majority of individuals (n = 98, 73.1%) had stopped using cannabis before clinical presentation (n = 98, 73.1%) (Valmaggia et al., 2014). In the North American Prodrome Longitudinal Study (NAPLS) Phase 1 project, CHR individuals (n = 340) were followed up for > 2 years. In order to examine the relationship between cannabis use and risk of transition to psychosis, individuals were categorized into three groups: No Use (n = 211); Cannabis Use without impairment (n = 63); and Cannabis Abuse/Dependence (n = 67). The cannabis abuse/dependence group had higher rates of conversion to psychosis than those without any use and those with cannabis use without impairment. Adjusting for alcohol use weakened this relationship (HR = 1.875, CI = 0.963–3.651, $p = 0.064$). While the authors interpreted this finding as alcohol use confounding the association between cannabis use and risk to transition, it is also possible that a true relationship exists but that the study was underpowered to adjust for multiple confounders (Auther et al., 2015). Participants (n = 283) were followed for $\geq$ 2 years to determine psychosis conversion.

The risk of transition to psychosis may be greater among those who experience cannabis-induced attenuated psychotic symptoms. In a study of 190 UHR individuals (76 males), those who reported a history of cannabis-induced attenuated psychotic symptoms (APS) were found to be at 4.90 (95% CI = 1.93–12.44) times greater risk of transition to a psychotic disorder at mean five-year follow-up. Greater severity of cannabis use was also found to increase the risk of transition to psychosis. However, this relationship was mediated by greater severity of cannabis use among those with a history of cannabis-induced APS (McHugh et al., 2017).

Kraan et al. (2016)conducted a meta-analysis of seven studies published between 1996 to 2015, identifying seven prospective studies reporting on lifetime cannabis use in UHR subjects (n = 1,171); and five that also examined current cannabis abuse or dependence. While lifetime cannabis use was not significantly associated with transition to psychosis, current cannabis abuse or dependence was associated with 1.75 times higher odds of transition to psychosis (95% CI = 1.14–2.71).

14.4.4 Effect of Cannabis Use on Psychosis Expression in General Population Samples

As outlined in Section 14.2, there is increasing recognition that psychosis exists as a continuum in the general population, with approximately 5–15% of the population self- or interview-based reporting one or more symptoms of psychosis (Johns et al., 2004; van Os et al., 2000). The ability to measure psychosis expression in the general population paved the way for a deeper understanding of the factors that lead to the evolution and persistence of psychosis. General population samples are also of larger sample size and provide an opportunity to examine the interactive role of environmental risk factors.

Longitudinal studies such as The Netherlands Mental Health Survey and Incidence Study (NEMESIS) and the Christchurch Health and Development Study (CHDS) (in New Zealand) have consistently shown that cannabis use is associated with increased rates of psychosis expression (Fergusson et al., 2003; Verdoux et al., 2003). In the first wave of the NEMESIS longitudinal study (1997–1999), baseline cannabis use predicted the presence of psychotic symptoms (adjusted odds ratio (OR) = 2.76, 95% CI = 1.18–6.47), the severity of psychotic symptoms (OR = 24.17, 95% CI = 5.44–107.46), and the need for treatment for psychotic symptoms as assessed by a clinician (OR = 12.01,

95% CI = 2.24–64.34), at follow-up (van Os et al., 2002). The CHDS is a longitudinal birth cohort comprising 1,265 children followed-up from birth to age 21. Those with cannabis dependence (DSM-IV criteria) had significantly higher rates of psychotic symptoms at age 18 years (rate ratio = 3.7; 95% CI = 2.8–5) and 21 years (rate ratio = 2.3; 95% CI = 1.7–3.2). This relationship was consistent even after adjusting for confounders (Fergusson et al., 2003).

The picture that emerges from general population samples suggests that cannabis use interacts with other environmental risk factors such as childhood trauma and urbanicity; and genetic risk to lead to the expression of psychosis. There is evidence to suggest that the contribution of these risk factors is additive, that is, the greater the number of risk factors, the greater is the odds of psychosis expression (Pries et al., 2018).

Emerging evidence also suggests the role of affective dysregulation in contributing to the risk of psychosis emerging from cannabis use and other environmental risk factors – the so-called affective pathway to psychosis (Myin-Germeys et al., 2003). In data from three waves of the second Netherlands Mental Health Survey and Incidence Study (NEMESIS-2), cannabis use and childhood trauma, and to a lesser extent urbanicity, showed greater-than-additive risk when there was a family history of affective dysregulation. In addition, the interaction contrast ratio grew progressively greater across severity levels of psychosis (none, attenuated psychosis, clinical psychosis) in the presence of affective dysregulation (Radhakrishnan et al., 2019). Even when other symptom dimensions are included in the analysis, after controlling for age, sex, and education, only affective dysregulation was found to be a significant moderator of psychosis expression (Pries et al., 2018). The role of affective dysregulation was also noted in an experience sampling study in a general population sample of 514 women. This study examined the moment-to-moment dynamics between negative affect and paranoia in daily life. Using time-lagged analysis, the study found that moments of increased negative affect resulted in a significant increase in paranoia over the subsequent 180 minutes, and psychotic symptoms at follow-up. The transfer from negative effect to paranoia was moderated by stress-sensitivity, while persistence of paranoia was moderated by depressive symptoms (Myin-Germeys et al., 2003).

More recently, Guloksuz et al. (2019) examined the independent and interactive effects of cannabis use and genetic risk for schizophrenia (captured by polygenic risk score for schizophrenia (PRS-SCZ)) in data from the European Network of National Networks studying Gene-Environment Interactions in Schizophrenia (EUGEI) and the Genetic Risk and Outcome of Psychosis (GROUP) study within the EUGEI. Using PRS-SCZ defined by the 75th percentile (PRS-SCZ$_{75}$) in Caucasian patients with schizophrenia (n = 1,699) and healthy, unrelated controls (n = 1,542), they compared the risk of schizophrenia among regular cannabis users, that is, those who used cannabis once or more per week. The analysis revealed that, while both regular cannabis use (OR = 3.96, 95% CI = 3.16–4.97) and genetic risk (PRS-SCZ$_{75}$) (OR = 2.85, 95% CI = 2.43–3.35) independently increased the risk of schizophrenia, there was also an additive interaction between PRS-SCZ75 and regular cannabis use (relative excess risk due to interaction (RERI) = 5.60; 95% CI = 0.88–10.33; p = 0.020) (Figure 14.1).

14.4.5 Is the Relationship between Cannabis Use and Psychosis Expression 'Causal'?

Whether cannabis is causally related to psychosis expression has been widely debated in the field (see Chapter 17). In a study using the Swedish national registry database, cannabis use was strongly associated with later schizophrenia (OR = 10.44, 95% CI = 8.99–12.11). While this association was reduced when controlling for increasing degrees of familial confounding, it continued to be significant (Giordano et al., 2015). Mendelian randomization studies, a type of instrumental variable analysis where single-nucleotide polymorphisms (SNPs) are used to enable randomization to experimental and control conditions, have been performed to interrogate the question of causality. While one study found that genetic liability for lifetime cannabis use was associated with a significant 37% increase in the risk of schizophrenia (Vaucher et al., 2018), two other studies found that genetic liability for schizophrenia was associated with increased risk of lifetime cannabis use (Gage et al., 2017; Pasman et al., 2018), suggesting that the relationship is bidirectional. Of note, these studies relied on lifetime cannabis use and not the frequency/severity of cannabis use.

Linkage disequilibrium score regression (LDSR) and polygenic risk scores (PRSs) studies have also demonstrated significant genome-wide genetic correlation between lifetime cannabis use/misuse and

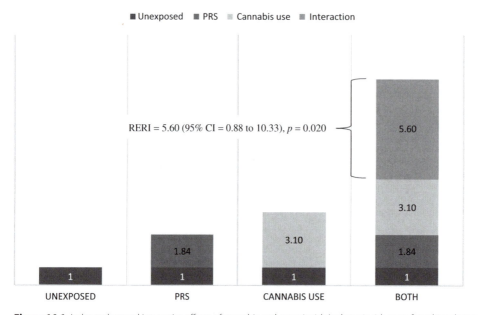

■ Unexposed ■ PRS ■ Cannabis use ■ Interaction

RERI = 5.60 (95% CI = 0.88 to 10.33), $p = 0.020$

5.60

3.10

1.84

1

3.10

1

1.84

1

1

UNEXPOSED   PRS   CANNABIS USE   BOTH

Figure 14.1 Independent and interactive effects of cannabis and genetic risk (polygenic risk score for schizophrenia (PRS)) on schizophrenia. Compared to unexposed (i.e., those without cannabis use), those with genetic risk (PRS) and cannabis use show increased risk of schizophrenia outcomes. Those with both cannabis use and genetic risk (PRS) show a greater risk suggestive of additive interaction between cannabis use and PRS. Adapted from Guloksuz et al. (2019) RERI = relative excess risk due to interaction.

schizophrenia (genetic r range = 0.22–0.25) (Pasman et al., 2018; Verweij et al., 2017), and that high PRSs for schizophrenia significantly predicted greater cannabis use (Verweij et al., 2017), respectively.

van Os et al. (2021) examined the question of causality in a within-subject study – which obviates confounding by genetic risk – from two general population cohorts (Early Developmental Stages of Psychopathology Study (EDSP), n = 1,395; Netherlands Mental Health Survey and Incidence Study-2 (NEMESIS-2), n = 6,603). In an adjusted fixed-effects model, prior cannabis use was associated with psychotic experiences (adjusted OR = 7.03, 95% CI = 2.39–20.69), whereas prior psychotic experiences were not associated with cannabis use (adjusted OR = 0.59, 95% CI = 0.21–1.71). This study suggests that the relationship between cannabis use and subsequent psychosis expression is likely causal (van Os et al., 2021).

The TRacking Adolescents' Individual Lives Survey (TRAILS) study, a large prospective population study of Dutch adolescents (n = 2,120), examined the direction of association between vulnerability for psychosis and cannabis use throughout adolescence using cross-lagged path analysis, while controlling for gender, family psychopathology, alcohol use, and tobacco use. Cannabis use in the past year was

documented according to self-report at all three waves of the study. The study found significant associations (r = 0.12–0.23) between psychosis vulnerability and cannabis use. Cannabis use at age 16 predicted psychosis vulnerability at age 19. Furthermore, psychosis vulnerability at ages 13 and 16 predicted cannabis use at ages 16 and 19 years, respectively. This study suggests that the association between cannabis use and psychosis is bidirectional causal (Griffith-Lendering et al., 2013). This conclusion of bidirectionality gains general support from the literature. A recent study also showed that the bidirectional association between cannabis use and psychosis is mediated by affective dysregulation, suggesting that there may be an affective pathway from cannabis use to psychosis (Radhakrishnan et al, 2022).

14.5 Biological Mechanisms Underlying the Effects of Cannabis on Psychosis Proneness

The precise biological mechanisms underlying the effects of cannabis use on psychosis proneness remain to be elucidated (see Chapters 10 and 16). A small study that included relatives of patients with schizophrenia found an increase in striatal dopamine release in schizophrenia patients and their relatives following administration of delta-9-tetrahydrocannabinol, the main psychoactive ingredient in cannabis (Kuepper et al., 2013). This suggested that striatal dopamine release following exposure to cannabis may reflect an underlying genetic risk for psychosis. Other studies have suggested that constructs such as aberrant salience (O'Tuathaigh et al., 2020), jumping-to-conclusions, and deficits in working memory (Reininghaus et al., 2019) may underlie the effects of cannabis on psychosis expression. Interestingly, cannabis use and schizotypy have been shown to be associated with abnormalities in face processing. In a study that measured evoked response (ERPs) during a visual face perception task among 97 individuals, those with high cannabis use and high schizotypy had significantly reduced N170 ERPs compared to the control group. Cannabis use (measured using Cannabis Experience Questionnaire (CEQ)) was also found to be correlated with schizotypy scores (measured using SPQ) (Brooks and Brenner, 2018). Recently, people with cannabis use disorder (D'Souza et al., 2021) and schizophrenia (Radhakrishnan et al., 2021) have also been shown to have lower brain synaptic density, consistent with the finding of the deficits in information processing.

14.6 Conclusion

Although the definition of psychosis proneness has undergone change over time, the association with cannabis use and psychosis has been consistent across definitions (i.e., schizotypy, CHR/UHR, and genetic high risk). Psychosis proneness is also associated with higher rates of cannabis use. Studies from general population samples show that cannabis use interacts with other environmental and genetic risk factors in an additive fashion to increase the risk of psychosis expression and that affective dysregulation plays an important role in mediating this risk. Whether the association between cannabis use and psychosis is causal remains debated, with studies suggesting that the relationship may be bidirectional with genetic risk for psychosis also increasing the risk of cannabis use. Finally, the biological mechanisms underlying the association between cannabis use and psychosis remain to be elucidated.

References

Airey, N. D., Hammersley, R., and Reid, M. (2020). Schizotypy but not cannabis use modestly predicts psychotogenic experiences: A cross-sectional study using the Oxford–Liverpool Inventory of Feelings and Experiences (O-LIFE). *J Addict*, **2020**, 5961275.

Albert, N., Glenthoj, L. B., Melau, M., et al. (2017). Course of illness in a sample of patients diagnosed with a schizotypal disorder and treated in a specialized early intervention setting. Findings from the 3.5 year follow-up of the OPUS II study. *Schizophr Res*, **182**, 24–30.

Albertella, L., Le Pelley, M. E., Yucel, M., et al. (2018). Age moderates the association between frequent cannabis use and negative schizotypy over time. *Addict Behav*, **87**, 183–189.

Auther, A. M., Cadenhead, K. S., Carrion, R. E., et al. (2015). Alcohol confounds relationship between cannabis misuse and psychosis conversion in a high-risk sample. *Acta Psychiatr Scand*, **132**, 60–68.

Auther, A. M., McLaughlin, D., Carrion, R. E., et al. (2012). Prospective study of cannabis use in adolescents at clinical high risk for psychosis: impact on conversion to psychosis and functional outcome. *Psychol Med*, **42**, 2485–2497.

Brooks, G. A., and Brenner, C. A. (2018). Is there a common vulnerability in cannabis phenomenology and schizotypy? The role of the N170 ERP. *Schizophr Res*, **197**, 444–450.

Carney, R., Cotter, J., Firth, J., et al. (2017). Cannabis use and symptom severity in individuals at ultra high risk for psychosis: A meta-analysis. *Acta Psychiatr Scand*, **136**, 5–15.

Castle, D. J., and Buckley, P. F. (2015). *Schizophrenia*, 2nd ed. Oxford: Oxford University Press.

Chapman, L. J., Chapman, J. P., and Raulin, M. L. (1976). Scales for physical and social anhedonia. *J Abnorm Psychol*, **85**, 374–382.

Claridge, G. (1994). Single indicator of risk for schizophrenia: probable fact or likely myth? *Schizophr Bull*, **20**, 151–168.

Claridge, G., and Broks, P. (1984). Schizotypy and hemisphere function—I: Theoretical considerations and the measurement of schizotypy. *Pers Individ Differ*, **5**, 633–648.

D'Souza, D. C., Radhakrishnan, R., Naganawa, M., et al. (2021). Preliminary in vivo evidence of lower hippocampal synaptic density in cannabis use disorder. *Mol Psychiatry*, **26**, 3192–3200.

Di Forti, M., Quattrone, D., Freeman, T. P., et al. (2019). The contribution of cannabis use to variation in the incidence of psychotic disorder across Europe (EU-GEI): A multicentre case-control study. *Lancet Psychiatry*, **6**, 427–436.

Eckblad, M., and Chapman, L. J. (1983). Magical ideation as an indicator of schizotypy. *J Consult Clin Psychol*, **51**, 215–225.

Eysenck, H. J. (1992). The definition and measurement of psychoticism. *Pers Individ Differ*, **13**, 757–785.

Fergusson, D. M., Horwood, L. J., and Swain-Campbell, N. R. (2003). Cannabis dependence and psychotic symptoms in young people. *Psychol Med*, **33**, 15–21.

Freeman, A. M., Mokrysz, C., Hindocha, C., et al. (2021). Does variation in trait schizotypy and frequency of cannabis use influence the acute subjective, cognitive and psychotomimetic effects of delta-9-tetrahydrocannabinol? A mega-analysis. *J Psychopharmacol*, **35**, 804–813.

Gage, S. H., Jones, H. J., Burgess, S., et al. (2017). Assessing causality in associations between cannabis use and schizophrenia risk: A two-sample Mendelian randomization study. *Psychol Med*, **47**, 971–980.

Ganesh, S., Cortes-Briones, J., Ranganathan, M., et al. (2020). Psychosis-relevant effects of intravenous delta-9-tetrahydrocannabinol: A mega analysis of individual participant-data from human laboratory studies. *Int J Neuropsychopharmacol*, **23**, 559–570.

Genetic Risk and Outcome in Psychosis (GROUP) Investigators. (2011). Evidence that familial liability for psychosis is expressed as differential sensitivity to cannabis: An analysis of patient-sibling and sibling-control pairs. *Arch Gen Psychiatry*, **68**, 138–147.

Giordano, G. N., Ohlsson, H., Sundquist, K., et al. (2015). The association between cannabis abuse and subsequent schizophrenia: A Swedish national co-relative control study. *Psychol Med*, **45**, 407–414.

Griffith-Lendering, M. F., Wigman, J. T., Prince van Leeuwen, A., et al. (2013). Cannabis use and vulnerability for psychosis in early adolescence: A TRAILS study. *Addiction*, **108**, 733–740.

Guloksuz, S., Pries, L. K., Delespaul, P., et al. (2019). Examining the independent and joint effects of molecular genetic liability and environmental exposures in schizophrenia: Results from the EUGEI study. *World Psychiatry*, **18**, 173–182.

Hindley, G., Beck, K., Borgan, F., et al. (2020). Psychiatric symptoms caused by cannabis constituents: A systematic review and meta-analysis. *Lancet Psychiatry*, **7**, 344–353.

Hjorthoj, C., Albert, N., and Nordentoft, M. (2018). Association of substance use disorders with conversion from schizotypal disorder to schizophrenia. *JAMA Psychiatry*, **75**, 733–739.

Johns, L. C., Cannon, M., Singleton, N., et al. (2004). Prevalence and correlates of self-reported psychotic symptoms in the British population. *Br J Psychiatry*, **185**, 298–305.

Johnson, E. C., Hatoum, A. S., Deak, J. D., et al. (2021). The relationship between cannabis and schizophrenia: A genetically informed perspective. *Addiction*, **116**, 3227–3234.

Kendler, K. S., Lieberman, J. A., and Walsh, D. (1989). The structured interview for schizotypy (SIS): A preliminary report. *Schizophr Bull*, **15**, 559–571.

Kraan, T., Velthorst, E., Koenders, L., et al. (2016). Cannabis use and transition to psychosis in individuals at ultra-high risk: review and meta-analysis. *Psychol Med*, **46**, 673–681.

Kuepper, R., Ceccarini, J., Lataster, J., et al. (2013). Delta-9-tetrahydrocannabinol-induced dopamine release as a function of psychosis risk: 18F-fallypride positron emission tomography study. *PLoS ONE*, **8**, e70378.

Linscott, R. J., and van Os, J. (2013). An updated and conservative systematic review and meta-analysis of epidemiological evidence on psychotic experiences in children and adults: On the pathway from proneness to persistence to dimensional expression across mental disorders. *Psychol Med*, **43**, 1133–1149.

Marconi, A., Di Forti, M., Lewis, C. M., et al. (2016). Meta-analysis of the association between the level of cannabis use and risk of psychosis. *Schizophr Bull*, **42**, 1262–1269.

Mason, O., and Claridge, G. (2006). The Oxford-Liverpool Inventory of Feelings and Experiences (O-LIFE): Further description and extended norms. *Schizophr Res*, **82**, 203–211.

McHugh, M. J., McGorry, P. D., Yung, A. R., et al. (2017). Cannabis-induced attenuated psychotic symptoms: Implications for prognosis in young people at ultra-high risk for psychosis. *Psychol Med*, **47**, 616–626.

Meehl, P. E. (1962). Schizotaxia, schizotypy, schizophrenia. *Am Psychologist*, **17**, 827–838.

Minor, K. S., Firmin, R. L., Bonfils, K. A., et al. (2014). Predicting creativity: The role of psychometric schizotypy and cannabis use in divergent thinking. *Psychiatry Res*, **220**, 205–210.

Myin-Germeys, I., Krabbendam, L., Delespaul, P., et al. (2003). The affective pathway to psychosis. *Schizophr Res*, **60**, 47.

Nordentoft, M., Thorup, A., Petersen, L., et al. (2006). Transition rates from schizotypal disorder to psychotic disorder for first-contact patients included in the OPUS trial. A randomized clinical trial of integrated treatment and standard treatment. *Schizophr Res*, **83**, 29–40.

O'Tuathaigh, C. M. P., Dawes, C., Bickerdike, A., et al. (2020). Does cannabis use predict psychometric schizotypy via aberrant salience? *Schizophr Res*, **220**, 194–200.

van Os, J., Bak, M., Hanssen, M., et al. (2002). Cannabis use and psychosis: A longitudinal population-based study. *Am J Epidemiol*, **156**, 319–327.

van Os, J., Hanssen, M., Bijl, R. V., et al. (2000). Strauss (1969) revisited: A psychosis continuum in the general population? *Schizophr Res*, **45**, 11–20.

van Os, J., Pries, L. K., Ten Have, M., et al. (2021). Schizophrenia and the environment: Within-person analyses may be required to yield evidence of unconfounded and causal association: The example of cannabis and psychosis. *Schizophr Bull*, **47**, 594–603.

Parnas, J., Raballo, A., Handest, P., et al. (2011). Self-experience in the early phases of schizophrenia: 5-year follow-up of the Copenhagen Prodromal Study. *World Psychiatry*, **10**, 200–204.

Pasman, J. A., Verweij, K. J. H., Gerring, Z., et al. (2018). GWAS of lifetime cannabis use reveals new risk loci, genetic overlap with psychiatric traits, and a causal influence of schizophrenia. *Nat Neurosci*, **21**, 1161–1170.

Pearson, J. S., and Kley, I. B. (1957). On the application of genetic expectancies as age-specific base rates in the study of human behavior disorders. *Psychol Bull*, **54**, 406–420.

Pries, L. K., Guloksuz, S., Ten Have, M., et al. (2018). Evidence that environmental and familial risks for psychosis additively impact a multidimensional subthreshold psychosis syndrome. *Schizophr Bull*, **44**, 710–719.

Quattrone, D., Reininghaus, U., Richards, A. L., et al. (2021). The continuity of effect of schizophrenia polygenic risk score and patterns of cannabis use on transdiagnostic symptom dimensions at first-episode psychosis: Findings from the EU-GEI study. *Transl Psychiatry*, **11**, 423.

Radhakrishnan, R., Addy, P. H., Sewell, R. A., et al. (2014a). Cannabis, cannabinoids, and the association with psychosis. In Madras, B., and Kuhar, M. (eds.), *The Effects of Drug Abuse on the Human Nervous System* (pp. 423–458). Amsterdam: Academic Press.

Radhakrishnan, R., Guloksuz, S., Ten Have, M., et al. (2019). Interaction between environmental and familial affective risk impacts psychosis admixture in states of affective dysregulation. *Psychol Med*, **49**, 1879–1889.

Radhakrishnan, R., Pries, L-K., Erzin, G., et al. Bidirectional relationships between cannabis use, anxiety and depressive symptoms in mediation of the association with psychotic experience: further support for an affective pathway to psychosis. *Psychol Med*, 1–7 doi: 10.1017/S0033291722002756 (Online ahead of print).

Radhakrishnan, R., Skosnik, P. D., Ranganathan, M., et al. (2021). In vivo evidence of lower synaptic vesicle density in schizophrenia. *Mol Psychiatry*, **26**, 7690–7698.

Radhakrishnan, R., Wilkinson, S. T., and D'Souza, D. C. (2014b). Gone to pot: A review of the association between cannabis and psychosis. *Front Psychiatry*, **5**, 54.

Rado, S. (1953). Dynamics and classification of disordered behavior. *Am J Psychiatry*, **110**, 406–416.

Raine, A. (1991). The SPQ: A scale for the assessment of schizotypal personality based on DSM-III-R criteria. *Schizophr Bull*, **17**, 555–564.

 (2006). Schizotypal personality: Neurodevelopmental and psychosocial trajectories. *Annu Rev Clin Psychol*, **2**, 291–326.

Reininghaus, U., Rauschenberg, C., Ten Have, M., et al. (2019). Reasoning bias, working memory performance and a transdiagnostic phenotype of affective disturbances and psychotic experiences in the general population. *Psychol Med*, **49**, 1799–1809.

Schafer, G., Feilding, A., Morgan, C. J., et al. (2012). Investigating the interaction between schizotypy, divergent thinking and cannabis use. *Conscious Cogn*, **21**, 292–298.

Stefanis, N. C., Hanssen, M., Smirnis, N. K., et al. (2002). Evidence that three dimensions of psychosis have a distribution in the general population. *Psychol Med*, **32**, 347–358.

Szoke, A., Galliot, A. M., Richard, J. R., et al. (2014). Association between cannabis use and schizotypal dimensions: A meta-analysis of cross-sectional studies. *Psychiatry Res*, **219**, 58–66.

Vadhan, N. P., Corcoran, C. M., Bedi, G., et al. (2017). Acute effects of smoked marijuana in marijuana smokers at clinical high-risk for psychosis: A preliminary study. *Psychiatry Res*, **257**, 372–374.

Valmaggia, L. R., Day, F. L., Jones, C., et al. (2014). Cannabis use and transition to psychosis in people at ultra-high risk. *Psychol Med*, **44**, 2503–2512.

Vaucher, J., Keating, B. J., Lasserre, A. M., et al. (2018). Cannabis use and risk of schizophrenia: A Mendelian randomization study. *Mol Psychiatry*, **23**, 1287–1292.

Verdoux, H., Sorbara, F., Gindre, C., et al. (2003). Cannabis use and dimensions of psychosis in a nonclinical population of female subjects. *Schizophr Res*, **59**, 77–84.

Verweij, K. J., Abdellaoui, A., Nivard, M. G., et al. (2017). Short communication: Genetic association between schizophrenia and cannabis use. *Drug Alcohol Depend*, **171**, 117–121.

Wuthrich, V. M., and Bates, T. C. (2006). Confirmatory factor analysis of the three-factor structure of the schizotypal personality questionnaire and Chapman schizotypy scales. *J Pers Assess*, **87**, 292–304.

Chapter

15

Which Cannabis Users Develop Psychosis?

Edoardo Spinazzola, Marta Di Forti, and Robin M. Murray

15.1 Introduction

The fact that not all cannabis users will develop psychosis suggests that cannabis may exert its causal role only in individuals in some way predisposed (Di Forti and Murray, 2005; Henquet et al., 2005). However, since the number of people who use cannabis worldwide is so high, those who will eventually develop psychosis, while still a minority, represent a large number. Indeed, a multisite study has shown that 12% of first episode of psychosis cases across Europe can be attributed to the use of high-potency cannabis; this figure increases to 50% in Amsterdam and 30% in London (Di Forti et al., 2019a). Cannabis use can also impact on the incidence of psychotic disorders over time. In Denmark and Portugal, over recent decades, there has been an increase in the number of cases of schizophrenia and psychosis, respectively, that may be attributable to cannabis use disorder (Gonçalves-Pinho et al., 2020; Hjorthøj et al., 2021a).

Given the complex nature of the association between cannabis use and psychosis, it is hard to determine which cannabis users will eventually develop psychosis. The link between cannabis use and schizophrenia is unlikely to be just the result of a genetic pre-disposition, it is more likely the result of Gene × Environment inter-play (Henquet et al., 2008; van Os et al., 2010). Already there is enough evidence to indicate that some factors – both on an individual-level and from the external environment – determine an individual's vulnerability to develop psychosis.

15.2 Age at First Cannabis Use and the Risk for Psychosis

The first epidemiological evidence clearly indicating that, among cannabis users, those who start smoking earlier have higher odds of developing psychosis came from the Dunedin study. This longitudinal prospective study indicated that cannabis users who started

their use in their early teens had a greater risk for later schizophreniform psychosis compared to those who started at age 18 years or later (Arseneault et al., 2002). Consistent with the developmental risk factor model of schizophrenia, these findings suggest that exposing the brain to cannabis while it is undergoing important developmental changes can contribute to increased risk to psychosis later in life (Murray and Lewis, 1987; Murray et al., 2017a). Exposure to cannabis may disrupt the endocannabinoid system, which plays a central role in neurodevelopment, thus negatively impacting on neurotransmitter function (Sideli et al., 2020; Volkow et al., 2014). Some neuroimaging evidence indicates that the use of cannabis during adolescence can have a detrimental impact on striatal dopaminergic activity (Urban et al., 2012). Furthermore, starting to use cannabis in adolescence is associated with an earlier appearance of a range of symptoms in individuals at clinical high risk for psychosis. These symptoms include anxiety, social withdrawal, derealization, memory impairment, and weakness of thinking and concentration (Dragt et al., 2012).

Not only does early cannabis use increase the risk of developing psychosis but, among patients with psychosis, on average those who have used cannabis experience the onset of the illness earlier. The largest meta-analysis to date reported that the age of onset of psychosis in cannabis users is almost three years younger than in non-users (Large et al., 2011). When considering daily users of high-potency cannabis, their onset was on average six years earlier compared to non-cannabis users (Di Forti et al., 2014). This latter study also showed that early age at first use and high-potency cannabis use are independently associated with a significantly higher hazard of developing a psychotic disorder; this finding conflicts with a hypothesis which suggested that age of first onset was determined just by the duration of cannabis use (Stefanis et al., 2013).

15.3 Frequency of Cannabis Use, Its Potency, and the Risk for Psychosis

The earliest study to draw attention to the dose–response effect between cannabis and psychosis dates back to 1987 and was carried out by Andréasson and colleagues. In this longitudinal cohort study, they found that Swedish military conscripts who had used cannabis more than 50 times in their life were 6 times more at risk of developing psychosis compared to their non-cannabis using counterparts (Andréasson et al., 1987). A later follow-up analysis of the same cohort at 27 years confirmed that cannabis was associated with the risk of developing schizophrenia in a dose-dependent fashion (Zammit, 2002). Other cohort studies, such as NEMESIS, confirmed these findings, also highlighting the importance of the dose of cannabis to which subjects were exposed (van Os et al., 2002). A case-control study of 280 patients with first-episode psychosis and 174 healthy controls reported that, in South London, patients preferentially used high-potency cannabis preparations of the skunk variety, and they reportedly used cannabis for longer and with greater frequency than their healthy control counterparts (Di Forti et al., 2009).

The potency of cannabis refers to the amount of Δ9-THC it contains. High-potency cannabis is particularly harmful for mental health (Smith, 2005); the Δ9-THC content of cannabis varies considerably in different strains of cannabis plants (Radhakrishnan et al., 2014), as well as Cannabidiol, CBD, which has been suggested to counteract some (Bhattacharyya et al., 2010; Englund et al., 2013) – but not all (Black et al., 2019) – of the negative effects of THC. Traditional UK cannabis resin contained 2–4% of Δ9-THC and had approximately the same amount of CBD, whereas some strains of herbal cannabis (termed skunk in the United Kingdom) contained much higher levels of Δ9-THC with virtually no CBD (Potter et al., 2008). In the United Kingdom, THC content in 'skunk' has remained constant over the last decade while it has increased in resin types of cannabis alongside a reduction in CBD (Potter et al., 2018). Consistently with the UK data, over the last few decades there has been an increase in the average content of THC, but not in CBD, in both herbal and resin types of cannabis in most Western countries, with increases primarily attributable to a greater market share of high-potency strains such as skunk (Freeman et al., 2021).

In 2015, a South London study, from a bigger sample of 410 patients with first-episode psychosis and 370 population controls, found that people using skunk-like cannabis on a daily basis were five times more likely to develop psychosis compared to those who had never used cannabis. The population attributable fraction of first-episode psychosis was 24%, indicating that high-potency cannabis use alone was responsible for 24% of people presenting to the psychiatric services in South London with a first episode of psychosis (Di Forti et al., 2015). Furthermore, variation in the daily use of high-potency cannabis was found responsible for contributing to the variation in the incidence of psychotic disorders across Europe (Di Forti et al., 2019a). More recently it has been shown how the incidence of psychosis can be influenced by variations in cannabis use across time, which was measured by assessing the proportion of schizophrenia patients with cannabis use disorder (Hjorthøj et al., 2021a).

A meta-analysis of the association between the extent of cannabis use and the risk of psychosis confirmed a dose–response relationship: the heaviest cannabis users have an almost four-fold increased risk of psychosis compared with non-users (Marconi et al., 2016). However, since that time, much more potent cannabis has become available in some countries. For example, in Canada and in those US States that have legalized recreational cannabis, a range of products such as oil, wax dabs, shatter, and crumble have become available which have THC levels up to 80–90%, and carry a greater risk of psychosis (Goodman et al., 2020).

15.4 Family History of Psychosis and Cannabis Use

Despite all this evidence, some have questioned the suitability of cohort studies to determine the extent to which cannabis use causes psychotic disorders (Gillespie and Kendler, 2021), suggesting that the predictions of the cases of schizophrenia that might be prevented by reducing cannabis consumption based on these studies are greatly inflated (Giordano et al., 2015). Given the high heritability of schizophrenia, they suggested that genetic epidemiological studies – together with other genetic designs – are best able to address the nature of this association (Gillespie and Kendler, 2021). However, genetic epidemiological studies, even though they can be easy to conceptualize, are difficult to conduct (Baselmans et al., 2021). Twin studies large enough to examine this mechanism are rare (Agrawal and Lynskey, 2014); their findings suggest that shared genetic/familial factors do contribute to this association, but do not explain it away, with contradictory results regarding the causal impact of cannabis use on the risk for psychosis (Giordano et al., 2015; Schaefer et al., 2021).

More studies have focused on family history of psychosis and cannabis use rather than on twins. An early case-control study indicated that cannabis users with psychosis were more likely to have a positive family history for psychotic disorders compared to non-cannabis using patients with psychosis (McGuire et al., 1995). Another study confirmed these findings (Bersani et al., 2002); Boydell et al. (2007) showed that 15% of cases of first onset schizophrenia with cannabis use had a positive family history for schizophrenia compared to a similar proportion, 12%, among the control group of non-cannabis using patients with schizophrenia.

A nationwide sample of individuals born in Denmark between 1955 and 1990 found a 2.5-fold increased risk of developing cannabis-induced psychosis in children with a mother with schizophrenia, but the risk of developing schizophrenia following a cannabis-induced psychosis diagnosis was not related to familial pre-disposition (Arendt et al., 2008). Likewise, more recently, the results of a Swedish national sample indicated that subjects with cannabis-induced psychosis who developed schizophrenia have the same familial risk for this disorder as the other individuals with schizophrenia. The authors concluded that the association between cannabis use and schizophrenia is in part the result of some sharing of familial risk for cannabis consumption and schizophrenia (Kendler et al., 2019).

Of course, it needs to be borne in mind that the presence of a family member with schizophrenia does not necessarily imply genetic transmission. It could be that the relative also abused cannabis or indeed had introduced the proband to cannabis.

The Genetic Risk and Outcome of Psychosis (GROUP) study showed that, in the sibling-control comparison, siblings presented more than 15 times greater sensitivity to positive schizotypy associated with current cannabis consumption than controls, with similar results for negative schizotypy. Self-reported sub-clinical psychotic symptoms were assessed with the Community Assessment of Psychic Experiences (CAPE) questionnaire. There was a significant association in the positive symptoms dimension between cannabis-using siblings and their relatives with psychosis compared with non-cannabis using siblings. No significant association was found on the negative domains of the CAPE scale (Genetic Risk and Outcome in Psychosis Investigators, 2011).

15.5 Schizophrenia Polygenic Risk Score (PRS-SZ), Cannabis Use, and Risk for Psychosis

The first studies investigating genetic factors that may confer vulnerability to psychotic disorders following cannabis exposure tested gene × environment interactions based on single candidate genes. Findings from the Dunedin cohort reported that the COMT (Catechol-methyl-transferase) gene moderated the effect of adolescent cannabis use on developing adult psychosis. More specifically, individuals who carried both valine alleles (Val/Val individuals) of the COMT gene were at greater risk of developing schizophreniform disorder in adulthood (OR = 10.9; 95% CI = 2.2–54.1) and, to a lesser extent, also those who carried just one valine allele (Val/Met individuals) (OR = 2.5; 95% CI = 0.78–8.2) (Caspi et al., 2005). The COMT gene codes for the homonymous enzyme which is involved in the metabolism of dopamine in the prefrontal cortex; disturbances in dopaminergic transmission are well known to be implicated in the pathogenesis of schizophrenia. These reports, however, were not replicated (Zammit et al., 2007). Initial promising data (Di Forti et al., 2012; Morgan et al., 2016; Van Winkel et al., 2011) implicated another dopaminergic candidate gene, AKT1 as a potential moderator of the effect of cannabis use on risk of psychosis. Other studies did not replicate these initial reports, with one recent study reporting that variation in AKT1, COMT, or FAAH was neither associated with psychotic-like experiences nor with euphoric experiences (Hindocha et al., 2020).

The advent of Genome Wide Association Studies (GWAS) – which have shown that many hundreds of thousands of common alleles influence susceptibility to various psychiatric disorders – have been used to investigate this association more accurately compared with previous studies based on specific candidate genes. GWAS findings can be summarized in a risk score, Polygenic Risk Score (PRS), constructed as the sum of the weighted effect of all the genetic markers together; this score describes the polygenic nature of complex disorders such as psychiatric disorders. Many studies have started to examine the link between psychosis proneness, measured by the PRS for schizophrenia (PRS-SZ) and cannabis use (Sideli et al., 2020).

Some studies found that the PRS-SZ explains a small but significant proportion of the variance for cannabis use ($R^2 = 0.47\%$, $p = 2.6 \times 10^{-4}$), suggesting that part of the association between cannabis use and schizophrenia is due to a shared genetic liability (Power et al., 2014). A recent study suggested that this relationship is not mediated through other phenotypic manifestations of genetic risk for schizophrenia during childhood, such as lower IQ, victimization, antisocial behaviour, emotional difficulties, impulsivity, or poorer social relationships (Jones et al., 2020). However, it should be noted that these studies are characterized by several flaws, which limit the generalizability of their findings. First, as was previously noted, liability to SZ explains only a small portion of the variance in cannabis use (Sideli et al., 2021). Second, these studies have been relatively small, and they have rarely considered other PRSs than schizophrenia (Hjorthøj et al., 2021b). Lastly, it is worth noting that one of these studies also reports that the genetic risk for schizophrenia plays the most important role in explaining late-onset cannabis use (Jones et al., 2020). The fact that this link is stronger for late-onset cannabis use compared to early onset indirectly confirms the importance of the role played by the non-genetic factors in young cannabis users' risk for psychosis.

One very large study found that PRS-SZ was not associated with cannabis use disorder (CUD) in either controls or patients with other psychiatric conditions, but there was a small increase in the risk of CUD among patients with schizophrenia. Therefore, the authors concluded that the leading theory to explain the association between cannabis use and psychosis is still the theory of causation (Hjorthøj et al., 2021b). Another recent study – which analysed a sample of 109,308 UK biobank participants cross-sectionally – tried to examine how PRS-SZ modulates the relationship between cannabis use and different types of self-reported psychotic experiences. Whilst reporting that individuals genetically predisposed to schizophrenia may be at higher risk of developing psychotic

symptoms as a result of cannabis use, it also showed that persecutory delusions have a particularly pronounced association with cannabis use frequency, but delusions of reference seem to interact with PRS-SZ beyond cannabis use. This seems to indicate that delusions of reference may be more directly modulated by genetic factors, whilst persecutory delusions may be more specifically the result of the harmful effects of cannabis on other brain regions (Wainberg et al., 2021). However, this finding needs to be replicated.

Overall, it appears more likely that genetic risk for schizophrenia exerts an additive interaction on some of the well-known environmental risk factors for psychotic disorders including cannabis use (Guloksuz et al., 2019). Indeed, Di Forti et al. (2019b) reported evidence supporting an independent effect of PRS-SZ and heavy cannabis use on risk for psychotic disorders, with those individuals with a high PRS-SZ who also used cannabis heavily having the greater risk of developing psychosis. More recently, Elkrief et al. (2021) reported comparable findings in a similar study aimed at assessing whether the relationship between PRS-SZ and psychotic-like experiences (PLEs) is either mediated or moderated by lifetime cannabis use at age 16. The authors concluded that cannabis use is a risk factor for PLEs, over and above genetic risk for schizophrenia.

15.6 What Are the Characteristics of Cannabis Users Who Are Psychotic?

Cannabis users with psychosis have a higher premorbid IQ and better pre-morbid social functioning compared to non-cannabis using first-episode psychosis patients (Ferraro et al., 2013, 2020, 2021). They are also less likely to show neurological soft signs than other psychotic patients (Ruiz-Veguilla et al., 2012). A possible explanation for this is that, on average in cannabis users, onset of psychosis is driven primarily by the pharmacological effects of cannabis, while, in non-cannabis using patients with psychosis, early neurodevelopmental disruption may play a more important role; this is confirmed by the evidence that cannabis users who will develop psychosis are more socially skilful and therefore able to obtain the substance (Murray et al., 2017b).

It has been suggested that people start using cannabis in order to seek relief from prodromal psychotic symptoms (Archie et al., 2013; Ferdinand et al., 2005).

This is the so-called self-medication hypothesis, which suggests a form of reverse causality in the interaction between cannabis use and psychosis, as it posits that psychotic symptoms in adolescents act as a risk factor for future cannabis use. However, this hypothesis has been rejected by the bulk of the literature, which indicates that cannabis use is a contributory cause of schizophrenia. The evidence indicates that patients with first-episode psychosis use cannabis for the same hedonic reasons as the general population (Kolliakou et al., 2011).

Recently, some evidence pointed out that cannabis may be a 'modifier' factor that affects symptom presentation of psychotic disorders. More specifically, first-episode psychosis patients with a history of daily use of high-potency cannabis present with more positive symptoms compared with those who never used cannabis or used low-potency types (B = 0.35; 95% CI = 0.14–0.56). Conversely, negative symptoms are more common in those first-episode psychosis patients who never used cannabis compared with all other groups (B = –0.22; 95% CI = –0.37 to –0.07) (Quattrone et al., 2020). Moreover, the effect of cannabis use on positive symptomatology is independent from the effect conferred by the genetic risk (Quattrone et al., 2021).

The interactive effects of childhood adversity and cannabis use have been examined by several studies. In 2008 Houston and colleagues found that subjects with a history of sexual abuse who used cannabis prior to age 16 were roughly 12 times more likely to develop psychosis (OR = 11.96; 95% CI = 2.10–68.22) (Houston et al., 2008). The additive interaction between childhood adversity and cannabis use was clearly pointed out by another study which reported that the presence of both these risk factors increased the odds for psychotic symptoms beyond the risk posed by each factor alone (Harley et al., 2010). The relationship between childhood adversity and psychosis was also more specifically affected by the pattern of cannabis use (Sideli et al., 2018).

The negative effects of cannabis continue to impact on patients' lives also after their first episode of illness. Patients who continue to use cannabis after the onset of psychosis, especially high-potency types and with higher frequency, have higher relapse rates, longer hospital admissions, and more intense psychiatric care compared to former users who discontinued or never-users (Schoeler et al., 2016; Zammit et al., 2008). Another study, while confirming that patients with psychosis who continue to use cannabis have a worse prognosis compared to other groups of patients, also assessed the mediation role played by medication adherence in this association. It was found that between 20% and 36% of the adverse effects of continued cannabis use on outcome in psychosis might be mediated through the effects of cannabis use on medication adherence (Schoeler et al., 2017). In other words, patients with psychosis who continue to use cannabis are less likely to comply with antipsychotic prescriptions, and this contributes to their clinical outcome. Another study showed that both nicotine dependence and cannabis use after psychosis onset predicted poor medication adherence and non-remission (Colizzi et al., 2016).

References

Agrawal, A., and Lynskey, M. T. (2014). Cannabis controversies: How genetics can inform the study of comorbidity. *Addiction*, **109**, 360–370.

Andréasson, S., Engström, A., Allebeck, P., et al. (1987). Cannabis and schizophrenia: A longitudinal study of Swedish conscripts. *Lancet*, **330**, 1483–1486.

Archie, S., Boydell, K. M., Stasiulis, E., et al. (2013). Reflections of young people who have had a first episode of psychosis: What attracted them to use alcohol and illicit drugs? *Early Interv Psychiatry*, **7**, 193–199.

Arendt, M., Mortensen, P. B., Rosenberg, R., et al. (2008). Familial predisposition for psychiatric disorder. *Arch Gen Psychiatry*, **65**, 1269.

Arseneault, L., Cannon, M., Poulton, R., et al. (2002). Cannabis use in adolescence and risk for adult psychosis: longitudinal prospective study. *BMJ*, **325**, 1212–1213.

Baselmans, B. M. L., Yengo, L., Van Rheenen, W., et al. (2021). Risk in relatives, heritability, SNP-based heritability, and genetic correlations in psychiatric disorders: A review. *Biol Psychiatry*, **89**, 11–19.

Bersani, G., Orlandi, V., Kotzalidis, G. D., et al. (2002). Cannabis and schizophrenia: Impact on onset, course, psychopathology and outcomes. *Eur Arch Psychiatry Clin Neurosci*, **252**, 86–92.

Bhattacharyya, S., Morrison, P. D., Fusar-Poli, P., et al. (2010). Opposite effects of delta-9-tetrahydrocannabinol and cannabidiol on human brain function and psychopathology. *Neuropsychopharmacology*, **35**, 764–774.

Black, N., Stockings, E., Campbell, G., et al. (2019). Cannabinoids for the treatment of mental disorders and symptoms of mental disorders: A systematic review and meta-analysis. *Lancet Psychiatry*, **6**, 995–1010.

Boydell, J., Dean, K., Dutta, R., et al. (2007). A comparison of symptoms and family history in schizophrenia with and without prior cannabis use: Implications for the concept of cannabis psychosis. *Schizophr Res*, **93**, 203–210.

Caspi, A., Moffitt, T. E., Cannon, M., et al. (2005). Moderation of the effect of adolescent-onset cannabis use on adult psychosis by a functional polymorhpism in the cathecol-O-methiltransferase gene: Longitudinal evidence of a gene x environment interaction. *Biol Psychiatry*, **57**, 1117–1127.

Colizzi, M., Carra, E., Fraietta, S., et al. (2016). Substance use, medication adherence and outcome one year following a first episode of psychosis. *Schizophr Res*, **170**, 311–317.

Di Forti, M., Iyegbe, C., Sallis, H., et al. (2012). Confirmation that the AKT1 (rs2494732) genotype influences the risk of psychosis in cannabis users. *Biol Psychiatry*, **72**, 811–816.

Di Forti, M., Marconi, A., Carra, E., et al. (2015). Proportion of patients in south London with first-episode psychosis attributable to use of high potency cannabis: a case-control study. *Lancet Psychiatry*, **2**, 233–238.

Di Forti, M., Morgan, C., Dazzan, P., et al. (2009). High-potency cannabis and the risk of psychosis. *Br J Psychiatry*, **195**, 488–491.

Di Forti, M., and Murray, R. M. (2005). Cannabis consumption and risk of developing schizophrenia: Myth or reality? *Epidemiol Psychiatric Sci*, **14**, 184–187.

Di Forti, M., Quattrone, D., Freeman, T. P., et al. (2019a). The contribution of cannabis use to variation in the incidence of psychotic disorder across Europe (EU-GEI): A multicentre case-control study. *Lancet Psychiatry*, **6**, 427–436.

Di Forti, M., Sallis, H., Allegri, F., et al. (2014). Daily use, especially of high-potency cannabis, drives the earlier onset of psychosis in cannabis users. *Schizophr Bull*, **40**, 1509–1517.

Di Forti, M., Wu-Choi, B., Quattrone, D., et al. (2019b). *The Independent and Combined Influence of Schizophrenia Polygenic Risk Score and Heavy Cannabis Use on Risk for Psychotic Disorder: A Case-Control Analysis from the EUGEI Study.* Cold Spring Harbor Laboratory.

Dragt, S., Nieman, D. H., Schultze-Lutter, F., et al. (2012). Cannabis use and age at onset of symptoms in subjects at clinical high risk for psychosis. *Acta Psychiatr Scand*, **125**, 45–53.

Elkrief, L., Lin, B., Marchi, M., et al. (2021). Independent contribution of polygenic risk for schizophrenia and cannabis use in predicting psychotic-like experiences in young adulthood: Testing gene × environment moderation and mediation. *Psychol Med*, 1–11.

Englund, A., Morrison, P. D., Nottage, J., et al. (2013). Cannabidiol inhibits THC-elicited paranoid symptoms and hippocampal-dependent memory impairment. *J Psychopharmacol*, **27**, 19–27.

Ferdinand, R. F., Sondeijker, F., Van Der Ende, J., et al. (2005). Cannabis use predicts future psychotic symptoms, and vice versa. *Addiction*, **100**, 612–618.

Ferraro, L., La Cascia, C., La Barbera, D., et al. (2021). The relationship of symptom dimensions with premorbid adjustment and cognitive characteristics at first episode psychosis: Findings from the EU-GEI study. *Schizophr Res*, **236**, 69–79.

Ferraro, L., La Cascia, C., Quattrone, D., et al. (2020). Premorbid adjustment and IQ in patients with first-episode psychosis: A multisite case-control study of their relationship with cannabis use. *Schizophr Bull*, **46**, 517–529.

Ferraro, L., Russo, M., O'Connor, J., et al. (2013). Cannabis users have higher premorbid IQ than other patients with first onset psychosis. *Schizophr Res*, **150**, 129–135.

Freeman, T. P., Craft, S., Wilson, J., et al. (2021). Changes in delta-9-tetrahydrocannabinol (THC) and cannabidiol (CBD) concentrations in cannabis over time: Systematic review and meta-analysis. *Addiction*, **116**, 1000–1010.

Genetic Risk and Outcome in Psychosis (GROUP) Investigators. (2011). Evidence that familial liability for psychosis is expressed as differential sensitivity to cannabis: An analysis of patient-sibling and sibling-control pairs. *Arch Gen Psychiatry*, **68**, 138–147.

Gillespie, N. A., and Kendler, K. S. (2021). Use of genetically informed methods to clarify the nature of the association between cannabis use and risk for schizophrenia. *JAMA Psychiatry*, **78**, 467–468.

Giordano, G. N., Ohlsson, H., Sundquist, K., et al. (2015). The association between cannabis abuse and subsequent schizophrenia: A Swedish national co-relative control study. *Psychol Med*, **45**, 407–414.

Gonçalves-Pinho, M., Bragança, M., and Freitas, A. (2020). Psychotic disorders hospitalizations associated with cannabis abuse or dependence: A nationwide big data analysis. *Int J Methods Psychiatr Res*, **29**, e1813.

Goodman, S., Wadsworth, E., Leos-Toro, C., et al. (2020). Prevalence and forms of cannabis use in legal vs. illegal recreational cannabis

153

markets. *Int J Drug Policy*, **76**, 102658.

Guloksuz, S., Pries, L. K., Delespaul, P., et al. (2019). Examining the independent and joint effects of molecular genetic liability and environmental exposures in schizophrenia: Results from the EUGEI study. *World Psychiatry*, **18**, 173–182.

Harley, M., Kelleher, I., Clarke, M., et al. (2010). Cannabis use and childhood trauma interact additively to increase the risk of psychotic symptoms in adolescence. *Psychol Med*, **40**, 1627–1634.

Henquet, C., Di Forti, M., Morrison, P., et al. (2008). Gene–environment interplay between cannabis and psychosis. *Schizophr Bull*, **34**, 1111–1121.

Henquet, C., Murray, R., Linszen, D., et al. (2005). The environment and schizophrenia: The role of cannabis use. *Schizophr Bull*, **31**, 608–612.

Hindocha, C., Quattrone, D., Freeman, T. P., et al. (2020). Do AKT1, COMT and FAAH influence reports of acute cannabis intoxication experiences in patients with first episode psychosis, controls and young adult cannabis users? *Transl Psychiatry*, **10**, 143.

Hjorthøj, C., Larsen, M. O., Starzer, M. S. K., et al. (2021a). Annual incidence of cannabis-induced psychosis, other substance-induced psychoses and dually diagnosed schizophrenia and cannabis use disorder in Denmark from 1994 to 2016. *Psychol Med*, **51**, 617–622.

Hjorthøj, C., Uddin, M. J., Wimberley, T., et al. (2021b). No evidence of associations between genetic liability for schizophrenia and development of cannabis use disorder. *Psychol Med*, **51**, 479–484.

Houston, J. E., Murphy, J., Adamson, G., et al. (2008). Childhood sexual

abuse, early cannabis use, and psychosis: Testing an interaction model based on the National Comorbidity Survey. *Schizophr Bull*, **34**, 580–585.

Jones, H. J., Hammerton, G., Mccloud, T., et al. (2020). Examining pathways between genetic liability for schizophrenia and patterns of tobacco and cannabis use in adolescence. *Psychol Med*, 1–8.

Kendler, K. S., Ohlsson, H., Sundquist, J., et al. (2019). Prediction of onset of substance-induced psychotic disorder and its progression to schizophrenia in a Swedish national sample. *Am J Psychiatry*, **176**, 711–719.

Kolliakou, A., Joseph, C., Ismail, K., et al. (2011). Why do patients with psychosis use cannabis and are they ready to change their use? *Int J Dev Neurosci*, **29**, 335–346.

Large, M., Sharma, S., Compton, M. T., et al. (2011). Cannabis use and earlier onset of psychosis: A systematic meta-analysis. *Arch Gen Psychiatry*, **68**, 555–561.

Marconi, A., Di Forti, M., Lewis, C. M., et al. (2016). Meta-analysis of the association between the level of cannabis use and risk of psychosis. *Schizophr Bull*, **42**, 1262–1269.

McGuire, P. K., Jones, P., Harvey, I., et al. (1995). Morbid risk of schizophrenia for relatives of patients with cannabis-associated psychosis. *Schizophr Res*, **15**, 277–281.

Morgan, C. J. A., Freeman, T. P., Powell, J., et al. (2016). AKT1 genotype moderates the acute psychotomimetic effects of naturalistically smoked cannabis in young cannabis smokers. *Translat Psychiatry*, **6**, e738–e738.

Murray, R. M., Bhavsar, V., Tripoli, G., et al. (2017a). 30 Years on: How the neurodevelopmental hypothesis of schizophrenia morphed into the developmental risk factor model of psychosis. *Schizophr Bull*, **43**, 1190–1196.

Murray, R. M., Englund, A., Abi-Dargham, A., et al. (2017b). Cannabis-associated psychosis: Neural substrate and clinical impact. *Neuropharmacology*, **124**, 89–104.

Murray, R. M., and Lewis, S. W. (1987). Is schizophrenia a neurodevelopmental disorder? *BMJ*, **295**, 681–682.

van Os, J., Bak, M., Hanssen, M., et al. (2002). Cannabis use and psychosis: A longitudinal population-based study. *Am J Epidemiology*, **156**, 319–327.

van Os, J., Kenis, G., and Rutten, B. P. F. (2010). The environment and schizophrenia. *Nature*, **468**, 203–212.

Potter, D. J., Clark, P., and Brown, M. B. (2008). Potency of delta 9-THC and other cannabinoids in cannabis in England in 2005: Implications for psychoactivity and pharmacology. *J Forensic Sci*, **53**, 90–94.

Potter, D. J., Hammond, K., Tuffnell, S., et al. (2018). Potency of Delta (9) -tetrahydrocannabinol and other cannabinoids in cannabis in England in 2016: Implications for public health and pharmacology. *Drug Test Anal*, **10**, 628–635.

Power, R. A., Verweij, K. J., Zuhair, M., et al. (2014). Genetic predisposition to schizophrenia associated with increased use of cannabis. *Mol Psychiatry*, **19**, 1201–1204.

Quattrone, D., Ferraro, L., Tripoli, G., et al. (2020). Daily use of high-potency cannabis is associated with more positive symptoms in first-episode psychosis patients: The EU-GEI case-control study. *Psychol Med*, **51**, 1–9.

Quattrone, D., Reininghaus, U., Richards, A. L., et al. (2021). The continuity of effect of schizophrenia polygenic risk score and patterns of cannabis use on transdiagnostic symptom dimensions at first-episode psychosis: findings from the

EU-GEI study. *Transl Psychiatry*, **11**, 423.

Radhakrishnan, R., Wilkinson, S. T., and D'Souza, D. C. (2014). Gone to pot: A review of the association between cannabis and psychosis. *Front Psychiatry*, **5**, 54.

Ruiz-Veguilla, M., Callado, L. F., and Ferrin, M. (2012). Neurological soft signs in patients with psychosis and cannabis abuse: A systematic review and meta-analysis of paradox. *Curr Pharm Des*, **18**, 5156–5164.

Schaefer, J. D., Jang, S. K., Vrieze, S., et al. (2021). Adolescent cannabis use and adult psychoticism: A longitudinal co-twin control analysis using data from two cohorts. *J Abnorm Psychol*, **130**, 691–701.

Schoeler, T., Petros, N., Di Forti, M., et al. (2016). Effects of continuation, frequency, and type of cannabis use on relapse in the first 2 years after onset of psychosis: An observational study. *Lancet Psychiatry*, **3**, 947–953.

(2017). Poor medication adherence and risk of relapse associated with continued cannabis use in patients with first-episode psychosis: A prospective analysis. *Lancet Psychiatry*, **4**, 627–633.

Sideli, L., Fisher, H. L., Murray, R. M., et al. (2018). Interaction between cannabis consumption and childhood abuse in psychotic disorders: Preliminary findings on the role of different patterns of cannabis use. *Early Interv Psychiatry*, **12**, 135–142.

Sideli, L., Quigley, H., La Cascia, C., et al. (2020). Cannabis use and the risk for psychosis and affective disorders. *J Dual Diagn*, **16**, 22–42.

Sideli, L., Trotta, G., Spinazzola, E., et al. (2021). Adverse effects of heavy cannabis use: Even plants can harm the brain. *Pain*, **162**, S97–S104.

Smith, N. (2005). High potency cannabis: The forgotten variable. *Addiction*, **100**, 1558–1560.

Stefanis, N. C., Dragovic, M., Power, B. D., et al. (2013). Age at initiation of cannabis use predicts age at onset of psychosis: The 7- to 8-year trend. *Schizophr Bull*, **39**, 251–254.

Urban, N. B. L., Slifstein, M., Thompson, J. L., et al. (2012). Dopamine release in chronic cannabis users: A [11C]Raclopride positron emission tomography study. *Biol Psychiatry*, **71**, 677–683.

Van Winkel, R., Van Beveren, N. J. M., and Simons, C. (2011). AKT1 moderation of cannabis-induced cognitive alterations in psychotic disorder.

Neuropsychopharmacology, **36**, 2529–2537.

Volkow, N. D., Wang, G. J., Telang, F., et al. (2014). Decreased dopamine brain reactivity in marijuana abusers is associated with negative emotionality and addiction severity. *Proc Natl Acad Sci*, **111**, E3149–E3156.

Wainberg, M., Jacobs, G. R., Di Forti, M., et al. (2021). Cannabis, schizophrenia genetic risk, and psychotic experiences: A cross-sectional study of 109,308 participants from the UK Biobank. *Transl Psychiatry*, **11**, 211.

Zammit, S. (2002). Self reported cannabis use as a risk factor for schizophrenia in Swedish conscripts of 1969: Historical cohort study. *BMJ*, **325**, 1199.

Zammit, S., Moore, T. H. M., Lingford-Hughes, A., et al. (2008). Effects of cannabis use on outcomes of psychotic disorders: Systematic review. *Br J Psychiatry*, **193**, 357–363.

Zammit, S., Spurlock, G., Williams, H., et al. (2007). Genotype effects of CHRNA7, CNR1 and COMT in schizophrenia: Interactions with tobacco and cannabis use. *Br J Psychiatry*, **191**, 402–407.

Cannabis Causes Positive, Negative, and Cognitive Symptoms and Produces Impairments in Electrophysiological Indices of Information Processing

Ashley M. Schnakenberg Martin, Mohini Ranganathan, and Deepak Cyril D'Souza

16.1 Cannabis Intoxication and Psychotic Symptoms

Several anecdotal reports, dating as far back as 1235, describe a sudden onset of psychotic symptoms (i.e., paranoid ideation, delusions, hallucinations, and deficits in attention and memory) that occur immediately following exposure to recreational or medicinal cannabis, last only the period of intoxication and self-remit without intervention (reviewed by Sewell et al., 2010; and see Chapters 1 and 2). In one of the largest collections of case reports (N = 200), Chopra and Smith (1974) reported that common symptoms included confusion and psychosis-like effects such as visual hallucinations and paranoia.

16.1.1 Epidemiological Studies on Cannabis, Cannabinoids, and Psychosis

Over the past several decades a number of case series, cross-sectional, prospective, and retrospective longitudinal studies have better characterized several distinct patterns of association between cannabis and psychosis, including (1) acute and transient psychosis limited to the period of intoxication; (2) acute and transient psychosis that outlasts the period of intoxication and that may or may not require intervention including hospitalization; and (3) late onset, persistent psychosis associated with a history of chronic cannabis exposure which lasts well beyond the acute effects of intoxication and meeting criteria for a psychotic disorder, such as schizophrenia. The latter has been best studied in the published epidemiological literature (Murray et al., 2017; Patel et al., 2020; Radhakrishnan et al., 2014; and see Chapters 10 and 15).

Longitudinal data describe an elevated risk for the subsequent development of psychosis after acute cannabis-induced psychosis (Arendt et al., 2005; Niemi-Pynttäri et al., 2013). Specifically, Niemi-Pynttäri et al. (2013) found that 50% of the patients were later re-diagnosed with a schizophrenia spectrum disorder and that, when they included any psychotic outcome, the proportion climbed to 75% (Niemi-Pynttäri et al., 2013), suggesting that the acute psychotic response may be a harbinger of a psychotic illness. The acute psychotic reaction may be influenced by cannabinoid potency, that is, higher concentration of THC or the absence or lower concentration of other cannabinoids such as cannabidiol (CBD) in herbal cannabis. This relationship to potency is highlighted by the relatively recent phenomenon of synthetic cannabinoid use and psychosis (Seely et al., 2012). Synthetic cannabinoids, commonly referred to as Spice or K2, are potent agonists and have been so widely connected to paranoid and psychotic reactions that the effects have been coined 'spico-phrenia' (Murray et al., 2014). This is in contrast to herbal cannabis, that is made up of various amounts of psychoactive THC (a partial cannabinoid agonist) and potentially protective CBD (Spaderna et al., 2013).

Cannabis, Cannabinoids, and Cognition: As detailed in Chapter 9, the literature on the influence of long-term cannabis use on cognition is mixed depending on the population being studied. It has been suggested that chronic and heavy (daily) cannabis use leads to cognitive dysfunction in areas of short-term memory, attention, executive function, intelligence, and working memory (Broyd et al., 2016b; Meier et al., 2012). These deficits greatly overlap with the cognitive impairments of schizophrenia

(CIAS), although, interestingly, in those with a psychotic disorder, moderate (compared to high and low) lifetime cannabis use has been associated with fewer neurocognitive deficits (Schnakenberg Martin et al., 2016) and is not related to superior social cognition (Helle et al., 2017), as had been previously suggested. These differences may be related to confounds including the impact of chronic illness, medications, variability in cognition among those with serious mental illness, and failure to consider biological sex as a potentially moderating variable, as recent research has suggested that otherwise healthy males with regular cannabis use may be more adversely affected (Hirst et al., 2021; Schnakenberg Martin et al., 2021). Further studies are needed to carefully examine the neurobiological underpinnings of the complex dose–response relationship in patient populations, keeping in mind the bidirectional relationship between risk for psychosis and cannabis use which in turn may affect the relationship between psychosis and cognition.

Cannabis, Cannabinoids, and Electrophysiological Indices of Information Processing: Electroencephalography (EEG) and event-related potentials (ERP; averaged EEG responses time-locked to stimuli) serve as objective and proximal measures of information processing that complement more distal measures of brain function, such as cognitive performance and subjective effects. EEG may be particularly sensitive to the effects of cannabis and its relationship with cognition, given that cannabinoids may disrupt cognition through altered neural synchrony (Skosnik et al., 2006, 2012, 2014), which is critical for sensory registration and integration, associative learning, conscious awareness, and organization of brain networks. In addition to altered neural synchrony, regular cannabis use has been associated with alterations in ERPs reflecting deficits in information processing (Radhakrishnan et al., 2014). For example, chronic cannabis use has been associated with alterations in the P50, reflecting altered sensory gating (Patrick and Struve, 2000), as well as mixed findings regarding the P300, an ERP that reflects context updating and automatic attention orientation (Morie et al., 2021; Radhakrishnan et al., 2014). Finally, because it is found to be predominately reduced in schizophrenia (Umbricht et al., 2003), the mismatch negativity (MMN) ERP requires particular consideration. The MMN is a negative deflecting waveform approximately 100–200 ms after an auditory stimulus that deviates in frequency, duration, or intensity from a series of standard stimuli, thus requiring the comparison of incoming auditory information to recent auditory sensory memory of the general, repeated, stimuli (Näätänen et al., 2007). Similar to people with schizophrenia, reduced frequency MMN amplitude in chronic ($\geq$ 8 years) and heavy ($\geq$ 15 joints/week) cannabis users compared to short-term users has been observed (Roser et al., 2010), with frequency amplitude in heavy cannabis users positively correlated with duration and quantity of cannabis exposure. Greenwood et al. (2014) later replicated these findings, observing a decrease in frequency MMN amplitude in chronic cannabis users compared to non-using controls (Greenwood et al., 2014). Long-term cannabis users were unique in that they differed in duration MMN amplitude compared to both controls and short-term cannabis users and, further, the decrease in duration MMN amplitude was correlated with an increase in duration of cannabis exposure and psychotic-like experience while under the influence of cannabis.

In a study of cannabis using and non-using individuals with schizophrenia, compared to cannabis using and non-using healthy controls, Rentzsch et al. (2011) found that cannabis using controls had decreased MMN compared to non-using peers, while individuals with schizophrenia and cannabis use had increased MMN compared to non-using peers with schizophrenia (Rentzsch et al., 2011). These findings suggest that persistent cannabis use may have differential effects on pre-attentive cognitive functioning in individuals with a psychotic disorder, compared to healthy controls. The authors also suggest that findings may be related to pre-existing endocannabinoid system differences between those with and without a psychotic disorder. Future research is needed to replicate these findings and further explore how alterations in MMN amplitude may predict the later development of psychosis in cannabis-using individuals.

Alarmingly, a growing body of evidence suggests that deficits in ERPs, such as the MMN, appear to persist even after periods of abstinence from cannabis (Broyd et al., 2016a). Additional evidence in support of the connection between cannabis, cannabinoids, and psychosis comes from experimental human laboratory studies of cannabinoids (Sherif et al., 2016) which are summarized in Section 16.1.2.

16.1.2 Experimental Studies of Cannabis, Cannabinoids, and Psychosis

Human Laboratory Studies as a Tool for the Study of Cannabinoids in Humans: Several exhaustive reviews have been published on human laboratory studies (HLS) with cannabis and cannabinoids such as delta-9-tetrahydrocannabinol (THC) (Bloomfield et al., 2019; Ganesh et al., 2020; Sherif et al., 2016). HLS directly establish the connection between acute cannabinoid exposure and psychosis without intervening events that often confound epidemiological data. HLS have demonstrated psychosis outcomes tightly time locked to cannabinoid exposure and have the advantage of precise knowledge of doses (including placebo) and controlled routes of administration. These benefits of HLS address the problem of variability in the THC content of recreational cannabis and the typical practice of sharing cannabis that make it challenging to establish precise dose–response relationships in epidemiological studies. Further, HLS facilitate testing the effects of individual cannabinoids (e.g., THC and CBD or their interactions), as well as examining interactions with drugs or other factors that may alter the risk for cannabinoid-related psychosis. This has allowed testing the benefits of antipsychotic medications in this model as well as examining how alterations in other neurotransmitter systems impact the overall risk of cannabinoid effects (Gupta et al., 2019; Kleinloog et al., 2012; O'Tuathaigh et al., 2012; Radhakrishnan et al., 2015; Ranganathan et al., 2019). Finally, HLS permit collection of objective data, such as cognitive outcomes and psychophysiological measures time locked to cannabinoid exposure, which can help identify underlying mechanisms of action and biomarkers; this can inform the development of tools for stratification of the risk of psychosis associated with cannabis (Cortes-Briones et al., 2015a; Skosnik et al., 2016).

Cannabinoid-Induced Acute Psychotomimetic Effects: In experimental studies both cannabis plant and a number of individual cannabinoids have been shown to produce a range of transient, psychotic-like symptoms in healthy individuals. These effects are influenced by the dose and route of administration such that inhaled and intravenous (IV) routes are associated with a rapid onset of effects (within minutes) with a peak at approximately 20–40 minutes and offset approximately 1.5–2 hours post-drug administration. The oral route of administration has a slower and more variable onset of subjective effects, peaking at approximately two hours but with high inter- and intra-individual variability.

These acute psychosis-like effects include suspiciousness, paranoid and grandiose delusions, conceptual disorganization, fragmented thinking, and perceptual alterations measured on standardized rating scales such as the Positive and Negative Syndrome Scale (PANSS), Clinician Administered Dissociative Symptoms Scale (CADSS), Psychotomimetic States Inventory (PSI), and Brief Psychiatric Rating Scale (BPRS) (Bhattacharyya et al., 2010b; Cortes-Briones et al., 2015b; D'Souza et al., 2004; Freeman et al., 2015; Morrison and Stone, 2011; Morrison et al., 2009). Psychotomimetic effects are accompanied by a distinct pattern of cognitive and psychophysiological deficits, as reviewed in the following section.

Several HLS have examined the acute interaction between THC and CBD to examine how CBD modulates the THC response. CBD pre-treatment is associated with lower THC-induced psychotomimetic effects, cognitive deficits, and psychophysiological effects without affecting THC-induced intoxication (Englund et al., 2013; Fusar-Poli et al., 2009a; Iseger and Bossong, 2015; Pennypacker and Romero-Sandoval, 2020). CBD also produces opposite effects to THC on blood oxygen-level dependent responses in tasks of verbal recall, response-inhibition, processing fearful facial expressions, auditory processing, and visual processing (Bhattacharyya et al., 2010a; Fusar-Poli et al., 2009b). For a fuller discussion of the potential antipsychotic effects of CBD, see Chapter 20.

Further, in addition to phytocannabinoids and their extracts, synthetic THC analogues nabilone and dronabinol also produce a similar profile of subjective effects and disrupt performance on a visual information-processing task (binocular depth inversion illusion), a marker of psychosis.

Cannabinoid-Induced Acute Cognitive Deficits: HLS demonstrate that THC has a clear detrimental impact on cognition in healthy humans as well as those with psychotic disorders, generating acute, transient, and dose-related impairments in working and verbal memory, executive function, abstract ability, time perception, and decision-making (Bloomfield et al., 2019; Radhakrishnan et al., 2014; Ranganathan and D'Souza, 2006; Sewell et al., 2013; Sherif et al., 2016; Volkow et al., 2016). Further, THC administration in healthy humans induces psycho-motor dysfunction as evidenced by decreased psycho-motor velocity, loss of balance and coordination, and visual tracking (Chang et al., 2006; Kurzthaler et al., 1999; Liguori et al., 2002; Stoller et al., 1976; Weinstein et al., 2008), as well as worse reaction time, divided attention, and impaired tracking performance (Asbridge et al., 2012; Bosker et al., 2012; Liguori et al., 2002; Weinstein et al., 2008).

THC-induced verbal learning deficits are particularly robust and have been replicated in several studies (D'Souza et al., 2004; Henquet et al., 2006; Morrison and Stone, 2011; Morrison et al., 2009; Ranganathan and D'Souza, 2006). Interestingly, THC-induced deficits in verbal learning, attention, and working memory were found to be unrelated to the psychotomimetic effects.

Importantly, unlike the observation of fewer cognitive deficits amongst cannabis using individuals with a psychotic disorder as described in Section 16.1.1, D'Souza et al. (2005) found that IV THC was associated with significantly greater deficits in attention, working memory, and verbal learning in individuals with schizophrenia compared to healthy controls (D'Souza et al., 2005).

16.1.3 Cannabinoid-Induced Alterations in Electrophysiological Indices of Information Processing

Acute THC administration generates neurophysiological abnormalities that are consistent with findings considered to be potential biomarkers for schizophrenia. Similar to studies on persistent cannabis use, HLS have demonstrated a robust relationship between THC and altered neural synchrony, neural noise, and other ERP components related to information processing such as the P50, P300 (P300a and P300b), and mismatch-negativity (MMN). For additional description of these EEG components, see the above section on Cannabis, Cannabinoids, and Electrophysiological Indices of Information Processing.

Acute administration of THC has been observed to reduce gamma (γ) oscillations (Cortes-Briones et al., 2015b), which are important for conscious awareness, sensory integration, and associative learning. Disruption in gamma synchrony was also related to THC-induced psychotic symptoms (Cortes-Briones et al., 2015b). In pre-clinical and human

studies, cannabinoids also disrupt theta (θ)-band (4–8 Hz) oscillations (Morrison and Stone, 2011; Skosnik et al., 2018), which are critical for cognition and potentially the moderation of gamma synchrony. THC-induced theta deficits have also been associated with memory performance (Böcker et al., 2010). Neural noise, or task-irrelevant random neural activity, has been shown to be increased in people with psychotic disorders (Yang et al., 2014), as well as – in a dose-dependent manner – in response to THC (Cortes-Briones et al., 2015a). THC-induced neural noise was also correlated with THC-induced positive but not negative symptoms. Findings suggest that increases in neural noise may be one pathway by which cannabis generates psychosis-like effects. These findings align with the hypothesis that alteration in synchronized neural activity may be a potential mechanism whereby cannabinoids induce psychosis (Skosnik et al., 2016).

Deficits in P50, an index of sensory gating, have also been observed in pre-clinical models exposed to cannabinoids (Dissanayake et al., 2008; Skosnik et al., 2018) and during THC administration in humans (Skosnik et al., 2018). Several studies have also found, similar to psychosis, that THC decreases in the amplitude of the P300, an ERP that reflects context updating and automatic attention (Radhakrishnan et al., 2014). Notably, the THC induced P300 decreases have been observed to be dose-dependent, which suggests that the cannabinoid system is involved in the regulation of cortical processing responsible for context updating and automatic attention orientation, in both a top down (P300b) and bottom-up (P300a) manner (D'Souza et al., 2012).

Regarding sensory encoding and memory, a study of acute oral THC administration found that THC alone did not impact MMN amplitude; however, in the same study a combination of THC and CBD was found to increase MMN amplitude (Juckel et al., 2007). While the authors proposed that the increased amplitude was due to the protective nature of CBD, it should be acknowledged that the oral route of administration has slower absorption and lower bioavailability than other routes (e.g., IV) and thus the oral administration may have accounted for the lack of observed effects. In contrast, acute administration of the synthetic cannabinoid agonist, nabilone, decreased duration and intensity MMN amplitudes compared to placebo (de la Salle et al., 2019). Notably, a recent randomized controlled trial by

Greenwood et al. (2021) observed that, compared to placebo, vaporized THC and CBD increased duration and intensity MMN amplitude in less-frequent compared to frequent cannabis users. These findings stand in contrast to the previous work of this group in the context of persistent cannabis use (Greenwood et al., 2014). The authors suggest that the conflicting findings may be due to comparably less cannabis exposure in participants in their follow-up study. Collectively, findings provide support for differential effects of acute and chronic THC exposure on the MMN (O'Donnell and Mackie, 2014).

Experimental THC administration in healthy humans induces psychotic symptoms, cognitive deficits, and electrophysiological outcomes analogous to psychosis and worsens psychotic symptoms and cognitive deficits in individuals with schizophrenia. It is important to acknowledge that these pro-psychotic effects of THC are not unique since other pharmacological agents such as ketamine (an N-methyl-D-aspartate receptor antagonist) can also produce transient psychotic symptoms. Moreover, these acute psychosis-like effects do not capture the often intractable and life-long alterations of neural structure and function and psychosocial impairment commonly associated with schizophrenia. Therefore, this analogy to psychosis must be interpreted with extreme caution as, biologically, these two states may differ. It must also be emphasized that experimental studies have largely concentrated on pharmacological challenge studies with THC. As detailed in Chapter 5, there are ≥ 70 additional cannabinoids, such as CBD, in the cannabis plant that act in parallel either in entourage, synergistically, or conversely with THC; therefore, the existing experimental literature is limited to the interpretation of the effects of THC alone. However, these experimental models provide an important translational tool bridging pre-clinical data and epidemiological studies in our understanding of the role of cannabinoids in psychosis.

16.1.4 Understanding Factors That Influence the Risk of Psychosis Associated with Cannabinoids

It is now well-established that cannabis use is associated with psychosis but also that this association is neither causal nor sufficient (see Chapter 17). This association is further complicated by genetic data suggesting a bidirectional causal influence between the polygenic risk score for schizophrenia and lifetime cannabis exposure (Gage et al., 2017; Stringer et al., 2016; Vaucher et al., 2018). Genetic risk for schizophrenia is associated with a greater likelihood of using cannabis which may interact with the genetic risk for the development of psychosis. Thus, investigations into risk factors, especially modifiable factors, remains an area of active research with several emerging leads. Broadly, these risk factors can be separated into those pertaining to cannabis (dose, frequency, potency, type of cannabinoids, etc.) and the individual (age of onset of cannabis use, sex, psychiatric or medical illness in self or family, etc.).

Higher potency of herbal cannabis is associated with greater immediate and long-term risk of psychosis (Murray et al., 2017; and see Chapter 15). Herbal cannabis contains numerous cannabinoids and, while not all of them have been studied carefully, they may influence the overall risk of psychosis. For instance, a higher concentration of CBD and/or lower THC concentration appears to lower the risk of psychosis in experimental as well as epidemiological data (see Chapter 20).

In acute experimental studies, when controlling for dose, stronger acute psychotomimetic effects are observed in less frequent recreational users (likely related to absence of tolerance), those with a pre-existing psychotic illness, and in those with clinical or genetic high risk for psychosis. In epidemiological studies of chronic cannabis exposure, an earlier onset of regular use, heavier, longer use of more potent cannabis, as well as a personal or familial history of psychotic disorder are associated with a greater risk of psychosis.

Collectively, this growing body of research suggests that risk for cannabinoid-induced psychosis can be mitigated through cannabis-related factors, such as use of lower potency (high CBD low THC) cannabis and avoidance of synthetic cannabinoids; as well as individual-related factors, such as avoiding cannabis use during critical periods of brain development (intra-uterine or before age 23); if one has a personal or family history of a psychotic disorder; and/or the presence of biomarkers indicative of increased risk, such as elevated polygenic risk score.

16.1.5 Future Directions

To expand our understanding of the relationship between cannabinoids and psychosis, there are several critical future directions for research that may clarify (1) potential mechanisms of action, (2) those at greatest risk for developing cannabis-induced psychosis, as well as (3) discrepancies in existing findings.

As described in this chapter, much of the literature has focused on the singular impact of THC and high potency cannabis (high THC concentration). However, given the numerous other constituents of cannabis, it is imperative that future research explores the impact of other constituents, such as CBD, as well as the potential interaction between THC and CBD. While high potency cannabis is linked with increased psychotomimetic symptoms, cognitive dysfunction, and risk for the development of psychosis, it is possible that CBD may have neuroprotective effects in specific sub-groups (i.e., early psychosis) that have not been thoroughly evaluated. Similarly, additional work is needed to discern differences in cannabinoid effects based on variation in routes of administration (e.g., smoked, vaped/vaporized, ingested), and when cannabis or cannabinoids are used in combination with other substances, such as the common practice of using cannabis with tobacco and/or alcohol.

Many discrepancies in the literature describing the neural impact of cannabis may be due to important methodological inconsistencies across studies, such as variations across subjects in age of initiation and frequency of cannabis use, sex, age, and polysubstance use as well as differing parameters in electrophysiological and neuroimaging assessments and analysis. One of the main differences across studies likely contributing to the lack of replicable findings is the high variability in definitions used for cannabis 'exposure'. For example, some studies considered cannabis use as subjects with any lifetime history, while others only included those actively using cannabis. Further, some studies defined heavy cannabis use as once a month, while others defined it as once a week or even up to five or more exposures a week. Future research would also benefit from mindful reporting of the time since last use of cannabis/cannabinoids and the potential influence of cannabis withdrawal syndrome on study outcomes. Therefore, it is imperative that future research attempts to use more transparent reporting and consistent definitions and/or interprets findings in the context of these limitations. This change moving forward could lead to considerable impact, helping to address methodological inconsistencies which, optimistically, could lead to increased replicability across findings.

There has also been limited work on the potential differential effects of cannabis based on sex. A growing literature suggests that males with regular cannabis use may be more susceptible to the cognitive effects of cannabis compared to their female cannabis-using peers. However, much of this work requires replication with larger samples, replication from independent research teams, and systematic evaluation of the relationship between menstrual cycle and the effects of cannabinoids. It is also unknown whether there are differences in acute versus chronic effects of cannabis based on sex.

While not reviewed in detail here, it is also important to acknowledge the small and mixed emerging literature on whether observed deficits resolve with sustained abstinence. Future research that addresses this question regarding the neuropsychiatric impact of cannabinoids will be pivotal for public health, and the development of novel clinical interventions for cannabis use disorder in the future.

Finally, there is also an urgent need for the development of dissemination strategies to increase public awareness of the relationship between cannabis and symptoms of psychosis (e.g., risk of cannabinoid-induced psychosis for clinical high-risk individuals, psychomotor dysfunction and danger of driving under the influence, cognitive impact of cannabis use in school-age adolescents and young adults, etc.). As discussed in Chapter 6, this is particularly important given the rapidly changing legislation around cannabis and cannabinoids and increasing rates of use and problematic use likely related to a decreased perception of risk.

16.2 Fact Boxes

Persistent cannabis use and psychotic illness:

- Development of a psychotic illness is related to early/heavy cannabis use in pre-adolescence.
- There is a positive association between elevated cannabis use and symptoms of schizotypy.
- Cannabis use in psychotic disorders is related to a worsening of symptoms and course of illness.

Acute cannabinoid exposure and symptoms of psychosis:

- THC and other cannabinoid agonists generate acute symptoms of psychosis that are transient and self-relenting.

- THC-induced psychotomimetic effects are dose-related.
- Cannabidiol does not induce psychotomimetic effects and may attenuate THC-related effects.
- History of a psychotic disorder results in an exaggerated response to THC, while a history of regular cannabis use results in a blunted response to THC.

Cognition and cannabinoids:

- Acute cannabinoid exposure and chronic cannabis use is associated with cognitive deficits in domains such as verbal learning, attention, and working memory.
- A growing body of literature suggests a possible differential cognitive impact in females and males with persistent cannabis use.

- Data is mixed on the resolution of cognitive deficits after sustained abstinence from cannabis.

Electrophysiological (EEG) indices of information processing and cannabis:

- EEG may be particularly sensitive to the effects of cannabis, given that cannabinoids appear to alter neural synchrony.
- Cannabinoids have been observed to increase neural noise, which may be a biomarker for psychosis.
- Acute and chronic cannabinoid exposure generate alterations in event-related potentials related to information processing, such as the P50, P300 (P300a and P300b), and mismatch-negativity (MMN).
- Acute and chronic cannabinoid exposure may have differential electrophysiological effects.

References

Arendt, M., Rosenberg, R., Foldager, L., et al. (2005). Cannabis-induced psychosis and subsequent schizophrenia-spectrum disorders: Follow-up study of 535 incident cases. *Br J Psychiatry*, **187**, 510–515.

Asbridge, M., Hayden, J. A., and Cartwright, J. L. (2012). Acute cannabis consumption and motor vehicle collision risk: Systematic review of observational studies and meta-analysis. *BMJ*, **344**, e536.

Bhattacharyya, S., Morrison, P. D., Fusar-Poli, P., et al. (2010a). Opposite effects of delta-9-tetrahydrocannabinol and cannabidiol on human brain function and psychopathology. *Neuropsychopharmacology*, **35**, 764–774.

(2010b). Opposite effects of Δ-9-tetrahydrocannabinol and cannabidiol on human brain function and psychopathology. *Neuropsychopharmacology*, **35**, 764–774.

Bloomfield, M. A. P., Hindocha, C., Green, S. F., et al. (2019). The neuropsychopharmacology of cannabis: A review of human imaging studies. *Pharmacol Ther*, **195**, 132–161.

Böcker, K. B., Hunault, C. C., Gerritsen, J., et al. (2010). Cannabinoid modulations of resting state EEG theta power and working memory are correlated in humans. *J Cogn Neurosci*, **22**, 1906–1916.

Bosker, W. M., Kuypers, K. P., Theunissen, E. L., et al. (2012). Medicinal Δ9-tetrahydrocannabinol (dronabinol) impairs on-the-road driving performance of occasional and heavy cannabis users but is not detected in standard field sobriety tests. *Addiction*, **107**, 1837–1844.

Broyd, S. J., Greenwood, L.-M., Van Hell, H. H., et al. (2016a). Mismatch negativity and P50 sensory gating in abstinent former cannabis users. *Neural Plasticity*, **2016**, 6526437.

Broyd, S. J., Van Hell, H. H., Beale, C., et al. (2016b). Acute and chronic effects of cannabinoids on human cognition: A systematic review. *Biol Psychiatry*, **79**, 557–567.

Chang, L., Yakupov, R., Cloak, C., et al. (2006). Marijuana use is associated with a reorganized visual-attention network and cerebellar hypoactivation. *Brain*, **129**, 1096–1112.

Chopra, G. S., and Smith, J. W. (1974). Psychotic reactions following cannabis use in East Indians. *Arch Gen Psychiatry*, **30**, 24–27.

Cortes-Briones, J., Cahill, J. D., Skosnik, P. D., et al. (2015a). The psychosis-like effects of Δ(9)-tetrahydrocannabinol are associated with increased cortical noise in healthy humans. *Biol Psychiatry*, **78**, 805–13.

Cortes-Briones, J., Skosnik, P. D., Mathalon, D., et al. (2015b). Δ 9-THC disrupts gamma (γ)-band neural oscillations in humans. *Neuropsychopharmacology*, **40**, 2124–2134.

D'Souza, D. C., Abi-Saab, W. M., Madonick, S., et al. (2005). Delta-9-tetrahydrocannabinol effects in schizophrenia: Implications for cognition, psychosis, and addiction. *Biol Psychiatry*, **57**, 594–608.

D'Souza, D. C., Fridberg, D. J., Skosnik, P. D., et al. (2012). Dose-related modulation of event-related potentials to novel and target stimuli by intravenous [delta]9-THC in humans. *Neuropsychopharmacology*, **37**, 1632–1646.

D'Souza, D. C., Perry, E., MacDougall, L., et al. (2004). The psychotomimetic effects of intravenous delta-9-tetrahydrocannabinol in healthy individuals: Implications for psychosis. *Neuropsychopharmacology*, **29**, 1558–1572.

Dissanayake, D. W., Zachariou, M., Marsden, C. A., et al. (2008). Auditory gating in rat hippocampus and medial prefrontal cortex: Effect of the cannabinoid agonist WIN55, 212-2. *Neuropharmacology*, **55**, 1397–1404.

Englund, A., Morrison, P. D., Nottage, J., et al. (2013). Cannabidiol inhibits THC-elicited paranoid symptoms and hippocampal-dependent memory impairment. *J Psychopharmacol*, **27**, 19–27.

Freeman, D., Dunn, G., Murray, R. M., et al. (2015). How cannabis causes paranoia: Using the intravenous administration of Δ-9-tetrahydrocannabinol (THC) to identify key cognitive mechanisms leading to paranoia. *Schizophr Bull*, **41**, 391–399.

Fusar-Poli, P., Crippa, J. A., Bhattacharyya, S., et al. (2009a). Distinct effects of {delta}9-tetrahydrocannabinol and cannabidiol on neural activation during emotional processing. *Arch Gen Psychiatry*, **66**, 95–105.

(2009b). Distinct effects of Δ9-tetrahydrocannabinol and cannabidiol on neural activation during emotional processing. *Arch Gen Psychiatry*, **66**, 95–105.

Gage, S. H., Jones, H. J., Burgess, S., et al. (2017). Assessing causality in associations between cannabis use and schizophrenia risk: A two-sample Mendelian randomization study. *Psychol Med*, **47**, 971–980.

Ganesh, S., Cortes-Briones, J., Ranganathan, M., et al. (2020). Psychosis-relevant effects of intravenous delta-9-tetrahydrocannabinol: A mega

analysis of individual participant-data from human laboratory studies. *Int J Neuropsychopharmacol*, **23**, 559–570.

Greenwood, L.-M., Broyd, S. J., Croft, R., et al. (2014). Chronic effects of cannabis use on the auditory mismatch negativity. *Biol Psychiatry*, **75**, 449–458.

Greenwood, L.-M., Broyd, S. J., Van Hell, H. H., et al. (2021). Acute effects of Δ9-tetrahydrocannabinol and cannabidiol on auditory mismatch negativity. *Psychopharmacology*, **239**, 1409–1424.

Gupta, S., De Aquino, J. P., D'Souza, D. C., et al. (2019). Effects of haloperidol on the delta-9-tetrahydrocannabinol response in humans: A responder analysis. *Psychopharmacology*, **236**, 2635–2640.

Helle, S., Løberg, E.-M., Gjestad, R., et al. (2017). The positive link between executive function and lifetime cannabis use in schizophrenia is not explained by current levels of superior social cognition. *Psychiatry Res*, **250**, 92–98.

Henquet, C., Rosa, A., Krabbendam, L., et al. (2006). An experimental study of catechol-O-methyltransferase Val158Met moderation of Δ-9-tetrahydrocannabinol-induced effects on psychosis and cognition. *Neuropsychopharmacology*, **31**, 2748–2757.

Hirst, R., Vaughn, D., Arastu, S., et al. (2021). Female sex as a protective factor in the effects of chronic cannabis use on verbal learning and memory. *J Int Neuropsychol Soc*, **27**, 581–591.

Iseger, T. A., and Bossong, M. G. (2015). A systematic review of the antipsychotic properties of cannabidiol in humans. *Schizophr Res*, **162**, 153–161.

Juckel, G., Roser, P., Nadulski, T., et al. (2007). Acute effects of Δ 9-tetrahydrocannabinol and standardized cannabis extract on the auditory evoked mismatch negativity. *Schizophr Res*, **97**, 109–117.

Kleinloog, D., Liem-Moolenaar, M., Jacobs, G., et al. (2012). Does olanzapine inhibit the psychomimetic effects of Δ9-tetrahydrocannabinol? *J Psychopharmacol*, **26**, 1307–1316.

Kurzthaler, I., Hummer, M., Miller, C., et al. (1999). Effect of cannabis use on cognitive functions and driving ability. *J Clin Psychiatry*, **60**, 395–399.

Liguori, A., Gatto C. P., and Jarrett, D. B. (2002). Separate and combined effects of marijuana and alcohol on mood, equilibrium and simulated driving. *Psychopharmacology*, **163**, 399–405.

Meier, M. H., Caspi, A., Ambler, A., et al. (2012). Persistent cannabis users show neuropsychological decline from childhood to midlife. *Proc Natl Acad Sci*, **109**, E2657–E2664.

Morie, K. P., Wu, J., Potenza, M. N., et al. (2021). Daily cannabis use in adolescents who smoke tobacco is associated with altered late-stage feedback processing: A high-density electrical mapping study. *J Psychiatr Res*, **139**, 82–90.

Morrison, P., and Stone, J. (2011). Synthetic delta-9-tetrahydrocannabinol elicits schizophrenia-like negative symptoms which are distinct from sedation. *Human Psychopharmacol Clin Exp*, **26**, 77–80.

Morrison, P., Zois, V., McKeown, D., et al. (2009). The acute effects of synthetic intravenous Δ 9-tetrahydrocannabinol on psychosis, mood and cognitive functioning. *Psychol Med*, **39**, 1607–1616.

Murray, R. M., Englund, A., Abi-Dargham, A., et al. (2017). Cannabis-associated psychosis: Neural substrate and clinical impact. *Neuropharmacology*, **124**, 89–104.

Murray, R. M., Mehta, M., and Di Forti, M. (2014). Different dopaminergic abnormalities underlie cannabis dependence and cannabis-induced psychosis. *Biol Psychiatry*, **6**, 430–431.

Näätänen, R., Paavilainen, P., Rinne, T., et al. (2007). The mismatch negativity (MMN) in basic research of central auditory processing: a review. *Clin Neurophysiol*, **118**, 2544–2590.

Niemi-Pynttäri, J. A., Sund, R., Putkonen, H., et al. (2013). Substance-induced psychoses converting into schizophrenia: A register-based study of 18,478 Finnish inpatient cases. *J Clin Psychiatry*, **74**, 20155.

O'Donnell, B. F., and Mackie, K. (2014). The mismatch negativity: A translational probe of auditory processing in cannabis users. *Biol Psychiatry*, **75**, 428–429.

O'Tuathaigh, C. M., Clarke, G., Walsh, J., et al. (2012). Genetic vs. pharmacological inactivation of COMT influences cannabinoid-induced expression of schizophrenia-related phenotypes. *Int J Neuropsychopharmacol*, **15**, 1331–1342.

Patel, S., Khan, S., Saipavankumar, M., et al. (2020). The association between cannabis use and schizophrenia: Causative or curative? A systematic review. *Cureus*, **12**, e9303.

Patrick, G., and Struve, F. A. (2000). Reduction of auditory P50 gating response in marihuana users: Further supporting data. *Clin Electroencephalogr*, **31**, 88–93.

Pennypacker, S. D., and Romero-Sandoval, E. A. (2020). CBD and THC: Do they complement each other like yin and yang? *Pharmacotherapy*, **40**, 1152–1165.

Radhakrishnan, R., Skosnik, P. D., Cortes-Briones, J., et al. (2015). GABA deficits enhance the psychotomimetic effects of Δ9-THC. *Neuropsychopharmacology*, **40**, 2047–2056.

Radhakrishnan, R., Wilkinson, S. T., and D'Souza, D. C. (2014). Gone to pot: A review of the association between cannabis and psychosis. *Front Psychiatry*, **5**, 54.

Ranganathan, M., and D'Souza, D. (2006). The acute effects of cannabinoids on memory in humans: A review. *Psychopharmacology*, **188**, 425–444.

Ranganathan, M., De Aquino, J. P., Cortes-Briones, J. A., et al. (2019). Highs and lows of cannabinoid-dopamine interactions: Effects of genetic variability and pharmacological modulation of catechol-O-methyl transferase on the acute response to delta-9-tetrahydrocannabinol in humans. *Psychopharmacology*, **236**, 3209–3219.

Rentzsch, J., Buntebart, E., Stadelmeier, A., et al. (2011). Differential effects of chronic cannabis use on preattentional cognitive functioning in abstinent schizophrenic patients and healthy subjects. *Schizophr Res*, **130**, 222–227.

Roser, P., Della, B., Norra, C., et al. (2010). Auditory mismatch negativity deficits in long-term heavy cannabis users. *Eur Arch Psychiatry Clin Neurosci*, **260**, 491–498.

de la Salle, S., Inyang, L., Impey, D., et al. (2019). Acute separate and combined effects of cannabinoid and nicotinic receptor agonists on MMN-indexed auditory deviance detection in healthy humans. *Pharmacol Biochem Behav*, **184**, 172739.

Schnakenberg Martin, A. M., Bonfils, K. A., Davis, B. J., et al. (2016). Compared to high and low cannabis use, moderate use is associated with fewer cognitive deficits in psychosis. *Schizophr Res Cogn*, **6**, 15–21.

Schnakenberg Martin, A. M., D'Souza, D. C., Newman, S. D., et al. (2021). Differential cognitive performance in females and males with regular cannabis use. *J Int Neuropsychol Soc*, **27**, 570–580.

Seely, K. A., Lapoint, J., Moran, J. H., et al. (2012). Spice drugs are more than harmless herbal blends: A review of the pharmacology and toxicology of synthetic cannabinoids. *Prog Neuro-Psychopharmacol Biol Psychiatry*, **39**, 234–243.

Sewell, R. A., Schnakenberg, A., Elander, J., et al. (2013). Acute effects of THC on time perception in frequent and infrequent cannabis users. *Psychopharmacology*, **226**, 401–413.

Sewell, R. A., Skosnik, P. D., Garcia-Sosa, I., et al. (2010). Behavioral, cognitive and psychophysiological effects of cannabinoids: Relevance to psychosis and schizophrenia. *Revista Brasileira de Psiquiatria*, **32**, 515–530.

Sherif, M., Radhakrishnan, R., D'Souza, D. C., et al. (2016). Human laboratory studies on cannabinoids and psychosis. *Biol Psychiatry*, **79**, 526–538.

Skosnik, P. D., Cortes-Briones, J. A., and Hajós, M. (2016). It's all in the rhythm: The role of cannabinoids in neural oscillations and psychosis. *Biol Psychiatry*, **79**, 568–577.

Skosnik, P. D., D'Souza, D. C., Steinmetz, A. B., et al. (2012). The effect of chronic cannabinoids on broadband EEG neural oscillations in humans. *Neuropsychopharmacology*, **37**, 2184–2193.

Skosnik, P. D., Hajós, M., Cortes-Briones, J. A., et al. (2018). Cannabinoid receptor-mediated disruption of sensory gating and neural oscillations: A translational study in rats and humans. *Neuropharmacology*, **135**, 412–423.

Skosnik, P. D., Krishnan, G. P., Aydt, E. E., et al. (2006). Psychophysiological evidence of altered neural synchronization in cannabis use: Relationship to schizotypy. *Am J Psychiatry*, **163**, 1798–1805.

Skosnik, P. D., Krishnan, G. P., D'Souza, D. C., et al. (2014). Disrupted gamma-band neural oscillations during coherent motion perception in heavy cannabis users. *Neuropsychopharmacology*, **39**, 3087–3099.

Spaderna, M., Addy, P. H., and D'Souza, D. C. (2013). Spicing things up: Synthetic cannabinoids. *Psychopharmacology*, **228**, 525–540.

Stoller, K., Swanson, G. D., and Bellville, J. W. (1976). Effects on visual tracking of δ9-tetrahydrocannabinol and pentobarbital. *J Clin Pharmacol*, **16**, 271–275.

Stringer, S., Minică, C., Verweij, K. J., et al. (2016). Genome-wide association study of lifetime cannabis use based on a large meta-analytic sample of 32 330 subjects from the International Cannabis Consortium. *Transl Psychiatry*, **6**, e769.

Umbricht, D., Koller, R., Schmid, L., et al. (2003). How specific are deficits in mismatch negativity generation to schizophrenia? *Biol Psychiatry*, **53**, 1120–1131.

Vaucher, J., Keating, B. J., Lasserre, A. M., et al. (2018). Cannabis use and risk of schizophrenia:

A Mendelian randomization study. *Mol Psychiatry*, **23**, 1287–1292.

Volkow, N. D., Swanson, J. M., Evins, A. E., et al. (2016). Effects of cannabis use on human behavior, including cognition, motivation, and psychosis: A review. *JAMA Psychiatry*, **73**, 292–297.

Weinstein, A., Brickner, O., Lerman, H., et al. (2008). Brain imaging study of the acute effects of Δ9-tetrahydrocannabinol (THC) on attention and motor coordination in regular users of marijuana. *Psychopharmacology*, **196**, 119–131.

Yang, G. J., Murray, J. D., Repovs, G., et al. (2014). Altered global brain signal in schizophrenia. *Proc Natl Acad Sci USA*, **111**, 7438–7443.

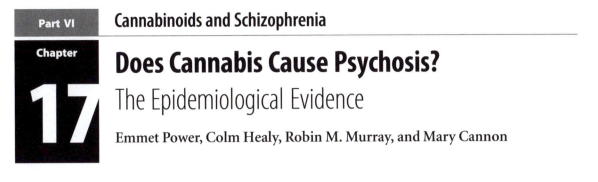

17

Does Cannabis Cause Psychosis?
The Epidemiological Evidence

Emmet Power, Colm Healy, Robin M. Murray, and Mary Cannon

17.1 Introduction

In the past 20 years, cannabis use has gone through a remarkable change in legal status in numerous countries across both sides of the Atlantic. Canada, Uruguay, and many states in America have legalized possession of cannabis for recreational use (Murray and Hall, 2020). Although in the United States it is still illegal federally, its acceptance for medical and recreational use has been broadly unchallenged with a decrease in perceived risk of use by adults and adolescents (Carliner et al., 2017). This shift in public opinion poses the question of whether cannabis is harmful? From a psychiatric standpoint, cannabis has a long-standing history of association with severe mental illness. For example, in late nineteenth-century colonial India, the Indian Hemp Drug Commission was established over concerns about the number of asylum patients with cannabis-induced insanity (Hall, 2019). In 1894, the commission's voluminous report highlighted that heavy cannabis use was associated with serious mental illness and was considered a contributing factor in 7–12% of cases (Ayonrinde, 2020). Two years later, hashish was reported to be responsible for 16% of psychiatric admissions to a Cairo asylum (Clouston, 1896).

Nearly a century later, a new series of studies documented a similar phenomenon, indicating that cannabis use may be a risk factor for schizophrenia, as use mostly preceded the onset of the disease (Allebeck et al., 1993; Linszen et al., 1994). However, these studies are limited as they likely have sampling and recall biases. A seminal cohort study of 45,570 Swedish conscripts indicated that high consumers of cannabis were six times more likely to have schizophrenia than non-users (Andréasson et al., 1987). However, the debate of whether this is actually a causal relationship still continues. So, what is the evidence that cannabis causes psychosis? Within this chapter we aim to address this question. We will also discuss some alternative hypotheses that have been put forward to explain the relationship between cannabis and psychosis, such as genetic pre-disposition to cannabis use and psychosis and other sources of confounding.

17.2 Assessing Causality from Observational Data

Assessing causality from observational data is challenging. This is particularly the case when the outcome is a complex disease, such as psychosis, with a multifactorial origin. Most environmental risk factors do not fit well with the common-sense requirements for causal relationships; necessary, sufficient, and immediate. For example, exposure to cannabis is not required for someone to develop a psychotic disorder nor does everyone who smoke cannabis develop a psychotic disorder. The immediate reaction to smoking cannabis isn't an acute psychotic episode (although this can happen). So, does this categorically indicate that cannabis in not causally related to psychosis? No; even the most well documented environmental risk factors, such as smoking tobacco in the case of lung cancer, would not meet this criterion.

What can we extrapolate from epidemiological studies investigating the relationship between cannabis and psychosis? We cannot say with certainty that if a specific individual smokes cannabis they will develop a psychotic disorder. What we can say, or what the evidence indicates, is that there is a 'highly suggestive' link between smoking cannabis and psychotic disorder (Arango et al., 2021). Those who smoke cannabis frequently have a 3.9-fold increased odds of a schizophrenia spectrum disorder relative to those who do not smoke cannabis (Marconi et al., 2016). To contextualize this association, the relative risk (RR) of lung cancer between those who are ex-smokers and those who never smoked is 4.3 (Lee et al., 2012).

Table 17.1 The Bradford–Hill criteria for causal association and description

Criteria	Description	Verdict and Evidence
Strength	Effect size of the association	Consistence evidence with substantial effect sizes, see Marconi et al. (2016); Moore et al. (2007); and Semple et al. (2005).
Consistency	Consistency across studies	Consistent evidence across a variety of studies, see Marconi et al. (2016); Moore et al. (2007); and Semple et al. (2005).
Temporality	Direction of the effect and Reverse Causality	Consistent evidence, see Marconi et al. (2016) and Moore et al. (2007).
Biological Gradient	Dose–Response Effect	Strong evidence, see Di Forti et al. (2019a); Marconi et al. (2016); and Moore et al. (2007).
Biological Plausibility	Plausible mechanisms between the exposure and the outcomes	Plausible but precise mechanisms are still unclear, see Murray et al. (2017).
Specificity	The effect is specific to that outcome	Unlikely given the overlapping nature of psychiatric disorder, see Gobbi et al. (2019).
Coherence	Comparison between epidemiological findings and experimental findings in humans and non-humans	The observational and experimental findings do not contradict one another, particularly in relation to THC (see Hindley et al., 2020). Suggestive alignment between human and animal studies (Rubino and Parolaro, 2016).
Experiment	Experimental study design	Strong evidence that THC can induce transient psychotic experiences (see Hindley et al., 2020; Morrison et al., 2009). Some suggestive evidence that CBD has anti-psychotic properties (McGuire et al., 2018).
Analogy	The similarity between the observed association and other similar associations	Unclear as there are limited comparative risk factors that would surpass cannabis use on the Hill criteria.

Having said this, association is not causation and this is particularly the case with observational studies where there are problems of sampling bias, confounding, and measurement error and, in the context of psychosis, a low disease prevalence. For these reasons, epidemiological investigations require a triangulation of the evidence and other criteria to assess causality. The Bradford-Hill criteria for assessing causality between the environment and disease has been a staple of epidemiology for the last 60 years (Hill, 1965). It provides nine criteria (Strength, Consistency, Temporality, Biological Gradient, Biological Plausibility, Specificity, Coherence, Experiment, and Analogy) by which to assess the plausibility of a causal relationship between an exposure and an outcome (see Table 17.1 for criteria and description). The criteria are not without critics and some criteria appear to be more directly related to causality than others (see Ioannidis, 2016; Rothman and Greenland, 1998; Susser, 1991) but

they have provided a useful framework for assessing the plausibility of a causal relationship. Within this chapter, we examine the relationship between cannabis use and psychosis through the lens of each of the criteria. We will draw as much as possible from meta-analytical evidence as it provides some degree of a consensus framework for the state of the literature.

17.3 Bradford-Hill Criteria

Three of the Bradford-Hill criteria (strength, consistency, and temporality) have been grouped together as they are intrinsically linked. A synthesis of the evidence between cannabis and psychotic disorder was published by Marconi et al. (2016). Since its publication, two umbrella reviews and a meta-umbrella have made direct reference to these results (Arango et al., 2021; Belbasis et al., 2018; Radua et al., 2018). Here, we discuss their findings along with other previous meta-analytical findings and other more recently single study work as they relate to the criteria.

17.3.1 Strength

The strength of the association refers to the size of the effect or increased risk of the outcome posed by reporting the exposure. Within this context it refers to the increased risk or effect size that smoking cannabis is associated with psychosis. An effect size of OR = 3.90 (CI = 284–5.34) was derived from a meta-analyses which includes data from 10 observational studies with 66,816 individuals (Marconi et al., 2016). Due to between-study discrepancies in how cannabis was measured, the OR refers to the risk in those heavy cannabis users who had smoked the greatest amount (top group of any ordinal variable composition: frequency in time, lifetime number of joints smoked, or most recent use). The data for these individual studies were from Europe (n = 6), Australia (n = 2), New Zealand (n = 1), and the United States (n = 1), and with varying follow-up times in longitudinal studies. This effect size is higher than previously reported meta-analyses (Moore et al., 2007; Semple et al., 2005). For example, Moore et al. (2007) examined seven observation studies covering similar cohorts and found an increased risk of OR = 1.41 (CI = 1.20–1.65). The discrepancy was considered largely attributed to how cannabis use was categorized, with Marconi and colleagues having a more nuanced approach. Shifting the criteria to median cannabis-use resulted in an OR of 1.97 which is more in line with the previous findings and also speaks to a dose–response effect (see Section 17.3.4).

Since the publication of Marconi et al. (2016) a number of studies on the relationship between cannabis use disorder and psychotic disorder have been published. For example, Bechtold et al. (2016) found that adolescent boys who had used cannabis weekly for three or more years had an increased risk of a psychotic disorder relative to those who never used cannabis. Kendler et al. (2019) found that cannabis-induced psychotic disorder was associated with a cumulative hazard rate for subsequent diagnosis of schizophrenia of 18%. In a Danish nationwide register-based cohort study, Hjorthøj et al. (2021a) elegantly demonstrated the changing population attributable risk fraction (PARF) that cannabis use disorder had on schizophrenia between 1972 and 2016. Their results suggested that, from 1972 to 1995, the percentage of cases of schizophrenia attributable to cannabis was stable, at around 2%; however, between 1995 and 2010, the PARF increased to 6–8% and has remained relatively stable since then. They largely attribute this change to an increase in the potency of cannabis in the region (Thomsen et al., 2019). Interestingly, a previous meta-analysis estimated that cannabis accounted for approximately 8% of the population incidence of schizophrenia (Arseneault et al., 2004). In another meta-analysis based on data from 35 case-control studies, 27% and 16% of patients with schizophrenia had lifetime or a current diagnosis of cannabis use disorder, respectively (Koskinen et al., 2010).

In all meta-analyses published to date there is still a noticeable absence of cohort data from outside of western countries, which is problematic. However, there is a suggestion that the particularly low prevalence of cannabis use in areas such as southern and eastern Asia may account for some of the discrepancies in the prevalence of clinical high risk for psychosis, which have been observed to be less than 0.5% (United Nations Office on Drugs and Crime, 2006). A few retrospective studies of psychiatric or substance use patients have been conducted in Africa and South America (Libuy et al., 2018; Rolfe et al., 1993). For example, using Chilean registry data, Libuy et al. (2018) reported an increased prevalence of schizophrenia among cannabis users attending addiction clinics. However, these studies may be subject to sampling and/or recall biases. There is a need for prospective cohort studies in these regions to see if the strength of the relationship between cannabis and psychosis is moderated by the region of investigation.

17.3.2 Consistency

The consistency of the results refers to the frequency by which the effect is observed across studies. This criterion helps triangulate the evidence from as many sources as possible. While there was heterogeneity in the effect size between the studies published in Marconi et al. (2016), all 10 studies included in the meta-analysis individually indicated a significant increased risk of cannabis use on psychosis (OR range = 1.85–7.45).

Perhaps a concern with relying on any meta-analytic investigation is that the results may have a publication bias as only investigations with significant effects would get published. However, Marconi et al.

(2016) did not find evidence of publication bias. Similarly, neither of the other meta-analyses found evidence to support the presence of publication bias (Moore et al., 2007; Semple et al., 2005).

A further consideration is the discrepancy in metrics of each of the studies within Marconi et al. (2016). What criteria were used to classify a participant as experiencing psychosis? Some studies used measured psychotic symptoms while others were measured using a diagnosis of schizophrenia or a psychotic disorder. A sensitivity analysis indicated relatively that both measurement types were associated with an increased risk of psychosis with overlapping confidence intervals, suggesting that the measurement type did not moderate the observed effect. One final unavoidable consideration is that all data on cannabis use is self-report, which may have some degree of error in estimation.

17.3.3 Temporality

The direction of effect is an important consideration if only to rule out the possibility of reverse causality. For example, has a person already been experiencing psychosis prior to smoking cannabis? This of course is only possible in longitudinal prospective studies that can remove such individuals from the analysis. This was explicitly examined in both the Marconi et al. (2016) and Moore et al. (2007) meta-analyses by conducting stratified analysis on just the longitudinal samples. Marconi et al. (2016) specifically excluded studies enrolling subjects with symptoms at baseline, while Moore et al. (2007) conducted secondary analyses with statistical adjustment or excluded participants and the results were consistent with their main findings. Both analyses suggest reverse causality is not likely to explain the relationship between cannabis use and psychosis. Since the publication of the meta-analyses, another study has provided additional support for the temporality criterion, even after stringent adjustment for confounding. Mustonen et al. (2018) examined 6,534 adolescents and found that cannabis use was associated with increased risk of psychosis even after adjustment for baseline prodromal symptoms, parental psychosis, and other substance use.

Having said this, it is important to state that temporality in causality is a complex issue, particularly when genetic effects are considered. This is discussed further in Sections 17.5 and 17.6. It should be noted that, even when adjustments are made for genetic confounding, there appears to be a considerable relationship between cannabis and psychosis (Giordano et al., 2015).

One final consideration related to temporality is the relationship between cannabis usage and age of onset of psychosis. A meta-analysis demonstrated that those who smoke cannabis had a 2.7 year earlier age at onset of psychosis than those who did not smoke cannabis (Large et al., 2011). Again, these results were not subject to publication bias.

17.3.4 Biological Gradient

The biological gradient refers to the dose–response effect of cannabis use on psychosis. This can be considered in a number of ways. One could consider the frequency at which someone is smoking cannabis, with the expectation that increased usage may be more indicative of a higher risk of psychosis. Another gradient may be the potency of the drug itself, as perhaps as expressed by the percentage of THC or the ratio of THC:CBD. Furthermore, as we have already mentioned, one might consider the age of onset of psychosis in those who reported using and not using cannabis (Large et al., 2011). Here we discuss some evidence for a biological gradient.

(a) **Frequency of Use:** Meta-analyses from Marconi et al. (2016) and Moore et al. (2007) report that the higher frequency users had an increased risk of psychosis. In Marconi et al. (2016), heavy cannabis users had an almost four-fold increased odds of psychosis. Moore et al. (2007), based on six studies, reported that the most frequent cannabis users (as defined as daily users, weekly users, those with dependence or those who have smoked cannabis more than 50 times) had a 2.09 increased odds of developing a psychotic disorder. Both of these results were higher than the effect sizes produced from the median user or lifetime user, suggesting that those who use cannabis more frequently are at greater risk of psychosis.

(b) **Cannabis Potency:** Acquiring data on the potency of cannabis that a participant is using is challenging for many reasons. To our knowledge, no observational study to date has successfully navigated these ethical and legal issues to acquire individual level data on the potency of the cannabis (however, see biological plausibility). However, regional analysis by the European Monitoring Centre for Drug and

Drug Addiction of 28 European Union member states, plus Norway and Turkey, have indicated that cannabis resin and herbal cannabis THC potency had more than doubled from 2006 to 2016 (Resin: 8.14%–17.22%; and Herbal: 5.00%–10.22%, respectively) (European Monitoring Centre for Drugs and Drug Addiction, 2018). For example, at a national level, Denmark's cannabis potency, as estimated from confiscated samples, increased three-fold from 2008 to 2017 (Thomsen et al., 2019).

How does this relate to psychosis and a biological gradient? The EU-GEI study, an international multi-site incidence study, was set up to estimate the incidence of psychotic disorder in each of 17 sites. The crude incidence of psychotic disorder was 21.4 per 100,000 person-years but there was also an 8-fold variability across the sites ranging from 6 per 100,000 person-years in Santiago, Spain to 46.1 per 100,000 person-years in Paris, France (Jongsma et al., 2018). Cleverly, Di Forti et al. (2019a) utilized the report from the European Monitoring Centre for Drugs and Drug Addiction as well as supplementary data from other countries to estimate the broad cannabis potency in 11 sites of the EU-GEI study. They report that those who used cannabis, were currently using cannabis, or had begun to use cannabis younger than age 15 had an increased incidence of psychosis relative to controls. Daily use was associated with a 2.6–3.1 increased odds of incidence of first episode psychosis. Interestingly, when they looked at the population attributable risk of high potency cannabis use (> 10% THC based on the EU report) to the incidence of first episode psychosis, 12.2% of the total cases could be attributable to high potency cannabis use. This was highest in sites with the highest THC content (30.3% in London, 50.3% in Amsterdam, and 18.9% in Paris). The adjusted incidence rate of psychotic disorder and the prevalence of high-potency cannabis in controls were strongly correlated (r = 0.7). These results seem to indicate a remarkable relationship between high potency cannabis use and the incidence of first episode psychosis and mirrored findings from some of the authors previous work in a London catchment area alone (population attributable fraction for skunk-like cannabis: 24%, Di Forti et al., 2015). As can be expected, these results drew a lot of attention (for comment and authors response see Clark, 2019; Di Forti et al., 2019a, 2019b; Gillespie et al., 2019; Linnman, 2019; and Sommer and van den Brink, 2019) but nevertheless appear to indicate that the potency of cannabis is strongly related to the risk of first episode psychosis. Moreover, a subsequent follow-up study indicated that the gradient of cannabis exposure, as expressed by the interaction between frequency of use and the estimated potency of the cannabis, was linearly related to positive symptom score among patients with psychosis (Quattrone et al., 2021).

17.3.5 Biological Plausibility

Addressing biological plausibility is a challenging prospect for observational studies, particularly when we consider all of the possible biological mechanisms associated with smoking cannabis. Most of the evidence for the biological plausibility comes from experimental studies. Elucidating the neural substrates has been very challenging and to date the mechanisms are not entirely clear but some progress has been made. It is not possible to discuss all results in this chapter, but see Murray et al. (2017) for an overview of the evidence. The two most heavily investigated cannabinoids are delta-9-tetrahydrocannabinol (Δ9-THC) and cannabidiol (CBD) and these appear to have opposing effects on psychotic phenomena. For example, a review paper of both randomized and non-randomized controlled trials in healthy people indicated that there is a strong transient effect for THC to increase total, positive, and negative symptoms of psychosis (Hindley et al., 2020). One study has shown that CBD, when administered to patients with schizophrenia in very high doses, has been associated with lower levels of positive psychotic symptoms, suggesting it may have some anti-psychotic properties (McGuire et al., 2018). Gunasekera et al. (2021) reviewed the active or resting state functional substrates of being administered THC and/or CBD. They reported that six articles from only two samples have examined the effect of THC and CBD relative to placebo. These studies found opposing effects of THC and CBD on BOLD hemodynamic response in the striatum during a range of cognitive tasks. CBD appeared to increase regional response, whereas THC decreased regional response.

The possible cellular mechanisms of cannabinoids are likely to involve the endocannabinoid system. It has been shown in animal models that the chronic administration of THC can have a significant effect on CB1 receptors causing down-regulation and desensitization, notably in the prefrontal cortex. Alterations in the endocannabinoid system have a number of downstream effects on GABAergic and glutamatergic transmission in the cortex, particularly the PFC. This presentation is similar to those seen in patients with schizophrenia (Rubino and Parolaro, 2016); however, there is only evidence of a weak relationship between THC and striatal dopamine in human studies (Murray et al., 2017).

17.3.6 Specificity

This criterion is often challenging. Cannabis has been associated with many other psychiatric phenomena such as depression, suicidal ideation, and suicidal attempts (Gobbi et al., 2019). Psychosis is associated with considerable comorbidities over a lifetime (Caspi et al., 2020). The NEMESIS-II study has indicated that, of the predictors of the clinical incidence of psychosis, depression was the strongest and prior psychopathology had a population attributable fraction of 85.5% (Guloksuz et al., 2020). Many individuals who are diagnosed with schizophrenia have a history of psychiatric disorder (Plana-Ripoll et al., 2019). Thus, there is a strong overlap between psychotic and non-psychotic disorders. Sir Austin Bradford Hill, himself, suggested that 'we must not, however, over-emphasize the importance of the characteristic. One-to-one relationships are not frequent. Indeed, I believe that a multi-causation is generally more likely than causation though possibly if we knew all the answer we might get back to a single factor' (Ioannidis, 2016, p. 1755).

17.3.7 Coherence and Experiment

Coherence, as a criterion, suggests that a proposed causal relationship shouldn't contradict firmly established evidence ('known facts') about the nature of a disease. This suggests that there should be an alignment between the epidemiological findings with experimental findings from humans and animals. Given the overlap in content we will discuss the evidence for the coherence and experiment criteria simultaneously.

Obviously, for ethical and legal reasons, it is not possible to conduct a randomized controlled trial of heavy cannabis use to see if this results in increased rates of psychosis. But, as discussed in Section 17.3.5, administration of THC can induce psychotic symptoms in healthy volunteers. Hindley et al. (2020) provided a clear synthesis of the experimental

evidence that the administration of THC results in a strong but transient increase (standard mean change score, SMC) in the total (SMC: 1.10), positive (SMC: 0.91), and negative (SMC: 0.78) symptom severity of psychosis. One small experimental study in patients with schizophrenia and controls demonstrated that the administration of THC transiently increased the positive, negative, and general symptoms of psychosis, and that patients were particularly susceptible to these effects (D'Souza et al., 2005). Animal models (rodent) of cannabinoid exposure indicate that chronic administration of THC or synthetic cannabinoids during adolescence decreases social behaviour in later life (Laviolette, 2021; Rubino and Parolaro, 2016). However, animal experimental studies specifically examining psychotic symptoms are challenging, particularly attempting to infer positive symptoms of psychosis. Most studies have used proxy measures such as pre-pulse inhibition (PPI) which is observable in animals and humans and among the most widely used physiological markers for schizophrenia (for review evidence of PPI dysregulations see San-Martin et al., 2020). The evidence for PPI dysregulation in rodent models after chronic exposure to cannabinoids has been mixed, with some studies reporting a disrupted sensorimotor gating while others did not observe a significant effect (Rubino and Parolaro, 2016).

17.3.8 Analogy

Analogy refers to the idea that the risk factor is similar to another factor that has a known increased risk of the disease. The meta-umbrella review by Arango et al. (2021) indicated that there were only three convincing prospective risk factors for psychosis with class I or class II evidence; clinical high risk status, cannabis use, and adversity in childhood. Considering these two other risk factors it is unclear how they would be comparable with cannabis use. Individuals with clinical high risk status (CHR) have a strongly increased risk of psychosis, with a 23% transition rate at 36 months (De Pablo et al., 2020); however, it has been suggested that CHR may be best conceptualized as an antecedent condition (similar to pre-diabetic condition) rather than a risk factor, as CHR may be the consequence of many risk factors for psychosis (potentially including cannabis). There is a long-standing relationship between adversity in childhood and psychosis, with many investigations also showing a dose–response relationships (Varese et al., 2012). However, there is arguably a better understanding of the biological plausibility and the experimental criteria for the role of cannabis in the aetiology of psychosis when compared with adversity. Interestingly, it has been reported that cannabis use and adversity may act synergistically on the risk of psychotic phenomena (Harley et al., 2010; Konings et al., 2012). The lack of analogous risk factors appears to simply reflect the limited evidence of risk factors available to date and the complex nature of the origins of psychosis.

17.4 Bradford-Hill Criteria Conclusions

What is clear from the evidence above is that cannabis use would meet the vast majority of the Bradford-Hill criteria, which suggest that it can be causally implicated in psychosis. The strength of the evidence for each of the criteria ranges from consistent in the context of strength, consistency, and temporality; strong in the context of biological gradient and experimental evidence; plausible in the context of biological plausibility and coherence; unlikely in the context of specificity; and unclear in the context of analogy. This evidence suggests that cannabis, particularly high potency cannabis, is a contributing factor to the incidence of psychosis in the population. However, the degree of its involvement is still debated by some. We will discuss some of the caveats to this conclusion in the remainder of this chapter.

17.5 Confounding of Association

One of the criticisms of the meta-analysis published on the relationship between cannabis and psychosis is that the estimated effect sizes in the studies are derived from unadjusted odds ratios (Marconi et al., 2016). This, while probably used for practical reasons to have similar comparisons across all studies, leaves open the possibility that the results may be explained by confounding. Many demographic, social, and clinical characteristics, such as male gender, urbanicity, socio-economic status, smoking tobacco, and exposure to trauma, may explain a proportion of the relationship between cannabis and psychosis, however it is highly unlikely that variability in these characteristics would entirely attenuate this relationship. The previous meta-analysis by Moore et al. (2007) reported more modest effect sizes post-adjustment, with variability in the degree of the attenuation (range

= 10–65% effect change). Several studies have adjusted for such characteristics and this did little to attenuate the relationship between cannabis and psychosis (Davis et al., 2013; Di Forti et al., 2009; Hjorthøj et al., 2021a; Jones et al., 2018; Mustonen et al., 2018; Vaucher et al., 2018). In an innovative analysis, Hjorthøj et al. (2021a) reported that, to completely attenuate the relationship, an unmeasured confounder would have to be associated with both cannabis use disorder and schizophrenia at a relative risk well above 5 and sometimes even above 10 beyond the other variables already included in the adjusted analysis. Such a large effect size for an unmeasured (or unknown) confounder or even cumulative effects of several unmeasured confounders seems unlikely.

17.6 Genetic Confounding

Currently, the most common argument against an environmental causal relationship between cannabis use and psychosis is that the result of observational studies, even those accounting for temporality, could be due to familial confounding (Gillespie and Kendler, 2021). There are strong genetic components to both schizophrenia and cannabis use (Sullivan et al., 2003; Tsuang et al., 1996). Even the most enthusiastic proponents of the environmental cause hypothesis would not deny that the risk that cannabis poses for psychosis may be modified (but not attenuated) by the familial pre-disposition to psychosis (Giordano et al., 2015; Kendler et al., 2019). To the authors knowledge, this has been explored twice using a co-relative design (Giordano et al., 2015; McGrath et al., 2010). In both of these articles the results indicated that there was a relationship between cannabis use/abuse and psychosis (delusional disorder and/or schizophrenia) even beyond the co-relative design. The registry-based family study (Giordano et al., 2015) went a step further and demonstrated the attenuation of the effect size was dependent on the degree of relatedness to subjects who were labelled discordant for cannabis abuse. They report that medically or legally documented problematic cannabis abuse was associated with a 10-fold increase in the odds of subsequent schizophrenia in the general population. Notably, even with the substantially attenuated risk in the full-sibling pair analysis, there was still over four-fold odds of risk of schizophrenia. This effect was partially attenuated further based on the time between the exposure and diagnosis. The use of registrar-based data likely leaves open the potential for misclassification error as most people who use cannabis, including those who do so regularly, would not have medically documented cannabis abuse. Nevertheless, even with the complex adjustment for relative design, the environmental effect of cannabis on psychosis was retained with a relatively large, albeit attenuated, effect size.

Other approaches to tackle this question, such as Mendelian randomization studies, have produced mixed results. The largest study to investigate the relationship between the genetic liabilities for schizophrenia (as based on a polygenic risk score (PRS)) and cannabis use disorder did not find a significant increased risk in controls, which partially counters the narrative that those with high PRS for schizophrenia are more likely to use cannabis (Hjorthøj et al., 2021b). The authors did find a small increased risk of cannabis use disorder in patients with schizophrenia based on their PRS. This differs from Gage et al. (2017) and Pasman et al. (2018), who both found bi-directional evidence indicating that genetic risk of cannabis initiation/use was associated with schizophrenia but that there was a stronger association between genetic risks of schizophrenia associated with cannabis initiation/ use. Vaucher et al. (2018) found evidence that PRS for lifetime cannabis use was associated with increased risk of schizophrenia. It is worth noting that Mendelian randomization studies are not free from bias themselves and the use of lifetime cannabis use as a phenotype for 'significant risk' is problematic, but a cautious weighing of these results would suggest the possibly of a bi-directional relationship between genetic risk of cannabis and psychosis as well as a genetic risk of psychosis for cannabis initiation.

17.7 Conclusion

The shift and change in the legal and illegal cannabis market, particularly in relation to high potency cannabis and its potential risks, have not been reflected in the public discourse around the harms of cannabis. From a research perspective, the epidemiological, experimental, and genetic evidence has resulted in a clear shift in the argument from 'whether there is a causal relationship between cannabis and psychosis' to the magnitude of this relationship. The potential harms of high potency cannabis use, especially during development and particularly in those with a family history of psychosis, need to be clearly explained to the public to address the imbalance in the narrative that cannabis is a harmless drug. The decision about what to do with that information is then for both the public and policymakers to consider.

References

Allebeck, P., Adamsson, C., Engström, A., et al. (1993). Cannabis and schizophrenia: A longitudinal study of cases treated in Stockholm County. *Acta Psychiatr Scand*, **88**, 21–24.

Andréasson, S., Engström, A., Allebeck, P., et al. (1987). Cannabis and schizophrenia: A longitudinal study of Swedish conscripts. *Lancet*, **330**, 1483–1486.

Arango, C., Dragioti, E., Solmi, M., et al. (2021). Risk and protective factors for mental disorders beyond genetics: An evidence-based atlas. *World Psychiatry*, **20**, 417–436.

Arseneault, L., Cannon, M., Witton, J., et al. (2004). Causal association between cannabis and psychosis: Examination of the evidence. *Br J Psychiatry*, **184**, 110–117.

Ayonrinde, O. A. (2020). Cannabis and psychosis: Revisiting a nineteenth century study of 'Indian Hemp and Insanity' in Colonial British India. *Psychol Med*, **50**, 1164–1172.

Bechtold, J., Hipwell, A., Lewis, D. A., et al. (2016). Concurrent and sustained cumulative effects of adolescent marijuana use on subclinical psychotic symptoms. *Am J Psychiatry*, **173**, 781–789.

Belbasis, L., Köhler, C. A., Stefanis, N., et al. (2018). Risk factors and peripheral biomarkers for schizophrenia spectrum disorders: An umbrella review of meta-analyses. *Acta Psychiatr Scand*, **137**, 88–97.

Carliner, H., Brown, Q. L., Sarvet, A. L., et al. (2017). Cannabis use, attitudes, and legal status in the US: A review. *Prev Med*, **104**, 13–23.

Caspi, A., Houts, R. M., Ambler, A., et al. (2020). Longitudinal assessment of mental health disorders and comorbidities across 4 decades among participants in the Dunedin birth cohort study. *JAMA Netw Open*, **3**, e203221.

Clark, C. S. (2019). High-potency cannabis and incident psychosis: Correcting the causal assumption. *Lancet Psychiatry*, **6**, e14.

Clouston, T. S. (1896). The Cairo Asylum: Dr. Warnock on hasheesh insanity. *J Mental Sci*, **42**, 790–795.

D'Souza, D. C., Abi-Saab, W. M., Madonick, S., et al. (2005). Delta-9-tetrahydrocannabinol effects in schizophrenia: Implications for cognition, psychosis, and addiction. *Biol Psychiatry*, **57**, 594–608.

Davis, G. P., Compton, M. T., Wang, S., et al. (2013). Association between cannabis use, psychosis, and schizotypal personality disorder: Findings from the National Epidemiologic Survey on Alcohol and Related Conditions. *Schizophr Res*, **151**, 197–202.

De Pablo, G. S., Catalan, A., and Fusar-Poli, P. (2020). Clinical validity of DSM-5 attenuated psychosis syndrome: Advances in diagnosis, prognosis, and treatment. *JAMA Psychiatry*, **77**, 311–320.

Di Forti, M., Marconi, A., Carra, E., et al. (2015). Proportion of patients in south London with first-episode psychosis attributable to use of high potency cannabis: A case-control study. *Lancet Psychiatry*, **2**, 233–238.

Di Forti, M., Morgan, C., Dazzan, P., et al. (2009). High-potency cannabis and the risk of psychosis. *Br J Psychiatry*, **195**, 488–491.

Di Forti, M., Morgan, C., Selten, J. P., et al. (2019a). High-potency cannabis and incident psychosis: Correcting the causal assumption – authors' reply. *Lancet Psychiatry*, **6**, 466–467.

Di Forti, M., Quattrone, D., Freeman, T. P., et al. (2019b). The contribution of cannabis use to variation in the incidence of psychotic disorder across Europe (EU-GEI): A multicentre case-control study. *Lancet Psychiatry*, **6**, 427–436.

European Monitoring Centre for Drugs and Drug Addiction. (2018). *European Drug Report 2018: Trends and Developments*. Luxembourg: Office for Official Publications of the European Communities.

Gage, S. H., Jones, H. J., Burgess, S., et al. (2017). Assessing causality in associations between cannabis use and schizophrenia risk: A two-sample Mendelian randomization study. *Psychol Med*, **47**, 971–980.

Gillespie, N. A., and Kendler, K. S. (2021). Use of genetically informed methods to clarify the nature of the association between cannabis use and risk for schizophrenia. *JAMA Psychiatry*, **78**, 467–468.

Gillespie, N. A., Pasman, J. A., Treur, J. L., et al. (2019). High-potency cannabis and incident psychosis: Correcting the causal assumption. *Lancet Psychiatry*, **6**, 464.

Giordano, G. N., Ohlsson, H., Sundquist, K., et al. (2015). The association between cannabis abuse and subsequent schizophrenia: A Swedish national co-relative control study. *Psychol Med*, **45**, 407–414.

Gobbi, G., Atkin, T., Zytynski, T., et al. (2019). Association of cannabis use in adolescence and risk of depression, anxiety, and suicidality in young adulthood: A systematic review and meta-analysis. *JAMA Psychiatry*, **76**, 426–434.

Guloksuz, S., Pries, L. K., Ten Have, M., et al. (2020). Association of preceding psychosis risk states and non-psychotic mental disorders with incidence of clinical psychosis in the general population: A prospective study in the NEMESIS-2 cohort. *World Psychiatry*, **19**, 199–205.

Gunasekera, B., Davies, C., Martin-Santos, R., et al. (2021). The yin and yang of cannabis: A systematic review of human neuroimaging evidence of the differential effects of Δ9-tetrahydrocannabinol and cannabidiol. *Biol Psychiatry Cogn Neurosci Neuroimaging*, **6**, 636–645.

Hall, W. (2019). The Indian Hemp Drugs Commission 1893–1894. *Addiction*, **114**, 1679–1682.

Harley, M., Kelleher, I., Clarke, M., et al. (2010). Cannabis use and childhood trauma interact additively to increase the risk of psychotic symptoms in adolescence. *Psychol Med*, **40**, 1627–1634.

Hill, A. B. (1965). The environment and disease: Association or causation? *Proc R Soc Med*. **58**, 295–300.

Hindley, G., Beck, K., Borgan, F., et al. (2020). Psychiatric symptoms caused by cannabis constituents: A systematic review and meta-analysis. *Lancet Psychiatry*, **7**, 344–353.

Hjorthøj, C., Posselt, C. M., and Nordentoft, M. (2021a). Development over time of the population-attributable risk fraction for cannabis use disorder in schizophrenia in Denmark. *JAMA Psychiatry*, **78**, 1013–1019.

Hjorthøj, C., Uddin, M. J., Wimberley, T., et al. (2021b). No evidence of associations between genetic liability for schizophrenia and development of cannabis use disorder. *Psychol Med*, **51**, 479–484.

Ioannidis, J. P. (2016). Exposure-wide epidemiology: Revisiting Bradford Hill. *Stat Med*, **35**, 1749–1762.

Jones, H. J., Gage, S. H., Heron, J., et al. (2018). Association of combined patterns of tobacco and cannabis use in adolescence with psychotic experiences. *JAMA Psychiatry*, **75**, 240–246.

Jongsma, H. E., Gayer-Anderson, C., Lasalvia, A., et al. (2018). Treated incidence of psychotic disorders in the multinational EU-GEI study. *JAMA Psychiatry*, **75**, 36–46.

Kendler, K. S., Ohlsson, H., Sundquist, J., et al. (2019). Prediction of onset of substance-induced psychotic disorder and its progression to schizophrenia in a Swedish national sample. *Am J Psychiatry*, **176**, 711–719.

Konings, M., Stefanis, N., Kuepper, R., et al. (2012). Replication in two independent population-based samples that childhood maltreatment and cannabis use synergistically impact on psychosis risk. *Psychol Med*, **42**, 149–159.

Koskinen, J., Löhönen, J., Koponen, H., et al. (2010). Rate of cannabis use disorders in clinical samples of patients with schizophrenia: A meta-analysis. *Schizophr Bull*, **36**, 1115–1130.

Large, M., Sharma, S., Compton, M. T., et al. (2011). Cannabis use and earlier onset of psychosis: A systematic meta-analysis. *Arch Gen Psychiatry*, **68**, 555–561.

Laviolette, S. R. (2021). Exploring the impact of adolescent exposure to cannabinoids and nicotine on psychiatric risk: Insights from translational animal models. *Psychol Med*, **51**, 940–947.

Lee, P. N., Forey, B. A., and Coombs, K. J. (2012). Systematic review with meta-analysis of the epidemiological evidence in the 1900s relating smoking to lung cancer. *BMC Cancer*, **12**, 1–90.

Libuy, N., de Angel, V., Ibáñez, C., et al. (2018). The relative prevalence of schizophrenia among cannabis and cocaine users attending addiction services. *Schizophr Res*, **194**, 13–17.

Linnman, C. (2019). High-potency cannabis and incident psychosis: Correcting the causal assumption. *Lancet Psychiatry*, **6**, 465–466.

Linszen, D. H., Dingemans, P. M., and Lenior, M. E. (1994). Cannabis abuse and the course of recent-onset schizophrenic disorders. *Arch Gen Psychiatry*, **51**, 273–279.

Marconi, A., Di Forti, M., Lewis, C. M., et al. (2016). Meta-analysis of the association between the level of

cannabis use and risk of psychosis. *Schizophr Bull*, **42**, 1262–1269.

McGrath, J., Welham, J., Scott, J., et al. (2010). Association between cannabis use and psychosis-related outcomes using sibling pair analysis in a cohort of young adults. *Arch Gen Psychiatry*, **67**, 440–447.

McGuire, P., Robson, P., Cubala, W. J., et al. (2018). Cannabidiol (CBD) as an adjunctive therapy in schizophrenia: A multicenter randomized controlled trial. *Am J Psychiatry*, **175**, 225–231.

Moore, T. H., Zammit, S., Lingford-Hughes, A., et al. (2007). Cannabis use and risk of psychotic or affective mental health outcomes: A systematic review. *Lancet*, **370**, 319–328.

Morrison, P. D., Zois, V., McKeown, D. A., et al. (2009). The acute effects of synthetic intravenous Δ9-tetrahydrocannabinol on psychosis, mood and cognitive functioning. *Psychol Med*, **39**, 1607–1616.

Murray, R. M., Englund, A., Abi-Dargham, A., et al. (2017). Cannabis-associated psychosis: Neural substrate and clinical impact. *Neuropharmacology*, **124**, 89–104.

Murray, R. M., and Hall, W. (2020). Will legalization and commercialization of cannabis use increase the incidence and prevalence of psychosis? *JAMA Psychiatry*, **77**, 777–778.

Mustonen, A., Niemelä, S., Nordström, T., et al. (2018). Adolescent cannabis use, baseline prodromal symptoms and the risk of psychosis. *Br J Psychiatry*, **212**, 227–233.

Pasman, J. A., Verweij, K. J., Gerring, Z., et al. (2018). GWAS of lifetime cannabis use reveals new risk loci, genetic overlap with psychiatric traits, and a causal effect of schizophrenia liability. *Nature Neurosci*, **21**, 1161–1170.

Plana-Ripoll, O., Pedersen, C. B., Holtz, Y., et al. (2019). Exploring comorbidity within mental disorders among a Danish national population. *JAMA Psychiatry*, **76**, 259–270.

Quattrone, D., Ferraro, L., Tripoli, G., et al. (2021). Daily use of high-potency cannabis is associated with more positive symptoms in first-episode psychosis patients: The EU-GEI case–control study. *Psychol Med*, **51**, 1329–1337.

Radua, J., Ramella-Cravaro, V., Ioannidis, J. P., et al. (2018). What causes psychosis? An umbrella review of risk and protective factors. *World Psychiatry*, **17**, 49–66.

Rolfe, M., Tang, C. M., Sabally, S., et al. (1993). Psychosis and cannabis abuse in The Gambia: A case-control study. *Br J Psychiatry*, **163**, 798–801.

Rothman, K. J., and Greenland, S. (1998). Types of epidemiologic studies. *Mod Epidemiol*, **3**, 95–97.

Rubino, T., and Parolaro, D. (2016). The impact of exposure to cannabinoids in adolescence: Insights from animal models. *Biol Psychiatry*, **79**, 578–585.

San-Martin, R., Castro, L. A., Menezes, P. R., et al. (2020). Meta-analysis of sensorimotor gating deficits in patients with schizophrenia evaluated by prepulse inhibition test. *Schizophr Bull*, **46**, 1482–1497.

Semple, D. M., McIntosh, A. M., and Lawrie, S. M. (2005). Cannabis as a risk factor for psychosis: Systematic review. *J Psychopharmacol*, **19**, 187–194.

Sommer, I., and van den Brink, W. (2019). High-potency cannabis and incident psychosis: Correcting the causal assumption. *Lancet Psychiatry*, **6**, 464–465.

Sullivan, P. F., Kendler, K. S., and Neale, M. C. (2003). Schizophrenia as a complex trait: Evidence from a meta-analysis of twin studies. *Arch Gen psychiatry*, **60**, 1187–1192.

Susser, M. (1991). What is a cause and how do we know one? A grammar for pragmatic epidemiology. *Am J Epidemiol*, **133**, 635–648.

Thomsen, K. R., Lindholst, C., Thylstrup, B., et al. (2019). Changes in the composition of cannabis from 2000–2017 in Denmark: Analysis of confiscated samples of cannabis resin. *Exp Clin Psychopharmacol*, **27**, 402.

Tsuang, M. T., Lyons, M. J., Eisen, S. A., et al. (1996). Genetic influences on abuse of illicit drugs: A study of 3,297 twin pairs. *Am J Med Genet*, **67**, 473–477.

United Nations Office on Drugs and Crime (2006). *World Drug Report* (Vol. 1). Amsterdam: Boom Koninklijke Uitgevers.

Varese, F., Smeets, F., Drukker, M., et al. (2012). Childhood adversities increase the risk of psychosis: A meta-analysis of patient-control, prospective-and cross-sectional cohort studies. *Schizophr Bull*, **38**, 661–671.

Vaucher, J., Keating, B. J., Lasserre, A. M., et al. (2018). Cannabis use and risk of schizophrenia: A Mendelian randomization study. *Mol Psychiatry*, **23**, 1287–1292.

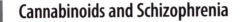

Chapter

18

Post-mortem Studies of the Brain Cannabinoid System in Schizophrenia

Suresh Sundram, Brian Dean, and David Copolov

18.1 Introduction

As outlined elsewhere in this book, epidemiological, clinical and genetic approaches have linked cannabis to schizophrenia from etiological, contributory, and exacerbating perspectives (see Chapters 17, 21, and 22). These studies implicate cannabis use as deleterious in schizophrenia either in increasing its incidence, precipitating illness onset, or worsening its outcomes (Chapter 23). This suggests that inhaled or ingested components of cannabis may interact directly with biological systems relevant to schizophrenia. Much work has focused on the main psychoactive component of cannabis, delta-9-tetrahydrocannabinol (Δ9-THC), which appears to induce psychotic symptoms in both healthy controls and those with schizophrenia (D'Souza et al., 2005). However, there are at least 60 other bioactive components that could mediate the effects of cannabis in humans (Mechoulam and Hanus, 2000; see Chapters 15 and 16). Hence, one explanation for the association of cannabis with schizophrenia is that the human endocannabinoid (eCB) system (ECS) may be disrupted in vulnerable individuals, pre-disposing them to the risk of developing, precipitating, or exacerbating schizophrenia when exposed to cannabis.

The human ECS is detailed elsewhere (see Chapters 1 and 2) and consists of a number of eCBs, their synthetic, degradative, and transport pathways, and the receptors to which they bind, principally the cannabinoid CB1 and CB2 receptors. The two major endocannabinoids are anandamide and 2-arachidonoyl glycerol (2-AG), with the latter predominating in the human central nervous system (CNS) (Piomelli, 2003). In addition to the CB1 and CB2 receptors, the endocannabinoids also activate other receptors in the CNS, including vanilloid (VR1), peroxisome proliferator-activated receptors, orphan G-protein coupled receptors (e.g., GPR55), and transmitter-gated ion channels (Pertwee, 2010). Although it is possible that any

component of the ECS may be altered in individuals vulnerable to developing schizophrenia, methodological constraints have restricted investigation to a number of key elements.

One methodological approach is to use post-mortem human brain tissue from people with schizophrenia and matched controls who did not have schizophrenia. This allows direct examination of some elements of the ECS in brain regions plausibly implicated in schizophrenia. This direct advantage is nevertheless compromised by a number of potentially confounding variables, such as mode of death, agonal state, post-mortem interval (PMI), symptom state at time of death, and medication and substance exposure, of which only some may be partially controlled. Moreover, post-mortem investigation is best restricted to those components least subject to autolytic change, such as membrane-bound receptors, in contrast to eCBs, which are susceptible to post-mortem degradation (Palkovits et al., 2008) For these reasons studies examining the ECS in schizophrenia using post-mortem human brain tissue have focused upon the CB1 receptor, given that it is the predominant CB receptor sub-class and its central role in mediating eCB function in the human brain.

18.2 The Cannabinoid CB1 Receptor in the Brain

The CB1 receptor was the first component of the human endogenous cannabinoid system to be identified (Herkenham et al., 1990). Its gene in humans is located on region q14–q15 of chromosome 6 (Hoehe et al., 1991) and encodes for a 472-amino acid protein (Matsuda et al., 1990). The CB1 receptor has seven trans-membrane spanning domains and interacts with guanine nucleotide binding proteins (G-proteins) as part of its signal transduction mechanism, placing it within the superfamily of G-protein

(A) 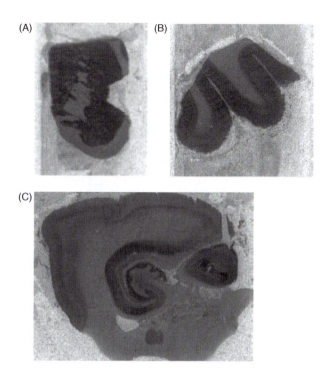 (B)

(C)

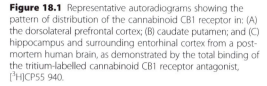

Figure 18.1 Representative autoradiograms showing the pattern of distribution of the cannabinoid CB1 receptor in: (A) the dorsolateral prefrontal cortex; (B) caudate putamen; and (C) hippocampus and surrounding entorhinal cortex from a post-mortem human brain, as demonstrated by the total binding of the tritium-labelled cannabinoid CB1 receptor antagonist, [³H]CP55 940.

coupled receptors (GPCRs). Two post-transcriptional splice isoforms of the CB1 receptor have been identified, termed the CB1a and CB1b receptors (Ryberg et al., 2005; Shire et al., 1995), and multiple polymorphic variants (Howlett and Abood, 2017). Both splice variants are found in the brain, with the CB1a having a 61 amino acid truncation to 411 amino acids and the Cb1b having a 33 amino acid truncation to 439 amino acids (Ryberg et al., 2005; Shire et al., 1995). The isoforms are co-expressed with the CB1 receptor in the brain at much lower levels (Bagher et al., 2013) and show similar membrane trafficking, but different signalling properties (Bagher et al., 2013; Straiker et al., 2012). These differences include an inverse agonist response to 2-AG (Howlett and Abood, 2017), suggesting a modulating effect on the CB1 receptor.

The distribution of the CB1 receptor has been mapped in the human brain (Figure 18.1) (Glass et al., 1997; Herkenham et al., 1990; Westlake et al., 1994; and see Chapter 2). There is a very high density of CB1 receptors in the globus pallidus, substantia nigra pars reticulata, subiculum, Ammon's horn, and the molecular layers of the dentate gyrus in the hippocampus and cerebellum, with a dense but lower level of binding in the neocortex, the remainder of the

hippocampus, entorhinal cortex, amygdaloid complex, and striatum. Neocortical binding is laminated, with highest levels in laminae I, V, and VI, a thin dense band in IV(b), and low binding in II, III, and IV (a and c). The regional density of cortical CB1 receptor also varies, with the densest binding being in the association areas of the frontal, temporal, and limbic lobes, and lowest densities in the primary motor and sensory cortices. Thalamic CB1 receptor binding anatomically corresponds to cortical binding, with moderate binding in the mediodorsal and anterior complex nuclei that connect to cortical associational areas, and very low levels in the geniculate bodies, ventral posterior and ventrolateral nuclei that connect to the primary sensory and motor cortices. The hypothalamus, nucleus solitarius, and central grey substance exhibit moderate levels of CB1 receptor binding, whereas there are minimal levels in the brainstem and area postrema.

In areas of very dense CB1 receptor binding, levels are of the same order of magnitude as that of striatal dopamine, cortical benzodiazepine, and whole brain glutamate receptor densities (Herkenham et al., 1990). These comparisons, however, need to be viewed in light of the physiological activity of the cannabinoid agonist, R-(+)-WIN55 212 in CB1 receptor-knockout mice (Breivogel et al., 2001; Di Marzo et al., 2000). This raises the possibility of non-CB1 cannabinoid receptors in the CNS that, although estimated to be small (Elphick and Egertova, 2001), may confound estimates of CB1 receptor density.

Low levels of the cannabinoid CB2 receptor have been identified in the CNS, in microglia, astrocytes, astrocytomas, and brain stem neurons (Nunez et al., 2004; Stella, 2010; Van Sickle et al., 2005) where they play a role in CNS inflammatory processes (Benito et al., 2008). However, their presence in healthy adult human neuronal tissue remains under discussion (Atwood and Mackie, 2010).

The distribution of mRNA for the CB1 receptor follows a pattern of distribution closely paralleling that of CB1 receptor binding (Mailleux et al., 1992; Westlake et al., 1994). The localization of the mRNA in the cortex is densest in laminae I and II and in the deep laminae IV, V, and VI, with variation between cortical regions. However, both in the hippocampus and cerebral cortex, the mRNA is extremely dense in some neurons surrounded by low-to-moderate densities in the majority of cells. This contrasts with other regions, for example the cerebellum, where mRNA distribution is relatively uniform across neurons. Equivalent levels of mRNA and binding are not maintained in the molecular layer of the hippocampal dentate gyrus, globus pallidus, substantia nigra, and entopeduncular nucleus, where binding is high with minimal levels of mRNA, and conversely in the dentate hilus and medial habenula with high mRNA signal and low binding levels. These differences between mRNA and binding levels may indicate gene transcription of CB1 receptors in cell bodies remote from the receptors' terminal axonal locations.

Relative to the density of the mRNA for the CB1 receptor, the mRNA for the CB1a receptor shows a variable pattern of brain regional densities (between 1 and 20% of the CB1 receptor) (Shire et al., 1995). The physiological significance of this variable difference between the distributions of the mRNA for the CB1 and CB1a receptors remains to be determined (Elphick and Egertova, 2001; Matsuda, 1997).

The temporal gene expression profile of the CB1 receptor across the human lifespan has recently been described in a large series (Tao et al., 2020). Highest expression levels were measured in the foetus during the second trimester, with a subsequent decrease noted in the hippocampus and prefrontal cortex.

This was for the full length CB1 receptor, as well as a 99 nucleotide truncated transcript (Tao et al., 2020).

The neural localization of CB1 receptors is primarily at axon terminals, which strongly suggests a role in modulating synaptic transmission (Katona et al., 2006). The functional properties of the CB1 receptor are detailed in Chapters 1 and 2, where they are proposed to inhibit synaptic neurotransmitter release (Castillo et al., 2012; Schlicker and Kathmann, 2001). In the prefrontal cortex, where the majority of human post-mortem studies have focused, CB1 receptors are principally located on GABA inhibitory basket inter-neurons and a lower proportion of excitatory glutamate pyramidal neurons (Volk and Lewis, 2016). The basket neurons are predominantly cholecystokinin (CCK) containing cells and target both pyramidal neurons and parvalbumin-positive inter-neurons. Thus, retrograde signalling of 2-AG released by pyramidal neurons activating CB1 receptors on CCK positive basket inter-neurons will suppress release of GABA and result in depolarization-induced suppression of inhibition (Volk and Lewis, 2016).

18.3 Post-mortem Human Brain Studies

Post-mortem human brain studies allow clear regional localization of changes in stable components of the endogenous cannabinoid system. A number of methods have been used to quantify changes in the CB1 receptor in schizophrenia: in-situ radioligand binding and quantitative autoradiography; in-situ hybridization; and immunohistochemistry. In addition, expression of mRNA for the CB1 and CB2 receptors and some ECS enzymes as well as functional enzymatic, receptor, and eCB studies have been reported.

18.3.1 In-situ Radioligand Binding and Quantitative Autoradiography Studies

A number of studies have used in-situ radioligand binding and quantitative auto-radiography to measure CB1 receptor density in post-mortem human brain tissue from people with schizophrenia and healthy controls; some studies have also incorporated other patient groups (Dalton et al., 2011; Dean et al., 2001; Deng et al., 2007; Jenko et al., 2012; Newell et al., 2006; Volk et al., 2014; Zavitsanou et al., 2004). The first published study (Dean et al., 2001) compared binding of the CB1 receptor agonist [^{3}H]CP55940 in the dorsolateral prefrontal cortex (DLPFC), Brodmann's area 9 (BA9), caudate-putamen (C-P), and hippocampal formation of post-mortem tissue obtained from 14 subjects with schizophrenia and 14 non-psychiatric controls. Some subjects from both groups had consumed cannabis before death, allowing a comparison between recent cannabis users and those who had been abstinent. The methodology used was previously shown to provide a good measure of the density of the CB1 receptor (Herkenham et al., 1990) and the concentration of [^{3}H]CP55940 was likely to provide single-point saturation.

When all subjects with schizophrenia were compared with all control subjects, the mean CB1 receptor density was increased by approximately 19%, but only in the DLPFC ($p < 0.05$). There were no significant differences between the groups in receptor density in the C-P or hippocampal formation. In subjects who had recently consumed cannabis (as determined by GC/MS of post-mortem plasma), there was a 23% increase in CB1 receptor density in the C-P compared with non-users, independent of schizophrenia ($p < 0.05$); in this comparison there were no significant differences in the DLPFC nor, again, in the hippocampus. The differences in the DLPFC between control and schizophrenia subjects and in the C-P between users and non-users could not be accounted for by post-mortem interval (PMI), brain pH, age, or gender. There were also no significant correlations between [^{3}H]CP55940 binding and duration of illness or final recorded antipsychotic drug dose in those with schizophrenia or with plasma THC levels in the cannabis users.

Another study, also using in-situ binding with [^{3}H]CP55940 and quantitative autoradiography, demonstrated increased CB1 receptor density in schizophrenia in the posterior cingulate cortex (PCC) (Newell et al., 2006). The study comprised post-mortem human brain tissue from 16 male subjects, eight controls and eight with schizophrenia matched for age and PMI, none of whom had used cannabis in the time preceding death. The pattern of [^{3}H]CP55940 binding in the PCC showed a laminar distribution with highest binding in superficial layers compared with deep layers. From adjacent Nissl-stained sections the authors concluded the superficial binding was in layers I and II and the deep binding in layers III–VI. The CB1 receptor density was increased

by 25% only in the superficial laminar and was not different in the lower laminar compared with the control group. The increased binding was not accounted for by suicide or final recorded antipsychotic drug dose.

Partially consistent with these studies using [^{3}H]CP55940 and measuring CB1 receptor density in the DLPFC, specifically, Brodmann's Area 46 (BA46), Dalton et al. (2011) found a selective 22% increase in schizophrenia. This study used a larger cohort of schizophrenia (n = 37) and control (n = 37) cases and was able to control for age, brain pH, and post-mortem interval. The larger sample enabled a split of the schizophrenia group into those with paranoid (n = 16) and non-paranoid (n = 21) features. The increase was seen only in those with paranoid schizophrenia, suggesting diagnostic specificity.

An alternative radioligand to [^{3}H]CP55940 is the CB1 receptor antagonist [^{3}H]SR141716A, which overcomes the limitation of agonist-induced affinity changes in the receptor (Price et al., 2005) and also does not bind the cannabinoid CB2 receptor. [^{3}H]SR141716A was used by Zavitsanou et al. (2004) to measure CB1 receptor density in the anterior cingulate cortex (ACC) in schizophrenia (n = 10) compared with controls (n = 9). This study found that [^{3}H]SR141716A binding was homogenous across all cortical layers, a finding different from the other studies detailed in this section. This study also found CB1 receptor density was increased in schizophrenia in the ACC by 64% and this was not associated with PMI. Moreover, like Dean et al. (2001), Zavitsanou et al. (2004) also noted no difference in CB1 receptor binding in the cortex between cannabis users and non-users and no relationship with antipsychotic drug dose.

Using another inverse agonist, [^{3}H]MePPEP, which also had the advantage of avoiding agonist-induced affinity change, Jenko et al. (2012) measured CB1 receptor binding in the DLPFC from schizophrenia (n = 47) and control (n = 43) samples. After having found no differences in CB1 receptor affinity (Kd) or density (Bmax) in a sub-set of the sample, they did show an overall increase using a 2-point binding assay of 20% which increased in significance after controlling for group differences in cigarette smoking, age at death, brain weight, brain pH, and time frozen (Jenko et al., 2012). A smaller study (21 schizophrenia and 21 control) using a tritiated analogue of the inverse agonist, rimonabant

(SR141716A), [³H]-OMAR, measured CB1 receptor binding in the prefrontal cortex (Volk et al., 2014) and also found a significant (8%) increase in binding.

In contrast to the studies already reviewed in this section, one quantitative autoradiography study used both CB1 receptor radioligands, [³H]CP55940 and [³H]SR141716A (Deng et al., 2007), and found no differences in receptor density in schizophrenia in the superior temporal gyrus (STG). This suggests that changes in CB1 receptor density in schizophrenia may be brain region specific. The study used tissue from 16 subjects, 8 with schizophrenia and 8 controls matched for age, sex (all male), and PMI. [³H]CP55 940 showed a trilaminar pattern of binding, with the upper band corresponding to cortical layers I and II, the middle band to layers III and IV, and the deepest band corresponding to layers V and VI, with the middle band having a lower level of binding compared with the other two. There were no significant differences between schizophrenia and control subjects in [³H]CP55940 binding in any of the bands. [³H]SR141716A demonstrated a homogenous pattern of binding through the STG and, again, no difference between schizophrenia and control subjects was demonstrated. Recent cannabis use did not alter binding significantly in the schizophrenia group and there was no effect of antipsychotic drug treatment. Fifteen of the 16 subjects in the study of Deng et al. (2007) had also been included in the study of Newell et al. (2006), where there was an increase in CB1 receptor density in the ACC, supporting regional specificity.

The use of the two radioligands also demonstrated that the amount of CB1 receptor protein measured was different between the two compounds. The [³H]CP55940 assay showed levels of at least 97 fmol/mg tissue equivalents (TE) compared to [³H]SR141716A levels of approximately 35 fmol/mg TE. This discrepancy may be due to sub-optimal assay conditions that may not have resulted in binding saturation, [³H]CP55940 binding to other receptors, or [³H]CP55940 inducing affinity change in the CB1 receptor.

18.3.2 Immunohistochemical Studies

In contrast to the reported increase in CB1 receptor binding, in particular in the PFC in schizophrenia, studies using immunohistochemistry have found decreased or unchanged CB1 receptor levels (Eggan et al., 2008, 2010; Koethe et al., 2007; Uriguen et al.,

2009). The study by Koethe et al. (2007) measured CB1 receptor protein in the ACC in tissue from schizophrenia, bipolar disorder, major depression, and non-psychiatrically ill control (n = 15 in each group) subjects, although not matched on PMI, substance abuse, or suicide. There were no changes in the number of CB1 receptor immuno-positive cells in the ACC in schizophrenia. There were also no changes in cell numbers or apparent neuron density in any of the diagnostic groups compared with the control group. This contrasts with the striking increase in CB1 receptor density in the ACC, as measured by quantitative autoradiography (Zavitsanou et al., 2004). Two obvious factors are the methodological difference and the heterogeneity of the ACC (Vogt et al., 1987). Immunohistochemistry covers only small regions and the Koethe et al. (2007) study may have selected a sub-region of the ACC unaffected in schizophrenia.

A study with a larger sample (n = 77) used immunohistochemistry and in-situ hybridization to measure the protein and mRNA levels of the CB1, dopamine D2, and adenosine A2A receptors in the DLPFC in people with schizophrenia (n = 31); non-schizophrenia suicides (n = 13); and non-suicide, non-psychiatrically ill controls (n = 33) (Uriguen et al., 2009). Recent cannabis use was an exclusion criterion. There was no difference overall in CB1 receptor protein levels between the groups. However, when the schizophrenia group were divided into those who had received antipsychotic drug treatment in the period immediately preceding death and those who were antipsychotic-free (as determined by post-mortem toxicological assay), differences were noted. The antipsychotic drug-treated group (n = 11) had a 29% decrease in CB1 receptor protein density, whereas the antipsychotic drug-free and non-schizophrenia suicide groups did not differ significantly from control subjects. The decrease was not attributable to suicide or a decrease in total protein.

Two studies from the University of Pittsburgh used in-situ hybridization, radioimmunocytochemistry, and immunohistochemistry to ascertain levels of CB1 receptor mRNA and protein level in schizophrenia (Eggan et al., 2008, 2010). The first compared 23 pairs of schizophrenia and control samples matched on age, sex, and PMI using tissue from the DLPFC (BA9) (Eggan et al., 2008). The immunoreactivity of CB1 receptor protein showed a banded pattern with greatest density in layer IV, next highest in layers II and III, then layer VI and lowest in layer V. There was no comment on layer I binding that appears of a density between layer III and VI. Using a pairwise comparison, a significant overall decrease of 11.6% was noted in the schizophrenia subjects that was not significant in a whole-group unpaired comparison. Rather surprisingly given the discordant banding patterns observed, a significant correlation (rho = 0.67; $p < 0.001$) was noted between the pairwise change in CB1 receptor mRNA and protein levels. Using standard immunohistochemistry on 12 of the 23 subject pairs, an overall significant decrease of 13.9% was observed in the subjects with schizophrenia that was also noted in deep portions of layers III, IV, and VI (on both pairwise and unpaired comparisons). There was no effect on any of the CB1 receptor levels by sex, death by suicide, antidepressant exposure, sodium valproate, antipsychotic or benzodiazepine medication use, or any substance abuse or dependence (including cannabis).

A subsequent study by the same group examined another DLPFC region (BA46) in the same subjects and in tissue from a different cohort of subjects with schizophrenia (Eggan et al., 2010). CB1 receptor immunoreactivity was decreased by 19% in the same 12 pairs of subjects that had a 13.9% decrease in BA9, and there was a significant correlation (rho = 0.73; $p < 0.001$) between the two regions. In the new cohort, CB1 receptor immunoreactivity was decreased by 20% compared with control subjects and by 23% compared with subjects with major depression. The pattern of binding in this area was similar to that observed in BA9, with the subjects with schizophrenia from the new cohort having lower levels of CB1 receptor immunoreactivity in layers I–IV but not V or VI. The differences observed were not a function of sex, death by suicide, antidepressant exposure, benzodiazepine or antipsychotic drug use, substance use disorder diagnosis, or history of cannabis use (Eggan et al., 2010).

18.3.3 In-situ Hybridization and Expression of Messenger RNA Studies

A few studies have measured expression of CB1 receptor mRNA (Dalton et al., 2011; Eggan et al., 2008; Guillozet-Bongaarts et al., 2014; Muguruza et al., 2019; Tao et al., 2020; Uriguen et al., 2009) using RT-qPCR or, more recently, high through-put technologies. In line with the immunohistochemistry studies but opposite to the receptor binding studies, these expression studies have shown either decreased CB1 receptor mRNA expression or no change in similar brain regions in schizophrenia.

In the Eggan et al. (2008) study, similar to CB1 receptor immunoreactivity, the mRNA expression pattern in BA9 was banded. It was confined to neurons with greatest density in layer II and the superficial part of layer III, intermediate in layers IV, V, and VI, lowest in the deep part of layer III, and absent in layer I; this was similar in both groups. The subjects with schizophrenia had a mean overall decrease of 14.8% of CB1 receptor mRNA compared with controls and this applied to each band, similar to that observed for the CB1 receptor protein. These authors used the same tissue samples to measure CB1 receptor binding using [^{3}H]-OMAR (Volk et al., 2014), and found an 8% increase in schizophrenia.

Three other studies where the CB1 receptor was measured, along with its mRNA transcript (Dalton et al., 2011; Koethe et al., 2007; Uriguen et al., 2009), showed no change in expression. The study by Koethe et al. (2007) similarly showed no change in CB1 receptor immunoreactivity in the ACC, in contrast to a decrease in CB1 receptor protein in the DLPFC in the antipsychotic drug treated group with schizophrenia in the study by Uriguen et al. (2009). In variance, Dalton et al. (2011) found an increase in CB1 receptor binding in the DLPFC in schizophrenia, but only in people with the paranoid sub-type of schizophrenia.

The in-situ hybridization study by Guillozet-Bongaarts et al. (2014) measured, *inter alia*, CB1 receptor mRNA in BA9 and BA46 tissue from schizophrenia (n = 19) and healthy control (n = 33) cases. They found a decrease in schizophrenia only in layer VI in BA9 and no other changes. The comparably sized study by Muguruza et al. (2019) found a more extensive decrease in CB1 receptor mRNA in BA9 using high throughput RT-qPCR, which was independent of antipsychotic drug treatment status. They then measured the functional coupling of the CB1 receptor to G-proteins in cortical membranes from these samples. There was no difference in maximum efficacy or strength of CB1 receptor-mediated [^{35}S]GTPγS binding stimulation by the agonist WIN-55,212-2 between schizophrenia and control samples, indicating expression changes were not affecting canonical receptor signalling pathways (Muguruza et al., 2019).

The largest study (Tao et al., 2020) to date in schizophrenia of CB1 receptor expression, including the 99-nucleotide truncated transcript variant, measured mRNA from the DLPFC, caudate, and hippocampus from a total of 703 samples including 175 samples from people with schizophrenia and also major depression and bipolar disorder. Decreased expression at both gene and full-length transcript level in the DLPFC was found in schizophrenia and depression compared to healthy controls, but not in other brain regions and not with the truncated transcript.

The only investigation of CB2 receptor expression in the human brain in schizophrenia found no correlation between expression in BA9 and schizophrenia (Ishiguro et al., 2010). However, the study found a single nucleotide polymorphism (rs12744386) in the CB2 receptor gene to be associated with schizophrenia compared to healthy controls and with lower CB2 mRNA expression in the human brain. This suggests – indirectly – a decrease in the CB2 receptor in schizophrenia; however, this receptor is predominantly if not exclusively expressed on immune cells in the CNS.

18.3.4 Quantification of Non-Receptor Components of the Brain Endocannabinoid System

Given accurate measurement of endogenous cannabinoids (eCBs) in post-mortem human brain tissue is compromised by rapid degradation, most studies looking at non-receptor components of the endocannabinoid system have focused on the enzymatic machinery (Muguruza et al., 2019; Volk et al., 2010, 2013). The one study to have attempted eCB quantification (Muguruza et al., 2013) used quantitative liquid chromatography with triple quadrupole mass spectrometric detection to measure 2-AG, anandamide, and four other related molecules in the DLPFC, hippocampus, and cerebellum in schizophrenia and matched control (n = 19) samples. Significantly increased 2-AG levels in the DLPFC and hippocampus were found, along with decreased anandamide levels in all regions (albeit only at trend level in the DLPFC in schizophrenia compared to healthy controls). Using the same case samples, these investigators showed there was no change in the levels or functional activity of the two main degradative enzymes, fatty acid amide hydrolase (FAAH) and monoacylglycerol lipase (MAGL) in schizophrenia,

although there was a small increase in the Vmax of FAAH (Muguruza et al., 2019). The lack of change was also observed in an earlier study (Volk et al., 2010) in DLPFC from schizophrenia samples (n = 42) where expression of FAAH, MAGL, and diacylglycerol lipase alpha and beta isoform mRNA were not different between schizophrenia and healthy controls. A follow-up study with an overlapping sample did identify an increase in mRNA in another degrading enzyme, alpha-beta-hydrolase domain 6 (ABHD6) but only in cases under the age of 40 and with a shorter duration of illness (<15 years) (Volk et al., 2013).

18.4 Summary, Limitations, and Interpretation

The majority of studies reviewed here have concentrated on the most functionally relevant and stable post-mortem component of the endocannabinoid system – the CB1 receptor – and have focused on highly implicated regions for schizophrenia such as the dorsolateral prefrontal cortex and hippocampus. The studies measuring CB1 receptor binding repeatedly report increased binding in the DLPFC and other frontal cortical regions in schizophrenia, in the range of 20%. These changes may be associated with diagnostic or other illness characteristics, and similar changes have been reported in unipolar depression (for a review see Garani et al., 2021). However, the changes do not seem to extend to other brain regions such as the hippocampus, caudate, or superior temporal gyrus. Moreover, the increase in binding is modest compared with the decrease described in Huntington's disease (97.5% in the substantia nigra pars reticulata) where there is specific degeneration of striatonigral terminals (Glass et al., 1993).

The general increase contrasts with those few studies measuring CB1 receptor immunoreactivity and mRNA where receptor protein and mRNA are unchanged or decreased in schizophrenia compared to healthy controls across the same brain regions. The two groups that have measured receptor binding and receptor protein and/or mRNA (Dalton et al., 2011; Volk et al., 2014) support this discordance, that may be due to an increase in the affinity of the receptor for ligand in the absence of a true change in receptor number. However, the common finding across a range of agonist, inverse agonist, and antagonist ligands make this less likely and similarly neuron numbers in the frontal cortex are unchanged in schizophrenia (Thune et al., 2001). More plausibly it could reflect a change in CB1 receptor trafficking where more receptor is cell surface membrane bound in schizophrenia. A testable alternate proposition could be that the CB1 receptor is altered differentially in different cells. For example, in CCK-GABA interneurons within the DLPFC there could be comparatively unchanged expression of CB1 receptors but on excitatory efferents an increase in CB1 receptors, where they are transcribed outside the DLPFC and transported to axon terminals within the DLPFC. These changes would also be consistent with the reported increase in 2-AG in the DLPFC in schizophrenia (Muguruza et al., 2013).

Post-mortem human brain studies in schizophrenia are plagued by a number of potential confounds, including antipsychotic and other psychotropic drug treatment, substance use, mode of death (especially suicide), and other illness-related factors that complicate interpretation of between-group differences. The use of non-schizophrenia psychiatric control groups such as those with major depression and bipolar disorder, toxicological analyses to exclude recent substance use and antipsychotic drug adherence, and sample matching have been used by various investigators in an attempt to ameliorate these confounds. Additionally, animal treatment studies with cannabinoids and antipsychotic drugs can assist in parcellating pathophysiological processes from those exogenously related.

The studies described in this chapter report an absence of any relationship between antipsychotic drug doses and CB1 receptor levels and one study (Uriguen et al., 2009) reported a decrease in CB1 receptor immunoreactivity in the DLPFC only in subjects with schizophrenia who had been treated with antipsychotic medication. These are, however, indirect measures of chronic antipsychotic drug effects on brain CB1 receptor levels. Chronic and sub-chronic animal treatment studies using in-situ radioligand binding and quantitative autoradiography studies in rats did not show changes in CB1 receptor binding in the cerebral cortex, caudate-putamen, or hippocampus (Sundram et al., 2005; Wiley et al., 2008); and a small-scale monkey treatment study also did not report changes in CB1 receptor protein or mRNA levels in the frontal cortex (Eggan et al., 2008, 2010). Therefore, from these limited data it would seem unlikely that antipsychotic treatment exerts a major effect on CB1 receptor levels in the frontal cortex of mammals.

It is possible that exogenous cannabinoids may influence CB1 receptor levels in schizophrenia, especially given the high rate of cannabis use in this group. The reported studies controlled for this variable by excluding subjects with recent cannabis use or demonstrating no effect on binding in cortical regions when comparing users and non-users. One study (Dean et al., 2001) did show an effect of cannabis consumption in the caudate-putamen, but not hippocampus or DLPFC. Therefore, there appear to be functional effects of cannabis on CB1 receptor density and downstream consequences in schizophrenia that are region-specific. The regional differences are consistent with animal studies in rodents and monkeys that show variable effects dependent on cannabinoid type, dose, duration, and brain region examined. Hence, cannabis use, or withdrawal remains a possible factor in explaining some of the variance between studies in schizophrenia. It is also possible that other exogenous agents such as alcohol, caffeine, or nicotine may influence CB1 receptor levels (Basavarajappa and Hungund, 2002; Marco et al., 2007) and this may have contributed to within- and between-study differences.

18.5 Conclusion

There are robust post-mortem human brain data supporting dysregulation of the endocannabinoid system in schizophrenia. These changes point to dorsolateral prefrontal cortical pathology with increased CB1 receptor binding but unchanged or possibly decreased mRNA expression and CB1 receptor immunoreactivity. The changes appear to be regionally and plausibly laminar specific and possibly accompanied by an increase in the major CNS ligand, 2-AG. It is premature to speculate on the possible functional sequelae of these changes until we better understand the discordant findings which may be alluding to receptor affinity changes, specific cell-type effects, compensatory or other unknown factors. Moreover, the possible impacts of confounding variables, such as chronic antipsychotic treatment and withdrawal, chronic cannabis use and withdrawal, and nicotine, alcohol, or caffeine use also need to be understood. Nevertheless, speculative impacts on depolarization-induced suppression of excitation and inhibition are possible (Volk and Lewis, 2016), as are influences on long-term depression and potentiation

(Morrison and Murray, 2020). Focusing investigations at a dendritic spine level, in particular in the functional relationship between CCK positive GABA inter-neurons and excitatory glutamate pyramidal cortical neurons, is warranted to better understand the pathological implications for schizophrenia of the multi-faceted dysfunctions in endocannabinoid neurotransmission reported thus far.

References

Atwood, B. K., and Mackie, K. (2010). CB2: A cannabinoid receptor with an identity crisis. *Br J Pharmacol*, **160**, 467–479.

Bagher, A. M., Laprairie, R. B., Kelly, M. E. M., et al. (2013). Co-expression of the human cannabinoid receptor coding region splice variants (hCB$_1$) affects the function of hCB$_1$ receptor complexes. *Eur J Pharmacol*, **721**, 341–354.

Basavarajappa, B. S., and Hungund, B. L. (2002). Neuromodulatory role of the endocannabinoid signaling system in alcoholism: An overview. *Prostaglandins Leukot Essent Fatty Acids*, **66**, 287–299.

Benito, C., Tolon, R. M., Pazos, M. R., et al. (2008). Cannabinoid CB2 receptors in human brain inflammation. *Br J Pharmacol*, **153**, 277–285.

Breivogel, C. S., Griffin, G., Di, M. V., and Martin, B. R. (2001). Evidence for a new G protein-coupled cannabinoid receptor in mouse brain. *Mol Pharmacol*, **60**, 155–163.

Castillo, P. E., Younts, T. J., Chávez, A. E., et al. (2012). Endocannabinoid signaling and synaptic function. *Neuron*, **76**, 70–81.

D'Souza, D. C., Abi-Saab, W. M., Madonick, S., et al. (2005). Delta-9-tetrahydrocannabinol effects in schizophrenia: Implications for cognition, psychosis, and addiction. *Biol Psychiatry*, **57**, 594–608.

Dalton, V. S., Long, L. E., Weickert, C. S., et al. (2011). Paranoid schizophrenia is characterized by increased CB1 receptor binding in the dorsolateral prefrontal cortex. *Neuropsychopharmacology*, **36**, 1620–1630.

Dean, B., Sundram, S., Bradbury, R., et al. (2001). Studies on [3H]CP-55940 binding in the human central nervous system: Regional specific changes in density of cannabinoid-1 receptors associated with schizophrenia and cannabis use. *Neuroscience*, **103**, 9–15.

Deng, C., Han, M., and Huang, X. F. (2007). No changes in densities of cannabinoid receptors in the superior temporal gyrus in schizophrenia. *Neurosci Bull*, **23**, 341–347.

Di Marzo, V., Breivogel, C. S., Tao, Q., et al. (2000). Levels, metabolism, and pharmacological activity of anandamide in CB(1) cannabinoid receptor knockout mice: Evidence for non-CB(1), non-CB(2) receptor- mediated actions of anandamide in mouse brain. *J Neurochem*, **75**, 2434–2444.

Eggan, S. M., Hashimoto, T., and Lewis, D. A. (2008). Reduced cortical cannabinoid 1 receptor messenger RNA and protein expression in schizophrenia. *Arch Gen Psychiatry*, **65**, 772–784.

Eggan, S. M., Stoyak, S. R., Verrico, C. D., et al. (2010). Cannabinoid CB1 receptor immunoreactivity in the prefrontal cortex: Comparison of schizophrenia and major depressive disorder. *Neuropsychopharmacology*, **35**, 2060–2071.

Elphick, M. R., and Egertova, M. (2001). The neurobiology and evolution of cannabinoid signalling. *Phil Trans R Soc Lond B*, **356**, 381–408.

Garani, R., Watts, J. J., and Mizrahi, R. (2021). Endocannabinoid system in psychotic and mood disorders, a review of human studies. *Prog Neuropsychopharmacol Biol Psychiatry*, **106**, 110096.

Glass, M., Dragunow, M., and Faull, R. L. (1997). Cannabinoid receptors in the human brain: A detailed anatomical and quantitative autoradiographic study in the foetal, neonatal and adult human brain. *Neuroscience*, **77**, 299–318.

Glass, M., Faull, R. L., and Dragunow, M. (1993). Loss of cannabinoid receptors in the substantia nigra in Huntington's disease. *Neuroscience*, **56**, 523–527.

Guillozet-Bongaarts, A. L., Hyde, T. M., Dalley, R. A., et al. (2014). Altered gene expression in the dorsolateral prefrontal cortex of individuals with schizophrenia. *Mol Psychiatry*, **19**, 478–485.

Herkenham, M., Lynn, A. B., Little, M. D., et al. (1990). Cannabinoid receptor localization in brain. *Proc Natl Acad Sci USA*, **87**, 1932–1936.

Hoehe, M. R., Caenazzo, L., Martinez, M. M., et al. (1991). Genetic and physical mapping of the human cannabinoid receptor gene to chromosome 6q14–q15. *New Biol*, **3**, 880–885.

Howlett, A. C., and Abood, M. E. (2017). CB1 and CB2 receptor pharmacology. *Adv Pharmacol*, **80**, 169–206.

Ishiguro, H., Horiuchi, Y., Ishikawa, M., et al. (2010). Brain cannabinoid CB2 receptor in schizophrenia. *Biol Psychiatry*, **67**, 974–982.

Jenko, K. J., Hirvonen, J., Henter, I. D., et al. (2012). Binding of a tritiated inverse agonist to cannabinoid CB1 receptors is increased in patients with schizophrenia. *Schizophr Res*, **141**, 185–188.

Katona, I., Urbán, G. M., Wallace, M., et al. (2006). Molecular composition of the endocannabinoid system at glutamatergic synapses. *J Neurosci*, **26**, 5628–5637.

Koethe, D., Llenos, I. C., Dulay, J. R., et al. (2007). Expression of CB1 cannabinoid receptor in the anterior cingulate cortex in schizophrenia, bipolar disorder, and major depression. *J Neural Transm*, **114**, 1055–1063.

Mailleux, P., Parmentier, M., and Vanderhaeghen, J. J. (1992). Distribution of cannabinoid receptor messenger RNA in the human brain: An in situ hybridization histochemistry with oligonucleotides. *Neurosci Lett*, **143**, 200–204.

Marco, E. M., Granstrem, O., Moreno, E., et al. (2007). Subchronic nicotine exposure in adolescence induces long-term effects on hippocampal and striatal cannabinoid-CB1 and mu-opioid receptors in rats. *Eur J Pharmacol*, **557**, 37–43.

Matsuda, L. A. (1997). Molecular aspects of cannabinoid receptors. *Crit Rev Neurobiol*, **11**, 143–166.

Matsuda, L. A., Lolait, S. J., Brownstein, M. J., et al. (1990). Structure of a cannabinoid receptor and functional expression of the cloned cDNA. *Nature*, **346**, 561–564.

Mechoulam, R., and Hanus, L. (2000). A historical overview of chemical research on cannabinoids. *Chem Phys Lipids*, **108**, 1–13.

Morrison, P. D., and Murray, R. M. (2020). Cannabis points to the synaptic pathology of mental disorders: How aberrant synaptic components disrupt the highest psychological functions. *Dialogues Clin Neurosci*, **22**, 251–258.

Muguruza, C., Lehtonen, M., Aaltonen, N., et al. (2013). Quantification of endocannabinoids in postmortem brain of schizophrenic subjects. *Schizophr Res*, **148**, 145–150.

Muguruza, C., Morentin, B., Meana, J. J., et al. (2019). Endocannabinoid system imbalance in the postmortem prefrontal cortex of subjects with schizophrenia. *J Psychopharmacol*, **33**, 1132–1140.

Newell, K. A., Deng, C., and Huang, X. F. (2006). Increased cannabinoid receptor density in the posterior cingulate cortex in schizophrenia. *Exp Brain Res*, **172**, 556–560.

Nunez, E., Benito, C., Pazos, M. R., et al. (2004). Cannabinoid CB2 receptors are expressed by perivascular microglial cells in the human brain: An immunohistochemical study. *Synapse*, **53**, 208–213.

Palkovits, M., Harvey-White, J., Liu, J., et al. (2008). Regional distribution and effects of postmortem delay on endocannabinoid content of the human brain. *Neuroscience*, **152**, 1032–1039.

Pertwee, R. G. (2010). Receptors and channels targeted by synthetic cannabinoid receptor agonists and antagonists. *Curr Med Chem*, **17**, 1360–1381.

Piomelli, D. (2003). The molecular logic of endocannabinoid signalling. *Nat Rev Neurosci*, **4**, 873–884.

Price, M. R., Baillie, G. L., Thomas, A., et al. (2005). Allosteric modulation of the cannabinoid CB1 receptor. *Mol Pharmacol*, **68**, 1484–1495.

Ryberg, E., Vu, H. K., Larsson, N., et al. (2005). Identification and characterisation of a novel splice variant of the human CB1 receptor. *FEBS Lett*, **579**, 259–264.

Schlicker, E., and Kathmann, M. (2001). Modulation of transmitter release via presynaptic cannabinoid receptors. *Trends Pharmacol Sci*, **22**, 565–572.

Shire, D., Carillon, C., Kaghad, M., et al. (1995). An amino-terminal variant of the central cannabinoid receptor resulting from alternative splicing. *J Biol Chem*, **270**, 3726–3731.

Stella, N. (2010). Cannabinoid and cannabinoid-like receptors in microglia, astrocytes, and astrocytomas. *Glia*, **58**, 1017–1030.

Straiker, A., Wager-Miller, J., Hutchens, J., et al. (2012). Differential signalling in human cannabinoid CB1 receptors and their splice variants in autaptic hippocampal neurones. *Br J Pharmacol*, **165**, 2660–2671.

Sundram, S., Copolov, D., and Dean, B. (2005). Clozapine decreases [3H] CP 55940 binding to the cannabinoid 1 receptor in the rat nucleus accumbens. *Naunyn Schmiedebergs Arch Pharmacol*, **371**, 428–433.

Tao, R., Li, C., Jaffe, A. E., et al. (2020). Cannabinoid receptor CNR1 expression and DNA methylation in human prefrontal cortex, hippocampus and caudate in brain development and schizophrenia. *Transl Psychiatry*, **10**, 158.

Thune, J. J., Uylings, H. B. M., and Pakkenberg, B. (2001). No deficit in total number of neurons in the prefrontal cortex in schizophrenics. *J Psychiatr Res*, **35**, 15–21.

Uriguen, L., Garcia-Fuster, M. J., Callado, L. F., et al. (2009). Immunodensity and mRNA expression of A2A adenosine, D2 dopamine, and CB1 cannabinoid receptors in postmortem frontal cortex of subjects with schizophrenia: Effect of antipsychotic treatment. *Psychopharmacology (Berl)*, **206**, 313–324.

Van Sickle, M. D., Duncan, M., Kingsley, P. J., et al. (2005). Identification and functional characterization of brainstem cannabinoid CB2 receptors. *Science*, **310**, 329–332.

Vogt, B. A., Pandya, D. N., and Rosene, D. L. (1987). Cingulate cortex of the rhesus monkey: I. Cytoarchitecture and thalamic afferents. *J Comp Neurol*, **262**, 256–270.

Volk, D. W., Eggan, S. M., Horti, A. G., et al. (2014). Reciprocal alterations in cortical cannabinoid receptor 1 binding relative to protein immunoreactivity and transcript levels in schizophrenia. *Schizophr Res*, **159**, 124–129.

Volk, D. W., Eggan, S. M., and Lewis, D. A. (2010). Alterations in metabotropic glutamate receptor 1α and regulator of G protein signaling 4 in the prefrontal cortex in schizophrenia. *Am J Psychiatry*, **167**, 1489–1498.

Volk, D. W., and Lewis, D. A. (2016). The role of endocannabinoid signaling in cortical inhibitory neuron dysfunction in schizophrenia. *Biol Psychiatry*, **79**, 595–603.

Volk, D. W., Siegel, B. I., Verrico, C. D., et al. (2013). Endocannabinoid metabolism in the prefrontal cortex in schizophrenia. *Schizophr Res*, **147**, 53–57.

Westlake, T. M., Howlett, A. C., Bonner, T. I., et al. (1994). Cannabinoid receptor binding and messenger RNA expression in human brain: An in vitro receptor autoradiography and in situ hybridization histochemistry study of normal aged and Alzheimer's brains. *Neuroscience*, **63**, 637–652.

Wiley, J. L., Kendler, S. H., Burston, J. J., et al. (2008). Antipsychotic-induced alterations in CB1 receptor-mediated G-protein signaling and in vivo pharmacology in rats. *Neuropharmacology*, **55**, 1183–1190.

Zavitsanou, K., Garrick, T., and Huang, X. F. (2004). Selective antagonist [3H]SR141716A binding to cannabinoid CB1 receptors is increased in the anterior cingulate cortex in schizophrenia. *Prog Neuropsychopharmacol Biol Psychiatry*, **28**, 355–360.

The Endocannabinoid System in Schizophrenia

Paul D. Morrison

It must be recognised that the brain is not a chemical factory . . .

In order to bring all the forthcoming biochemical observations into a meaningful framework it will prove necessary to emphasise more strongly aspects of neuro-circuits and connectivity and to do so both at the microscopic and macroscopic level . . .
(Carlsson, 2001, Nobel Lecture*)*

19.1 Introduction

Arvid Carlsson can be regarded as the originator of *wetware* hypotheses to explain major mental illness. This is the straightforward idea that an excess, or deficit, of a particular neurotransmitter or receptor is the core difference between the mentally ill and the healthy brain.

At the time when Carlsson first articulated the hypothesis, in regard to dopamine of course, neuropharmacology was focused on clarifying two main themes. First, the mechanics of neurotransmitter release. And, second, the actual *visualization* of receptors, which had hitherto only existed in the imagination of pharmacologists.

By the mid-1970s, both themes had been clarified, albeit at a fairly blurred level of resolution, with additional Nobel recognition (Katz and Miledi, 1970). But not even Carlsson could have anticipated how the molecular era, a decade or so later, would accelerate knowledge at such a bewildering rate. Having been able to construct a model synapse with two or three components at most, the pharmacologist was now required to accommodate hundreds of densely packed, precisely localized, inter-connected components; growth factors, scaffolding proteins, and cell death pathways, to name a few. Complexity accrued further with the realization that the individual pre- and post-synaptic components are not static, but are in flux, regarding shape, location, and

numbers, and that the majority of components, if not directly involved in synaptic transmission, function to adjust the sensitivity of individual synapses within the network, over various timescales.

In the quote above, Carlsson points back to an earlier, more fundamental neuroscience, the neuroscience of Ramón Y. Cajal, who concluded that neuro-circuits are electrical and plastic (DeFelipe, 2006). A wetware hypothesis tends to make a leap from the biochemical (an excess or deficit of a component) to the psychological, apparently oblivious to neurophysiology and electrical signalling. This represents a shortcut but, despite the gap, the biochemical observations have interest in their own right, perhaps not in terms of revealing a long-sought pathophysiology, but in the service of diagnostics or prognostics. Here we review the literature on alterations of endocannabinoid components in schizophrenia.

19.2 Endocannabinoid Components

Studies examining the endocannabinoid (eCB) system in schizophrenia have focused on two areas, endocannabinoid levels and CB1 receptor numbers. In both cases, deviations from normality have been observed (Ibarra-Lecue et al., 2018; Minichino et al., 2019; Sloan et al., 2019).

Specifically, there have been consistent reports of increased anandamide (AEA) concentrations in the cerebrospinal fluid (CSF) from schizophrenic patients (Minichino et al., 2019). Rather than being pathological, it has been postulated that raised AEA serves to limit psychosis and provide protection. There is some evidence to support a positive effect of excess anandamide on general wellbeing, but the data at present does not indicate that AEA limits positive psychotic symptoms. Furthermore, in one study which analysed brain tissue directly, schizophrenic patients actually had less AEA compared to matched controls (Muguruza et al., 2013).

In regard to CB1 receptors, findings have been inconsistent, according to the methods employed (Ibarra-Lecue et al., 2018; Sloan et al., 2019). Post-mortem studies using radiotracers have generally shown increased CB1 receptor availability in brain tissue from schizophrenic patients compared to controls. In stark contrast, and somewhat confusingly, CB1 protein and CB1 RNA levels have been typically reported as lower in schizophrenic patients compared to controls. In-vivo imaging of CB1 receptor availability in humans has emerged but, again, the picture is inconsistent. Two early in-vivo studies suggested that, compared to healthy controls, schizophrenic patients have increased central CB1 receptors, whereas two more recent, and perhaps methodologically superior studies, have reported decreased central CB1 receptors in the patient group (Sloan et al., 2019).

Overall, there is increasing evidence that, in biochemical terms, the endocannabinoid system is altered in schizophrenia, although the direction of change is inconsistent. Whether such changes are part of the pathology in schizophrenia, a compensatory response aimed at restoring health, or insignificant within a whole sea of molecular changes is unclear. And, of course, the effect of any particular change on electrical signalling in neuronal circuits and connectivity is unknown.

19.3 Endocannabinoid Concentrations in Schizophrenia

Studies to date have focused mainly on anandamide (AEA). Very few studies have reported 2-arachidonoylglycerol (2AG) levels. This is a limitation for the field, as 2-AG is believed to be the retrograde signal, mediating plastic adaptations at glutamate and GABA synapses in the CNS and altering neuronal network dynamics. One study in post-mortem brain tissue reported increased 2-AG levels from schizophrenic patients versus healthy controls (Muguruza et al., 2013).

Several studies have reported increased AEA concentrations in blood samples from schizophrenic patients (De Marchi et al., 2003). These findings carry the drawback that AEA is synthesized in peripheral tissues, as well as centrally, making identification of the source of excess AEA impossible. Indeed, CNS and blood-derived concentrations are thought to be unrelated. Increased blood concentrations are not thought to be a consequence of overflow from the CNS (Hillard, 2018). To circumvent this problem, some studies have used cerebrospinal fluid (CSF) sampling. Generally, elevated AEA concentrations in schizophrenia have been observed (Table 19.1).

Giuffrida et al. (2004) measured CSF anandamide levels in a sample of first-episode, antipsychotic naive schizophrenic patients (n = 47), medicated schizophrenic patients (34 typical, 37 atypical), patients suffering from an affective disorder (n = 22), or dementia (n = 13), and healthy controls (n = 84). The major finding was that AEA levels were approximately eight times higher in the CSF of schizophrenics compared to healthy controls. In contrast, AEA levels were not elevated in affective disorders or in dementia. AEA levels appeared to 'normalize' in the group of schizophrenic patients who were prescribed typical D2 blocking drugs (haloperidol, phenothiazenes) but remained elevated in those treated with atypical antipsychotics (risperidone, olanzapine, quetiapine, clozapine). That said, the typical versus atypical distinction is now regarded as having no basis in receptor or clinical pharmacology, so the latter finding carries uncertain weight (Morrison et al., 2019).

Stemming from previous animal work suggesting that AEA serves as a negative feedback signal on dopaminergic drive, it was hypothesized that, in schizophrenic patients, AEA levels would show an inverse relationship with psychosis as rated by the PANSS scale (Giuffrida et al., 2004). Overall, following the removal of three outliers, AEA levels were inversely related to cumulative PANSS scores (r = −0.4), negative symptom scores (r = −0.3), and general symptom scores (r = −0.4), but showed *no* relationship with ratings of positive psychotic symptoms. So, although elevations in CSF AEA appeared to be beneficial for patients, most significantly on the general PANSS scale, the findings did not support negative-feedback inhibition of dopamine-driven positive psychotic symptoms.

Two additional studies have been in general agreement. Leweke et al. (2007) found that CSF AEA concentrations in schizophrenic patients were inversely related to negative, but not positive symptom scores, while Potvin et al. (2020) reported that AEA concentrations (*albeit blood-derived*) were inversely related to depressive, but not positive symptoms scores.

Koethe et al. (2009) compared CSF AEA levels between prodromal patients (n = 27) and healthy controls (n = 81). AEA concentrations were found to be approximately six times greater in the

Table 19.1 Anandamide levels in schizophrenia

Measure	Sample Population	Main Findings	Reference
CSF Anandamide (AEA)	Schizophrenic patients (10) vs healthy controls (11) Comorbid substance use excluded.	↑AEA in schizophrenic patients.	Leweke et al. (1999)
Blood-derived AEA	Schizophrenic patients (12) vs healthy controls (20).	↑AEA in schizophrenic patients, which decreased after clinical remission.	De Marchi et al. (2003)
CSF AEA	First episode psychosis (AP naïve 47, typical AP 34, atypical AP 37) vs affective disorder (22) vs dementia (13) vs healthy controls (84). Urine drug screen +ve excluded.	↑ AEA in AP naïve psychotic patients and those treated with atypical APs. No relationship between AEA levels and positive psychotic symptoms. An inverse correlation between AEA levels and general and negative symptom scores.	Giuffrida et al. (2004)
CSF AEA and Blood-derived AEA	First episode psychosis (AP naïve 47) vs healthy controls (81). Both groups sub-divided into high and low frequency cannabis users. Urine drug screen +ve excluded.	↑ AEA in CSF of low frequency cannabis using patients versus the other three groups. An inverse correlation between AEA levels in low frequency cannabis using patients and negative symptom scores. No differences in blood AEA between the four groups.	Leweke et al. (2007)
Blood-derived AEA	Co-morbid substance abuse disorder + schizophrenia patients (29) vs healthy controls (17).	↑ AEA in CSF of co-morbid patients compared to healthy controls.	Potvin et al. (2008)
CSF AEA Blood-derived AEA	Prodromal patients (27) vs healthy controls (81). Urine drug screen +ve excluded.	↑ AEA in CSF of prodromal patients. Trend for lower transition to psychosis in prodromal patients with higher AEA. No differences in blood AEA between groups.	Koethe et al. (2009)
Blood-derived AEA	Substance abuse disorder (38) vs Schizophrenic patients (25) vs healthy controls (27).	↓ AEA in blood of substance abuse disorder compared to healthy controls. No differences in blood AEA between schizophrenic patients and healthy controls.	Desfossés et al. (2012)
Brain tissue AEA and 2-AG	Schizophrenic patients (19) vs matched controls (19).	↑2-AG in the prefrontal cortex, hippocampus, and cerebellum from schizophrenic patients. ↓ AEA in the prefrontal cortex, hippocampus, and cerebellum from schizophrenic patients.	Muguruza et al. (2013)
Blood-derived AEA	Twin pairs discordant for schizophrenia (25) vs discordant for bipolar (6) vs healthy twin pairs.	↑ AEA in both patient groups compared to healthy controls. No differences in blood AEA between schizophrenic patients and their non-affected co-twin. A higher risk of subsequent transition to illness in co-twin with ↓ AEA.	Koethe et al. (2019)

Table 19.1 (cont.)

Measure	Sample Population	Main Findings	Reference
Blood-derived AEA	Schizophrenic patients (115) vs healthy controls (109).	↑AEA in schizophrenic patients, which decreased after treatment.	Wang et al. (2018)
Blood-derived AEA in an emergency setting	Schizophrenia spectrum patients(107) vs healthy controls (36).	↑ AEA in patients in the emergency setting, which decreased after stabilization. No relationship between AEA levels and positive psychotic symptoms. An inverse correlation between AEA levels and depression scores.	Potvin et al. (2020)
mRNA for endocannabinoid synthesizing and metabolizing enzymes	Tissue from schizophrenic patients (14) vs matched controls (14).	No differences between the dorsolateral prefrontal cortex from schizophrenic patients and healthy controls in mRNA levels for endocannabinoid synthesizing and metabolizing enzymes.	Volk et al. (2010)

prodromal group. In a subsequent step, the prodromal group were split at the median into high versus low AEA groups. The relative risk of transition into frank psychosis was smaller in the high AEA group (0.33, 95% CI = 0.09–1.29), although only at a trend level ($p = 0.09$). The authors suggested that AEA mobilization may play a protective role in at least a sub-group of patients with early stage schizophrenia. In an elegant, subsequent study, Koethe et al. (2019) recruited twins, one of whom suffered from schizophrenia. Initially unaffected co-twins who went on to develop schizophrenia had lower AEA levels (*albeit blood-derived*) compared to co-twins who remained well.

Several studies have indicated that blood-derived AEA levels are elevated in schizophrenic patients during acute episodes and return to normal following treatment (De Marchi et al., 2003; Potvin et al., 2020; Wang et al., 2018). However, increased circulating AEA has also been associated with a number of pathophysiological conditions (stress, inflammation, obesity) and physiological states (following food presentation and exercise) (Hillard, 2018). As such, increased blood-derived AEA concentrations cannot be regarded as a specific biomarker for psychosis or for schizophrenia.

Direct brain tissue measurement of AEA and 2-AG from schizophrenic patients (n = 19) and matched controls (n = 19) was carried out by Muguruza et al. (2013). In stark contrast to the studies already mentioned, AEA levels were decreased in the prefrontal cortex, hippocampus, and cerebellum of patients. Levels of 2-AG, on the other hand, were higher in the patient group, in the same brain regions.

Several studies have measured the enzymes which synthesize and metabolize the two main endocannabinoids; N-acyl phosphatidylethanolamine phospholipase (NAPE) and diacylglycerol lipase (DGL), for the synthesis of AEA and 2-AG, respectively, and fatty acid amide hydrolase (FAAH) and monoacylglycerol lipase (MGL) for their respective metabolism. Changes in schizophrenic patients versus controls have been reported in some, but not all studies using peripheral immune cells (Ibarra-Lecue et al., 2018), which in any case have major limitations, being remote from CNS tissue. One study measured prefrontal cortex-derived DGL, MGL, and FAAH levels from schizophrenic patients (n = 14) versus matched controls (n = 14), and found no differences (Volk et al., 2010).

Overall, the most consistent finding is of increased AEA in the CSF and blood-derived samples of schizophrenic patients. But it appears to be the case that increased AEA represents a protective response to stress in general, rather than having a specific relationship with psychotic illness. Given the multitude of possible confounds and also the extent of the crossover between data from healthy controls and patient groups, it is highly unlikely that AEA measurements will turn out to have diagnostic or prognostic utility for the individual psychiatric patient.

Table 19.2 CB1 receptor numbers in schizophrenia: Post-mortem findings

Measure	Sample Population	Main Findings	Reference
CB1 density	Tissue from schizophrenic patients (14) vs controls (14)	↑ CB1 in the dorsolateral prefrontal cortex (BA9) of schizophrenic patients	Dean et al. (2001)
CB1 density	Tissue from schizophrenic patients (10) vs controls (9)	↑ CB1 in the L-anterior cingulate cortex of schizophrenic patients	Zavitsanou et al. (2004)
CB1 density	Tissue from schizophrenic patients (8) vs controls (8)	↑ CB1 in the posterior cingulate cortex of schizophrenic patients	Newell et al. (2006)
CB1 density & CB1 mRNA	Tissue from schizophrenic patients (37) vs controls (37)	↑ CB1 density in the dorsolateral prefrontal cortex (BA46) of schizophrenic patients No differences in CB_1 mRNA	Dalton et al. (2011)
CB1 density	Tissue from schizophrenic patients (47) vs controls (43)	↑ CB1 in the dorsolateral prefrontal cortex (BA9,46) of schizophrenic patients	Jenko et al. (2012)
CB1 density	Tissue from schizophrenic patients (8) vs controls (8)	No differences in CB1 in the superior temporal gyrus	Deng et al. (2007)
CB1 protein	Tissue from schizophrenic patients (15) vs bipolar patients (15) vs controls (15)	No differences in CB1 in the anterior cortex from schizophrenic patients, bipolar patients, and controls	Koethe et al. (2007)
CB1 mRNA & CB1 protein	Tissue from schizophrenic patients (23) vs controls (23)	↓ CB1 protein & ↓ CB1 mRNA in the dorsolateral prefrontal cortex (BA9) of schizophrenic patients	Eggan et al. (2008)
CB1 protein	Tissue from schizophrenic patients (26) vs major depressives (26) vs controls (26)	↓ CB1 protein in the dorsolateral prefrontal cortex (BA46) of schizophrenic patients compared to major depressives and controls	Eggan et al. (2010)
CB1 mRNA & CB1 protein	Tissue from schizophrenic patients (25) vs controls (25)	↓ CB1 protein in the dorsolateral prefrontal cortex of anti-psychotic treated, but not anti-psychotic free schizophrenic patients. No differences in CB1 mRNA	Urigüen et al. (2009)

19.4 CB1 Receptors in Schizophrenia: Post-mortem Findings

Five of six post-mortem studies using radiotracers have reported an increase in central CB1 receptor density in schizophrenic patients compared to matched controls. In contrast, and somewhat perplexingly, three of four studies using immunological methods to measure CB1 receptor protein have, in general, found changes in the opposite direction (Table 19.2).

19.5 Quantitative Autoradiography

Dean et al. (2001) found a 23% increased binding of the CB1 radiotracer [³H]CP-55940 in the dorsolateral prefrontal cortex (DLPFC) from schizophrenic patients (n = 14) compared to matched controls (n = 14). In a larger sample (2 matched groups of 37), using the same radiotracer, Dalton et al. (2011) obtained a similar result (22% increased binding) in the DLPFC from schizophrenic patients. Again in agreement, Jenko et al. (2012) found 20% increased binding of the CB1 radiotracer [3H]MePPEP in the DLPFC from schizophrenic patients (n = 47) versus controls (n = 43).

Zavitsanou et al. (2004) found a 64% increased binding of the CB1 radiotracer [³H]SR141716A in the left anterior cingulate cortex (ACC) from patients with schizophrenia (n = 10) compared to controls (n = 9). Newell et al. (2006) reported a 25% increased binding of [³H]CP-55940 in the posterior cingulate cortex (PCC) from schizophrenic patients (n = 8) versus controls (n = 8).

One radiotracer study was negative. Deng et al. (2007) found no differences in the binding of [^{3}H]SR141716A or [^{3}H]CP-55940 in the superior temporal gyrus from schizophrenic patients (n = 8) versus controls (n = 8).

19.6 Quantification of CB1 Protein

Using in-situ hybridization and immunochemistry, the Pittsburgh group of Lewis and colleagues measured CB1 mRNA and CB1 protein in the DLPFC from schizophrenic subjects versus controls (n = 23 in each group). In contrast to the findings above, CB1 mRNA and CB$_1$ protein levels were decreased in DLPFC tissue from schizophrenic patients by 15% and 10–14%, respectively. The authors proposed that CB1 down-regulation constitutes a compensatory mechanism in schizophrenia aimed at restoring 'normal' network dynamics (Eggan et al., 2008).

In a subsequent study, the Pittsburgh group found that CB1 protein levels were decreased by 20–23% in DLPFC tissue from schizophrenic patients versus controls and patients with major depression (n = 26 in each group) (Eggan et al., 2010).

Urigüen et al. (2009) measured CB1 mRNA and protein in the DLPFC from schizophrenic patients (n = 31) and controls (n = 46). Anti-psychotic status was established by toxicological screening at post-mortem. The major finding was that CB1 protein was significantly decreased in anti-psychotic-treated schizophrenic patients, but not in drug-free subjects. No differences in mRNA amounts encoding for CB1 receptors were found. The authors suggested that anti-psychotics induce down-regulation of CB1 receptors in the brain (Urigüen et al., 2009).

One study using immunological methods was negative. Koethe et al. (2007) quantified CB1 receptors in the ACC using immunochemistry. *No differences* in CB1 density were found in tissue from schizophrenic patients, bipolar patients, and controls (n = 15 in all groups).

19.7 CB1 Receptors in Schizophrenia: In-Vivo Findings

Four studies have used positron emission tomography (PET) neuroimaging to measure the availability of the CB1 receptor in schizophrenic patients versus healthy controls (see Table 19.3). There is no CNS region devoid of CB1 receptors, which precludes the use of the relatively straightforward reference method, forcing researchers to use other methods which are less clear and incorporate non-specific binding, although good test–re-test validity has brought some reassurance (Sloan et al., 2019). Two studies have reported an increased availability of brain CB1 receptors in schizophrenic patients compared to controls, while two have reported decreases.

Table 19.3 CB1 receptor numbers in schizophrenia: In-vivo findings

Measure	Sample Population	Main Findings	Reference
Binding of [^{11}C]OMAR	Schizophrenic patients (9) vs healthy controls (10)	↑CB1 availability in the pons.	Wong et al. (2010)
Binding of [^{18}F]MK-9470	Antipsychotic-treated schizophrenic patients (51) and antipsychotic-free schizophrenic patients (16) vs healthy controls (12)	↑CB1 availability in treated and untreated schizophrenic patients compared to controls in the parietal, inf. frontal, insular, and cingulate cortices, medial temporal lobe, and ventral striatum.	Ceccarini et al. (2013)
Binding of [^{11}C]OMAR	Antipsychotic-treated schizophrenic patients (18) and antipsychotic-free schizophrenic patients (7) vs healthy controls (18)	↓CB1 availability in schizophrenic patients compared to controls in the insular and cingulate cortices, medial temporal lobe, caudate nucleus, and hypothalamus.	Ranganathan et al. (2016)
Binding of [^{18}F]FMPEP-d$_2$ and [^{11}C]MePPEP	Study 1: First episode psychosis patients (7) vs healthy controls (11) First episode psychosis patients (20) vs healthy controls (20)	↓CB1 availability in first episode psychosis patients compared to controls in the anterior cingulate cortex, hippocampus, striatum, and thalamus.	Borgan et al. (2019)

Wong et al. (2010) used the CB1 radiotracer [^{11}C]OMAR to estimate CB1 receptor availability in a sample of antipsychotic treated schizophrenic patients (n = 9) versus healthy controls (n = 10). They reported increased binding in schizophrenic patients across all brain regions studied, although the increase was only significant in the pons. The schizophrenic group was, on average, almost nine years older than the control group, raising the possibility that group differences stemmed from age rather than psychotic illness.

Ceccarini et al. (2013) investigated schizophrenic patients and controls who were matched for age; a proportion of the patients (16 of 67) were antipsychotic free. In agreement with the study by Wong et al. (2010), Ceccarini et al. (2013) found increased binding of the CB1 receptor ligand [^{18}F]MK-9470 in schizophrenic patients across all brain regions studied, which reached significance in the cerebral cortex, medial temporal lobe, and ventral striatum.

Ranganathan et al. (2016) used the same radiotracer as Wong et al. (2010), [^{11}C]OMAR, in a sample of schizophrenic patients (25) and healthy controls (18). In contrast to the previous PET studies, they reported decreased CB1 receptor availability in the insula and cingulate cortices, the medial temporal lobe, caudate nucleus, and hypothalamus (Ranganathan et al., 2016).

The most recent report combined a study from Turku (in 7 psychotic patients versus 11 healthy controls) and a study from London (in 20 psychotic patients versus 20 healthy controls) using the CB1 radiotracers [^{18}F]FMPEP-d$_2$ and [^{11}C]MePPEP, respectively. In general agreement with the findings of Ranganathan et al. (2016), Borgan et al. (2019) found decreased CB1 receptor availability in the anterior cingulate, hippocampus, striatum, and thalamus.

19.8 CB1 Receptors in Schizophrenia: Summary

It is unclear from post-mortem studies and from in-vivo PET imaging how CB1 receptor numbers are altered in schizophrenia. Studies using post-mortem schizophrenic brain tissue have consistently shown increased CB1 receptor density. But the measurement of CB1 protein using immunological methods shows consistent changes in the opposite direction, which is very puzzling. Findings from in-vivo PET imaging has been inconsistent, with individual studies reporting changes in both directions.

Some authors have attempted to resolve the inconsistency, pointing to possible confounding variables, such as antipsychotic treatment, tobacco use, and cannabis use (Mihov, 2016). Three out of three PET studies comparing cannabis users to controls have shown a decrease of central CB1 receptors in cannabis users, in keeping with down-regulation of the receptor from agonist exposure (Ceccarini et al., 2015; D'Souza et al., 2016; Hirvonen et al., 2012). At present, this is the most consistent finding across the field (Sloan et al., 2019).

Changes in CB1 receptor numbers have also been reported in other psychiatric syndromes, including alcohol dependence, PTSD, major depression, and anorexia nervosa, using post-mortem studies (CB1 density, protein, and mRNA) and in-vivo PET studies (CB1 availability) (Ibarra-Lecue et al., 2018; Sloan et al., 2019). PET studies have tended to show an upregulation of CB1 receptors in PTSD (Sloan et al., 2019).

Overall, it remains uncertain if CB1 receptors are increased or decreased in the brain of schizophrenic patients. Given the multitude of possible confounds and also the extent of the crossover between data from healthy controls and patient groups, it is highly unlikely that CB1 receptor measurements will turn out to have diagnostic or prognostic utility for the individual psychiatric patient.

19.9 Neuronal Circuits and Connectivity

In the quote which began this chapter, Carlsson points the wetware enthusiast towards neurophysiology, emphasizing that an excess or deficit in a particular transmitter or receptor must be understood in the context of neuronal circuits. The necessary insight is that a direct leap from the wetware to the psychological realm, grabbing at metaphor for support, will not suffice as a complete pathophysiological explanation for mental illness. This applies to all wetware hypotheses, aside from those hormonal disorders in which the difference between patients and controls is vast, with no overlap at all, by definition. Clearly, the quantification of a single component (whether an endocannabinoid or other) within a sea of changes cannot yield adequate detail into the pathological structure of mental illness.

The classic 'wetware' molecules, such as serotonin and dopamine, and new arrivals such as the endocannabinoids, may or may not represent 'the wind of psychotic fire', 'aberrant salience', or 'the final common pathway', but they certainly signal to synaptic components which modulate network dynamics in higher centres. It is beyond argument that dopamine, serotonin, and the endocannabinoids all regulate the strength of individual connections within neuronal networks, a conclusion based on neurophysiology (Bailey et al., 2000; Chevaleyre et al., 2006; Lisman, 2017) and not metaphor.

Neurons are electrical components. And it is the rich connectivity between neurons that supports the most basic sensory and motor functions as well as the higher faculties; a connectivity that supports coherence, in which neurons involved in processing the same object fire in synchrony, within the millisecond range (Buzsáki and Draguhn, 2004; Engel and Singer, 2001), and a connectivity which is plastic, sculpted by the environment, according to learning rules predicted by Ramón Y. Cajal, then Hebb, and demonstrated by Bliss, Collingridge, Kandel, and others (Collingridge and Bliss, 1995; Kandel, 1998).

In the context of endocannabinoid signalling, the major advances have come, not from measuring levels of a single component such as AEA or CB1 receptors but from electrophysiological studies, at the microscopic scale (Chevaleyre et al., 2006; Katona and Freund, 2012). The function of 2-AG in long-term depression and spike-timing dependent plasticity at glutamate and GABA synapses within neuronal networks arose, not from neurochemical assays, but from intracellular recording and patch clamping (Kreitzer and Malenka, 2007; Shen et al., 2008; Wilson and Nicoll, 2001; Xu et al., 2018).

19.10 CB1 Agonists, Schizophrenia, and Disrupted Theta and Gamma Oscillations

The fine-grained dynamics of endocannabinoid signalling are disrupted in animals by exogenous CB1 agonists, such as delta-9-tetrahydrocannabinol (THC), impacting upon synchronized neuronal firing and network rhythms in the theta (4–8 Hz) and gamma band (30–80 Hz), manifesting as working memory impairments (Kucewicz et al., 2011; Robbe and Buzsáki, 2009; Robbe et al., 2006).

Similarly, in humans, exogenous CB1 agonists, such as THC, can elicit working memory impairments, a paranoid psychosis, and abnormal network rhythms in the theta and gamma band (Cortes-Briones et al., 2015; D'Souza et al., 2004; Morrison et al., 2011; Nottage et al., 2015; Stone et al., 2012).

Finally, disruption of network rhythms, particularly in the theta and gamma band, has been proposed as a fundamental feature of schizophrenic psychosis (Lewis et al., 2005; Pittman-Polletta et al., 2015; Uhlhaas and Singer, 2015) and, of course, working memory deficits are well recognized.

19.11 Conclusion

At present, the quantification of AEA or CB1 receptors adds nothing to our knowledge of the pathophysiology of mental illness. Inconsistency dominates the field. There is also no indication that the quantification of an isolated endocannabinoid component (or any neurochemical component for that matter) informs diagnostics, prognostics, or therapeutics for the individual psychiatric patient. Nothing on the horizon promises the emergence of an endocannabinoid or any other neurochemical biomarker with acceptable sensitivity and specificity. Larger samples will be proposed no doubt, but there is too much crossover between groups and too many confounds, in short – too much noise, even for the much-heralded machine-learning approaches. Finally, the need for meta-analysis to demonstrate consistent change in a particular component reveals that such change is unlikely to be of much relevance for the individual patient.

Somewhat ironically, Carlsson, the most decorated wetware hypothesist, directs students of mental illness away from the wetware to neuronal circuits. Carlsson was typically some years ahead of the field, but it may take some time before his advice is adhered to, given the beguiling simplicity of wetware hypotheses .

References

Bailey, C. H., Giustetto, M., Huang, Y. Y., et al. (2000). Is heterosynaptic modulation essential for stabilizing Hebbian plasticity and memory? *Nat Rev Neurosci*, **1**, 11–20.

Borgan, F., Laurikainen, H., Veronese, M., et al. (2019). In vivo availability of cannabinoid 1 receptor levels in patients with first-episode psychosis. *JAMA Psychiatry*, **76**, 1074–1084.

Buzsáki, G., and Draguhn, A. (2004). Neuronal oscillations in cortical Networks. *Science*, **304**, 1926–1929.

Carlsson, A. (2001). A half-century of neurotransmitter research: Impact on neurology and psychiatry.

Nobel lecture. *Biosci Rep*, **21**, 691–710.

Ceccarini, J., De Hert, M., Van Winkel, R., et al. (2013). Increased ventral striatal CB1 receptor binding is related to negative symptoms in drug-free patients with schizophrenia. *Neuroimage*, **79**, 304–312.

Ceccarini, J., Kuepper, R., Kemels, D., et al. (2015). [18F]MK-9470 PET measurement of cannabinoid CB1 receptor availability in chronic cannabis users. *Addict Biol*, **20**, 357–367.

Chevaleyre, V., Takahashi, K. A., and Castillo, P. E. (2006). Endocannabinoid-mediated synaptic plasticity in the CNS. *Annu Rev Neurosci*, **29**, 37–76.

Collingridge, G. L., and Bliss, T. V. P. (1995). Memories of NMDA receptors and LTP. *Trends Neurosci*, **18**, 54–56.

Cortes-Briones, J., Skosnik, P. D., Mathalon, D., et al. (2015). Δ9-THC disrupts gamma (γ)-band neural oscillations in humans. *Neuropsychopharmacology*, **40**, 2124–2134.

D'Souza, D. C., Cortes-Briones, J. A., Ranganathan, M., et al. (2016). Rapid changes in CB1 receptor availability in cannabis dependent males after abstinence from cannabis. *Biol Psychiatry Cogn Neurosci Neuroimaging*, **1**, 60–67.

D'Souza, D. C., Perry, E., MacDougall, L., et al. (2004). The psychotomimetic effects of intravenous delta-9-tetrahydrocannabinol in healthy individuals: Implications for psychosis. *Neuropsychopharmacology*, **29**, 1558–1572.

Dalton, V. S., Long, L. E., Weickert, C. S., et al. (2011). Paranoid schizophrenia is characterized by increased CB1 receptor binding in the dorsolateral prefrontal cortex. *Neuropsychopharmacology*, **36**, 1620–1630.

De Marchi, N., De Petrocellis, L., Orlando, P., et al. (2003). Endocannabinoid signalling in the blood of patients with schizophrenia. *Lipids Health Dis*, **2**, 5.

Dean, B., Sundram, S., Bradbury, R., et al. (2001). Studies on [3H]CP-55940 binding in the human central nervous system: regional specific changes in density of cannabinoid-1 receptors associated with schizophrenia and cannabis use. *Neuroscience*, **103**, 9–15.

DeFelipe, J. (2006). Brain plasticity and mental processes: Cajal again. *Nat Rev Neurosci*, **7**, 811–817.

Deng, C., Han, M., and Huang, X.-F. (2007). No changes in densities of cannabinoid receptors in the superior temporal gyrus in schizophrenia. *Neurosci Bull*, **23**, 341–347.

Desfossés, J., Stip, E., Bentaleb, L. A., et al. (2012). Plasma endocannabinoid alterations in individuals with substance use disorder are dependent on the 'mirror effect' of schizophrenia. *Front Psychiatry*, **3**, 85.

Eggan, S. M., Hashimoto, T., and Lewis, D. A. (2008). Reduced cortical cannabinoid 1 receptor messenger RNA and protein expression in schizophrenia. *Arch Gen Psychiatry*, **65**, 772–784.

Eggan, S. M., Stoyak, S. R., Verrico, C. D., et al. (2010). Cannabinoid CB1 receptor immunoreactivity in the prefrontal cortex: Comparison of schizophrenia and major depressive disorder. *Neuropsychopharmacology*, **35**, 2060–2071.

Engel, A. K., and Singer, W. (2001). Temporal binding and the neural correlates of sensory awareness. *Trends Cogn Sci*, **5**, 16–25.

Giuffrida, A., Leweke, F. M., Gerth, C. W., et al. (2004). Cerebrospinal anandamide levels are elevated in acute schizophrenia and are inversely correlated with psychotic symptoms. *Neuropsychopharmacology*, **29**, 2108–2114.

Hillard, C. J. (2018). Circulating endocannabinoids: From whence do they come and where are they going? *Neuropsychopharmacology*, **43**, 155–172.

Hirvonen, J., Goodwin, R. S., Li, C.-T., et al. (2012). Reversible and regionally selective downregulation of brain cannabinoid CB1 receptors in chronic daily cannabis smokers. *Mol Psychiatry*, **17**, 642–649.

Ibarra-Lecue, I., Pilar-Cuéllar, F., Mugaruza, C., et al. (2018). The endocannabinoid system in mental disorders: Evidence from human brain studies. *Biochem Pharmacol*, **157**, 97–107.

Jenko, K. J., Hirvonen, J., Henter, I. D., et al. (2012). Binding of a tritiated inverse agonist to cannabinoid CB1 receptors is increased in patients with schizophrenia. *Schizophr Res*, **141**, 185–188.

Kandel, E. R. (1998). A new intellectual framework for psychiatry. *Am J Psychiatry*, **155**, 457–469.

Katona, I., and Freund, T. F. (2012). Multiple functions of endocannabinoid signaling in the brain. *Annu Rev Neurosci*, **35**, 529–558.

Katz, B., and Miledi, R. (1970). Membrane noise produced by acetylcholine. *Nature*, **226**, 962–963.

Koethe, D., Giuffrida, A., Schreiber, D., et al. (2009). Anandamide elevation in cerebrospinal fluid in initial prodromal states of psychosis. *Br J Psychiatry*, **194**, 371–372.

Koethe, D., Llenos, I. C., Dulay, J. R., et al. (2007). Expression of CB1 cannabinoid receptor in the anterior cingulate cortex in schizophrenia, bipolar disorder, and major depression. *J Neural Transm (Vienna)*, **114**, 1055–1063.

Koethe, D., Pahlisch, F., Hellmich, M., et al. (2019). Familial abnormalities of endocannabinoid signaling in schizophrenia. *World J Biol Psychiatry*, **20**, 117–125.

Kreitzer, A. C., and Malenka, R. C. (2007). Endocannabinoid-mediated rescue of striatal LTD and motor deficits in Parkinson's disease models. *Nature*, **445**, 643–647.

Kucewicz, M. T., Tricklebank, M. D., Bogacz, R., et al. (2011). Dysfunctional prefrontal cortical network activity and interactions following cannabinoid receptor activation. *J Neurosci*, **31**, 15560–15568.

Leweke, F. M., Giuffrida, A., Koethe, D., et al. (2007). Anandamide levels in cerebrospinal fluid of first-episode schizophrenic patients: Impact of cannabis use. *Schizophr Res*, **94**, 29–36.

Leweke, F. M., Giuffrida, A., Wurster, U., et al. (1999). Elevated endogenous cannabinoids in schizophrenia. *NeuroReport*, **10**, 1665–1669.

Lewis, D. A., Hashimoto, T., and Volk, D. W. (2005). Cortical inhibitory neurons and schizophrenia. *Nat Rev Neurosci*, **6**, 312–324.

Lisman, J. (2017). Glutamatergic synapses are structurally and biochemically complex because of multiple plasticity processes: Long-term potentiation, long-term depression, short-term potentiation and scaling. *Phil Trans R Soc Lond B Biol Sci*, **372**, 20160260.

Mihov, Y. (2016). Positron emission tomography studies on cannabinoid receptor type 1 in schizophrenia. *Biol Psychiatry*, **79**, e97–e99.

Minichino, A., Senior, M., Brondino, N., et al. (2019). Measuring disturbance of the endocannabinoid system in psychosis: A systematic review and meta-analysis. *JAMA Psychiatry*, **76**, 914–923.

Morrison, P. D., Nottage, J., Stone, J. M., et al. (2011). Disruption of frontal θ coherence by Δ9-tetrahydrocannabinol is associated with positive psychotic symptoms. *Neuropsychopharmacology*, **36**, 827–836.

Morrison, P. D., Taylor, D., and McGuire, P. (2019). *The Maudsley Guidelines on Advanced Prescribing in Psychosis*. Hoboken, NJ: Wiley.

Muguruza, C., Lehtonen, M., Aaltonen, N., et al. (2013). Quantification of endocannabinoids in postmortem brain of schizophrenic subjects. *Schizophr Res*, **148**, 145–150.

Newell, K. A., Deng, C., and Huang, X.-F. (2006). Increased cannabinoid receptor density in the posterior cingulate cortex in schizophrenia. *Exp Brain Res*, **172**, 556–560.

Nottage, J. F., Stone, J., Murray, R. M., et al. (2015). Delta-9-tetrahydrocannabinol, neural oscillations above 20 Hz and induced acute psychosis. *Psychopharmacology (Berl)*, **232**, 519–528.

Pittman-Polletta, B. R., Kocsis, B., Vijayan, S., et al. (2015). Brain rhythms connect impaired inhibition to altered cognition in schizophrenia. *Biol Psychiatry*, **77**, 1020–1030.

Potvin, S., Kouassi, E., Lipp, O., et al. (2008). Endogenous cannabinoids in patients with schizophrenia and substance use disorder during quetiapine therapy. *J Psychopharmacol*, **22**, 262–269.

Potvin, S., Mahrouche, L., Assaf, R., et al. (2020). Peripheral endogenous cannabinoid levels are increased in schizophrenia patients evaluated in a psychiatric emergency setting. *Front Psychiatry*, **11**, 628.

Ranganathan, M., Cortes-Briones, J., Radhakrishnan, R., et al. (2016). Reduced brain cannabinoid receptor availability in schizophrenia. *Biol Psychiatry*, **79**, 997–1005.

Robbe, D., and Buzsáki, G. (2009). Alteration of theta timescale dynamics of hippocampal place cells by a cannabinoid is associated with memory impairment. *J Neurosci*, **29**, 12597–12605.

Robbe, D., Montgomery, S. M., Thome, A., et al. (2006). Cannabinoids reveal importance of spike timing coordination in hippocampal function. *Nat Neurosci*, **9**, 1526–1533.

Shen, W., Flajolet, M., Greengard, P., et al. (2008). Dichotomous dopaminergic control of striatal synaptic plasticity. *Science*, **321**, 848–851.

Sloan, M. E., Grant, C. W., Gowin, J. L., et al. (2019). Endocannabinoid signaling in psychiatric disorders: A review of positron emission tomography studies. *Acta Pharmacol Sin*, **40**, 342–350.

Stone, J. M., Morrison, P. D., Brugger, S., et al. (2012). Communication breakdown: Delta-9 tetrahydrocannabinol effects on pre-speech neural coherence. *Mol Psychiatry*, **17**, 568–569.

Uhlhaas, P. J., and Singer, W. (2015). Oscillations and neuronal dynamics in schizophrenia: The search for basic symptoms and translational opportunities. *Biol Psychiatry*, **77**, 1001–1009.

Urigüen, L., García-Fuster, M. J., Callado, L. F., et al. (2009). Immunodensity and mRNA expression of A2A adenosine, D2 dopamine, and CB1 cannabinoid receptors in postmortem frontal cortex of subjects with schizophrenia: Effect of antipsychotic treatment. *Psychopharmacology (Berl)*, **206**, 313–324.

Volk, D. W., Eggan, S. M., and Lewis, D. A. (2010). Alterations in metabotropic glutamate receptor 1α and regulator of G protein signaling 4 in the prefrontal cortex in schizophrenia. *Am J Psychiatry*, **167**, 1489–1498.

Wang, D., Sun, X., Yan, J., et al. (2018). Alterations of eicosanoids and related mediators in patients with schizophrenia. *J Psychiatr Res*, **102**, 168–178.

Wilson, R. I., and Nicoll, R. A. (2001). Endogenous cannabinoids mediate retrograde signalling at hippocampal synapses. *Nature*, **410**, 588–592.

Wong, D. F., Kuwabara, H., Horti, A. G., et al. (2010). Quantification of cerebral cannabinoid receptors subtype 1 (CB1) in healthy subjects and schizophrenia by the novel PET radioligand [11C]OMAR. *Neuroimage*, **52**, 1505–1513.

Xu, H., Perez, S., Cornil, A., et al. (2018). Dopamine-endocannabinoid interactions mediate spike-timing-dependent

potentiation in the striatum. *Nat Commun*, **9**, 4118.

Zavitsanou, K., Garrick, T., and Huang, X. F. (2004). Selective antagonist [3H]SR141716A binding to cannabinoid CB1 receptors is increased in the anterior cingulate cortex in schizophrenia. *Prog Neuropsychopharmacol Biol Psychiatry*, **28**, 355–360.

Cannabidiol as a Potential Antipsychotic

20

F. Markus Leweke and Cathrin Rohleder

20.1 Introduction

Schizophrenia spectrum disorders are complex disorders with a heterogenous combination of symptoms such as perceptual alterations, delusional perception, hallucinations, disorganized speech and disorders of thought as well as delusions ('positive symptoms'), grossly disorganized or abnormal motor behaviour (including catatonia), 'negative symptoms' such as diminished emotional expression, alogia, avolition, social dysfunction, as well as affecting cognitive impairments (e.g., sensory information processing, attention, working memory, and executive functions) (DSM-V, American Psychiatric Association, 2013; Wong and Van Tol, 2003).

A recent systematic review and meta-analysis reported that the median point and median lifetime prevalence of psychotic disorders are about 3.89 and 7.49 per 1,000 persons, respectively (Moreno-Küstner et al., 2018). Despite this relatively low prevalence, the burden of these diseases is substantial. For instance, although the global age-standardized point prevalence of schizophrenia was estimated to be only 0.28% in 2016, it has been calculated that schizophrenia contributed 1.7% (or 13.4 million) of total years of life lived with disability (YLDs) to the burden of disease globally in 2016 (Charlson et al., 2018). Therefore, prevention and treatment of schizophrenia spectrum and other psychotic disorders is a major priority.

Currently available antipsychotic drugs are quite effective in treating positive symptoms. However, they induce a plethora of side-effects such as extrapyramidal symptoms, sedation, sexual dysfunction, or weight gain and associated metabolic complications, and do not sufficiently ameliorate negative symptoms and cognitive impairments in most cases (Leucht et al., 2013; Leweke et al., 2012a). Furthermore, 19.8% of patients with acute schizophrenia do not show any symptom improvement after four-to-six weeks of treatment with an antipsychotic drug, and

66.9% of patients do not reach symptomatic remission (Samara et al., 2019). Hence, novel antipsychotic drugs with improved efficacy (particularly regarding negative and cognitive symptoms) and fewer side-effects are urgently needed to improve treatment response and remission rates. As the currently available antipsychotics primarily act via dopaminergic or serotonergic receptors, recent research has focused on new pharmacological approaches (Mueller et al., 2016). CBD is one of these promising compounds, representing an entirely novel class of antipsychotic drugs (Leweke et al., 2016; Rohleder et al., 2016a).

20.2 Evidence from Animal Models

Although most of the symptoms observed in schizophrenia spectrum disorders are human-specific, features such as abnormal motor behaviour, negative symptoms, and cognitive impairments can be modelled in animals to investigate the potential therapeutic effects of CBD on specific aspects of psychosis.

Various animal models have been developed based on the different etiological factors of schizophrenia, including acute and chronic cannabinoid treatment, pharmacological and genetic glutamatergic models affecting the N-methyl-D-aspartic acid (NMDA) receptor, pharmacological dopaminergic models using amphetamine or apomorphine, pre-natal infection model (poly I:C model or maternal immune activation (MIA) model), disruption of neurogenesis by pre-natal treatment with methylazoxymethanol (MAM), and a spontaneously hypertensive rat (SHR) strain model (Kirby, 2016; Rohleder et al., 2016a).

20.2.1 Effects of CBD on Abnormal Motor Behaviour

As early as 1991, Zuardi et al. reported that CBD (60 mg/kg) reduced stereotypic motor behaviour

Table 20.1 Effects of CBD on abnormal motor behaviour in different animal models

Animal model	Behavioural paradigm	Treatment regimen and test procedure	Effective dose (mg/kg)	Reference
Apomorphine (acute, 6.4 mg/kg) male Wistar rats	Stereotypic biting and sniffing behaviour, catalepsy, palpebral ptosis	15, 30, or 60 mg/kg CBD, i.p. concomitant with apomorphine injection. Behavioural assessments started 30 min after the injection.	60	Zuardi et al. (1991)
D-amphetamine (acute 5 mg/kg), male Swiss mice	Open Field test	15, 30, or 60 mg/kg CBD, i.p. 20 min prior to amphetamine injection. Behavioural assessments started 30 min after the injection.	30, 60	Moreira and Guimaraes (2005)
D-amphetamine (acute 5 mg/kg, on day 21, 45 min after CBD injection), male adult C57BL/6JArc mice	Open Field test	1, 5, 10, or 50 mg/kg, i.p. over 21 days,	50	Long et al. (2010)
Ketamine (acute 60 mg/kg), male Swiss mice	Open Field test	15, 30, or 60 mg/kg CBD, i.p. 10 min prior to amphetamine injection. Behavioural assessments started 30 min after the injection.	30	Moreira and Guimaraes (2005)
MK-801 (acute, 0.3 mg/kg), male Sprague Dawley rats	Locomotor activity in an experimental box	1 or 3 mg/kg CBD, i.p. injection 20 min prior to MK-801 administration. A modified social interaction test started 20 min after the last injection	1	Gururajan et al. (2012)
Spontaneously hypertensive rats (SHR)	Locomotion and rearing frequency during a social interaction task	1, 5, 15, 30, or 60 mg/kg CBD, i.p. injection 30 min prior to social interaction test	–	Almeida et al. (2013)

induced by the dopaminergic agonist apomorphine in rats. This effect was comparable to the impact of the antipsychotic haloperidol. Similarly, acute pre-treatment with CBD (30 and 60 mg/kg) or the antipsychotic clozapine as well as chronic CBD treatment (50 mg/kg) attenuated the hyperlocomotion induced by the dopaminergic agonist amphetamine in mice (Long et al., 2010; Moreira and Guimaraes, 2005). Furthermore, both CBD (30 or 1 mg/kg) and clozapine pre-treatment inhibited the hyperlocomotion induced by the NMDA-receptor antagonists ketamine and MK-801 in rodents (Gururajan et al., 2012; Moreira and Guimaraes, 2005). However, CBD did not alter the hyperlocomotion observed in SHR rats (Almeida et al., 2013). Nevertheless, these data (summarized in Table 20.1) suggest that CBD has antipsychotic-like properties and may reduce grossly disorganized or abnormal motor behaviour in patients with schizophrenia spectrum and other psychotic disorders.

20.2.2 Effects of CBD on Altered Social Behaviour

Altered social behaviour is a crucial negative symptom (American Psychiatric Association, 2013), and deficits in social functioning and cognition are among the most impairing and therapeutically challenging characteristics of schizophrenia (Bellack et al., 1990; Bucci et al., 2018; Nikolaides et al., 2016).

Pre-clinical studies investigating the effects of CBD on social behaviour (Table 20.2) showed that CBD could restore social interaction behaviors in some rodent models for schizophrenia. Thus, CBD may also improve social functioning in the schizophrenia spectrum and other psychotic disorders.

Table 20.2 Effects of CBD on social interaction behaviour in different animal models

Animal model	Behavioural paradigm	Treatment regimen and test procedure	Effective dose (mg/kg)	Reference
Pre-natal infection model/ Maternal immune activation (poly I:C, i.v. 4 mg/kg, GD15) model, male Sprague Dawley rats	Social interaction	10 mg/kg, i.p., twice daily over 3 weeks (PND 56–PND 80). Social interaction test conducted on PND 79	10 twice daily	Osborne et al. (2017)
Pre-natal infection model/ Maternal immune activation (poly I:C, i.v. 10 mg/kg on GD9) model, C57Bl/6J	Social interaction	1 mg/kg, i.p., PND 30–60, Social interaction assessment on PND 90	–	Peres et al. (2016)
Pre-natal Methylazoxymethanol acetate (MAM, 22 mg/kg, ip on GD 17), Sprague Dawley rats	Social interaction	10 or 30 mg/kg, i.p., PND 19–39, Social interaction assessment was conducted at adulthood from PND 100	30	Stark et al. (2019)
Spontaneously hypertensive rats (SHR)	Social interaction	1, 5, 15, 30, or 60 mg/kg CBD, i.p. injection 30 min prior to social interaction test	–	Almeida et al. (2013)
Spontaneously hypertensive rats (SHR)	Social interaction	0.5, 1, or 5 mg/kg CBD, i.p. PND 30–60, PPI assessment on PND 90	–	Peres et al. (2018)
Δ^9-THC (1 mg/kg, single dose), male Sprague Dawley rats	Social interaction	5 or 20 mg/kg CBD, i.p. injection 20 min prior to Δ^9-THC administration. Social interaction test started 20min after the second injection	20	Malone et al. (2009)
Δ^9-THC (3 mg single dose and ascending doses 1, 3, and 10 mg/kg over 21 days), male Wistar rats	Social interaction	3 mg CDB (single dose) or ascending doses of CBD (1, 3, and 10 mg/kg) over 21 days, i.p., 20 min prior to Δ^9-THC injection	3 (worsening of Δ^9-THC induced impairments)	Klein et al. (2011)
MK-801 (acute, 0.3 or 0.6 mg/ kg), male Sprague Dawley rats	Social interaction	MK-801 (acute, 0.3 or 0.6 mg/kg), male Sprague Dawley rats. Social interaction test started 20 min after the last injection	3, 10 (partially)	Gururajan et al. (2011)
MK-801 (acute, 0.3 mg/kg), male Sprague Dawley rats	Social interaction	1 or 3 mg/kg CBD, i.p. injection 20 min prior to MK-801 administration. A modified social interaction test started 20 min after the last injection	3	Gururajan et al. (2012)
MK-801 (acute, 0.08 mg/kg), male Wistar rats	Social recognition	5, 12, or 30 mg/kg CBD, i.p. injection 30 min prior to MK-801 administration. Social recognition test started 30 min after the last injection	–	Deiana et al. (2015)
MK-801 (chronic: 1 mg/kg, 28 days), male C57BL/6J mice	Social interaction	30 or 60 mg/kg CBD, i.p. injection 30 min prior to social interaction test	60	Gomes et al. (2015b)

GD, gestational day; PND, post-natal day; poly I:C, polyinosinic–polycytidilic acid.

In a pre-natal infection (or maternal immune activation [MIA]) model, chronic adult CBD treatment (10 mg/kg twice daily, post-natal days (PND) 56–80) reversed the social interaction impairments in male offspring of female rats treated with polyinosinic–polycytidylic acid (poly I:C, 4 mg/kg) during pregnancy (Osborne et al., 2017), while peri-adolescent (PND days 30–60) treatment with 1 mg/kg CBD was not effective in an MIA mouse model (Peres et al., 2016). However, peri-adolescent CBD treatment (30 mg/kg, PND 19–39) was found to reverse social interaction impairments in rats that underwent pre-natal exposure to methylazoxymethanol acetate (MAM), an effect that was not observed after treatment with a lower CBD dose (10 mg/kg) or the antipsychotic drug haloperidol (Stark et al., 2019).

Although CBD showed some promising effects in these two neurodevelopmental models (MIA, MAM), it did not affect social interaction in the spontaneously hypertensive rat (SHR) model (Almeida et al., 2013; Peres et al., 2018). On the other hand, the majority of studies using a pharmacological intervention to induce impairments of social interaction reported that CBD was able to attenuate or reverse the altered social behaviour. In the cannabinoid model, cannabidiol pre-treatment (20 mg/kg) reversed the effects of 1 mg/kg Δ^9-THC on the social interaction behaviour of Sprague Dawley rats (Malone et al., 2009). Interestingly, pre-treatment with a lower dose of CBD (3 mg/kg) exacerbated the Δ^9-THC effects (3 mg/kg) on social interaction in Wistar rats (Klein et al., 2011). These contradicting results might be caused by the different CBD/Δ^9-THC ratios (20/1 versus 1:1) used in the two studies.

Furthermore, CBD inhibited the acute effects of the NMDA antagonist MK-801 in two different social interaction paradigms in rats (Gururajan et al., 2011, 2012), and reversed the social interaction behaviour in mice chronically treated with MK-801 (Gomes et al., 2015b). However, CBD did not restore the social recognition impairments induced by acute low-dose injection of MK-801 in Wistar rats (Deiana et al., 2015).

Although CBD did not restore social interaction impairments in the SHR model and contradictory results were reported for the cannabinoid and the MIA model, the MAM and glutamatergic model results are promising, in particular against the backdrop that the antipsychotic clozapine also inhibited MK-801 effects on social behaviour (Gomes et al., 2015b; Gururajan et al., 2012).

20.2.3 Effects of CBD on Sensorimotor Gating Deficits

Pre-pulse inhibition (PPI) of the acoustic startle response (ASR) is a measure of sensorimotor gating (a pre-attentive filter mechanism), in which a weak sensory stimulus ('pre-pulse') attenuates the amplitude of a motor response ('startle reaction') to an intense startling stimulus, occurring within a certain time frame after the pre-pulse (Braff et al., 1978; Rohleder et al., 2016b). Reduced PPI in schizophrenia patients was first described in 1978 (Braff et al., 1978) and has been repeatedly reported since then (Braff et al., 2001; Swerdlow et al., 2018). Although PPI impairments are not specific to schizophrenia, PPI is considered an endophenotype of schizophrenia (Swerdlow et al., 2018). As PPI can be reliably assessed in animals, it is frequently used as a behavioural measure of aspects of schizophrenia in different animal models (Rohleder et al., 2016a).

Several studies reported that CBD reversed PPI deficits in different rodent models; however, CBD was not effective in all animal models (Table 20.3). In male *Swiss* mice, acute and chronic CBD pre-treatment attenuated the amphetamine-disruptive effects on PPI after intra-accumbens (60 nmol) and systemic administration (15, 30, or 60 mg/kg), respectively (Pedrazzi et al., 2015). Furthermore, acute (100 mg/kg) but not chronic CBD treatment (1, 50, 100 mg/kg; 21 days) increased PPI levels in *Nrg1* TM HET (Long et al., 2012). On the other hand, animal models using a pharmacological approach to mimic the glutamatergic deficits in schizophrenia showed that both acute pre-treatment (5 mg/kg) and chronic CBD treatment (30 or 60 mg/kg) reverse the MK-801 (NMDA receptor antagonist) induced PPI impairments in mice (Gomes et al., 2015a; Long et al., 2006). Interestingly, despite CBD's efficacy in mice, pre-treatment with CBD (3, 10, or 30 mg/kg) did not prevent the PPI deficits induced by acute MK-801 injection in Sprague Dawley rats (Gururajan et al., 2011). However, in the SHR model, CBD (single dose, 30 mg/kg) reversed PPI deficits in adult rats (Levin et al., 2014) and prevented the emergence of PPI impairments in rats treated during peri-adolescence (PND 30–60; 0.5, 1, and 5 mg/kg) (Peres et al., 2018).

In summary, despite some contradictory findings, these studies point to a potential efficacy of cannabidiol for the treatment of sensorimotor gating impairments observed in schizophrenia patients.

Table 20.3 Effects of CBD on PPI in different animal models

Animal model	Treatment regimen and test procedure	Effective dose (mg/kg)	Reference
Amphetamine (acute, 10 mg/kg) male Swiss mice	15, 30, or 60 mg/kg CBD, i.p. 30 min prior to amphetamine injection. PPI paradigm started 30 min after the last injection And intra-accumbens microinjection of CBD (60 nmol; 0.2 μl) followed immediately by a systemic injection of amphetamine 10 mg/kg. PPI paradigm started 10 min after amphetamine injection	15, 30, 60	Pedrazzi et al. (2015)
Male *Nrg1* TM HET mice	1, 50 or 100 mg/kg CBD, i.p. over 21 days. PPI assessment 30–45 min after the first injection and on day 21	100 (acute)	Long et al. (2012)
MK-801 (chronic: 1 mg/kg, 28 days), male C57BL/6J mice	30 or 60 mg/kg CBD, i.p. treatment began on 6th day of MK-801 administration. PPI assessment on day 29	30, 60	Gomes et al. (2015a)
MK-801 (acute, 1 mg/kg), male C57BL/6J mice	5 mg/kg CBD, i.p. injection 20 min prior to MK-801 administration. PPI paradigm started 5 min after the last injection	5	Long et al. (2006)
MK-801 (acute, 0.3 or 0.6 mg/kg), male Sprague Dawley rats	MK-801 (acute, 0.3 or 0.6 mg/kg), male Sprague Dawley rats PPI paradigm started 20 min after the last injection	–	Gururajan et al. (2011)
Spontaneously hypertensive rats (SHR)	15, 30, or 60 mg/kg CBD, i.p. 30 min prior to PPI paradigm	30	Levin et al. (2014)
Spontaneously hypertensive rats (SHR)	0.5, 1, or 5 mg/kg CBD, i.p. PND 30–60, PPI assessment on PND 90	0.5 (significant difference compared to vehicle treated SHR rats), 1 and 5 (no significant difference compared to vehicle treated SHR rats, but also no difference to Wistar control rats)	Peres et al. (2018)

Nrg1 TM HET, heterozygous transmembrane *Neuregulin1* mutation; PND, post-natal day.

20.2.4 Effects of CBD on Working Memory

Neurocognitive dysfunction is a core feature of schizophrenia and, to a lesser extent, of other psychoses (Bowie et al., 2018; Díaz-Caneja et al., 2019; Kahn and Keefe, 2013; Lewandowski et al., 2011; Seidman et al., 2016; Sheffield et al., 2018). It often precedes the onset of the positive symptoms of psychosis by many years (Kahn and Keefe, 2013; Sheffield et al., 2018) and is associated with poorer therapeutic and psychosocial outcomes (Kahn and Keefe, 2013; Sheffield et al., 2018). Furthermore, current pharmacotherapies do not appear to ameliorate these cognitive impairments to any substantial degree (Kahn and Keefe, 2013; Sheffield et al., 2018).

The effects of CBD on cognition, in particular on working memory, have been investigated in pharmacological models targeting the endocannabinoid (Δ^9-THC administration) and glutamatergic system (ketamine and MK-801 administration) as well as in two neurodevelopmental models (MIA and pre-natal MAM). Various behavioural paradigms have been used for the assessment of induced cognitive impairments (Table 20.4). Although CBD did not reverse induced cognitive deficits in all models,

Table 20.4 Effects of CBD on cognition (working memory) in different animal models and behavioural paradigms

Animal model	Behavioural paradigm	Treatment regimen and test procedure	Effective dose (mg/kg)	Reference
Δ^9-THC (3 mg/kg, PND 28–48 or PND 69–89), male CD1 mice	NOR	3 mg/kg CBD (concurrent to Δ^9-THC treatment, PND 28–48 or PND 69–89), cognitive assessment was done on day 2 after treatment and after 44 drug-free days	3	Murphy et al. (2017)
Δ^9-THC (0.2, 0.5 mg/kg i.m.), male adult rhesus monkeys	vsPAL, SOSS	0.5 mg/kg CBD, i.m. concurrently with Δ^9-THC administration, cognitive assessment started 30 min after the injections	0.5 (vs PAL)	Wright et al. (2013)
Δ^9-THC rich and CBD-rich cannabis extracts, male, adult Lister rats	DMPT	CBD-rich cannabis extracts (0.5, 5, 10, or 50 mg/kg CBD and up to 4 mg/kg Δ^9-THC), i.p. 30 min prior to the cognitive assessment. In addition, CBD-rich cannabis extracts (containing 5 or 10 mg/Kg CBD) were simultaneously injected with Δ^9-THC-rich cannabis extracts (2 mg/kg Δ^9-THC)	50 (as the CBD-rich cannabis extract contained nearly 4 mg/kg Δ^9-THC in addition to 50 mg/kg CBD)	Fadda et al. (2004)
Ketamine (acute 20 mg/kg; sub-chronic 30 mg/kg i.p. over 10 days followed by 6 days wash-out), male Sprague Dawley rats	NOR	Acute: CBD (1.8, 3.7, 7.5, 15, or 30 mg/kg, i.p.) injection 30 min prior to ketamine injection, cognitive assessment started 45 min after ketamine injection; sub-chronic:CBD (7.5 mg twice daily, i.p.), over 6 days starting after ketamine washout	acute: 1.8, 3.7, 7.5, 15, or 30 (7.5 and 30 most effective) sub-chronic: 7.5 twice daily	Kozela et al. (2019)
MK-801 (chronic: 1 mg/kg, 28 days), male C57BL/6J mice	NOR	30 or 60 mg/kg CBD, i.p. injection 30 min prior to the cognitive assessment	30, 60	Gomes et al. (2015b)
MK-801 (0.1 mg/kg, acute), male, adult Lister rats	DMPT	CBD-rich cannabis extracts (5 or 10 mg/kg CBD), i.p. concurrently with MK-801 injection, 30 min prior to the cognitive assessment	–	Fadda et al. (2006)
Pre-natal infection model/ Maternal immune activation (poly I:C, i.v. 4 mg/kg, GD15) model, male Sprague Dawley rats	NOR, rewarded T-maze test	10 mg/kg, i.p., twice daily over 3 weeks (PND 56–PND 80). NOR task on PND 72 and rewarded T-maze test on PND 78	10 twice daily (NOR and rewarded T-maze test)	Osborne et al. (2017)

Table 20.4 (cont.)

Animal model	Behavioural paradigm	Treatment regimen and test procedure	Effective dose (mg/kg)	Reference
Pre-natal infection model/ Maternal immune activation (poly I:C, i.v. 4 mg/kg, GD15) model, female Sprague Dawley rats	NOR, rewarded T-maze test	10 mg/kg, i.p., twice daily over 3 weeks (PND 56–PND 80)	10 twice daily (NOR)	Osborne et al. (2019)
Pre-natal Methylazoxymethanol acetate (MAM, 22 mg/kg, ip on GD 17), Sprague Dawley rats	NOR	10 or 30 mg/kg, i.p., PND 19–39, cognitive assessment was conducted at adulthood from PND 100	30	Stark et al. (2019)

DMTP, Delayed Matching to Position; GD, gestational day; NOR, Novel Object Recognition, PND, post-natal day; poly I:C: polyinosinic-polycytidilic acid; SOSS, Self-Ordered Spatial Search; vsPAL, Visuospatial Paired Associates Learning.

species, and paradigms, promising effects on cognition have been reported, as outlined in Section 20.3.

In the Δ^9-THC model, concomitant chronic CBD administration (CBD/Δ^9-THC ratio 1/1) prevented intermediate and long-term impairments in working memory (object recognition) in mice (Murphy et al., 2017). Furthermore, acute simultaneous injection of CBD (CBD/Δ^9-THC ratio: 1/1 and 2.5/1) attenuated cognitive impairments in the visuospatial Paired Associates Learning Task but not in the Self-Ordered Spatial Search memory tasks in adult male rhesus monkeys (Wright et al., 2013). However, in rats, only higher ratios of simultaneous CBD and Δ^9-THC administration (12.5/1 but not 5/1 or lower) were able to prevent working memory impairments assessed with a Delayed Matching to Sample task (Fadda et al., 2004).

Object recognition deficits induced by the NMDA receptor antagonist ketamine were prevented by both acute CBD pre-treatment (7.5 and 30 mg/kg) and repeated CBD administration (7.5 mg/kg) after sub-chronic ketamine injections (Kozela et al., 2019). Similar beneficial effects were observed after repeated CBD treatment (30 and 60 mg/kg) in a mice model using the NMDA receptor antagonist MK-801 (Gomes et al., 2015b). However, single doses of CBD-rich cannabis extracts (containing 5 or 10 mg/kg CBD, respectively) simultaneously injected with MK-801 did not prevent MK-801 induced working memory impairments in rats (Fadda et al., 2006).

Interestingly, in neurodevelopmental rat models, peri-adolescent CBD treatment reversed the object recognition memory impairment induced by pre-natal MAM (Stark et al., 2019) or poly I:C exposure (Osborne et al., 2017, 2019). Furthermore, peri-adolescent CBD treatment attenuated the working memory impairments observed in the rewarded T-maze alternation test in male Sprague Dawley rats (Osborne et al., 2017).

20.2.5 Conclusion

Despite some conflicting results, a growing body of pre-clinical literature suggests that CBD does possess antipsychotic properties and may effectively reduce abnormal motor behaviour, negative symptoms (e.g., social dysfunction), and cognitive impairments (e.g., PPI and specific working memory impairments).

Apart from pre-clinical studies, CBD has been studied over the last three decades in patients with schizophrenia and Parkinson's Disease psychosis. Although only a few studies have been conducted so far, they substantiate the promising pre-clinical findings. Unfortunately, despite promising pre-clinical data, none of these studies investigated the effects of CBD on abnormal motor behaviour and PPI.

20.3 Evidence from Clinical Studies and Trials

The published literature on CBD in humans with schizophrenia encompass three case reports (Makiol and Kluge, 2019; Zuardi et al., 1995, 2006) and four randomized controlled trials (RCTs) – including one active-controlled clinical trial in acute schizophrenia (Leweke et al., 2012b, 2021), two placebo-controlled add-on studies in sub-acute (McGuire et al., 2018) and chronic (Boggs et al., 2018) schizophrenia spectrum patients on stable antipsychotic medication, as well as one single dose add-on study in non-acute schizophrenia patients (Hallak et al., 2010). In addition, a small open-label pilot study explored the antipsychotic efficacy of CBD in Parkinson's Disease patients with psychotic symptoms (Zuardi et al., 2009).

These study results (summarized in Table 20.5) indicate that CBD has, in particular, promising antipsychotic effects when administered for at least four weeks and a more favourable side-effect profile than currently available antipsychotics. However, more extensive randomized, controlled clinical trials are needed to confirm cannabidiol's antipsychotic efficacy and safety in larger cohorts.

20.3.1 Case Reports and Open-Label Studies

In 1995, Zuardi et al. reported CBD use in a 19-year old female patient diagnosed with schizophrenia who experienced severe side-effects with previous antipsychotic mediations. After a wash-out period, the young woman was treated over 26 days with increasing doses of up to 1,500 mg CBD per day. Overall, CBD markedly improved psychotic symptoms as indicated by reduced scores on the Brief Psychiatric Rating Scales (BPRS) and Interactive Observation Scale for Psychiatric Inpatients (IOSPI). Subsequent treatment with the first generation antipsychotic haloperidol did not further increase the CBD-associated clinical improvements (Zuardi et al., 1995).

Although this first monotherapy study with CBD was successful, an ensuing case series was published over a decade later (Zuardi et al., 2006). After a five-day wash-out period, three treatment-resistant schizophrenia patients received increasing doses of up to 1,280 mg CBD per day over 30 days. CBD was well tolerated, and no side-effects were observed. However, only one patient showed mild improvements in positive and negative symptoms evaluated by BPRS.

Recently, successful adjunctive CBD treatment in a case of severe treatment-resistant schizophrenia has been reported (Makiol and Kluge, 2019). A 57-year-old woman, with a 21-year history of schizophrenia, received – after several other unsuccessful treatment attempts – 1,000 mg CBD per day over seven weeks as an adjunct to her clozapine and lamotrigine medication. During that time, her positive and negative symptoms improved markedly; however, her auditory hallucinations did not disappear completely. After increasing the dose to 1,500 mg/day, the hallucinations gradually subsided, and by 2.5 weeks were no longer present. On discharge, the patient fulfilled remission criteria (based on the Positive and Negative Syndrome Scale (PANSS) scores) with only mild negative symptoms. Further, CBD was well tolerated, apart from a mild transient hand tremor.

Psychosis is a common feature in Parkinson's Disease (PD), with a prevalence of approximately 26% (Ffytche and Aarsland, 2017; Mack et al., 2012). Zuardi et al. (2009) explored the antipsychotic efficacy, tolerability, and safety of CBD in six patients with PD psychosis in an open-label pilot study. Patients received a flexible dose of up to 400 mg/day over four weeks as adjunctive therapy to their standard PD medication. CBD treatment was associated with a significant reduction in the psychotic symptoms assessed by the BPRS and the Parkinson Psychosis Questionnaire. Importantly, no decline in motor function or other adverse effects were observed during CBD treatment. Despite the small sample size and the absence of placebo control, these pilot data are indicative of CBD's potential antipsychotic efficacy in non-schizophrenia spectrum disorders and underline its good tolerability and safety. However, larger trials are needed to confirm these promising results in PD patients with psychosis.

20.3.2 Randomized Controlled Trials

The first double-blind, randomized, active-controlled, parallel-group clinical trial of CBD in people with schizophrenia was conducted by Leweke et al. (2012b). In this four-week trial of acutely unwell patients, 600–800 mg daily of CBD (n = 21) showed comparable antipsychotic efficacy to the selective dopamine D2/3 receptor antagonist amisulpride (600–800 mg/day; n = 21). Only lorazepam (up to 7.5 mg/day) was allowed as a rescue medication where needed. Both groups showed significant clinical improvement of positive and negative symptoms of psychosis as assessed by the PANSS and BPRS (change (mean ± SD) after CBD and amisulpride treatment, respectively, baseline to day 14 PANSS total: 18.8 ± 10.7 and 18.8 ± 19.9; BPRS: 14.5 ± 7.9 and 12.7 ± 12.0; baseline to day 28 PANSS total: 30.5 ± 16.4 and 30.8 ± 24.7, BPRS: 20.5 ± 12.3 and 19.4 ± 15.6). Importantly, CBD had a superior side-effect profile compared to amisulpride and did not induce

Table 20.5 Overview of studies investigating the effects of CBD in patients with psychosis

Study	Number of participants and sample characteristics	CBD regimen	Primary efficacy endpoint	Outcome	Side-effects
Single case report, open label (Zuardi et al., 1995)	1 (19 yrs, female), treatment-resistant schizophrenia (BPRS score = 50, blinded rating)	1,500 mg/day (gelatin capsules, dissolved in corn oil) as monotherapy over 26 days	Psychotic symptoms (BPRS)	Improvement of psychotic symptoms (BPRS score = 30, blinded rating); clinical improvement was not increased by treatment with haloperidol	Well tolerated
Case series, open label (Zuardi et al., 2006)	3 (22–23 yrs, male), treatment-resistant schizophrenia (BPRS score [median (min–max)] = 29 (19–30))	Increasing doses of up to 1,280 mg/day over 30 days	Psychotic symptoms (BPRS)	Mild improvements in one case (mild BPRS score reduction [3 points])	No side-effects
Single case report (Makiol and Kluge, 2019)	1 (57 yrs, female), treatment-resistant schizophrenia (PANSS total score = 117, PANSS negative score = 41)	Increasing doses of up to 1,500 mg/day as add-on to clozapine and lamotrigine; duration unclear, more than 9.5 weeks	Positive and negative symptoms (PANSS)	Remission with only mild negative symptoms (PANSS total score = 68, PANSS negative score = 21)	Well-tolerated apart from mild transient hand tremor
Open label pilot study (Zuardi et al., 2009)	6 (mean age 58.8 ± 14.9 yrs, 4 male), Parkinson's disease with psychosis for at least 3 months prior study entry (BPRS score (median [min–max]) = 18.5 [11–26])	Increasing doses of up to 400 mg/day (gelatin capsules, dissolved in corn oil) over 4 weeks as add-on to l-dopa treatment	Psychotic symptoms (BPRS/PPQ)	Significant decrease of psychotic symptoms (BPRS score (median [min–max]) = 5.5 [0–12])	Well-tolerated
Double-blind, randomized, active-controlled, parallel-group study (Leweke et al., 2012b)	42 (39 included in full analysis set; CBD group: 20; 29.7 ± 8.3 yrs, 15 male; amisulpride group: 19, 30.6 ± 9.4 yrs, 17 male), acute schizophrenia (PANSS total/BPRS score [mean ± SD] = 91.2 ± 14.0/58.1 ± 9.7 and 95.5 ± 17.1/ 57.7 ± 10.3 in the CBD and amisulpride group, respectively)	600–800 mg/day over 4 weeks	Primary outcome: Psychotic symptoms (PANSS/BPRS)	Significant improvement of symptoms compared to baseline on days 14 (Change in PANSS total score [mean ± SD] = 18.8 ± 10.7 and 18.8 ± 19.9 in the CBD and amisulpride group, respectively) and 28 (Change in PANSS total score [mean ± SD] = 30.5 ± 16.4 and 30.1 ± 24.7 in the CBD and amisulpride group, respectively) for both treatment groups	Superior side-effect profile of cannabidiol compared to amisulpride

Study	Sample	Intervention	Outcome	Results	Adverse effects
(Leweke et al., 2021)			Secondary outcome: Neurocognitive performance in the following domains: • Pattern recognition • Attention, • Working memory • Verbal and visual memory and learning • Processing speed • Verbal executive functions	No relevant difference in neurocognitive performance CBD and amisulpride (AMI) at baseline, and no post-treatment differences between both groups. Improvements within both groups from pre- to post-treatment (standardized differences reported as Cohen's d) in visual memory (CBD: 0.49, p = 0.015, AMI: 0.63, p = 0.018) and processing speed (CBD: 0.41, p = 0.004, AMI: 0.57, p = 0.023). CBD improved sustained attention (CBD: 0.47, p = 0.013), and visuomotor coordination (CBD: 0.32, p = 0.010). AMI enhanced working memory performance in the Subject Ordered Pointing Task (AMI: 0.53, p = 0.043) and the Letter Number Sequencing (AMI: 0.67, p = 0.017).	
Double blind, placebo-controlled, parallel-group, add-on study (Hallak et al., 2010)	28 (>18 yrs, CBD 600 group: 9, 5 male; CBD 300 group: 9, 6 male; placebo group 10, 7 male) schizophrenia, no acute psychotic episode PANSS/BPRS score [mean ± SD] = 20.2 ± 7.1/8.9 ± 5.1, 23.5 ± 9.4/ 11.3 ± 5.1, and 21.9 ± 5.8/8.6 ± 5.0 in the CBD 600, CBD 300, and placebo group, respectively)	Single dose of 300 or 600 mg (gelatin capsules) as add-on to antipsychotic mediation	Selective attention (SWCT) and electrodermal responsiveness to auditive stimuli	No significant effects on electrodermal measures and attention	Possible sedative effects of 600 mg CBD

Table 20.5 (cont.)

Study	Number of participants and sample characteristics	CBD regimen	Primary efficacy endpoint	Outcome	Side-effects
Randomized, placebo-controlled, parallel-group, add-on study (McGuire et al., 2018)	88 (CBD group: 43; 40.9 ± 12.5 yrs, 28 male; placebo group: 45, 40.8 ± 11.0 yrs, 23 male), schizophrenia or related psychotic disorder (PANSS total score [mean ± SD] = 79.3 ± 12.5 and 80.6 ± 14.9 in the CBD and placebo group, respectively)	1,000 mg/day (oral solution, GW42003) over 6 weeks as add-on to a stable dose of antipsychotic medication	Psychotic symptoms (PANSS)	Proportion of responders (improvement in PANSS total score >20%) higher on cannabidiol than placebo, greater reduction of positive PANSS score in the CBD group by trend	Well-tolerated, and rates of adverse events were similar between the CBD and placebo groups
Randomized, placebo-controlled, parallel-group, add-on study (Boggs et al., 2018)	39 (36 included in full analysis set; CBD group: 18, mean age 48.4 ± 9.3, 12 male; placebo group: 18, mean age 46.4 ± 9.5, 13 male) chronic schizophrenia (PANSS total score [mean ± SD] =76.6 ± 17.0 and 82.7 ± 8.8 in the CBD and placebo group, respectively)	600 mg/day over 6 weeks as add-on to a stable dose of antipsychotic medication	Cognition (MCCB)	No improvement in MCCB performance. No improvement in psychotic symptoms (PANSS, secondary outcome)	Side-effects were similar between the CBD and placebo groups except for sedation (20% and 5% in the CBD and placebo group, respectively)

BPRS, Brief Psychiatric Rating Scale; MCCB, MATRICS Consensus Cognitive Battery; PANSS, Positive and Negative Syndrome Scale; PPQ, Parkinson Psychosis Questionnaire; SWCT, Stroop Colour Word Test.

elevated prolactin levels, weight gain, or extrapyramidal symptoms. Most strikingly, in an analysis of secondary outcomes, Leweke et al. (2021) reported on the effects on neurocognitive performance in the study. At baseline, there was no relevant difference in neurocognitive performance between treatment groups, and both groups showed improvements from pre- to post-treatment (standardized differences reported as Cohen's d) in visual memory (CBD: 0.49, $p = 0.015$ versus AMI: 0.63, $p = 0.018$) and processing speed (CBD: 0.41, $p = 0.004$ versus AMI: 0.57, $p = 0.023$). In addition, CBD improved sustained attention (CBD: 0.47, $p = 0.013$ versus AMI: 0.52, $p = 0.085$) and visuomotor coordination (CBD: 0.32, $p = 0.010$ versus AMI: 0.63, $p = 0.088$), while AMI led to enhanced working memory performance in two different paradigms, the Subject Ordered Pointing Task (AMI: 0.53, $p = 0.043$ versus CBD: 0.03, $p = 0.932$) and the Letter Number Sequencing (AMI: 0.67, $p = 0.017$ versus CBD: 0.08, $p = 0.755$).

Two recent double-blind, randomized, placebo-controlled, parallel-group clinical trials investigated the efficacy of CBD as an add-on to stable antipsychotic medication in sub-acute and chronic schizophrenia spectrum patients (Boggs et al., 2018; McGuire et al., 2018). In one trial, 88 patients with schizophrenia (n = 83) or related disorders [e.g., schizoaffective (n = 3), schizophrenia-like disorder (n = 1) or delusional disorder (n = 1)] received 1,000 mg CBD per day (n = 43) or placebo (n = 45) over six weeks (McGuire et al., 2018). CBD treatment led to improved positive symptoms in the CBD group as compared to the placebo control group (PANSS treatment difference = −1.4, 95% CI = −2.5 to −0.2). Further, the patients in the CBD group felt less unwell and were more likely rated as clinically improved compared to the placebo group. In addition, patients who received CBD showed slightly improved cognitive performance compared to those who received placebo, but the differences did not reach statistical significance. As this study focused on sub-acute patients with a PANSS score ≥ 60 receiving a stable dose of an antipsychotic for at least four weeks (no treatment-resistance), the additional beneficial effect over that of the concomitant antipsychotic medication is promising, albeit the magnitude of the effects were modest. CBD was well tolerated, and rates of adverse events were similar between the CBD and placebo groups. However, numerically the levels of gastrointestinal disorders (diarrhoea or nausea) were marginally higher in the CBD group (potentially due to the pharmaceutical preparation), while somnolence was slightly more often observed in the placebo group.

In the second add-on study with a similar design, 39 chronic schizophrenia patients who had been on a stable dose of antipsychotic medications for at least three months (including first and generation antipsychotics as well as long-acting injectable antipsychotics) were treated with 600 mg CBD per day (n = 20) or placebo (n = 19) over six weeks (Boggs et al., 2018). CBD did not improve cognitive performance (primary endpoint) assessed by MATRICS Consensus Cognitive Battery (MCCB). PANSS total score decreased in both groups over time; that is, CBD had no beneficial effect on psychotic symptoms (secondary outcome). Furthermore, side-effects were similar in both groups, except for sedation, which was more prevalent in the CBD group. Methodological differences between this and the study of McGuire et al. (2018) may explain the differential outcomes. For example, 11% and 39% of the CBD and placebo groups ($p = 0.05$), respectively, were receiving multiple antipsychotics. Further, additional treatment with antidepressants, anticholinergic drugs, anticonvulsants/mood stabilizers, and benzodiazepine was allowed. The duration of illness (mean ± SD: 25.6 ± 12.7 and 28.2 ± 8.5 in the CBD and placebo group, respectively), the long-term polypharmaceutical treatment, the significantly higher proportion of patients being treated with multiple antipsychotics in the placebo group, as well as the lower CBD dose used (600 versus 1,000 mg/day) are also relevant differences across these studies.

Finally, Hallak et al. (2010) examined the acute effects of a single dose of CBD on selective attention (using the Stroop Colour Word Test) and electrodermal response to an auditory stimulus, in 28 individuals with schizophrenia. Neither 300 (n = 9) nor 600 mg (n = 9) of CBD improved selective attention compared to placebo (n = 10). The implications of these findings are limited, given only a single dose of CBD was administered.

20.3.3 Use of Cannabidiol in Early Intervention: Evidence from Randomized Clinical Trials in Clinical-High-Risk (CHR) Mental State for Psychosis

Recently, the use of CBD in individuals with a high risk of developing psychosis has come to the fore.

A randomized, placebo-controlled, double-blind fMRI study (Bhattacharyya et al., 2018) in 33 CHR and 19 healthy control individuals observed alterations in striatal, parahippocampal, and midbrain function in CHR individuals treated with placebo compared to controls. On the other hand, CHR individuals who received a single dose of CBD (600 mg) showed an intermediate level of activation compared to the placebo CHR group and healthy controls, leading the authors to conclude that a single dose of CBD may partially normalize dysfunctions in these brain regions. Thirty-two of the CHR patients included in the abovementioned study were also tested in the Trier Social Stress Test (TSST) after taking 600 mg CBD or placebo for one week (Appiah-Kusi et al., 2020). In addition, their serum cortisol, as well as anxiety and stress associated with public speaking, were assessed. Compared to healthy participants (n = 26) and the CHR placebo group, CHR individuals receiving CBD showed an intermediate cortisol and anxiety responses in association with experimental stress. Thus, CBD may positively affect the altered neuroendocrine and psychological responses to acute stress in CHR patients.

20.3.4 Conclusion

Pre-clinical studies investigating the antipsychotic properties of CBD in various animal models and behavioural paradigms indicate that CBD ameliorates abnormal motor behaviour, dysfunctional social behaviour, impaired sensorimotor gating, as well as certain aspects of cognitive impairments in rodents and rhesus monkeys. In humans, case studies and randomized, double-blind clinical trials have shown that CBD might have antipsychotic effects in some patients with schizophrenia spectrum disorders and PD psychosis. To date, studies have largely been of sub-acute patients on stable antipsychotic monotherapy, but some data suggest CBD may be particularly effective in the early stages of schizophrenia spectrum disorders, notably CHR populations. Furthermore, the published clinical trials suggest that CBD is safe, well-tolerated, and has a favourable side-effect profile compared to currently available antipsychotics. However, efficacy regarding cognition is equivocal. Based on the task-selective differences observed in pre-clinical studies, CBD might not improve impaired cognition per se, but only specific cognitive functions. The effects of CBD on reduced PPI (a pre-attentive filter mechanism, preventing sensory overload and cognitive fragmentation) have not yet been studied in humans, despite promising pre-clinical data.

Further high-quality, double-blind, randomized, controlled clinical trials are required to replicate the initial findings, investigate long-term efficacy and safety in larger cohorts, and explore its efficacy in individuals at CHR for psychosis.

References

Almeida, V., Levin, R., Peres, F. F., et al. (2013). Cannabidiol exhibits anxiolytic but not antipsychotic property evaluated in the social interaction test. *Prog Neuropsychopharmacol Biol Psychiatry*, **41**, 30–35.

American Psychiatric Association. (2013). *Diagnostic and Statistical Manual of Mental Disorders*. Arlington: American Psychiatric Association.

Appiah-Kusi, E., Petros, N., Wilson, R., et al. (2020). Effects of short-term cannabidiol treatment on response to social stress in subjects at clinical high risk of developing psychosis. *Psychopharmacology*, 237, 1121–1130.

Bellack, A. S., Morrison, R. L., Wixted, J. T., et al. (1990). An analysis of social competence in schizophrenia. *Br J Psychiatry*, **156**, 809–818.

Bhattacharyya, S., Wilson, R., Appiah-Kusi, E., et al. (2018). Effect of cannabidiol on medial temporal, midbrain, and striatal dysfunction in people at clinical high risk of psychosis: A randomized clinical trial. *JAMA Psychiatry*, **75**, 1107–1117.

Boggs, D. L., Surti, T., Gupta, A., et al. (2018). The effects of cannabidiol (CBD) on cognition and symptoms in outpatients with chronic schizophrenia: A randomized placebo controlled trial. *Psychopharmacology (Berl)*, **235**, 1923–1932.

Bowie, C. R., Best, M. W., Depp, C., et al. (2018). Cognitive and functional deficits in bipolar disorder and schizophrenia as a function of the presence and history of psychosis. *Bipolar Disord*, **20**, 604–613.

Braff, D., Stone, C., Callaway, E., et al. (1978). Prestimulus effects on human startle reflex in normals and schizophrenics. *Psychophysiology*, **15**, 339–343.

Braff, D. L., Geyer, M. A., and Swerdlow, N. R. (2001). Human studies of prepulse inhibition of startle: Normal subjects, patient groups, and pharmacological studies. *Psychopharmacology (Berl)*, **156**, 234–258.

Bucci, P., Galderisi, S., Mucci, A., et al. (2018). Premorbid academic and social functioning in patients with schizophrenia and its associations with negative symptoms and cognition. *Acta Psychiatr Scand*, **138**, 253–266.

Charlson, F. J., Ferrari, A. J., Santomauro, D. F., et al. (2018). Global epidemiology and burden of schizophrenia: Findings from the global burden of disease study 2016. *Schizophr Bull*, **44**, 1195–1203.

Deiana, S., Watanabe, A., Yamasaki, Y., et al. (2015). MK-801-induced deficits in social recognition in rats: Reversal by aripiprazole, but not olanzapine, risperidone, or cannabidiol. *Behav Pharmacol*, **26**, 748–765.

Díaz-Caneja, C. M., Cervilla, J. A., Haro, J. M., et al. (2019). Cognition and functionality in delusional disorder. *Eur Psychiatry*, **55**, 52–60.

Fadda, P., Robinson, L., Fratta, W., et al. (2004). Differential effects of THC- or CBD-rich cannabis extracts on working memory in rats. *Neuropharmacology*, **47**, 1170–1179.

(2006). Scopolamine and MK801-induced working memory deficits in rats are not reversed by CBD-rich cannabis extracts. *Behav Brain Res*, **168**, 307–311.

Ffytche, D. H., and Aarsland, D. (2017). Psychosis in Parkinson's disease. *Int Rev Neurobiol*, **133**, 585–622.

Gomes, F. V., Issy, A. C., Ferreira, F. R., et al. (2015a). Cannabidiol attenuates sensorimotor gating disruption and molecular changes induced by chronic antagonism of NMDA receptors in mice. *Int J Neuropsychopharmacol*, **18**, pyu041.

Gomes, F. V., Llorente, R., Del Bel, E. A., et al. (2015b). Decreased glial

reactivity could be involved in the antipsychotic-like effect of cannabidiol. *Schizophr Res*, **164**, 155–163.

Gururajan, A., Taylor, D. A., and Malone, D. T. (2011). Effect of cannabidiol in a MK-801-rodent model of aspects of schizophrenia. *Behav Brain Res*, **222**, 299–308.

(2012). Cannabidiol and clozapine reverse MK-801-induced deficits in social interaction and hyperactivity in Sprague-Dawley rats. *J Psychopharmacol*, **26**, 1317–1332.

Hallak, J. E., Machado-De-Sousa, J. P., Crippa, J. A., et al. (2010). Performance of schizophrenic patients in the Stroop Color Word Test and electrodermal responsiveness after acute administration of cannabidiol (CBD). *Rev Bras Psiquiatr*, **32**, 56–61.

Kahn, R. S., and Keefe, R. S. E. (2013). Schizophrenia is a cognitive illness: Time for a change in focus. *JAMA Psychiatry*, **70**, 1107–1112.

Kirby, B. P. (2016). Animal models of psychotic disorders: Dimensional approach modeling negative symptoms. In Pletnikov, M. V., and Waddington, J. L. (eds.) *Handbook of Behavioral Neuroscience* (pp. 55–67). London: Elsevier.

Klein, C., Karanges, E., Spiro, A., et al. (2011). Cannabidiol potentiates delta-tetrahydrocannabinol (THC) behavioural effects and alters THC pharmacokinetics during acute and chronic treatment in adolescent rats. *Psychopharmacology (Berl)*, **218**, 443–457.

Kozela, E., Krawczyk, M., Kos, T., et al. (2019). Cannabidiol improves cognitive impairment and reverses cortical transcriptional changes induced by ketamine, in schizophrenia-like model in rats. *Mol Neurobiol*, **57**, 1733–1747.

Leucht, S., Cipriani, A., Spineli, L., et al. (2013). Comparative efficacy and

tolerability of 15 antipsychotic drugs in schizophrenia: A multiple-treatments meta-analysis. *Lancet*, **382**, 951–962.

Levin, R., Peres, F. F., Almeida, V., et al. (2014). Effects of cannabinoid drugs on the deficit of prepulse inhibition of startle in an animal model of schizophrenia: The SHR strain. *Front Pharmacol*, **5**, 10.

Lewandowski, K. E., Cohen, B. M., and Ongur, D. (2011). Evolution of neuropsychological dysfunction during the course of schizophrenia and bipolar disorder. *Psychol Med*, **41**, 225–241.

Leweke, F. M., Mueller, J. K., Lange, B., et al. (2016). Therapeutic potential of cannabinoids in psychosis. *Biol Psychiatry*, **79**, 604–612.

Leweke, F. M., Odorfer, T. M., and Bumb, J. M. (2012a). Medical needs in the treatment of psychotic disorders. *Handb Exp Pharmacol*, **212**, 165–185.

Leweke, F. M., Piomelli, D., Pahlisch, F., et al. (2012b). Cannabidiol enhances anandamide signaling and alleviates psychotic symptoms of schizophrenia. *Transl Psychiatry*, **2**, e94.

Leweke, F. M., Rohleder, C., Gerth, C. W., et al. (2021). Cannabidiol and amisulpride improve cognition in acute schizophrenia in an explorative, double-blind, active-controlled, randomized clinical trial. *Front Pharmacol*, **12**, 614811.

Long, L. E., Chesworth, R., Huang, X. F., et al. (2010). A behavioural comparison of acute and chronic Delta9-tetrahydrocannabinol and cannabidiol in C57BL/6JArc mice. *Int J Neuropsychopharmacol*, **13**, 861–876.

(2012). Distinct neurobehavioural effects of cannabidiol in transmembrane domain neuregulin 1 mutant mice. *PLoS ONE*, **7**, e34129.

Long, L. E., Malone, D. T., and Taylor, D. A. (2006). Cannabidiol reverses MK-801-induced disruption of prepulse inhibition in mice. *Neuropsychopharmacology*, **31**, 795–803.

Mack, J., Rabins, P., Anderson, K., et al. (2012). Prevalence of psychotic symptoms in a community-based Parkinson disease sample. *Am J Geriatr Psychiatry*, **20**, 123–132.

Makiol, C., and Kluge, M. (2019). Remission of severe, treatment-resistant schizophrenia following adjunctive cannabidiol. *Aust NZ J Psychiatry*, **53**, 262.

Malone, D. T., Jongejan, D., and Taylor, D. A. (2009). Cannabidiol reverses the reduction in social interaction produced by low dose Delta(9)-tetrahydrocannabinol in rats. *Pharmacol Biochem Behav*, **93**, 91–96.

McGuire, P., Robson, P., Cubala, W. J., et al. (2018). Cannabidiol (CBD) as an adjunctive therapy in schizophrenia: A multicenter randomized controlled trial. *Am J Psychiatry*, **175**, 225–231.

Moreira, F. A., and Guimaraes, F. S. (2005). Cannabidiol inhibits the hyperlocomotion induced by psychotomimetic drugs in mice. *Eur J Pharmacol*, **512**, 199–205.

Moreno-Küstner, B., Martín, C., and Pastor, L. (2018). Prevalence of psychotic disorders and its association with methodological issues. A systematic review and meta-analyses. *PLoS ONE*, **13**, e0195687.

Mueller, J. K., Rohleder, C., and Leweke, F. M. (2016). What is the promise of nicotinergic compounds in schizophrenia treatment? *Future Med Chem*, **8**, 2009–2012.

Murphy, M., Mills, S., Winstone, J., et al. (2017). Chronic adolescent delta(9)-tetrahydrocannabinol treatment of male mice leads to long-term cognitive and behavioral dysfunction, which are prevented by concurrent cannabidiol treatment. *Cannabis Cannabinoid Res*, **2**, 235–246.

Nikolaides, A., Miess, S., Auvera, I., et al. (2016). Restricted attention to social cues in schizophrenia patients. *Eur Arch Psychiatry Clin Neurosci*, **266**, 649–661.

Osborne, A. L., Solowij, N., Babic, I., et al. (2017). Improved social interaction, recognition and working memory with cannabidiol treatment in a prenatal infection (poly I:C) rat model. *Neuropsychopharmacology*, **42**, 1447–1457.

(2019). Cannabidiol improves behavioural and neurochemical deficits in adult female offspring of the maternal immune activation (poly I:C) model of neurodevelopmental disorders. *Brain Behav Immun*, **81**, 574–587.

Pedrazzi, J. F., Issy, A. C., Gomes, F. V., et al. (2015). Cannabidiol effects in the prepulse inhibition disruption induced by amphetamine. *Psychopharmacology (Berl)*, **232**, 3057–3065.

Peres, F. F., Diana, M. C., Levin, R., et al. (2018). Cannabidiol administered during peri-adolescence prevents behavioral abnormalities in an animal model of schizophrenia. *Front Pharmacol*, **9**, 901.

Peres, F. F., Diana, M. C., Suiama, M. A., et al. (2016). Peripubertal treatment with cannabidiol prevents the emergence of psychosis in an animal model of schizophrenia. *Schizophr Res*, **172**, 220–221.

Rohleder, C., Muller, J. K., Lange, B., et al. (2016a). Cannabidiol as a potential new type of an antipsychotic. A critical review of the evidence. *Front Pharmacol*, **7**, 422.

Rohleder, C., Wiedermann, D., Neumaier, B., et al. (2016b). The functional networks of prepulse inhibition: Neuronal connectivity analysis based on FDG-PET in awake and unrestrained rats. *Front Behav Neurosci*, **10**, 148.

Samara, M. T., Nikolakopoulou, A., Salanti, G., et al. (2019). How many patients with schizophrenia do not respond to antipsychotic drugs in the short term? An analysis based on individual patient data from randomized controlled trials. *Schizophr Bull*, **45**, 639–646.

Seidman, L. J., Shapiro, D. I., Stone, W. S., et al. (2016). Association of neurocognition with transition to psychosis: Baseline functioning in the second phase of the North American prodrome longitudinal study. *JAMA Psychiatry*, **73**, 1239–1248.

Sheffield, J. M., Karcher, N. R., and Barch, D. M. (2018). Cognitive deficits in psychotic disorders: A lifespan perspective. *Neuropsychol Rev*, **28**, 509–533.

Stark, T., Ruda-Kucerova, J., Iannotti, F. A., et al. (2019). Peripubertal cannabidiol treatment rescues behavioral and neurochemical abnormalities in the MAM model of schizophrenia. *Neuropharmacology*, **146**, 212–221.

Swerdlow, N. R., Light, G. A., Thomas, M. L., et al. (2018). Deficient prepulse inhibition in schizophrenia in a multi-site cohort: Internal replication and extension. *Schizophr Res*, **198**, 6–15.

Wong, A. H. C., and Van Tol, H. H. M. (2003). Schizophrenia: From phenomenology to neurobiology. *Neurosci Biobehav Rev*, **27**, 269–306.

Wright, M. J., Jr., Vandewater, S. A., and Taffe, M. A. (2013). Cannabidiol attenuates deficits of visuospatial associative memory induced by Delta(9) tetrahydrocannabinol. *Br J Pharmacol*, **170**, 1365–1373.

Zuardi, A. W., Crippa, J. A., Hallak, J. E., et al. (2009). Cannabidiol for the treatment of psychosis in Parkinson's disease. *J Psychopharmacol*, **23**, 979–983.

Zuardi, A. W., Hallak, J. E., Dursun, S. M., et al. (2006). Cannabidiol monotherapy for treatment-resistant schizophrenia. *J Psychopharmacol*, **20**, 683–686.

Zuardi, A. W., Morais, S. L., Guimarães, F. S., et al. (1995). Antipsychotic effect of cannabidiol. *J Clin Psychiatry*, **56**, 485–486.

Zuardi, A. W., Rodrigues, J. A., and Cunha, J. M. (1991). Effects of cannabidiol in animal models predictive of antipsychotic activity. *Psychopharmacology (Berl)*, **104**, 260–264.

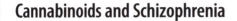
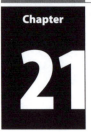

Chapter

21

Genetic Explanations for the Association between Cannabis and Schizophrenia

Sarah M. C. Colbert and Emma C. Johnson

21.1 Introduction

The relationship between cannabis and schizophrenia has long been a question of intense interest, with decades of cohort studies documenting increased rates of psychosis and schizophrenia in individuals who use cannabis (Andréasson et al., 1987; Di Forti et al., 2019a; Gage et al., 2016; van Os et al., 2002). The extent to which cannabis use causally increases the risk of developing schizophrenia is an important question, especially given changing sociocultural attitudes toward cannabis use and increased legalization (Hall et al., 2019). For example, one study found that the proportion of schizophrenia cases attributable to cannabis use disorder in Denmark has increased from 2% around 1995 to 8% in 2010; the authors speculate this is due to the increased use and potency of cannabis during that period (Hjorthøj et al., 2021a). However, it is difficult for epidemiologic studies to accurately estimate the causal effect of cannabis on schizophrenia due to the potential influence of confounding factors. Potential confounders of the relationship between cannabis and schizophrenia include shared environmental and genetic influences. For example, if there are genetic factors that increase a person's likelihood of heavy cannabis use, and some of those same factors also increase a person's risk of developing schizophrenia, this shared genetic pre-disposition may result in an *overestimate* of the causal link between cannabis use and higher rates of schizophrenia in a typical cohort study. For this reason, scientists have been interested in testing whether there is indeed evidence of shared genetic factors that contribute to both likelihood of cannabis use and schizophrenia risk.

In this chapter, we will review the evidence from studies that have tried to address the question of genetic overlap between cannabis use and schizophrenia (see Figure 21.1). First, we discuss the findings from twin and family studies, including discordant twin and sibling designs. Then, we move onto

molecular genetic studies (or studies that examine measured genotype data rather than similarity between relatives) which have used a variety of modern methods to test for genetic overlap; these include polygenic score approaches, the calculation of genetic correlations, and methods that attempt to parse causality in the presence of genetic pleiotropy. Throughout, we address limitations of all these various methods. Finally, we discuss what we may conclude from these genetically-informed studies and consider future directions in this area.

21.2 Evidence from Twin and Family Studies

There is substantial evidence for familial contributions to the relationship between schizophrenia and cannabis (McGuire et al., 1995), and family studies provide the perfect opportunity to account for familial confounding that may be due to either genetic factors, shared environmental factors, or both, which otherwise may go unmeasured. Family studies are frequently used in the field of behavioural genetics, with the specific study design depending on what level of familial relationships is available in the data. For example, when data between monozygotic twins are available, particularly for twin pairs in which a given phenotypic trait is only present in one of the twins, researchers can perform a discordant twin study (Vitaro et al., 2009). As monozygotic twins completely share their genetics as well as their family-level environment, any differences between the members of the twin pair (e.g., a schizophrenia case versus unaffected control) can be assumed to be due to unique environmental factors (e.g., cannabis use versus no cannabis use), enabling the identification of potentially causal relationships between the trait of interest (schizophrenia) and the unique environmental factors (cannabis use). In other samples where data may only exist for siblings, comparisons can still be

Genetic explanations for cannabis and schizophrenia: methods of assessment

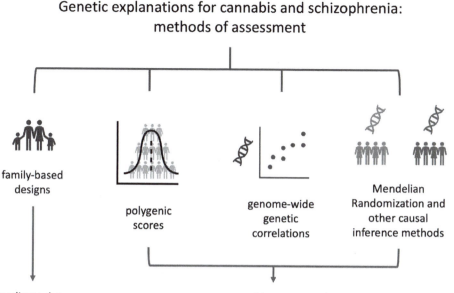

Figure 21.1 An overview of different methods for assessing whether cannabis use and schizophrenia have shared genetic overlap. Family-based designs leverage estimates of genetic sharing across different relationships (parent–child, siblings and dizygotic twins, monozygotic twins) to estimate shared genetic and environmental overlap of two traits; discordant relative designs can be used to determine whether there is evidence for causality. The remaining three methods rely on measured, genome-wide genotype data on common genetic variants. Polygenic scores represent an individual's genetic liability for a given trait and can be used to assess whether polygenic risk for schizophrenia, for example, is associated with cannabis use in an independent sample. Genetic correlations can be estimated from the summary statistics of two genome-wide association studies. Causal inference methods, like Mendelian randomization and latent causal variable analysis, use genetic variants as 'instruments' to try and assess whether there is evidence of causality. Latent causal variable analysis also estimates the genetic correlation between two traits and assesses the evidence for causality while accounting for this correlation.

made that account for familial confounding, as full siblings still share more genetic and environmental factors than two random non-relatives. Family studies are even able to utilize data from less related individuals, such as half siblings or cousins, to make comparisons between pairs of different degrees of relatedness, or between those with and without family history of a trait.

While there are plenty of family studies which examine cannabis use (Distel et al., 2011; Ellingson et al., 2021; Lynskey et al., 2003; Merikangas et al., 2009) and schizophrenia (Asarnow et al., 2001; Baron et al., 1985; Kendler et al., 1993; Maier et al., 1993) separately, few exist which look directly at the relationship between cannabis use and schizophrenia. However, there are family studies which consider the relationship between cannabis use and psychosis or psychotic-like experiences and, due to these traits close relatedness to schizophrenia (Andreasen, 1989; Yung et al., 2009), we choose to include these studies in our discussion as well. A leading explanation for

the genetic overlap between cannabis use and schizophrenia is that schizophrenia or psychosis may be caused by cannabis use (Arseneault et al., 2004; Degenhardt and Hall, 2006; Henquet et al., 2005; van Os et al., 2002). McGrath et al. (2010) used a sibling pair study to test whether the association between early cannabis use and psychosis-related outcomes within sibling pairs was significant, finding that, compared to their siblings, individuals with more years since first cannabis use did in fact score significantly higher on a questionnaire aimed to measure delusional-like experiences. Another sibling study found that individuals with schizophrenia used cannabis more frequently than their unaffected siblings and unrelated matched controls, yet sibling controls, with presumably a higher genetic predisposition for schizophrenia, and unrelated controls did not significantly differ in frequency of cannabis use (Veling et al., 2008). Further evidence that cannabis use may be a risk factor for psychosis comes from a co-twin control study performed by Nesvåg et al.

(2017), in which the latent risk of psychotic-like experiences was 3.5-times higher among individuals with cannabis use disorder symptoms, compared to their twin who experienced no symptoms of cannabis use disorder. Furthermore, a recent discordant twin/sibling study, which used twin and sibling pairs in which both members were cannabis exposed, found that psychotic-like experiences were more common in individuals who used cannabis more frequently compared to their twin or sibling (Karcher et al., 2019).

On the other hand, several family studies are contradictory, and find evidence to suggest that the relationship between cannabis use and schizophrenia or psychosis decreases after accounting for familial confounders, suggesting that overlap is more likely a result of common genetic pre-disposition or familial environmental factors. In a 2015 co-relative control study by Giordano et al., cannabis abuse was found to increase the likelihood of developing schizophrenia, however this association decreased as the level of genetic relatedness increased (Giordano et al., 2015). This decline observed in co-relative pairs of closer relatedness suggests a significant contribution of shared genetic components to the relationship between cannabis abuse and schizophrenia; however, the remaining 4-times higher risk for schizophrenia amongst cannabis abuse cases after controlling for familial contributions means causality, while not the only factor, could still partially underlie this association. More evidence for cannabis use alone being unlikely to cause schizophrenia or psychosis comes from a study by Proal et al. (2014), who found that individuals with a history of adolescent cannabis use had increased risk for schizophrenia because individuals with adolescent cannabis use were more likely to have a family history of schizophrenia compared to their non-using counterparts. A similar study was unable to detect any difference between cannabis users and non-users when measuring the proportion of individuals with a family history of schizophrenia (Boydell et al., 2007). Results of family studies likely differ according to the type of study design or the particular measures of cannabis use and schizophrenia/psychosis; however, while results of family studies do not converge on a common explanation underlying the relationship between cannabis use and schizophrenia, they point to a combination of causality and familial confounding, with cannabis use possibly exacerbating an individual's pre-existing liability toward schizophrenia (Karcher et al., 2019; Nesvåg et al., 2017).

21.3 Molecular Genetic Studies

Molecular genetic studies refer to studies that analyse individuals' measured genotypes and use that data to test hypotheses – including whether there are shared genetic factors that contribute to cannabis use and schizophrenia – rather than drawing inferences by studying family members with known degrees of genetic relatedness. Since genome-wide genotyping has become relatively cheap and efficient, there has been a proliferation of methods that can be applied to genome-wide data to assess not only the genetic factors underlying a single trait or disorder, but the simultaneous study of multiple disorders or traits as well. A genome-wide association study (GWAS), for example, tests whether any of the common single nucleotide polymorphisms (SNPs) that pass genotype quality control and imputation procedures in the study are statistically associated with the trait that is being studied. GWASs form the foundation for many of the other methods discussed in this chapter: polygenic scores, genome-wide genetic correlations, and causal inference methods using genetic instruments.

21.3.1 Polygenic Scores

A polygenic score is a method of aggregating the genetic signals for a trait across the genome and creating an individual 'genetic liability score' for each person in a study for whom genome-wide genotype data is available. To do this, we can simply take the effect sizes from a GWAS of, say, cannabis use, multiply those effect sizes by the number of risk alleles a person has at a given locus, and then sum those multiplications across all the genetic variants to create a polygenic score of cannabis use. This score would then represent an individual's genetic liability to use cannabis.

Polygenic scores are widely used for a number of reasons. First, for many complex, polygenic traits and disorders, GWAS sample sizes are still relatively small and under-powered. Because there are many common genetic variants that influence these traits and disorders and each genetic variant has a very small effect size, under-powered GWASs result in few genetic variants that pass the stringent statistical significance threshold of p-value $< 5e-8$. Polygenic scores skirt this issue by aggregating the genetic signal from more than just the few SNPs that pass the genome-wide significance threshold, thus including genetic contributions from many SNPs that may indeed be associated with the trait of interest but just missed the significance threshold. Second, polygenic scores can be used to examine cross-trait associations in samples where that type of examination otherwise would not be possible. For example, Power et al. (2014) used the largest GWAS of schizophrenia at the time to create a genetic risk score for schizophrenia in a small, independent sample and test whether polygenic liability for schizophrenia was associated with cannabis use. As schizophrenia is a relatively rare disorder, with an estimated population prevalence of 1% or less (Saha et al., 2005), most population-based samples, or even samples ascertained for other disorders, will have a very low occurrence of schizophrenia. However, a polygenic score approach allows researchers like Power et al. to leverage an existing GWAS of schizophrenia and examine cross-trait associations between liability to schizophrenia and whatever traits might be available in their smaller, independent samples.

Power et al. (2014) is one of the first examples of a study that used a polygenic score approach to examine whether there was evidence of shared genetic aetiology between schizophrenia and cannabis use. Using the largest GWAS of schizophrenia at the time ($N_{cases} = 13,833$, $N_{controls} = 18,310$), Power et al. tested whether a polygenic score for schizophrenia was associated with cannabis use, age of first use, and lifetime number of uses in a sample of 1,011 cannabis users and 1,071 non-users. They found that genetic risk for schizophrenia was significantly associated with likelihood of ever using cannabis and quantity of use but was not associated with age of initiation. These results suggest that, although the percent variance explained was quite small ($R^2 < 1\%$), some of the same alleles that contribute to schizophrenia risk also contribute to increased likelihood of cannabis use and quantity of use. Interestingly, they also saw this same pattern when they looked at a subset of twins: the authors found that twins who both used cannabis had the greatest burden of schizophrenia risk alleles, twin pairs where only one twin used cannabis had a moderate level of polygenic risk for schizophrenia, and twin pairs where neither used cannabis had the lowest levels of genetic risk for schizophrenia.

Reginsson et al. (2018) found similar results when they examined the association between polygenic scores for schizophrenia and bipolar and addiction phenotypes in a sample of 144,609 Icelandic individuals. Specifically, they found that polygenic liability for schizophrenia was significantly associated with increased risk of cannabis use disorder in the sample (OR = 1.23, $p = 1.1e{-}19$). Notably, individuals with schizophrenia diagnoses were excluded from the study, suggesting that cannabis use disorder and schizophrenia share risk alleles and this association was not driven by comorbid cases. Demontis et al. (2019) also found that a polygenic score for schizophrenia was significantly associated with cannabis use disorder in their sample ($N_{cases} = 2,387$).

Power et al. tested associations with cannabis *ever-use*, while Reginsson et al. and Demontis et al. looked at cannabis use *disorder* (a much more severe phenotype than whether someone has ever tried cannabis), but Carey et al. (2016) found significant, positive associations between a schizophrenia polygenic score and both non-problematic cannabis use *and* severe cannabis dependence. Similarly, Verweij et al. (2017) found that a polygenic score for schizophrenia was significantly associated with five of the eight cannabis use phenotypes they examined, including lifetime use, regular use, and quantity of use. This suggests that schizophrenia may share genetic factors with a range of stages of cannabis involvement.

There have also been a few studies that have found no significant association between polygenic liability for schizophrenia and cannabis use or use disorder. In a study of 88,637 individuals in the Danish registry system, Hjorthøj et al. (2021) found no evidence that a polygenic score for schizophrenia was associated with cannabis use disorder in controls, although the polygenic score *was* associated with cannabis use disorder in schizophrenia patients. Similarly, a pre-print from Di Forti et al. (2019b) reports that a polygenic score for schizophrenia does not significantly predict cannabis initiation, frequency of use, or the type of cannabis used (*p*-values > 0.06) in a sample of 492 first-episode psychosis patients and 787 controls.

While there is fairly strong evidence that the alleles that pre-dispose one to develop schizophrenia also contribute to likelihood of using cannabis, the literature on polygenic studies of cannabis use and schizophrenia is mixed; this may be due in part to heterogeneity across study samples, inconsistencies in polygenic score methodologies, and statistically under-powered GWAS samples. As GWASs of schizophrenia continue to grow, the true nature of genetic overlap between schizophrenia and cannabis use may become clearer.

21.3.2 SNP-based Genetic Correlations

While polygenic scores offer one method to estimate genetic overlap between traits, another approach to estimating shared genetic risks is to calculate the genome-wide genetic correlation between two traits. Published in 2015, a method called linkage disequilibrium score regression (LDSR) enabled the calculation of cross-trait genetic correlations without requiring individual-level genotype data (Bulik-Sullivan et al., 2015a, 2015b). This was a crucial advance; whereas individual-level genotype data in the target sample is required for the creation of polygenic scores, LDSR allows researchers to use what are called summary statistics – or in other words, the output of a GWAS – from two GWASs as input. As the summary statistics from a GWAS are much more easily shared among researchers than individual-level genotype data (which comes with restrictions due to identifiability and privacy concerns), LDSR has enabled many analyses that would not otherwise be possible.

Multiple studies have reported significant, positive genetic correlations between cannabis use (and cannabis use disorder) and schizophrenia, including the largest GWAS of lifetime cannabis use to date from Pasman et al. (2018) (N = 184,765). Using LDSR, Pasman et al. identified a modest but significant positive genetic correlation between lifetime cannabis use and schizophrenia ($r_g = 0.25$). Verweij et al. (2017) found very similar results in their LDSR analysis on schizophrenia and cannabis use ($r_g = 0.22$). A large GWAS of cannabis use disorder ($N_{cases} = 20,916$) also identified a significant positive correlation with schizophrenia ($r_g = 0.31$) (Johnson et al., 2020). Furthermore, a recent study by one of the current authors found that, even when accounting for the genetic effects of tobacco smoking and cannabis ever-use in the same model, the genetic association between cannabis use disorder and schizophrenia remains significant (Johnson et al., 2021). One recent study did not find a significant genetic correlation between cannabis use disorder and schizophrenia, but it should be noted that it was using a much smaller GWAS of cannabis use disorder ($N_{cases} = 2,387$) (Abdellaoui et al., 2021).

Overall, the findings from genetic correlation studies support the existence of genetic overlap between cannabis use and schizophrenia. As is the case for polygenic risk score studies, increasingly large and well-powered GWASs in the years to come may refine some of these estimates of genetic overlap.

21.3.3 Causal Inference Methods

Some studies have sought to use genetic data to estimate the causal relationship between cannabis use and schizophrenia while accounting for their shared genetic factors. These two possible mechanisms that may account for the comorbidity of cannabis use and schizophrenia – common genetic pre-disposition and causality – are not mutually exclusive. Still, to accurately estimate the causal effect of cannabis use on risk of developing schizophrenia, one must account for their shared genetic factors to the best of our ability.

One method for estimating causal relationships using genetic data is called Mendelian Randomization (MR). Briefly, this approach can be thought of as analogous to a randomized controlled trial (RCT); just as patients in an RCT are randomly assigned to either the treatment or placebo arm – thereby mitigating the influence of possible confounders – our genotypes are randomly 'assigned' at birth. Thus, if we consider the inheritance of a risk allele for, say, heavy cannabis use to be analogous to the 'treatment' arm of a RCT, we can then observe whether individuals with that risk allele tend to develop schizophrenia more often than individuals without that risk allele, and thus draw conclusions about the causal role of cannabis use on schizophrenia risk. Critically, one assumption that must be met in order for an MR study to be valid is that the risk allele(s), or genetic instruments, of interest must only be associated with the outcome (schizophrenia) via the exposure (cannabis use); that is, the genetic instruments must not be associated with the outcome through any pathway other than one mediated by the exposure. This assumption is difficult to meet for complex traits such as cannabis use and schizophrenia, as they are influenced by a range of genetic and environmental factors, some of which may overlap and/or interact in unknown ways.

The MR literature on cannabis and schizophrenia is rather mixed. One MR study from Vaucher et al. (2017) found evidence of a causal effect of genetic liability to cannabis ever-use on schizophrenia risk but two other MR studies found stronger evidence for a causal effect in the *opposite* direction: genetic liability to schizophrenia increasing the likelihood of cannabis use (Gage et al., 2017; Pasman et al., 2018). All of the above studies have looked at a measure of lifetime cannabis ever-use, and few MR studies have looked at heavy or problematic cannabis use. However, one of the current authors recently published a paper that included a type of MR called a multivariable MR analysis, which simultaneously accounts for additional risk factors in the model, to assess the causal relationship between cannabis use disorder and schizophrenia. We found some evidence that genetic liability to cannabis use disorder increases risk of schizophrenia ($\beta = 0.10$, 95% CI = 0.02–0.18), accounting for the genetic effects of cannabis ever-use, ever-smoked tobacco regularly, and nicotine dependence (Johnson et al., 2021). In univariate MR analyses, we found evidence of a *bidirectional* causal relationship, whereby genetic liability to cannabis use disorder causes increased risk of schizophrenia *and* genetic liability to schizophrenia causally increases risk of cannabis use disorder.

Given the evidence for widespread pleiotropy, or shared genetic influences, amongst complex traits (including cannabis use and schizophrenia), other methods have been developed that attempt to account for genetic correlation between traits while estimating their causal relationship. One such method is called latent causal variable (LCV) analysis, which estimates the 'genetic causality proportion' of two traits while simultaneously accounting for their genetic correlation and other potential confounders, like sample overlap between two studies (O'Connor and Price, 2018). In the same study referenced above (Johnson et al., 2021), we also performed an LCV analysis and found no evidence of genetic causality between cannabis use disorder and schizophrenia (genetic causality proportion = –0.08, *p*-value = 0.87). This finding is actually consistent with the bidirectional relationship estimated in the univariate MR analyses (i.e., liability to cannabis use disorder causing increased schizophrenia risk *and* liability to schizophrenia causing increased risk of cannabis use disorder), as LCV cannot account for a bidirectional relationship (the effects in opposite directions essentially cancel each other out).

While the results from MR and other causal inference methods are inconclusive in terms of a causal relationship between cannabis and schizophrenia, with most studies suggesting either bidirectionality or a relationship in the direction of schizophrenia liability causally increasing risk of cannabis use, better-powered GWAS that provide stronger genetic instruments may help to clarify these relationships. Triangulating across evidence from longitudinal cohort studies alongside MR and other genetic methods may prove helpful in discerning the degree to which the comorbidity of cannabis use and schizophrenia is due to shared genetic factors and/or a causal effect of cannabis use increasing one's risk of developing schizophrenia.

21.4 Conclusion

Overall, the evidence from family-based studies and more modern statistical genetic methods suggests that there *is* some shared genetic basis between cannabis use and schizophrenia, albeit modest, with most estimates of genetic correlation hovering around $r_g = 0.25 - 0.30$. This does *not* mean that anyone who uses cannabis is destined to develop schizophrenia because of their genetics, or vice versa. There are two key facts to keep in mind when interpreting the studies presented in this chapter:

- Each common genetic variant associated with a complex trait like cannabis use contributes a *very* small amount of risk, and there is no set number of or specific group of variants that are necessary and sufficient to express a complex trait; and

- All of the genetic correlations and associations reported here are population-level measures; this does *not* necessarily mean they are relevant at the level of individual risk prediction.

Furthermore, evidence of a shared genetic basis does not preclude the existence of a *causal* relationship between cannabis use and schizophrenia risk – this simply suggests that there are common genetic factors that contribute to both phenotypes, and this shared pre-disposition must be taken into account when analysing cross-sectional or longitudinal cohort data to estimate the causal effect of cannabis on the development of psychosis and schizophrenia.

Interestingly, schizophrenia appears to share genetic risk with multiple stages of cannabis involvement, from initiation to diagnostic levels of problem use. In contrast, much of the evidence for a causal influence of cannabis on psychosis and schizophrenia from epidemiologic studies has been found specifically for heavy cannabis use (Di Forti et al., 2014; Marconi et al., 2016), not just initiation or occasional use. It may be that the genetic variants which influence liability for both cannabis use and schizophrenia are related to openness to new experiences or some other trait that is shared across the different stages of cannabis involvement.

One key limitation of most genetically-informed studies of cannabis and schizophrenia, or at least those dealing with genome-wide data, is that there is often little data available on comorbid phenotypes in a GWAS focused on one particular trait. While this is not as much of a concern for a GWAS of cannabis use (because schizophrenia is relatively rare and thus less likely to be present in the GWAS samples), it is much more likely that individuals in a GWAS of schizophrenia will have comorbid cannabis use and maybe even cannabis use disorder. This could potentially lead to overestimates of the true genetic correlation between cannabis use and schizophrenia. Future efforts to track down and account for comorbid cases in GWAS must be made. As the majority of large GWAS are formed via extensive meta-analysis efforts, this will be a difficult task but extremely informative and important for future cross-disorder work.

In summary, the majority of family-based studies and molecular genetic studies point to evidence of a shared genetic overlap between cannabis use and schizophrenia. It seems likely that both common genetic pre-dispositions as well as a causal effect of heavy and high-potency cannabis use on psychosis contribute to the comorbidity between cannabis use and schizophrenia.

References

Abdellaoui, A., Smit, D. J. A., van den Brink, W., et al. (2021). Genomic relationships across psychiatric disorders including substance use disorders. *Drug Alcohol Depend*, **220**, 108535.

Andreasen, N. C. (1989). The American concept of schizophrenia. *Schizophr Bull*, **15**, 519–531.

Andréasson, S., Allbeck, P., Engström, A., et al. (1987). Cannabis and schizophrenia: A longitudinal study of Swedish conscripts. *Lancet*, **330**, 1483–1486.

Arseneault, L., Cannon, M., Witton, J., et al. (2004). Causal association between cannabis and psychosis: Examination of the evidence. *Br J Psychiatry*, **184**, 110–117.

Asarnow, R. F., Nuechterlein, K. H., Fogelson, D., et al. (2001). Schizophrenia and schizophrenia-spectrum personality disorders in the first-degree relatives of children with schizophrenia: The UCLA family study. *Arch Gen Psychiatry*, **58**, 581–588.

Baron, M., Gruen, R., Rainer, J. D., et al. (1985). A family study of schizophrenic and normal control probands: Implications for the spectrum concept of schizophrenia. *Am J Psychiatry*, **142**, 447–455.

Boydell, J., Dean, K., Dutta, R., et al. (2007). A comparison of symptoms and family history in schizophrenia with and without prior cannabis use: Implications for the concept of cannabis psychosis. *Schizophr Res*, **93**, 203–210.

Bulik-Sullivan, B. K., Finucane, H. K., Anttila, V., et al. (2015a). An atlas of genetic correlations across human diseases and traits. *Nat Genet*, **47**, 1236.

Bulik-Sullivan, B. K., Loh, P.-R., et al. (2015b). LD score regression distinguishes confounding from polygenicity in genome-wide association studies. *Nat Genet*, **47**, 291–295.

Carey, C. E., Agrawal, A., Bucholz, K. K., et al. (2016). Associations between polygenic risk for psychiatric disorders and substance involvement. *Front Genet*, **7**, 149.

Degenhardt, L., and Hall, W. (2006). Is cannabis use a contributory cause of psychosis? *Can J Psychiatry*, **51**, 556–565.

Demontis, D., Rajagopal, V. M., Thorgeirsson, T. E., et al. (2019). Genome-wide association study implicates CHRNA2 in cannabis use disorder. *Nat Neurosci*, **22**, 1066–1074.

Distel, M. A., Vink, J. M., Bartels, M., et al. (2011). Age moderates non-genetic influences on the initiation of cannabis use: A twin-sibling study in Dutch adolescents and young adults. *Addiction*, **106**, 1658–1666.

Ellingson, J. M., Ross, J. M., Winiger, E., et al. (2021). Familial factors may not explain the effect of moderate-to-heavy cannabis use on cognitive functioning in adolescents: A sibling-comparison study. *Addiction*, **116**, 833–844.

Di Forti, M., Quattrone, D., Freeman, T. P., et al. (2019a). The contribution of cannabis use to variation in the incidence of psychotic disorder across Europe (EU-GEI): A multicentre case-control study. *Lancet Psychiatry*, **6**, 427–436.

Di Forti, M., Sallis, H., Allegri, F., et al. (2014). Daily use, especially of high-potency cannabis, drives the earlier onset of psychosis in cannabis users. *Schizophr Bull*, **40**, 1509–1517.

Di Forti, M., Wu-Choi, B., Quattrone, D., et al. (2019b). The independent and combined influence of schizophrenia polygenic risk score and heavy cannabis use on risk for psychotic disorder: A case-control analysis from the EUGEI study. *bioRxiv*, 844803.

Gage, S. H., Hickman, M., and Zammit, S. (2016). Association between cannabis and psychosis: Epidemiologic evidence. *Biol Psychiatry*, **79**, 549–556.

Gage, S. H., Jones, H. J., Burgess, S., et al. (2017). Assessing causality in associations between cannabis use and schizophrenia risk:

A two-sample Mendelian randomization study. *Psychol Med*, **47**, 971–980.

Giordano, G. N., Ohlsson, H., Sundquist, K., et al. (2015). The association between cannabis abuse and subsequent schizophrenia: A Swedish national co-relative control study. *Psychol Med*, **45**, 407–414.

Hall, W., Stjepanović, D., Caulkins, J., et al. (2019). Public health implications of legalising the production and sale of cannabis for medicinal and recreational use. *Lancet*, **394**, 1580–1590.

Henquet, C., Murray, R., Linszen, D., et al. (2005). The environment and schizophrenia: The role of cannabis use. *Schizophr Bull*, **31**, 608–612.

Hjorthøj, C., Uddin, M. J., Wimberley, T., et al. (2021). No evidence of associations between genetic liability for schizophrenia and development of cannabis use disorder. *Psychol Med*, **51**, 479–484.

Johnson, E. C., Demontis, D., Thorgeirsson, T. E., et al. (2020). A large-scale genome-wide association study meta-analysis of cannabis use disorder. *Lancet Psychiatry*, **7**, 1032–1045.

Johnson, E. C., Hatoum, A. S., Deak, J. D., et al. (2021). The relationship between cannabis and schizophrenia: A genetically informed perspective. *Addiction*, **116**, 3227–3234.

Karcher, N. R., Barch, D. M., Demers, C. H., et al. (2019). Genetic predisposition vs individual-specific processes in the association between psychotic-like experiences and cannabis use. *JAMA Psychiatry*, **76**, 87–94.

Kendler, K. S., McGuire, M., Gruenberg, A. M., et al. (1993). The Roscommon Family Study: III. Schizophrenia-related personality disorders in relatives. *Arch Gen Psychiatry*, **50**, 781–788.

Lynskey, M. T., Heath, A. C., Bucholz, K. K., et al. (2003). Escalation of drug use in early-onset cannabis users vs co-twin controls. *JAMA*, **289**, 427–433.

Maier, W., Lichtermann, D., Minges, J., et al. (1993). Continuity and discontinuity of affective disorders and schizophrenia: Results of a controlled family study. *Arch Gen Psychiatry*, **50**, 871–883.

Marconi, A., Di Forti, M., Lewis, C. M., et al. (2016). Meta-analysis of the association between the level of cannabis use and risk of psychosis. *Schizophr Bull*, **42**, 1262–1269.

McGrath, J., Welham, J., Scott, J., et al. (2010). Association between cannabis use and psychosis-related outcomes using sibling pair analysis in a cohort of young adults. *Arch Gen Psychiatry*, **67**, 440–447.

McGuire, P. K., Jones, P., Harvey, I., et al. (1995). Morbid risk of schizophrenia for relatives of patients with cannabis-associated psychosis. *Schizophr Res*, **15**, 277–281.

Merikangas, K. R., Li, J. J., Stipelman, B., et al. (2009). The familial aggregation of cannabis use disorders. *Addiction*, **104**, 622–629.

Nesvåg, R., Reichborn-Kjennerud, T., Gillespie, N. A., et al. (2017). Genetic and environmental contributions to the association between cannabis use and psychotic-like experiences in young adult twins. *Schizophr Bull*, **43**, 644–653.

O'Connor, L. J., and Price, A. L. (2018). Distinguishing genetic correlation from causation across 52 diseases and complex traits. *Nat Genet*, **50**, 1728–1734.

van Os, J., Bak, M., Hanssen, M., et al. (2002). Cannabis use and psychosis: A longitudinal population-based study. *Am J Epidemiol*, **156**, 319–327.

Pasman, J. A., Verweij, K. J. H., Gerring, Z., et al. (2018). GWAS of lifetime cannabis use reveals new risk loci, genetic overlap with psychiatric traits, and a causal influence of schizophrenia. *Nat Neurosci*, **21**, 1161–1170.

Power, R. A., Verweij, K. J., Zuhair, M., et al. (2014). Genetic predisposition to schizophrenia associated with increased use of cannabis. *Mol Psychiatry*, **19**, 1201.

Proal, A. C., Fleming, J., Galvez-Buccollini, J. A., et al. (2014). A controlled family study of cannabis users with and without psychosis. *Schizophr Res*, **152**, 283–288.

Reginsson, G. W., Ingason, A., Euesden, J., et al. (2018). Polygenic risk scores for schizophrenia and bipolar disorder associate with addiction. *Addict Biol*, **23**, 485–492.

Saha, S., Chant, D., Welham, J., et al. (2005). A systematic review of the prevalence of schizophrenia. *PLoS Med*, **2**, e141.

Vaucher, J., Keating, B. J., Lasserre, A. M., et al. (2017). Cannabis use and risk of schizophrenia: A Mendelian randomization study. *Mol Psychiatry*, **23**, 1287.

Veling, W., Mackenbach, J. P., van Os, J., et al. (2008). Cannabis use and genetic predisposition for schizophrenia: A case-control study. *Psychol Med*, **38**, 1251–1256.

Verweij, K. J. H., Abdellaoui, A., Nivard, M. G., et al. (2017). Genetic association between schizophrenia and cannabis use. *Drug Alcohol Depend*, **171**, 117–121.

Vitaro, F., Brendgen, M., and Arseneault, L. (2009). The discordant MZ-twin method: One step closer to the holy grail of causality. *Int J Behav Dev*, **33**, 376–382.

Yung, A. R., Nelson, B., Baker, K., et al. (2009). Psychotic-like experiences in a community sample of adolescents: Implications for the continuum model of psychosis and prediction of schizophrenia. *Aust NZ J Psychiatry*, **43**, 118–128.

Chapter 22

The Acute Effects of Cannabinoids in Patients with Psychotic Illness

Suhas Ganesh, Cécile Henquet, R. Andrew Sewell, Rebecca Kuepper, Mohini Ranganathan, and Deepak Cyril D'Souza

22.1 Introduction

As discussed in other chapters in this book, the acute effects of cannabis and cannabinoids in healthy humans have been well-characterized. This chapter reviews the acute effects of cannabis and cannabinoids in people with psychotic illness, as well as those at clinical high risk (CHR).

People with schizophrenia have a higher lifetime risk of having substance use and substance use disorders than the general population (Cantor-Graae et al., 2001; Kessler et al., 2005; Khokhar et al., 2018; McCreadie, 2002; Regier et al., 1990; Ringen et al., 2008; Swartz et al., 2006). Data from 53 treatment studies of schizophrenia patients revealed that 12-month prevalence estimates of use and misuse of cannabis were 29% and 19%, respectively, while lifetime use and misuse estimates were 42% and 23%, respectively (Green et al., 2005). The rates of problematic cannabis use in people with schizophrenia and psychotic disorders aggregate around 25% (Koskinen et al., 2010) compared to ~3% in the general population (Hasin, 2018). The median rate of cannabis misuse has been shown to be higher in first-episode (current 28.6%, lifetime 44.4%) than chronic patients (current 22.0%, lifetime 12.2%).

Understanding the rates of cannabis use and misuse in individuals at risk for psychosis and with first episode psychosis is particularly important. A recent meta-analysis of 35 studies on the prevalence of cannabis use in first episode psychosis noted a pooled prevalence of 33.7% (Myles et al., 2016). Cannabis use amounting to abuse or dependence has been demonstrated to increase the odds of transition to psychosis in those at CHR for psychotic disorders (Kraan et al., 2016). Following the recent trends toward liberalization of cannabis use in many jurisdictions, during the period from 2002 to 2017, an increase in the rates of use (10.4%–15.3%) as well as daily use (1.9%–4.2%) has been noted among US adults

(Compton et al., 2019). However, the specific trends in people with schizophrenia spectrum disorders remain to be accurately determined. Given that cannabis use in psychotic patients is associated with exacerbation of symptoms, higher rates of hospitalization, and poorer functional outcomes (Lowe et al., 2019; Rabin and George, 2017), understanding the acute effects is important. Information about the acute effects of cannabis and cannabinoids on individuals with, without, or at risk for schizophrenia comes from retrospective self-reports, real-time self-reports, and experimental studies.

22.2 Effects of Cannabis in Clinical High-Risk Groups and Recently-Diagnosed Patients

22.2.1 Retrospective Self-Reports

Dimensional approaches to the understanding of psychosis are discussed in detail in Chapters 16 and 23. Barkus and Lewis (2008) investigated the effects of cannabis in individuals with high versus average 'psychosis-proneness'. Psychosis-proneness was determined psychometrically using the Schizotypal Personality Questionnaire (SPQ) (Raine, 1991), and the authors developed a self-report questionnaire, the Cannabis Experiences Questionnaire (CEQ), to investigate acute 'Pleasurable Experiences' and 'Psychosis-like Experiences', as well as 'After-Effects' following cannabis use (Barkus et al., 2006). They showed that individuals with high psychosis-proneness reported higher levels of both pleasurable experiences and psychosis-like experiences when smoking cannabis than did controls. These authors further investigated the effects of high schizotypy on Δ^9-THC sensitivity and found that high-scoring schizotypes were more likely to report psychosis-like experiences and unpleasant after-effects following cannabis exposure (Stirling et al., 2008).

Another study examined the effects of cannabis use in patients recently diagnosed with or at CHR for schizophrenia (Peters et al., 2009). The authors developed an in-house 'yes–no' questionnaire of acute effects of cannabis compiled from previous studies on subjective effects of cannabis or drugs in general in schizophrenia patients, and a list of chronic effects of cannabis relating to prodromal signs of schizophrenia from the literature on long-term effects of frequent cannabis use in subjects without major psychiatric illness. Recent-onset subjects (diagnosed using the Inventory for the Retrospective Assessment of the Onset of Schizophrenia) were asked to rate only those effects that they had experienced before the first onset of their psychosis. High-risk patients reported feeling more anxious, depressed, and suspicious soon after cannabis use, but some also felt less depressed. Recently diagnosed schizophrenia patients also reported increased visual and auditory hallucinations and confusion after cannabis use. Both patient groups reported the long-term effects of cannabis use to be depression, less control over thoughts, and social problems. Finally, a large proportion (37%) of recent-onset schizophrenia patients reported that their first psychotic symptoms occurred during cannabis intoxication.

One case report has described repeated paranoid psychosis precipitated by smoking 'Spice', a blend of the synthetic cannabinoids CP-47,497 and JWH-018 (see Chapter 3). The man (age 25 years) had a strong family history of schizophrenia and had experienced his first psychotic break at age 18 precipitated by smoking cannabis. He had several further psychotic episodes thereafter, all triggered by smoking cannabis. He subsequently smoked Spice on three separate occasions and developed an acute psychotic relapse on each occasion, with marked auditory command hallucinations and paranoid delusions, which were new symptoms for him (Muller et al., 2010). Another case series described four hospitalized patients with a known diagnosis of schizophrenia who used synthetic cannabinoid AM-2201 (confirmed with gas chromatography-mass spectrometry) while hospitalized for a psychotic episode. The use of the synthetic cannabinoid resulted in the appearance of new psychotic symptoms, along with worsening of mood and anxiety symptoms; the authors did not note worsening of pre-existing psychotic symptoms (Celofiga et al., 2014). Other reports have noted psychotic episodes induced by these synthetic cannabinoids in healthy

people (Missouri Department of Health and Senior Services, 2010; Vearrier and Osterhoudt, 2010) (Figure 22.1; Box 22.1).

22.2.2 Retrospective Clinical Data

Self-reported cannabis use is high among people with established schizophrenia, who describe positive effects from cannabis use, such as improved mood and sleep, and lessened social anxiety, even though cannabis use seems to worsen psychotic symptoms during the course of illness and negatively impacts the disease course (Grech et al., 2005; Linszen and van Amelsvoort, 2007). Most studies of first-episode patients demonstrate that substance misuse typically precedes psychosis onset, often by several years (Buhler et al., 2002; Mauri et al., 2006; Rabinowitz et al., 1998; Silver and Abboud, 1994), and this is particularly true of cannabis misuse (Allebeck et al., 1993; Linszen et al., 1994). The interval between the initiation of regular cannabis use and the age of onset of psychotic disorder has been estimated to be ~6.3 years (Myles et al., 2016). It is less clear the extent to which substance misuse precedes prodromal symptoms, albeit two studies reported that pre-prodromal substance misuse occurred in around a third (28% to 34%) of schizophrenia patients (Hambrecht and Hafner, 1996; Veen et al., 2004). In a study of first-episode psychosis, Compton et al. (2009) showed that *progression* to daily cannabis use increases the risk for prodromal symptoms and psychotic illness, although daily cannabis use in itself does not. The authors concluded that an increase in cannabis use may hasten the onset of prodromal as well as psychotic symptoms. Another meta-analysis noted that, while lifetime-cannabis use by itself did not increase the rates of conversion to psychosis in CHR individuals, cannabis abuse and dependence as per DSM-IV (currently equivalent of cannabis use disorder) increased the odds of conversion by 1.75 times, consistent with the earlier reports.

More recently, McHugh et al. (2017) examined the prognostic significance of experiencing attenuated psychotic symptoms (APS) induced by cannabis in CHR individuals. Cannabis abuse was noted in 58% of the 190 CHR individuals recruited for the study and cannabis-induced APS were present in 26%. The latter sub-group was 4.9 (95% CI = 1.93–12.44) times more likely to transition to psychosis over a mean duration of 5 years. The authors suggested that a sub-

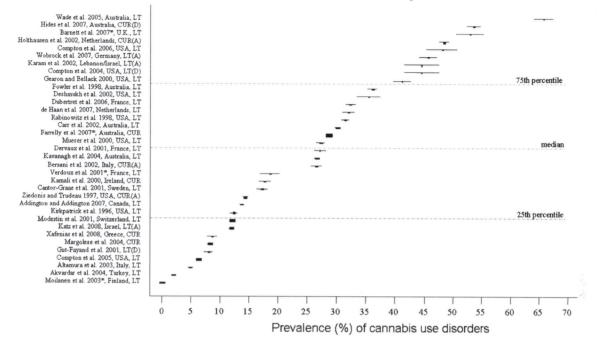

Cannabis Use Disorders in Schizophrenia

With permission from Koskinen et al., 2010

Figure 22.1 Meta-analysis of prevalence of cannabis use disorders in schizophrenia. With permission from Koskinen et al. (2010).

Box 22.1 Effects of cannabis in clinical high-risk groups and recently-diagnosed patients

- The prevalence of cannabis use and cannabis use disorder are higher among persons with psychosis.
- Many people with a psychotic illness or at risk thereof experience their first psychotic symptom under the influence of cannabis.
- In those at risk for psychosis, cannabis-induced attenuated psychotic symptoms increase the odds of conversion to psychosis by around 5-times.
- Both cannabis and synthetic cannabinoids have been described to precipitate psychotic episodes.

---

population of people at CHR for psychosis may be specifically vulnerable to the psychotomimetic properties of cannabis, possibly reflecting genetic vulnerability or other unmeasured factors. Wainberg et al. (2021) tested the relationship between self-reported cannabis use and psychosis-like experiences and the influence of schizophrenia Polygenic Risk Score, using data from the UK biobank. In addition to finding a strong association between self-reported cannabis use and self-reported psychosis-like experiences, the authors noted that those with higher schizophrenia polygenic risk score had higher risk

for particular psychotic symptoms such as auditory hallucinations, visual hallucinations, and delusions of reference. These data complement the results of a meta-analysis in UHR subjects that found that those who used cannabis experienced significantly more symptoms of unusual thought content and suspiciousness compared to non-users (Carney et al., 2017). Hindocha et al. (2020) examined the effects of polymorphisms in *AKT1* (rs2494732), *COMT* Val158Met (rs4680), and *FAAH* (rs324420) on cannabis experiences in a large cohort of first episode psychosis patients, cannabis using controls, and

227

non-using young adults. Patients experienced more cannabis-induced psychotic-like experiences compared to both control groups. Cannabis-induced euphoric experiences were more common in the young adult controls compared to the other two groups. None of the genetic polymorphisms tested had a significant interaction effects for either psychosis-like or euphoric experiences induced by cannabis (Hindocha et al., 2020).

Taken together, these results suggest that a subgroup of individuals who experience attenuated psychosis symptoms following cannabis exposure among those with CHR for psychosis may be particularly vulnerable to develop a persisting psychotic disorder. Furthermore, genetic risk for schizophrenia may specifically enhance the risk of developing positive symptoms such as hallucinations and delusions following acute cannabis exposure.

22.3 Acute Effects of Cannabis in People with Established Schizophrenia

22.3.1 Retrospective Self-Reports

Few studies have investigated schizophrenia patients' subjective experiences following cannabis use. Outcomes from such studies include no reported effects (Peralta and Cuesta, 1992); reductions in anxiety, depression, and negative symptoms; increased suspiciousness; and variable effects on hallucinations (Arndt et al., 1992; Dixon et al., 1990; Peralta and Cuesta, 1992). Dixon et al. (1990) assessed the self-reported acute effects of alcohol, cannabis, and cocaine in 40 patients with schizophrenia or schizophreniform psychosis. The majority reported decreased dysphoria in association with all three drugs, decreased anxiety with cannabis and alcohol, increased anxiety with cocaine, and increased paranoia and hallucinations with cannabis and cocaine but not from alcohol. Weil (1970) found that many patients reported derealization in association with cannabis. In contrast, Hekimian and Gershon (1968) described favourable subjective responses in cannabis using patients with schizophrenia. Knudsen and Vilmar (1984) found that patients reported feeling 'inspired, relaxed, energized, or active' following cannabis use, and also used cannabis to reverse the side-effects of antipsychotic medication. After these initial positive effects, however, patients described an exacerbation of positive psychotic symptoms and increases in dysphoria and aggression.

Reports of the subjective effect of cannabis use on psychotic symptoms have been contradictory. Cannabis was reported by some patients to be unpleasant and to cause adverse psychic effects (Negrete et al., 1986). Treffert (1978) followed four schizophrenia patients longitudinally and found severe exacerbations of psychosis and functional deterioration after periods of moderate cannabis use, while a later study found half of a group of patients felt cannabis increased their positive symptoms (Addington and Duchak, 1997). However, Knudsen and Vilmar (1984) had reported patients observing that cannabis helped to reverse neuroleptic effects and to inspire, energize, or relax. Gregg et al. (2009) found roughly half of 45 participants (50.9%) reported that they were using drugs (including cannabis) or alcohol to cope with or reduce auditory hallucinations; somewhat more (57.4%) were using drugs to abate feelings of suspiciousness or paranoia, and two out of five (38.7%) were using drugs when they were experiencing medication side-effects. In another study, chronically treated psychotic patients were asked a series of questions about how their antipsychotic medication affected their psychosis (Kapur et al., 2005). Among the most common reported effects was that the medication 'helps me stop thinking' so that 'the symptoms do not bother me so much'. It is possible that, from the patients' viewpoint, cannabis use is beneficial because it decreases their pre-occupation with psychotic symptoms, even as it increases symptoms as measured objectively. Alternatively, while cannabis may increase psychotic symptoms, cannabis may also reduce symptom-related distress, such that users may experience the overall effects of cannabis as 'beneficial'.

One area that remains largely unexplored is drug users' *stated reasons for drug use* – what they *believe* leads them to use. These perceptions, however inaccurate, may themselves drive drug-taking behaviour and thus merit further investigation (Dixon et al., 1991). Behaviour is often based on attitudes that are shaped by beliefs (Fishbein, 1980). Beliefs that are based on personal experience have a stronger influence in the formation of attitudes than information gained in other ways, and better predict later behaviour (Fazio and Zanna, 1981). Thus, what drug users believe are their reasons for using drugs may be a crucial determinant of their drug-use behaviour, including whether they continue to use or relapse (Box 22.2).

> **Box 22.2** Reported acute effects of cannabis in people with established schizophrenia
>
> - The self-medication hypothesis suggests that people with psychosis use cannabis to alleviate the psychotic symptoms and medication side-effects.
> - There is little support for this hypothesis as this is the least endorsed reason for use across many studies.
> - Commonly cited reasons for use are to enhance positive mood, to cope with negative emotion, and for social reasons.

Numerous qualitative studies have been conducted in North America, Australia, and Europe investigating self-reported reasons for drug use in patients with psychotic disorders. Some protocols involve patients selecting reasons for use from pre-determined lists (Addington and Duchak, 1997; Dixon et al., 1991; Test et al., 1989; Warner et al., 1994); others ask open-ended questions (Baigent et al., 1995; Fowler et al., 1998). Despite differences in methodology, results are similar. There are three main motives for drug use, regardless of the drug type:

1. To enhance positive mood or achieve intoxication –'get high' (Dixon et al., 1991) or 'feel good' (Fowler et al., 1998).
2. To cope with negative emotions – 'decrease depression' or 'relax' (Addington and Duchak, 1997; Baker et al., 2002; Dixon et al., 1991; Fowler et al., 1998; Gearon et al., 2001; Goswami et al., 2004; B. Green et al., 2004; Schofield et al., 2006; Spencer et al., 2002).
3. For social reasons – 'something to do with friends' (Test et al., 1989) and 'to face people better' (Fowler et al., 1998).

In a review of 14 studies specifically addressing self-reported reasons for cannabis use in patients with psychotic disorders, Dekker et al. (2009) concluded that these three reasons were the most cited, with only a minority (12.9%) reporting cannabis use as a means to relieve medication side-effects or symptoms of psychosis such as hallucinations and suspiciousness. People with psychosis appear more likely to use cannabis for mood elevation than for relaxation; less likely to use out of habit or for social reasons, and more likely to use to cope with boredom or other negative affective states (A. I. Green et al., 2004). In a study that examined the reasons for cannabis use in patients with first episode psychosis comparing non-psychosis cannabis users, the distinguishing reasons for use were 'to arrange thoughts' and 'to decrease hallucinations and suspiciousness' (Mane et al., 2015).

However, a study that examined five domains for reasons of use longitudinally at baseline, 3 months, and 12 months noted that 'relief of positive symptoms and side-effects' was the least endorsed reason at each time point. The most endorsed reasons were 'enhancement' followed by 'coping with negative affect' and 'social motive'. Interestingly, the strength of endorsement decreased for all five domains over the longitudinal follow-up (Kolliakou et al., 2015).

Of course, retrospective self-report data are subject to distortion. Individuals who misuse substances typically use denial and rationalization to justify their use. In addition, cannabis alters perception and has amnestic effects that may influence the interpretation of events and, therefore, interfere with the accurate recall of cannabis effects. Cannabis is often used in combination with nicotine, alcohol, and other illicit drugs, so it is difficult to attribute consequences solely to cannabis in naturalistic studies. Finally, it is possible that the positive and negative effects of cannabis may be dose-related, and dose–response relationships are almost impossible to assess in naturalistic studies because cannabis dose is seldom measured, and its principal psychoactive ingredient (Δ^9-THC) is not assayed. Some limitations of self-report can be addressed through experimental studies as well as experience sampling.

22.3.2 Experience Sampling

Although studies reviewed here have shown that patients are generally more sensitive to the acute negative effects of cannabis, the beneficial effects of cannabis use that patients themselves report often lead them to continue to use despite long-term negative consequences. Evidence that patients may use cannabis to 'self-medicate' distress associated with their illness comes from a population-based study that linked vulnerability for psychosis in cannabis-naïve individuals with future cannabis use (Ferdinand et al., 2005). However, other population-based studies found no such evidence for self-medication effects (Henquet et al., 2005; Stefanis et al., 2004). Henquet et al. (2010) conducted a *momentary assessment study* to explore the complicated dynamics of cannabis use and its varied effects in psychotic patients in the context of daily life by using the Experience Sampling Method (ESM) (Myin-Germeys et al., 2001, 2002).[1] The study investigated the acute effects of cannabis on mood and psychotic symptoms in the daily life of 42 patients with a psychotic disorder and 38 healthy controls who were all regular cannabis users. The frequency of cannabis use was significantly higher in patients than in controls, but there was no evidence for self-medication, as neither positive nor negative affect predicted cannabis use at the next sampling point. Similarly, no associations were found between delusions or hallucinations and subsequent cannabis use. Cannabis acutely induced hallucinatory experiences in patients but not healthy controls, while decreases in negative affect were observed after cannabis use in patients but not in controls, indicating that patients were also much more sensitive to the mood-enhancing effects of cannabis. In addition, patients were more sensitive to the increased sociability seen with cannabis: endorsed preference for being alone decreased under the influence of cannabis, while no such effect was observed in the control group.

More recent studies that employ mobile phone and web-based technology applications to profile psychosis like experiences in real-time following cannabis exposure are currently under way (Hides et al., 2020; Santesteban Echarri et al., 2021). Such applications used in longitudinal studies may bring a better understanding of psychosis like experiences resulting from cannabis use in CHR individuals, helping inform etiological and prognostic modelling.

The experience-sampling approach addresses some of the limitations of retrospective self-report. Experimental approaches address some of the limitations of the experience-sampling approach by using standardized doses, standardized delivery, objective assessments of symptoms, and performance-based measures of memory, attention, and executive function.

22.3.3 Experimental Data

22.3.3.1 Acute Effects of Cannabinoids in People at Risk for Schizophrenia

The acute effect of exposure to Δ^9-THC in persons at CHR for psychosis is relatively understudied in an experimental paradigm. A recent preliminary study examined the effect of smoking 5.5% Δ^9-THC or placebo in six regular cannabis users also ascertained to be at clinical high risk and six matched healthy controls (Vadhan et al., 2017). In the CHR group, there was an increase in subjective reports of paranoia, anxiety, slowed time perception, visual illusions, feelings of strangeness, and inattention; these effects were not observed in the control group. Objectively, the CHR group showed decreased performance on working memory and response inhibition tasks. The authors concluded that the psychosis-like effects of THC in this population could relate to the pre-existing risk for psychotic disorders (Box 22.3 and Figure 22.2).

22.3.3.2 Acute Effects of Cannabinoids in People Diagnosed with Schizophrenia

Only two published studies have administered Δ^9-THC to schizophrenia patients directly in order to study the acute effects on psychosis outcomes, cognition, and side-effects. D'Souza et al. (2005) conducted a randomized, double-blind, placebo-controlled study in order to investigate whether schizophrenia patients were more vulnerable than healthy controls to the effects of Δ^9-THC, in terms of cognition and psychotic symptoms. The study included subjects with past cannabis experience but without lifetime cannabis misuse or lifetime misuse of drugs (other than nicotine). Controls were healthy subjects; neither they nor their immediate family had any history of DSM-IV axis I disorders. Thirteen stable antipsychotic-medicated schizophrenia patients and 22 healthy controls were given 0 mg, 2.5 mg, and 5 mg Δ^9-THC intravenously in a three-day, double-blind, randomized, counterbalanced study. Test days were separated by at least a week (more than three times the elimination half-life of Δ^9-THC) in order to minimize carry-over effects. Subjects refrained from consuming caffeine, alcohol, and illicit drugs for two weeks

---

[1] ESM is a pseudo-random time-sampling self-assessment technique. Subjects receive a digital wristwatch and a paper-and-pen ESM booklet. Twelve times a day on six consecutive days, the watch beeps randomly once in each 90-minute time block between 7:30 a.m. and 12:30 p.m. After each beep, subjects complete 7-point Likert scales on affect, thoughts, symptom severity, and activity at the moment of the beep. This permits a systematic observation of recreational cannabis use in daily life. Previous studies using ESM have demonstrated its feasibility, validity, and reliability in schizophrenia patients.

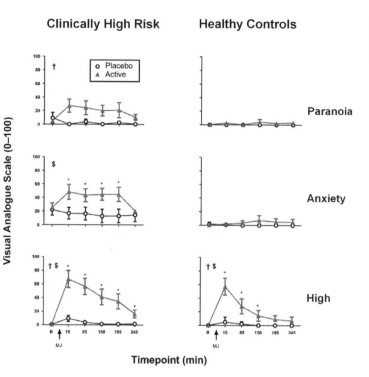

Figure 22.2 CHR group had a significant increase in subjective experience of anxiety and paranoia with THC compared to placebo. Adapted from Vadhan et al. (2017).

Box 22.3   Acute effects of cannabinoids in people at risk for schizophrenia

- In people at CHR for psychosis, experimental exposure to THC results in worsening of positive psychotic symptoms and anxiety.
- THC also worsens cognitive functions such as working memory and response inhibition in people at risk for psychosis.

---

before testing until study completion, and urinary testing confirmed self-reported abstinence. Symptoms of schizophrenia were assessed at several time points following Δ^9-THC or placebo administration by means of the Positive and Negative Syndrome Scale (PANSS) (Kay et al., 1986). A three-point or greater increase on the PANSS positive symptom sub-scale was considered a clinically significant response. Acute Δ^9-THC effects on neuropsychological functioning were tested using a verbal fluency test (Corkin et al., 1964), the Hopkins Verbal Learning Test (Brandt, 1991) for learning and immediate and delayed recall, and a continuous performance test (Gordon, 1986) to measure attention. Motor side-effects were measured using the Abnormal Involuntary Movement Scale (AIMS) for dyskinesias,

the Barnes Akathisia Scale for akathisia, and the Simpson Angus Scale (SAS) for Parkinsonism: see Figure 22.3.

There were similarities between the two groups, as well as differences. Δ^9-THC acutely impaired immediate recall, delayed free recall, and delayed cued recall in a dose-dependent fashion (Figure 22.4), as well as increasing omission errors in the attention task. Schizophrenia patients were more sensitive to the cognitive effects of cannabis, particularly impairment of memory and attention, although there were no significant group-by-dose interactive effects. Δ^9-THC had no effects on verbal fluency, nor did it make subjects more calm and relaxed. Δ^9-THC transiently increased positive symptoms in both schizophrenia patients and matched healthy controls. These effects

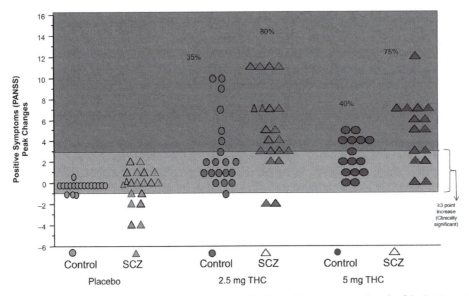

Figure 22.3 Peak increase in positive symptoms measured by the positive symptoms sub-scale of the Positive and Negative Symptoms Scale (PANNS) (group means 1 SD). Clinically significant increase = 3 points or greater increase in PANSSS positive symptom sub-scale score. Adapted from D'Souza et al. (2005). A black and white version of this figure will appear in some formats. For the colour version, please refer to the plate section.

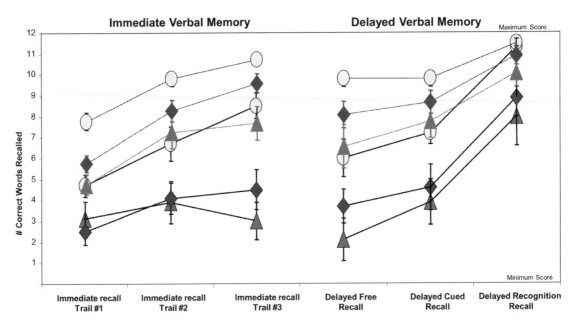

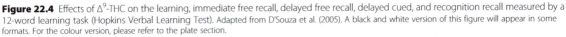

Figure 22.4 Effects of Δ[9]-THC on the learning, immediate free recall, delayed free recall, delayed cued, and recognition recall measured by a 12-word learning task (Hopkins Verbal Learning Test). Adapted from D'Souza et al. (2005). A black and white version of this figure will appear in some formats. For the colour version, please refer to the plate section.

were dose-related, occurred 10–20 minutes after Δ^9-THC administration, and resolved within 4 hours. Eighty percent of the schizophrenia patients but only 35% of control subjects had a clinically significant increase in psychotic symptoms in response to 2.5 mg Δ^9-THC, and 75% of schizophrenia patients but only 40% of control subjects had a suprathreshold response to 5 mg. There was no interaction between group, dose, and time, nor was there a difference between groups in the effects of Δ^9-THC on other measures, such as feeling high (VAS) or perceptual alterations (on the Clinician-Administered Dissociative States Scale). Δ^9-THC increased total scores on the AIMS (dyskinesia) as well as on the SAS (rigidity). Plasma Δ^9-THC and 11-nor-Δ^9-carboxy-THC levels were the same in both patient and control groups.

To summarize, Δ^9-THC transiently exacerbated a range of positive and negative psychotic symptoms, perceptual alternations, cognitive deficits, and medication side-effects associated with schizophrenia without producing clear beneficial effects. More schizophrenia patients than controls had clinically significant psychotic exacerbation in response to Δ^9-THC administration, and schizophrenia patients were more vulnerable to the negative effects of Δ^9-THC on learning and memory, despite maintenance on stable therapeutic doses of antipsychotic medications. This study indicated that individuals with an established psychotic disorder show abnormal sensitivity to the cognitive and the psychotomimetic effects of Δ^9-THC, a finding that has also been described in epidemiological studies (Henquet et al., 2005; van Os et al., 2002).

A second study also investigated differential sensitivity to the acute effects of Δ^9-THC in psychotic patients (Henquet et al., 2006). In this double-blind, placebo-controlled cross-over study, subjects smoked a tobacco cigarette containing either 300 μg/kg Δ^9-THC or 0 μg Δ^9-THC during two test sessions separated by one week. Thirty patients with a DSM-IV diagnosis of a psychotic disorder, 12 relatives of

patients with a psychotic disorder, and 32 healthy controls were enrolled; excluded were cannabis-naïve subjects, subjects with weekly use of drugs other than cannabis, and subjects drinking more than five units/day of alcohol. Fifteen minutes after cigarette inhalation, subjects took a neuropsychological test battery that included a visual verbal learning test and the Abstract Visual Patterns Learning test (which measures memory storage and retrieval of verbal information); a continuous performance test (CPT), the Stroop Colour-Word test (measuring attention), and the Digit Symbol Substitution Test (measuring speed). Transient psychotic experiences were assessed using the 40-item Community Assessment of Psychic Experiences (CAPE), a self-report instrument that was developed to capture variation in the positive and negative dimensions of psychotic experiences as well as variation in depression in the general population (Konings and Maharajh, 2006; http://cape42.homestead.com; last accessed 12 November 2022). As sub-clinical psychotic experiences measured with the CAPE show continuity with less severe states of psychosis seen in psychotic illness, and are transmitted in families, CAPE scores are considered a proxy for underlying psychosis liability. In this experimental study, the items of the CAPE were modified to measure momentary psychotic experiences during Δ^9-THC intoxication (CAPE-state). Catechol-O-methyltransferase (COMT) Val[158]Met genotypes were also measured (Box 22.4).

In both patients and controls, Δ^9-THC acutely impaired memory and attention. Interestingly, further comparison between patients and controls (unpublished data) showed only minor differences between groups in sensitivity to the cognitive effects of cannabis. In fact, patients seemed to be less sensitive to the verbal memory effects of Δ^9-THC than healthy controls, and there were no significant between-group differences in delayed free recall, delayed recognition, or visual memory. Only the acute effects of Δ^9-THC on attention were more

---

Box 22.4

- THC impairs performance on specific cognitive tasks in persons with schizophrenia.
- A much larger proportion of patients with schizophrenia experience worsening of psychosis with THC compared to controls (80% versus 35%).
- These effects are noted despite being on antipsychotic treatment.
- Most people with psychosis do not experience calming or relaxing effects with THC.
- Individual differences in sensitivity to the acute effects of Δ^9-THC may be due to differing genetic vulnerabilities.

pronounced in patients than in controls. Reaction time on a CPT increased (i.e., attention deteriorated) in patients (β = 1.25, 95% CI = 0.002–0.16, p = 0.04), but not in controls (β = 0.18, 95% CI = 0.35–2.15, p = 0.007). Patients also had a significantly larger increase in STROOP interference score (the time needed to complete Card III relative to Cards I and II) after Δ^9-THC exposure than did controls (β = 0.16, 95% CI = 0.05–0.27, p = 0.004 for patients and β = 0.01, 95% CI = –0.08–0.11, p = 0.8 for controls). In addition, the Val[158]Val genotype predicted increased sensitivity to the acute effects of Δ^9-THC on cognition. The Val[158]Met genotype moderated the acute effects of Δ^9-THC on psychotic symptoms, but only in individuals with pre-existing elevated scores on the CAPE-trait questionnaire.

These seemingly contradictory findings of the effects of Δ^9-THC on cognition may explain why only a minority of the individuals exposed to Δ^9-THC develop psychotic symptoms. In addition, available data seem to suggest that higher-order interactions are necessary to explain individual differences in sensitivity to the acute effects of Δ^9-THC on cognition and psychosis. Δ^9-THC sensitivity in patients and controls alike may be restricted to individuals with the Val[158]Val genotype or specific variations in other genes.

D'Souza et al. (2008) reported that chronic cannabis smoking affects acute responses to Δ^9-THC in healthy subjects. In a three-day, double-blind, placebo-controlled study, the dose-related effects of 0 mg, 2.5 mg, and 5 mg intravenous Δ^9-THC were studied in 30 frequent users of cannabis and 22 healthy controls. Frequent users showed the same euphoric effects as controls, but fewer psychotomimetic, perceptual altering, cognitive impairing, and anxiogenic effects. Their cortisol levels increased less, and their prolactin levels were lower. These data suggest that frequent cannabis users either are inherently tolerant to the psychotomimetic, perceptual altering, amnestic, endocrine, and other effects of cannabinoids; develop tolerance; or both. Similarly, Ramaekers et al. (2009) investigated the effects of high doses of Δ^9-THC (500 µg/kg) on neuropsychological performance in 12 heavy (more than four days a week) and 12 occasional (weekly use or less) users; deficits in performance were seen only in the occasional users. Di Forti et al. (2009) recently showed that patients are more likely to use cannabis for longer periods and with greater frequency than healthy controls; this increased use might actually mitigate the negative effects of

cannabis smoking in some patients. The authors investigated patterns of cannabis use in 280 patients with first-episode psychosis and 174 healthy controls. There were no between-group differences in age of first use, but patients were more likely to be current daily users and to have smoked cannabis for more than five years. In addition, the patient group used more 'skunk' (high-potency cannabis) than controls. Mason et al. (2009) also investigated the moderating effects of prior exposure to cannabis on psychosis outcome (PSI scores) and found, in line with D'Souza's work, that lower-frequency cannabis users manifested greater acute psychotomimetic responses to cannabis.

Schwarcz et al. (2009) administered dronabinol to six treatment-resistant schizophrenia patients who reported improvement in symptoms with past use of cannabis. Using a fixed schedule (5 mg dronabinol daily for the first week; 10 mg daily during the second week, and 20 mg daily during the third week), they documented clinical improvement on the Brief Psychiatric Rating Scale items of *conceptual disorganization, hallucinatory behaviour, suspiciousness,* and *unusual thought content,* as well as improvement in overall functioning measured with the Clinical Global Impression scale. In eight more chronic treatment-refractory schizophrenia patients treated with dronabinol, four showed no change, but four showed remarkable improvement in paranoia and agitation (Schwarcz, personal communication, 2010). Although the study lacked a control group, this suggests that there is a sub-set of schizophrenia patients for whom Δ^9-THC may not worsen symptomatology, and that patients differ in their sensitivity to the acute effects of Δ^9-THC.

The psychoactive effects of cannabis increase with Δ^9-THC content. It is important to note, however, that Δ^9-THC is not equivalent to cannabis, which contains >100 other cannabinoids (Elsohly and Slade, 2005; Thomas and Elsohly, 2016), of which Δ^9-THC is the most active. All the experimental studies administered Δ^9-THC, albeit using differing routes of administration: intravenous (D'Souza et al., 2005), smoked (Henquet et al., 2006), and oral (Schwarcz et al., 2009). However, more recently, some of the other constituents of cannabis are receiving greater attention. One such compound is cannabidiol.

22.4 Effects of Cannabidiol

Cannabidiol is covered in detail in Chapter 20. It is not pro-psychotic but actually appears to ameliorate the psychotomimetic effects of herbal cannabis (Morgan and Curran, 2008; Rottanburg et al., 1982; Solomons et al., 1990). Cannabidiol has been shown to have anxiolytic and antipsychotic effects (Leweke et al., 2005; Zuardi et al., 2006), leading to the suggestion that cannabidiol may offset some of the adverse effects of Δ^9-THC. In patients with psychotic illness, cannabidiol appears to act like an antipsychotic. Zuardi et al. (1995, 2006) reported that open-label cannabidiol treatment of four schizophrenia patients for four weeks resulted in a 50% response rate and the two patients who did not respond to cannabidiol were also refractory to clozapine. A double-blind, active-controlled, clinical trial comparing cannabidiol to the prototypical antipsychotic amisulpiride in the treatment of 40 schizophrenia patients suggested that cannabidiol was well tolerated, with antipsychotic efficacy equal to amisulpiride (Leweke et al., 2005) and, further, reduction in the positive symptoms are mediated by increase in serum anandamide levels (Leweke et al., 2012). Finally, a recent open-label four-week study in six outpatients with Parkinson's disease and psychosis showed that cannabidiol was well tolerated and markedly reduced psychosis (Zuardi et al., 2009). Thus, pre-clinical data and a small body of clinical data suggest that cannabidiol may be a well-tolerated and efficacious antipsychotic medication (Box 22.5).

More recently, experimental studies have investigated the acute neurobiological effects of cannabidiol administration in persons at CHR for psychosis. Bhattacharyya et al. (2018) reported that, compared to placebo, a single oral dose of cannabidiol partly normalized the reduced activation in right caudate during encoding, and the midbrain and para-hippocampal region during recall. Using the same paradigm, normalization of increased activation in the para-hippocampal region and reduced activation in the striatum during emotional processing of fearful face and normalization of reduced activation in the left insula/parietal operculum during a monetary incentive salience task have also been demonstrated (Davies et al., 2020; Wilson et al., 2019).

22.5 Conclusion

Cannabis use and misuse is common in people with psychotic disorder and individuals at CHR for psychosis. Individuals with a history of comorbid cannabis use may have an earlier age at onset of psychosis. Furthermore, an increase in cannabis use may hasten the onset of prodromal as well as psychotic symptoms.

Collectively, momentary assessment data, epidemiological findings, and laboratory experiments suggest that patients with a psychotic disorder show increased sensitivity to the pro-psychotic effects of cannabis and Δ^9-THC. Self-report data indicates that patients experience rewarding effects of cannabis immediately and negative effects on psychotic symptoms only later. The combination of delayed negative effects and increased sensitivity to immediate rewarding effects may explain psychotic patients' persistent cannabis use. According to this model, proposed by Spencer et al. (2002), use of cannabis is driven by expectations about the acute effects of cannabis. Sub-acute negative psychotic effects are then experienced as evidence that more use is necessary in order to bring about the anticipated rewarding effects. This motivation to improve mood reinforces use and promotes cannabis dependence, despite the long-term negative impact cannabis may have on functional outcome. There is little evidence to support the 'self-medication' hypothesis, at least in its original form.

Evidence suggests, unlike THC, cannabidiol may not exacerbate symptoms in those with established psychosis. Furthermore, there is emerging though tantalizing evidence that CBD may in fact have a role in the treatment of individuals with established psychosis or at higher risk for psychosis (Chapter 20).

With the liberalization of cannabis laws in many countries, cannabis and cannabis-based products will

---

Box 22.5 Acute effects of cannabidiol in contrast to THC

- Unlike THC, cannabidiol does not worsen the cognitive functions or induce psychotomimetic symptoms in persons with psychosis.
- On the contrary, cannabidiol may have antipsychotic properties.
- Experimental exposure to cannabidiol suggests that it normalizes some of the neurophysiological abnormalities relevant to psychosis.

be more accessible to both individuals with psychotic disorders and those at risk for psychosis. The potency of cannabis (THC content) and of cannabis-based products has increased. Given that the acute effects of cannabinoids are dose-related, the use of higher potency cannabis and cannabis-based products by individuals with psychotic disorders or at an increased risk for psychosis is a cause of concern. In addition, relative to smoked cannabis, the longer duration of effects of edible cannabinoids and the inability to titrate effects when using edibles could make for more adverse outcomes in individuals with established psychosis or higher risk for psychosis. Further research is necessary to understanding the neurobiology of why individuals with established psychosis or higher risk for psychosis are both more likely to use cannabis and are more vulnerable to cannabis. Lastly, further research is necessary to develop non-pharmacological and pharmacological treatments for problematic cannabis use in individuals with established psychosis or at higher risk for psychosis.

References

Addington, J., and Duchak, V. (1997). Reasons for substance use in schizophrenia. *Acta Psychiatr Scand*, **96**, 329–333.

Allebeck, P., Adamsson, C., Engstrom, A. et al. (1993). Cannabis and schizophrenia: A longitudinal study of cases treated in Stockholm County. *Acta Psychiatr Scand*, **88**, 21–24.

Arndt, S., Tyrrell, G., Flaum, M., et al. (1992). Comorbidity of substance abuse and schizophrenia: The role of pre-morbid adjustment. *Psychol Med*, **22**, 379–388.

Baigent, M., Holme, G., and Hafner, R. J. (1995). Self reports of the interaction between substance abuse and schizophrenia. *Aust NZ J Psychiatry*, **29**, 69–74.

Baker, A., Lewin, T., Reichler, H., et al. (2002). Motivational interviewing among psychiatric in-patients with substance use disorders. *Acta Psychiatr Scand*, **106**, 233–240.

Barkus, E., and Lewis, S. (2008). Schizotypy and psychosis-like experiences from recreational cannabis in a non-clinical sample. *Psychol Med*, **38**, 1267–1276.

Barkus, E., Stirling, J. Hopkins, R., et al. (2006). Cannabis-induced psychosis-like experiences are associated with high schizotypy. *Psychopathology*, **39**, 175–178.

Bhattacharyya, S., Wilson, R., Appiah-Kusi, E., et al. (2018). Effect of cannabidiol on medial temporal, midbrain, and striatal dysfunction in people at clinical high risk of psychosis: A randomized clinical trial. *JAMA Psychiatry*, **75**, 1107–1117.

Brandt, J. (1991). The Hopkins verbal learning test: Development of a new memory test with six equivalent forms. *Clin Neuropsychologist*, **5**, 125–142.

Buhler, B., Hambrecht, M., Loffler, W., et al. (2002). Precipitation and determination of the onset and course of schizophrenia by substance abuse: A retrospective and prospective study of 232 population-based first illness episodes. *Schizophr Res*, **54**, 243–251.

Cantor-Graae, E., Nordstrom, L., and McNeil, T. (2001). Substance abuse in schizophrenia: A review of the literature and a study of correlates in Sweden. *Schizophr Res*, **48**, 69–82.

Carney, R., Cotter, J., Firth, J., et al. (2017). Cannabis use and symptom severity in individuals at ultra high risk for psychosis: A meta-analysis. *Acta Psychiatr Scand*, **136**, 5–15.

Celofiga, A., Koprivsek, J., and Klavz, J. (2014). Use of synthetic cannabinoids in patients with psychotic disorders: case series. *J Dual Diagn*, **10**, 168–173.

Compton, M. T., Kelley, M. E., Ramsay, C. E., et al. (2009). Association of pre-onset cannabis, alcohol, and tobacco use with age at onset of prodrome and age at onset of psychosis in first-episode patients. *Am J Psychiatry*, **166**, 1251–1257.

Compton, W. M., Han, B., Jones, C. M., et al. (2019). Cannabis use disorders among adults in the United States during a time of increasing use of cannabis. *Drug Alcohol Depend*, **204**, 107468.

Corkin, S., Milner, B., and Rasmussen, T. (1964). Effects of different cortical excisions on sensory thresholds in man. *Trans Am Neurol Assoc*, **89**, 112–116.

D'Souza, D. C., Abi-Saab, W. M., Madonick, S., et al. (2005). Delta-9-tetrahydrocannabinol effects in schizophrenia: Implications for cognition, psychosis, and addiction. *Biol Psychiatry*, **57**, 594–608.

D'Souza, D. C., Ranganathan, M., Braley, G., et al. (2008). Blunted psychotomimetic and amnestic effects of delta-9-tetrahydrocannabinol in frequent users of cannabis. *Neuropsychopharmacology*, **33**, 2505–2516.

Davies, C., Wilson, R., Appiah-Kusi, E., et al. (2020). A single dose of cannabidiol modulates medial temporal and striatal function during fear processing in people at clinical high risk for psychosis. *Transl Psychiatry*, **10**, 311.

Dekker, N., Linszen, D., and De Haan, L. (2009). Reasons for cannabis use and effects of cannabis use as reported by patients with psychotic disorders. *Psychopathology*, **42**, 350–360.

Di Forti, M., Morgan, C., Dazzan, P., et al. (2009). High-potency cannabis and the risk of psychosis. *Br J Psychiatry*, **195**, 488–491.

Dixon, L., Haas, G., Weiden, P., et al. (1990). Acute effects of drug abuse in schizophrenic patients: Clinical observations and patients' self-reports. *Schizophr Bull*, **16**, 69–79.

Dixon, L., Haas, G., Weiden, P. J., et al. (1991). Drug abuse in schizophrenic patients: Clinical correlates and reasons for use. *Am J Psychiatry*, **148**, 224–230.

Elsohly, M. A., and Slade, D. (2005). Chemical constituents of marijuana: The complex mixture of natural cannabinoids. *Life Sci*, **78**, 539–548.

Fazio, R., and Zanna, M. (1981). Direct experience and attitude–behavior consistency. In Berkowitz, L. (ed.) *Advances in Experimental Social Psychology* (pp. 161–186). Chicago: University of Chicago Press.

Ferdinand, R. F., Sondeijker, F., van der Ende, J., et al. (2005). Cannabis use predicts future psychotic symptoms, and vice versa. *Addiction*, **100**, 612–618.

Fishbein, M. (1980). A theory of reasoned action: Some applications and implications. *Nebr Symp Motiv*, **27**, 65–116.

Fowler, I., Carr, V., Carter, N., et al. (1998). Patterns of current and lifetime substance use in schizophrenia. *Schizophr Bull*, **24**, 443–455.

Gearon, J. S., Bellack, A. S., Rachbeisel, J., et al. (2001). Drug-use behavior and correlates in people with schizophrenia. *Addict Behav*, **26**, 51–61.

Gordon, M. (1986). Microprocessor-based assessment of attention deficit disorders (ADD). *Psychopharmacol Bull*, **22**, 288–290.

Goswami, S., Mattoo, S. K., Basu, D., et al. (2004). Substance-abusing schizophrenics: Do they self-medicate? *Am J Addict*, **13**, 139–150.

Grech, A., Van Os, J., Jones, P. B., et al. (2005). Cannabis use and outcome of recent onset psychosis. *Eur Psychiatry*, **20**, 349–353.

Green, A. I., Tohen, M. F., Hamer, R. M., et al. (2004). First episode schizophrenia-related psychosis and substance use disorders: Acute response to olanzapine and haloperidol. *Schizophr Res*, **66**, 125–135.

Green, B., Kavanagh, D. J., and Young, R. M. (2004). Reasons for cannabis use in men with and without psychosis. *Drug Alcohol Rev*, **23**, 445–453.

Green, B., Young, R., and Kavanagh, D. (2005). Cannabis use and misuse prevalence among people with psychosis. *Br J Psychiatry*, **187**, 306–313.

Gregg, L., Barrowclough, C., and Haddock, G. (2009). Development and validation of a scale for assessing reasons for substance use in schizophrenia: The ReSUS scale. *Addict Behav*, **34**, 830–837.

Hambrecht, M., and Hafner, H. (1996). Substance abuse and the onset of schizophrenia. *Biol Psychiatry*, **40**, 1155–1163.

Hasin, D. S. (2018). U.S. epidemiology of cannabis use and associated problems. *Neuropsychopharmacology*, **43**, 195–212.

Hekimian, L. J., and Gershon, S. (1968). Characteristics of drug abusers admitted to a psychiatric hospital. *JAMA*, **205**, 125–130.

Henquet, C., Krabbendam, L., Spauwen, J., et al. (2005). Prospective cohort study of cannabis use, predisposition for psychosis, and psychotic symptoms in young people. *BMJ*, **330**, 11.

Henquet, C., van Os, J., Kuepper, R., et al. (2010). Psychosis reactivity to cannabis use in daily life: An experience sampling study. *Br J Psychiatry*, **196**, 447–453.

Henquet, C., Rosa, A., Krabbendam, L., et al. (2006). An experimental study of catechol-o-methyltransferase Val158Met moderation of delta-9-tetrahydrocannabinol-induced effects on psychosis and cognition. *Neuropsychopharmacology*, **31**, 2748–2757.

Hides, L., Baker, A., Norberg, M., et al. (2020). A web-based program for cannabis use and psychotic experiences in young people (keep it real): Protocol for a randomized controlled trial. *JMIR Res Protoc*, **9**, e15803.

Hindocha, C., Quattrone, D., Freeman, T. P., et al. (2020). Do AKT1, COMT and FAAH influence reports of acute cannabis intoxication experiences in patients with first episode psychosis, controls and young adult cannabis users? *Transl Psychiatry*, **10**, 143.

Kapur, S., Mizrahi, R., and Li, M. (2005). From dopamine to salience to psychosis: Linking biology, pharmacology and phenomenology of psychosis. *Schizophr Res*, **79**, 59–68.

Kay, S. R., Opler, L. A., and Fiszbein, A. (1986). Significance of positive and negative syndromes in chronic schizophrenia. *Br J Psychiatry*, **149**, 439–448.

Kessler, R. C., Chiu, W. T., Demler, O., et al. (2005). Prevalence, severity, and comorbidity of 12-month DSM-IV disorders in the National Comorbidity Survey Replication. *Arch Gen Psychiatry*, **62**, 617–627.

Khokhar, J. Y., Dwiel, L. L., Henricks, A. M., et al. (2018). The link between schizophrenia and substance use disorder: A unifying hypothesis. *Schizophr Res*, **194**, 78–85.

Knudsen, P., and Vilmar, T. (1984). Cannabis and neuroleptic agents in schizophrenia. *Acta Psychiatr Scand*, **69**, 162–174.

Kolliakou, A., Castle, D., Sallis, H., et al. (2015). Reasons for cannabis use in first-episode psychosis: Does strength of endorsement change over 12 months? *Eur Psychiatry*, **30**, 152–159.

Konings, M., and Maharajh, H. D. (2006). Cannabis use and mood disorders: Patterns of clinical presentations among adolescents in a developing country. *Int J Adolesc Med Health*, **18**, 221–233.

Koskinen, J., Lohonen, J., Koponen, H., et al. (2010). Rates of cannabis use disorders in clinical samples of patients with schizophrenia: A meta-analysis. *Schizophr Bull*, **36**, 1115–1124.

Kraan, T., Velthorst, E., Koenders, L., et al. (2016). Cannabis use and transition to psychosis in individuals at ultra-high risk: Review and meta-analysis. *Psychol Med*, **46**, 673–681.

Leweke, F., Koethe, D., and Gerth, C. (2005). Cannabidiol as an antipsychotic: A double-blind, controlled clinical trial of cannabidiol versus amisulpride in acute schizophrenia. *15th Annual Symposium on Cannabinoids*. Clearwater Beach, FL, Cannabinoid Research Society.

Leweke, F. M., Piomelli, D., Pahlisch, F., et al. (2012). Cannabidiol enhances anandamide signaling and alleviates psychotic symptoms of schizophrenia. *Transl Psychiatry*, **2**, e94.

Linszen, D., and van Amelsvoort, T. (2007). Cannabis and psychosis: An update on course and biological plausible mechanisms. *Curr Opin Psychiatry*, **20**, 116–120.

Linszen, D. H., Dingemans, P. M., and Lenior, M. E. (1994). Cannabis abuse and the course of recent-onset schizophrenic disorders. *Arch Gen Psychiatry*, **51**, 273–279.

Lowe, D. J. E., Sasiadek, J. D., Coles, A. S., et al. (2019). Cannabis and mental illness: A review. *Eur Arch Psychiat Clin Neurosci*, **269**, 107–120.

Mane, A., Fernandez-Exposito, M., Berge, D., et al. (2015). Relationship between cannabis and psychosis: Reasons for use and associated clinical variables. *Psychiatry Res*, **229**, 70–74.

Mason, O., Morgan, C. J., Dhiman, S. K., et al. (2009). Acute cannabis use causes increased psychotomimetic experiences in individuals prone to psychosis. *Psychol Med*, **39**, 951–956.

Mauri, M., Volonteri, L., De Gaspari, I., et al. (2006). Substance abuse in first-episode schizophrenic patients: A retrospective study. *Clin Pract Epidemiol Mental Health* **2**, 1–8.

McCreadie, R. G. (2002). Use of drugs, alcohol and tobacco by people with schizophrenia: Case-control study. *Br J Psychiatry*, **181**, 321–325.

McHugh, M. J., McGorry, P. D. Yung, A. R., et al. (2017). Cannabis-induced attenuated psychotic symptoms: Implications for prognosis in young people at ultra-high risk for psychosis. *Psychol Med*, **47**, 616–626.

Missouri Department of Health and Senior Services. (2010). *Health Advisory: K2 Synthetic Marijuana Use among Teenagers and Young Adults in Missouri*. Jefferson City, MO: Missouri Department of Health and Senior Services.

Morgan, C. J., and Curran, H. V. (2008). Effects of cannabidiol on schizophrenia-like symptoms in people who use cannabis. *Br J Psychiatry*, **192**, 306–307.

Muller, H., Sperling, W., Kohrmann, M., et al. (2010). The synthetic cannabinoid Spice as a trigger for an acute exacerbation of cannabis induced recurrent psychotic episodes. *Schizophr Res*, **118**, 309–310.

Myin-Germeys, I., Krabbendam, L., Jolles, J., et al. (2002). Are cognitive impairments associated with sensitivity to stress in schizophrenia? An experience sampling study. *Am J Psychiatry*, **159**, 443–449.

Myin-Germeys, I., van Os, J., Schwartz, J., et al. (2001). Emotional reactivity to daily life stress in psychosis. *Arch Gen Psychiatry*, **58**, 1137–1144.

Myles, H., Myles, N., and Large, M. (2016). Cannabis use in first episode psychosis: Meta-analysis of prevalence, and the time course of initiation and continued use. *Aust NZ J Psychiatry*, **50**, 208–219.

Negrete, J. C., Knapp, W. P., Douglas, D. E., et al. (1986). Cannabis affects the severity of schizophrenic symptoms: Results of a clinical survey. *Psychol Med*, **16**, 515–520.

van Os, J., Bak, M., Hanssen, M., et al. (2002). Cannabis use and psychosis: A longitudinal population-based study. *Am J Epidemiol*, **156**, 319–327.

Peralta, V., and Cuesta, M. J. (1992). Influence of cannabis abuse on schizophrenic psychopathology. *Acta Psychiatr Scand*, **85**, 127–130.

Peters, B., de Koning, P., Dingemans, P., et al. (2009). Subjective effects of cannabis before the first psychotic episode. *Aust NZ J Psychiatry*, **43**, 1155–1162.

Rabin, R. A., and George, T. P. (2017). Understanding the link between cannabinoids and psychosis. *Clin Pharmacol Ther*, **101**, 197–199.

Rabinowitz, J., Bromet, E. J. Lavelle, J., et al. (1998). Prevalence and severity of substance use disorders and onset of psychosis in first-admission psychotic patients. *Psychol Med*, **28**, 1411–1419.

Raine, A. (1991). The SPQ: A scale for the assessment of schizotypal personality based on DSM-III-R criteria. *Schizophr Bull*, 17, 555–564.

Ramaekers, J. G., Kauert, G., Theunissen, E. L., et al. (2009). Neurocognitive performance during acute THC intoxication in heavy and occasional cannabis users. *J Psychopharmacol*, 23, 266–277.

Regier, D., Farmer, M., Rae, D., et al. (1990). Comorbidity of mental disorders with alcohol and other drug abuse. Results from the Epidemiologic Catchment Area (ECA) Study [comment]. *JAMA*, 264, 2511–2518.

Ringen, P., Lagerberg, T., Birkenaes, A., et al. (2008). Differences in prevalence and patterns of substance use in schizophrenia and bipolar disorder. *Psychol Med*, 38, 1241–1249.

Rottanburg, D., Robins, A. H., Ben-Arie, O., et al. (1982). Cannabis-associated psychosis with hypomanic features. *Lancet*, 2, 1364–1366.

Santesteban Echarri, O., Kim, G., Haffey, P., et al. (2021). LooseLeaf, a mobile-based application to monitor cannabis use and cannabis-related experiences for youth at clinical high-risk for psychosis: Development and user acceptance testing. *Int J Hum–Comp Interact*, 37, 501–511.

Schofield, D., Tennant, C., Nash, L., et al. (2006). Reasons for cannabis use in psychosis. *Aust NZ J Psychiatry*, 40, 570–574.

Schwarcz, G., Karajgi, B., and McCarthy, R. (2009). Synthetic delta-9-tetrahydrocannabinol (dronabinol) can improve the symptoms of schizophrenia. *J Clin Psychopharmacol*, 29, 255–258.

Silver, H., and Abboud, E. (1994). Drug abuse in schizophrenia: Comparison of patients who began drug abuse before their first admission with those who began abusing drugs after their first admission. *Schizophr Res*, 13, 57–63.

Solomons, K., Neppe, V. M., and Kuyl, J. M. (1990). Toxic cannabis psychosis is a valid entity. *S Afr Med J*, 78, 476–481.

Spencer, C., Castle, D., and Michie, P. T. (2002). Motivations that maintain substance use among individuals with psychotic disorders. *Schizophr Bull*, 28, 233–247.

Stefanis, N. C., Delespaul, P., Henquet, C., et al. (2004). Early adolescent cannabis exposure and positive and negative dimensions of psychosis. *Addiction*, 99, 1333–1341.

Stirling, J., Barkus, E. J., Nabosi, L., et al. (2008). Cannabis-induced psychotic-like experiences are predicted by high schizotypy. Confirmation of preliminary results in a large cohort. *Psychopathology*, 41, 371–378.

Swartz, M., Wagner, H., Swanson, J., et al. (2006). Substance use in persons with schizophrenia: Baseline prevalence and correlates from the NIMH CATIE study. *J Nerv Ment Dis*, 194, 164–172.

Test, M. A., Wallisch, L. S., Allness, D. J., et al. (1989). Substance use in young adults with schizophrenic disorders. *Schizophr Bull*, 15, 465–476.

Thomas, B. F., and Elsohly, M. A. (2016). The botany of cannabis sativa L. In Thomas, B. F., and Elsohly, M. A. (eds.) *The Analytical Chemistry of Cannabis* (pp. 1–26). Amsterdam: Elsevier.

Treffert, D. A. (1978). Marijuana use in schizophrenia: A clear hazard. *Am J Psychiatry*, 135, 1213–1215.

Vadhan, N. P., Corcoran, C. M., Bedi, G., et al. (2017). Acute effects of smoked marijuana in marijuana smokers at clinical high-risk for psychosis: A preliminary study. *Psychiatry Res*, 257, 372–374.

Vearrier, D., and Osterhoudt, K. C. (2010). A teenager with agitation: Higher than she should have climbed. *Pediatr Emerg Care*, 26, 462–465.

Veen, N. D., Selten, J. P., van der Tweel, I., et al. (2004). Cannabis use and age at onset of schizophrenia. *Am J Psychiatry*, 161, 501–506.

Wainberg, M., Jacobs, G. R., di Forti, M., et al. (2021). Cannabis, schizophrenia genetic risk, and psychotic experiences: A cross-sectional study of 109,308 participants from the UK Biobank. *Transl Psychiatry*, 11, 211.

Warner, R., Taylor, D., Wright, J., et al. (1994). Substance use among the mentally ill: Prevalence, reasons for use, and effects on illness. *Am J Orthopsychiatry*, 64, 30–39.

Weil, A. T. (1970). Adverse reactions to marihuana. Classification and suggested treatment. *N Engl J Med*, 282, 997–1000.

Wilson, R., Bossong, M. G., Appiah-Kusi, E., et al. (2019). Cannabidiol attenuates insular dysfunction during motivational salience processing in subjects at clinical high risk for psychosis. *Transl Psychiatry*, 9, 203.

Zuardi, A., Crippa, J. A., Hallak, J., et al. (2009). Cannabidiol for the treatment of psychosis in Parkinson's disease. *J Psychopharmacol*, 23, 979–983.

Zuardi, A. W., Hallak, J. E. Dursun, S. M., et al. (2006). Cannabidiol monotherapy for treatment-resistant schizophrenia. *J Psychopharmacol*, 20, 683–686.

Zuardi, A. W., Morais, S. L. Guimaraes, F. S., et al. (1995). Antipsychotic effect of cannabidiol. *J Clin Psychiatry*, 56, 485–486.

Chapter

23

Cannabis and the Long-term Course of Psychosis

Tabea Schoeler

23.1 The Association between Continued Cannabis Use and Long-term Course of Psychosis

Numerous large-scale epidemiological studies in the general population have been conducted to scrutinize the role of cannabis use in the onset of psychosis, implicating that cannabis use constitutes a contributory cause of psychosis (Arseneault et al., 2004). If cannabis use is a causal factor involved in the development of psychosis, it seems likely that the use of cannabis perpetuates and aggravates symptoms in individuals with pre-existing psychosis. Since cannabis use is a factor amenable to treatment, detailed knowledge about its effects on the long-term course of psychosis is, therefore, paramount to allow healthcare providers to tackle the most harmful patterns of cannabis use, particularly in individuals that appear most sensitive to its adverse effects. While early cross-sectional studies assessing the link between cannabis use and illness course in individuals with psychosis were already conducted in the 1970s (Bowers, 1977), more rigorous longitudinal research monitoring cannabis intake in samples of first episode psychosis (FEP) patients has only emerged in more recent years. In particular, efforts have been made to assess in more detail how different cannabis use patterns affect illness outcomes, such as the trajectory of cannabis use following the onset (e.g., initiation, continuation, discontinuation of use), the frequency of cannabis use, or the potency of the consumed cannabis.

Although cannabis using FEP patients are routinely encouraged by their treating clinicians and carers to reduce their consumption after entering early intervention services, more than half continue using the drug following the onset of their illness (Myles et al., 2016). Since very few individuals initiate cannabis use following the onset of illness (Gonzalez-Pinto et al., 2011), research has mostly focused on questions concerning the impact of continued cannabis use on the illness course of psychosis. A piece of research summarizing data from more than 16,000 individuals diagnosed with a psychotic disorder assessed the impact of continued cannabis use on risk of relapse of psychosis (most commonly defined as re-emergence of psychotic symptoms leading to hospital admission) and related outcomes (e.g., positive symptoms at follow-up) (Schoeler et al., 2016b). It was found that continued cannabis users were more likely to relapse, to require longer hospital stays when treated for their relapse, and to show more severe positive symptomatology at follow-up when compared to non-using patients with psychosis. In contrast, individuals who discontinued cannabis use after the onset of illness did not differ from non-using individuals in their long-term clinical outcomes. Together, this pooled evidence highlights that the continuation of cannabis use following the onset of illness may be particularly harmful with respect to clinical outcomes, while abstaining from cannabis may prevent some of the harmful consequences associated with the drug. Recent studies building on this evidence have replicated such findings, providing further support for the notion of reversible effects of cannabis with respect to clinical outcomes in individuals with psychosis. For example, compared to FEP patients discontinuing cannabis use following the onset, individuals exposed to daily cannabis use throughout a two-year follow-up showed a more severe illness course, including higher risk of psychotic relapse and the need for more intensive care when treated for their relapse (Schoeler et al., 2016d). Similarly, a 10-year follow-up of FEP patients implicated that individuals abandoning cannabis use fared significantly better over the long-term when compared to those who continued using the drug (Setién-Suero et al., 2019).

For clinical care, it is also crucial to gain a more nuanced understanding of the impact of cannabis use across different levels of exposure, as effects on long-term outcome may vary as a function of frequency of use or the strain of the consumed cannabis. For example, daily cannabis users were at highest risk of poor clinical outcome when compared to FEP patients using cannabis in a less frequent manner (Schoeler et al., 2016d). Similarly, risk of relapse was predicted by the number of positive urine toxicology tests (Scheffler et al., 2021). Conversely, FEP patients using cannabis only in an infrequent manner did not show the poor outcome seen in daily cannabis users (Schoeler et al., 2016d). Together, these findings implicate that cannabis use may impact on illness course in a dose-dependent manner, highlighting that reductions in exposure to cannabis could prevent some of the long-term harms associated with frequent cannabis use in FEP patients. Another pertinent question concerns the impact of the type of the consumed cannabis on outcome in psychosis. For example, around one third of FEP patients in London reported using predominantly high-potency varieties of cannabis, such as 'skunk-type' forms (Di Forti et al., 2019). 'Skunk' has been shown to contain higher levels of delta-9-tetrahydrocannabinol (THC), the main psychoactive ingredient in cannabis, when compared to the traditional 'hash-type' varieties of cannabis (Potter et al., 2008). In this context, it has been reported that the use of high-potency forms of cannabis ('skunk-type') is particularly harmful with respect to clinical outcome in FEP patients, while the use of milder forms ('hash-type') appears to have less detrimental effects (Schoeler et al., 2016d). This finding is supported by experimental research, implicating that increasing levels of THC administration causes greater symptom manifestations in individuals with pre-existing psychosis (D'Souza et al., 2005).

In summary, longitudinal research exploring the role of different cannabis use patterns on long-term outcome of psychosis has been vital, as such efforts have highlighted that a frequent exposure to high-potency forms of cannabis may pose substantial risk for poor outcome in FEP patients. Conversely, on a more positive note, such research suggests that the effects of cannabis in FEP patients may indeed be reversible. Hence, interventional strategies aiming at reducing cannabis intake, while simultaneously encouraging the use of milder forms of cannabis, have the potential to improve the long-term prognosis in FEP patients.

23.2 The Effect of Continued Cannabis Use across Outcome Dimensions of Psychosis

While there is relatively consistent evidence implicating continued cannabis as a risk factor for poor illness course when defined in terms of exacerbation of positive symptoms (e.g., hallucinations, paranoia, delusions), its impact on other outcome dimensions is less clear. For example, a common observation is that continued cannabis use is not a prognostic factor for long-term negative symptoms (typically characterized by blunted affect, alogia, asociality, avolition, anhedonia) or psychosocial functioning in psychosis (Foti et al., 2010; Schoeler et al., 2016b; Setien-Suero et al., 2019). In contrast, other studies do report poor functional outcomes in FEP patients with heavy cannabis use (Schimmelmann et al., 2012), in line with studies documenting better functional outcomes in patients who discontinued cannabis use following the onset of illness (Gonzalez-Pinto et al., 2011; Setien-Suero et al., 2019). As such, adverse effects of cannabis on long-term functioning and negative symptoms in psychosis cannot be ruled out, especially if used heavily. However, positive psychotic symptomatology may be particularly susceptible to the influence of cannabis, while other outcome dimensions appear to be less severely affected by the use of the drug (Schimmelmann et al., 2012).

Paradoxically, there is also evidence suggesting that cannabis users with psychosis perform *better* on cognitive measures when compared to non-using individuals with psychosis (Schoeler et al., 2016a). This contradicts findings from studies assessing healthy long-term cannabis users, where adverse effects of cannabis on cognitive functioning are documented (Schoeler et al., 2016a). While further research is needed to elucidate the reasons underlying the seemingly differential effects of cannabis in users with and without a psychotic disorder, a number of explanations for this counter-intuitive finding have been expressed. For example, it has been suggested that cannabis using patients with psychosis represent a sub-group characterized by high levels of psychosocial functioning, as they are 'skilful' enough to obtain the illegal drug. This is, however, not supported by research conducted in countries where cannabis is readily accessible, that is, where social skills do not play a significant role in accessing the drug (Korver et al., 2010). The perhaps more convincing argument is that cannabis using patients represent a neurodevelopmentally less vulnerable group (Ferraro et al., 2013) when compared to non-using patients. In other words, psychosis in cannabis users would have occurred as a consequence of cannabis exposure, while psychosis outside the context of cannabis use would have resulted from a high genetic and neurodevelopmental vulnerability to psychosis.

In summary, the existing evidence suggests that continued cannabis use adversely impacts a number of outcome dimensions of psychosis. Although adverse effects associated with cannabis use seem to be most prominent with respect to positive symptomatology and related clinical measures (e.g., risk of relapse), reductions in heavy cannabis use after the onset of illness nevertheless appear to ameliorate functioning and negative symptoms in the long-run. Importantly, more longitudinal research assessing the effects of different levels of cannabis exposure across distinct outcome dimensions is needed, before drawing more definitive conclusions.

23.3 Continued Cannabis Use and Long-term Course of Psychosis: The Question of Causality

While evidence implicating cannabis use in an unfavourable illness course of psychosis is countless, the crux of the story concerns the causal nature of this association. Scrutinizing causality is an important step to take in this context; cannabis using patients with psychosis differ from non-users in a number of demographic and clinical characteristics that could also alter the course of the illness. As such, any difference seen in outcome between the two groups cannot be directly attributed to the cannabis use itself. However, well-designed prospective studies typically control for important factors that could explain the observed cannabis-outcome associations in psychosis, indicating that factors such as age of onset of psychosis, onset illness severity, duration of untreated psychosis, socioeconomic status, or gender are unlikely to fully explain the adverse outcomes seen in cannabis using FEP patients (Foti et al., 2010; Schoeler et al., 2016d). More challenging, however, is the control of unmeasured factors associated with both cannabis use and outcome in psychosis. For example, it is plausible that a shared genetic predisposition to both cannabis use and psychosis illness severity underlies the unfavourable illness course seen in cannabis using patients. To control for such unobserved patient characteristics, longitudinal studies have compared periods of cannabis use to periods of non-use following the onset of illness *within the same individual*, thereby accounting for all factors that precede the illness onset (e.g., familial and genetic factors, duration of untreated psychosis, pre-morbid

adjustment, childhood trauma). Using such design, it was found that periods of greater exposure to cannabis were characterized by higher risk of relapse of psychosis and more severe psychotic symptomatology (Foti et al., 2010; Schoeler et al., 2016c), in line with the notion of causality.

Another conceivable explanation for the cannabis–outcome association is that the poor outcome seen in cannabis using FEP patients is simply the result of reverse causation. More specifically, it is possible that cannabis use constitutes a form of self-medication (Khantzian, 1997) for negative and affective symptoms, higher illness burden, or the side-effects of antipsychotic medication in FEP patients. To evaluate if reverse causation explains the observed association between cannabis use and poor outcome in psychosis, a number of studies have assessed the bi-directional relationship between continued cannabis use and outcome in individuals with pre-existing psychosis. For example, in a 2-year follow-up of FEP patients, cannabis use predicted subsequent relapse, while there was little evidence in support of the reverse direction (Schoeler et al., 2016c). Similarly, studies using daily assessment techniques when assessing patients with psychosis showed that neither affective states nor psychotic symptoms were linked to subsequent increases in cannabis use (Henquet et al., 2010). Hence, such evidence indicates that self-medication due to affective symptoms or illness burden is unlikely to fully explain the association between cannabis use and risk of poor illness course in patients with psychosis.

To summarize, evidence exploiting more stringent statistical methods to address confounding and reverse causation has been instrumental when assessing causality of the cannabis–outcome association. Overall, this line of evidence supports the notion of causality, suggesting that continued cannabis use is likely to constitute a contributory cause for poor long-term outcome in psychosis.

23.4 The Inter-play between Cannabis Use and Other Factors Shaping the Long-term Course of Psychosis

Given the multifactorial nature of clinical outcome in psychosis, cannabis use represents only one among many potential modifiable risk factors altering the illness course of psychosis. Other notable risk factors implicated in poor outcome of psychosis include medication non-adherence and persistent substance use (Alvarez-Jimenez et al., 2012). A key question is, therefore, as to whether cannabis use has direct effects on outcome, or, alternatively, if intermediate risk factors explain the link between cannabis use and poor outcome of psychosis. For example, it has often been observed that cannabis use links to non-adherence to antipsychotic medication (Foglia et al., 2017), which, in turn, is one of the most predictive factors for long-term outcome in psychosis. This begs the question as to whether the unfavourable outcome seen in FEP patients with comorbid cannabis use may simply be the result of poor adherence to their pre-scribed medication. Indeed, a prospective study in FEP patients found that medication non-adherence mediated some of the adverse effects of continued cannabis use on risk of relapse (Schoeler et al., 2017). At the same time, a considerable proportion of the adverse effects associated with cannabis use remained unexplained, meaning that continued cannabis use predicted poor outcome even in individuals adhering to their medication. This is in line with research reporting deleterious effects of continued cannabis use on outcome in patients treated with long-acting injectable antipsychotics injections (whereby antipsychotic maintenance is ensured) (Emsley et al., 2020). In this context, it has been suggested that cannabis use may alter antipsychotic treatment response (Reid and Bhattacharyya, 2019), since cannabis using FEP patients appear to have an inadequate and slower response to treatment with antipsychotic medication (Pelayo-Terán et al., 2014). Nevertheless, despite the potentially reduced treatment response, it has been pointed out that antipsychotics are still effective in reducing psychotic symptoms in patients with comorbid cannabis use disorder (Wilson and Bhattacharyya, 2016). Experimental studies support this conclusion, showing that pre-treatment with antipsychotic medication (haloperidol) reduced some of the THC-induced psychosis-like symptoms in healthy volunteers (Liem-Moolenaar et al., 2010). Moreover, antipsychotic medication could also help in reducing craving and the consumption of cannabis (Wilson and Bhattacharyya, 2016). Hence, to mitigate cannabis-related harms, interventions should not only target problematic cannabis use patterns in patients with psychosis but should also aim to improve medication adherence in this group of patients.

Another documented factor influencing the long-term course of psychosis is the use of psychoactive substances other than cannabis (e.g., tobacco, alcohol, amphetamines, cocaine), which has been linked to a worsening of symptoms, functioning, and quality-of-life in FEP patients (Ouellet-Plamondon et al., 2017). In this context, a number of findings are worth discussing. First, research has shown that cannabis use predicts poor prognosis in FEP patients independent of co-occurring use of other illicit substances (Schoeler et al., 2016d). This suggests that the increased risk of poor outcome in cannabis using patients with psychosis is unlikely to be the result of a polysubstance use pattern commonly seen in cannabis users. Controlling for the effects of tobacco use poses, however, particular challenges, since cannabis is typically mixed with tobacco (e.g., in joints) in European countries (Hindocha et al., 2016). As such, it is virtually impossible to separate the effects of cannabis use from tobacco use in FEP patients residing in European countries. Nevertheless, studies conducted in countries where cannabis is typically not mixed with tobacco (e.g., United States) replicate aforementioned findings, implicating cannabis as a risk factor for poor outcome in psychosis (Foti et al., 2010). Second, research aiming to disentangle the effect of psychoactive substance use in patients with psychosis further highlight that cannabis is only one among a number of psychoactive substances that are likely to impact on outcome of psychosis. For example, the use of cigarettes and illicit substances remained a significant predictor for more frequent relapses of psychosis after accounting for cannabis use (Schoeler et al., 2016d). This suggests that the simultaneous use of cannabis and other psychoactive substances may be particularly harmful with respect to clinical outcome in FEP patients.

Overall, research has shown that continued cannabis use, as one factor potentially amendable to treatment, is one among a number of impactful risk factors for long-term outcome in psychosis. The reported magnitude of association between cannabis use and clinical outcomes is similar to other identified environmental risk factors shaping the illness course, such as antipsychotic treatment or the abuse of other psychoactive substances. This emphasizes the importance of cannabis use as a clinically relevant target for treatment in psychosis, alongside the targeting of other factors implicated in the illness course.

23.5 Conclusions

Given the existing evidence focusing on the role of cannabis use in the long-term course of psychosis, a key conclusion to be drawn is that FEP patients exposed to frequent use of high potency cannabis are at a particular risk of experiencing a severe illness course over the long-term. Detrimental effects of cannabis use are documented for a range of outcomes, notably increased risk of relapse and rehospitalization, exacerbation of positive psychotic symptoms, medication non-compliance, and likely poor functional outcome. While complete abstinence of cannabis may not always be feasible in this group of individuals, a switch to less harmful cannabis use patterns (e.g., use of milder forms of cannabis, less frequent cannabis use), while ensuring medication adherence, has the potential to significantly improve the prognosis of psychosis. The relationship between cannabis use and long-term outcome of psychosis remains, however, a complex one. Further research elucidating the more fine-grained mechanisms underlying cannabis-associated harms will be vital to better understand pathways leading to recovery from psychosis.

References

Alvarez-Jimenez, M., Priede, A., Hetrick, S. E., et al. (2012). Risk factors for relapse following treatment for first episode psychosis: A systematic review and meta-analysis of longitudinal studies. *Schizophr Res*, **139**, 116–128.

Arseneault, L., Cannon, M., Witton, J., et al. (2004). Causal association between cannabis and psychosis: Examination of the evidence. *Br J Psychiatry*, **184**, 110–117.

Bowers, M. B. (1977). Psychoses precipitated by psychotomimetic drugs: A follow-up study. *Arch Gen Psychiatry*, **34**, 832–835.

D'Souza, D. C., Abi-Saab, W. M., Madonick, S., et al. (2005). Delta-9-tetrahydrocannabinol effects in schizophrenia: Implications for cognition, psychosis, and addiction. *Biol Psychiatry*, **57**, 594–608.

Di Forti, M., Quattrone, D., Freeman, T. P., et al. (2019). The contribution of cannabis use to variation in the incidence of psychotic disorder across Europe (EU-GEI): A multicentre case-control study. *Lancet Psychiatry*, **6**, 427–436.

Emsley, R., Asmal, L., Rubio, J. M., et al. (2020). Predictors of psychosis breakthrough during 24 months of long-acting antipsychotic maintenance treatment in first episode schizophrenia. *Schizophr Res*, **225**, 55–62.

Ferraro, L., Russo, M., O'Connor, J., et al. (2013). Cannabis users have higher premorbid IQ than other patients with first onset psychosis. *Schizophr Res*, **150**, 129–135.

Foglia, E., Schoeler, T., Klamerus, E., et al. (2017). Cannabis use and adherence to antipsychotic medication: A systematic review and meta-analysis. *Psychol Med*, 47, 1691–1705.

Foti, D. J., Kotov, R., Guey, L. T., et al. (2010). Cannabis use and the course of schizophrenia: 10-year follow-up after first hospitalization. *Am J Psychiatry*, **167**, 987–993.

Gonzalez-Pinto, A., Alberich, S., Barbeito, S., et al. (2011). Cannabis and first-episode psychosis: Different long-term outcomes depending on continued or discontinued use. *Schizophr Bull*, 37, 631–639.

Henquet, C., van Os, J., Kuepper, R., et al. (2010). Psychosis reactivity to cannabis use in daily life: An experience sampling study. *Br J Psychiatry*, **196**, 447–453.

Hindocha, C., Freeman, T. P., Ferris, J. A., et al. (2016). No smoke without tobacco: A global overview of cannabis and tobacco routes of administration and their association with intention to quit. *Front Psychiatry*, 7, 104.

Khantzian, E. J. (1997). The self-medication hypothesis of substance use disorders: A reconsideration and recent applications. *Harvard Rev Psychiatry*, **4**, 231–244.

Korver, N., Nieman, D. H., Becker, H. E., et al. (2010). Symptomatology and neuropsychological functioning in cannabis using subjects at ultra-high risk for developing psychosis and healthy controls. *Aust NZ J Psychiatry*, **44**, 230–236.

Liem-Moolenaar, M., te Beek, E. T., de Kam, M. L., et al. (2010). Central nervous system effects of haloperidol on THC in healthy male volunteers. *J Psychopharmacol*, **24**, 1697–1708.

Myles, H., Myles, N., and Large, M. (2016). Cannabis use in first episode psychosis: Meta-analysis of prevalence, and the time course of initiation and continued use. *Aust NZ J Psychiatry*, **50**, 208–219.

Ouellet-Plamondon, C., Abdel-Baki, A., Salvat, É., et al. (2017). Specific impact of stimulant, alcohol and cannabis use disorders on first-episode psychosis: 2-year functional and symptomatic outcomes. *Psychol Med*, 47, 2461–2471.

Pelayo-Terán, J. M., Diaz, F. J., Pérez-Iglesias, R., et al. (2014). Trajectories of symptom dimensions in short-term response to antipsychotic treatment in patients with a first episode of non-affective psychosis. *Psychol Med*, **44**, 37–50.

Potter, D. J., Clark, P., and Brown, M. B. (2008). Potency of Δ 9-THC and other cannabinoids in cannabis in England in 2005: Implications for psychoactivity and pharmacology. *J Forens Sci*, **53**, 90–94.

Reid, S., and Bhattacharyya, S. (2019). Antipsychotic treatment failure in patients with psychosis and co-morbid cannabis use: A systematic review. *Psychiatry Res*, **280**, 112523.

Scheffler, F., Phahladira, L., Luckhoff, H., et al. (2021). Cannabis use and clinical outcome in people with first-episode schizophrenia spectrum disorders over 24 months of treatment. *Psychiatry Res*, **302**, 114022.

Schimmelmann, B. G., Conus, P., Cotton, S., et al. (2012). Prevalence and impact of cannabis use disorders in adolescents with early onset first episode psychosis. *Eur Psychiatry*, **27**, 463–469.

Schoeler, T., Kambeitz, J., Behlke, I., et al. (2016a). The effects of cannabis on memory function in users with and without a psychotic disorder: Findings from a combined meta-analysis. *Psychol Med*, **46**, 177–188.

Schoeler, T., Monk, A., Sami, M. B., et al. (2016b). Continued versus discontinued cannabis use in patients with psychosis: A systematic review and meta-analysis. *Lancet Psychiatry*, **3**, 215–225.

Schoeler, T., Petros, N., Di Forti, M., et al. (2016c). Association between continued cannabis use and risk of relapse in first-episode psychosis: A quasi-experimental investigation within an observational study. *JAMA Psychiatry*, **73**, 1173–1179.

et al. (2016d). Effects of continuation, frequency, and type of cannabis use on relapse in the first 2 years after onset of psychosis: An observational study. *Lancet Psychiatry*, **3**, 947–953.

et al. (2017). Effect of continued cannabis use on medication adherence in the first two years following onset of psychosis. *Psychiatry Res*, **255**, 36–41.

Setién-Suero, E., Neergaard, K., Ortiz-García de la Foz, V., et al. (2019). Stopping cannabis use benefits outcome in psychosis: Findings from 10-year follow-up study in the PAFIP-cohort. *Acta Psychiatr Scand*, **140**, 349–359.

Wilson, R., and Bhattacharyya, S. (2016). Antipsychotic efficacy in psychosis with co-morbid cannabis misuse: A systematic review. *J Psychopharmacol*, **30**, 99–111.

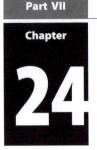

Treating Cannabis Use in Schizophrenia and Other Psychotic Disorders

Alexandria S. Coles, Ashley E. Kivlichan, David J. Castle, and Tony P. George

24.1 Cannabis Use in Psychosis

While the rates of problematic cannabis use (e.g., DSM-5 cannabis use disorder; CUD) are ~3% in the US population (Hasin, 2018), rates in people with schizophrenia have been estimated to be significantly higher (~25%) (Koskinen et al., 2010; see Chapters 4 and 17). Cannabis use in psychotic patients is associated with exacerbation of positive and negative symptoms of psychosis, higher rates of inpatient hospitalization, and poorer functional outcomes (Lowe et al., 2019; Rabin and George, 2017). Moreover, with legalization of recreational cannabis use in Western countries such as Canada, and in some American states, the prevalence of cannabis use and CUD is expected to increase (Hajizadeh, 2016), and this may disproportionately impact people with psychotic disorders including schizophrenia (George et al., 2018). Thus, the development of effective interventions to reduce use and promote abstinence from cannabis would be expected to improve the clinical course and quality-of-life of these patients.

24.2 Potential Neurobehavioural Mechanisms

As detailed in Chapters 14–18, cannabis use (notably containing delta-9-tetrahydrocannabinol, THC) increases positive symptoms of psychosis (D'Souza et al., 2005), which may be attributed to increased striatal dopaminergic activity (Guillin et al., 2007). Clinical data have been mixed on the effects of cannabis on negative symptoms, in part because patients report that cannabis reduces anxiety and depression (Bersani et al., 2002; Compton et al., 2004), possibly because of cannabinoids such as cannabidiol (CBD) or reversal of cannabis withdrawal symptoms. THC exposure has been associated with worsened negative symptoms, possibly due to disruption of frontal and striatal dopaminergic networks (Bloomfield et al., 2014). Moreover, the effects of cannabis on cognitive deficits in schizophrenia remain mixed (Rabin et al., 2011). However, intravenous THC administration has been found to impair verbal learning and memory (D'Souza et al., 2005), while extended cannabis abstinence improved these cognitive measures selectively in people with schizophrenia as compared to non-psychiatric cannabis using controls (Rabin et al., 2017). This is important given that cognition is a reliable predictor of functional outcomes in schizophrenia and psychotic disorders (Green, 2016) and supports the need for successful intervention strategies to address problematic cannabis use in these patients.

24.3 Clinical Assessment

The clinical assessment of people with co-occurring CUD and psychosis ideally requires an assessment of clinical stability, level of cannabis use (e.g., self-report plus confirmatory urine toxicology) and other addictive behaviours (e.g., alcohol, tobacco, and stimulants being the other most common co-morbidities in this population), as well as motivation to change cannabis use behaviours. Acutely psychotic patients are often unable and/or unwilling to engage in cannabis treatment, so clinical stabilization is important prior to initiating cannabis treatment. Given the long half-life of THC's metabolite carboxy-THC (~4–6 weeks; Schwilke et al., 2011), urine toxicology is often positive several weeks after cannabis use cessation. An assessment of cannabis use patterns, including frequency, method of use (e.g., smoking, vaporizer, edibles), as well as THC (and CBD) content is useful, as well as measures of cannabis addiction and impact on functioning. Measures include the Cannabis Use Disorders Identification Test (CUDIT) (Adamson et al., 2010) and the Addiction Severity Index (ASI), which assesses nine domains, including mental health, substance use, legal, psychosocial, and medical outcomes (McLellan et al., 1992). These assessments can be very useful for determining the level of treatment intensity and planning required by the patient. In addition, the DSM-IV global assessment of functioning (GAF) score can be very helpful, as cannabis and other substance misuse is a strong determinant of poor functional outcomes in psychosis (Longenecker et al., 2021). Motivation to quit cannabis is based on the Trans-theoretical (Stages of Change) Model (Krebs et al., 2018), and can be assessed by a number of scales including the Marijuana Contemplation Ladder (Slavet et al., 2006) and adaptations specifically for psychotic patients, such as the Reasons for Use Scale, which assesses motivations that maintain substance use among people with psychotic disorders (Kolliakou et al., 2012; Spencer et al., 2002).

Typically, those patients who indicate their willingness to quit or reduce cannabis use in the ensuing 30 days are most suitable to begin treatment; otherwise, motivational interviewing (MI) methods to engage patients into treatment are utilized (see Section 24.5). Most outpatient programmes typically require that patients not present for behavioural treatment when they are intoxicated; this can take six to eight hours of abstinence to remit.

24.4 Pharmacological Treatments

Managing co-morbid CUD in schizophrenia remains clinically challenging, with no approved treatments (Drake and Mueser, 2001). Nonetheless, similar to bipolar disorder (Coles et al., 2019), promising pharmacotherapies have been investigated in these patients. Two retrospective studies (Green et al., 2003; Tang et al., 2017), an observational study (Machielsen et al., 2012), an open-label trial (Potvin et al., 2006), and two randomized controlled trials (RCTs) (Brunette et al., 2011; Schnell et al., 2014) using the second-generation antipsychotics clozapine and ziprasidone found beneficial effects on psychosis and cannabis use. The rationale is that better management of positive, negative, and cognitive symptoms of psychosis may lead to a decrease in cannabis and other addictions (Kozak et al., 2017); clozapine may have putative effects on the drive to use a range of substances, but the precise mechanisms are unclear (Green, 2007). The first retrospective study by Green et al. (2003) examined data on alcohol and cannabis abstinence in 41 schizophrenia patients treated with

clozapine (n = 33) or risperidone (n = 8). Over a one-year period, abstinence rates were significantly higher for alcohol and cannabis in the clozapine versus risperidone groups (54% versus 13% respectively; $p < 0.05$). The second study was a retrospective chart review of youth with psychotic disorders and cannabis use exposed to clozapine (n = 13) versus those treated with other antipsychotic drugs (n = 14) over one-month periods between 2010 and 2012. Treatment with clozapine was associated with significant reductions in cannabis use (OR = 7.1; 95% CI = 2.3–22.3) and psychotic symptoms (OR = 3.7; 95% CI = 1.2–11.8) as compared to other antipsychotic drugs (Tang et al., 2017).

An observational study of 123 Dutch cannabis using patients with schizophrenia (Machielsen et al., 2012) found that clozapine (350 mg/day; n = 27) and olanzapine (13.8 mg/day; n = 60) were superior to risperidone (3.5 mg/day; n = 54) for reducing cannabis craving. In an open-label trial conducted in Montreal, Canada in 24 patients with schizophrenia spectrum disorders who were switched to quetiapine (mean dose 466 ± 227 mg/day) for 12 weeks (Potvin et al., 2006), there were reductions in cannabis, alcohol, and other substance use. In the study by Brunette et al. (2011) in New Hampshire, a total of 31 individual with schizophrenia were either switched to clozapine (n = 15) or remained on their existing antipsychotic treatment (n = 16). There were significant reductions in cannabis use by 4.5 joints per week using self-report with TLFB methods. However, there were no differences in clinical symptoms between groups. Another study from Germany compared treatment with clozapine versus ziprasidone for cannabis use in patients with schizophrenia (N = 30). Both antipsychotics were associated with reductions in cannabis use, and side-effects were lower and adherence improved in the ziprasidone group (Schnell et al., 2014). Interestingly, there is some evidence that problematic cannabis use is associated with treatment-resistant schizophrenia, both of which may respond to clozapine (Arsalan et al., 2019). Larger randomized controlled trials of clozapine and other second-generation antipsychotic drugs in cannabis misusing psychotic patients are warranted. A summary of pharmacotherapies that have been studied in people with CUD and psychosis is presented in Table 24.1.

It should be noted that non-adherence to antipsychotics is common in people with schizophrenia, and

Table 24.1 Pharmacological treatment for cannabis in schizophrenia (N = 6 studies; N = 276 participants)

Study	Sample	Treatment	Study Design	Results
Green et al. (2003)	N = 41 participants with Schizophrenia or Schizoaffective disorder AND alcohol or CUD	Clozapine (n = 33) OR Risperidone (n = 8)	1-year retrospective abstinence study	Abstinence rates were significantly higher in patients treated with clozapine compared those treated with risperidone (54% versus 13%, $p = 0.05$)
Potvin et al. (2006)	N = 24 patients with schizophrenia and CUD	Quetiapine (400 mg/day)	Open-label trial for 12 weeks	Reductions in cannabis and other substance use during the 12-week trial
Brunette et al. (2011)	N = 31 participants with schizophrenia or schizoaffective disorder and CUD	Clozapine (400 mg/day) OR maintain current antipsychotic treatment (control)	A 12-week, randomized, open-label trial	Clozapine group saw a significant reduction in cannabis use intensity compared to control
Machielsen et al. (2014)	N = 123 patients with schizophrenia and CUD	Clozapine (350 mg/day; n = 27) OR Olanzapine (13.8 mg/day; n = 60) OR Risperidone (3.5 mg/day; n = 54)	Observational study of antipsychotic drug treatment and craving assessments pre- and post-treatment	Clozapine and Olanzapine were superior to Risperidone for reducing cannabis craving in schizophrenia
Schnell et al. (2014)	N = 30 participants with schizophrenia and CUD	Ziprasidone (Average dose of 225 mg/day; n = 16) OR Clozapine (Average of 200 mg/day; n = 14)	A 12-month, randomized controlled pilot study	Cannabis use was reduced in both groups during follow-up, though Clozapine treatment resulted in significantly fewer positive symptoms, but more side-effects compared to the Ziprasidone group
Tang et al. (2017)	N = 27 adolescent participants with CUD and a psychotic disorder	Clozapine (n = 13) OR continued antipsychotic treatment (n = 14)	A retrospective cohort chart review	Individuals treated with Clozapine saw a significant reduction in cannabis use compared to those who maintained their current antipsychotic treatment

Abbreviations: CUD, cannabis use disorder; UDS, urine drug screen; NRT, transdermal patch nicotine replacement therapy; CBT, cognitive behavioural therapy; RP, relapse prevention; ND, no dose; MET, motivational enhancement therapy; MI, motivational interviewing; SUD, substance use disorder; CAP, cannabis and psychosis therapy; PE, psychoeducation; SMI, severe mental illness; AUD, alcohol use disorder; CM, contingency management.

even more so in those who use cannabis. Thus, part of the pharmacological treatment strategy in such individuals should include the use of long-acting injectable (LAI; depot) formulations of antipsychotic drugs. The evidence base, however, is sparse, in part due to challenges in engaging people with SUDs in clinical trials, but early studies in people with schizophrenia and SUDs treated with LAIs are promising (Abdel-Baki et al., 2020; Szerman et al., 2020; and reviewed by Coles et al., 2021).

24.4.1 Non-psychosis Medication Studies

In non-psychotic cannabis-using populations (see Table 24.2) there are several off-label pharmacotherapies that have been investigated for treating problematic cannabis use. These have included cannabinoids

Table 24.2 Pharmacological treatments for cannabis use disorder participants without psychosis (N = 29 studies; N = 2,119 participants)

Study	Sample	Treatment	Study Design	Results
Cannabinoid Agonists (6 studies, N = 508 participants)				
Levin et al. (2011)	N = 156 participants with CUD	Dronabinol (20 mg, 2×/day; n = 79) OR Placebo (n = 77) (1-week placebo lead-in for both groups)	A 12-week randomized, double-blind, placebo-controlled trial	No significant differences in abstinence between groups (Dronabinol: 17.7%; placebo 15.6%). Withdrawal symptoms were significantly lower in the Dronabinol group compared to placebo ($p = 0.02$).
Haney et al. (2013)	N = 11 participants with CUD	Nabilone (3 phase administration: 0 mg/day, 6 mg/day, 8 mg/day)	Three 8-day inpatient phases with 7 outpatient days between treatment administration	With increased dose, Nabilone administration decreased cannabis use compared to placebo ($p < 0.05$), and decreased withdrawal symptoms.
Allsop et al. (2014)	N = 51 participants with CUD	Nabiximols (n = 27) OR Placebo (n = 24)	A 9-day randomized, double-blind, inpatient trial with 28-day follow-up period	Nabiximols significantly reduced CWS scores by 66% compared to placebo ($p = 0.01$).
Levin et al. (2016)	N = 122 participants with CUD	Dronabinol (0.6 mg, 3×/day) AND Lofexidine (n = 61) OR Placebo (n = 61) (1-week placebo lead-in for all groups)	A 12-week double blind, placebo-controlled, randomized controlled trial	Treatment with combined Dronabinol–Lofexidine did not produce significantly different abstinence results compared to placebo (18/61 versus 17/61). Withdrawal scores were not significant within the treatment group ($p = 0.83$).
Trigo et al. (2018)	N = 40 participants with CUD	Nabiximols (n = 20) OR Placebo (n = 20) with combination MET/CBT intervention	A 12-week double-bind, randomized clinical trial	Decreased cannabis use in both groups ($p<0.001$), with no significant between-group differences.
Lintzeris et al. (2019)	N = 128 participants with CUD	Nabiximols (n = 61) OR Placebo (n = 67) AND weekly CBT-based individual counselling	A 12-week, multi-site, double-blind randomized clinical trial	Nabiximols significantly decreased the use of cannabis (35.0 days) compared to the placebo (53.1 days) during the 84-day clinical trial period ($p = 0.02$).
Antidepressants (5 studies, N = 359 participants)				
Carpenter et al. (2009)	N = 106 participants with CUD	SR Bupropion Hydrochloride (n = 40) OR Nefazodone (n = 36) OR Placebo (n = 30)	A 13-week double-blind, randomized, placebo controlled clinical trial	Limited reduction in cannabis dependence ($p = 0.14$). Participants having more severe cannabis dependence showed an increased reduction in dependence severity in the Bupropion SR and Nefazodone groups compared to placebo.

Table 24.2 (cont.)

Study	Sample	Treatment	Study Design	Results
Penetar et al. (2012)	N = 22 participants with CUD	Bupropion (n = 10) OR Placebo (n = 12)	A 3-week double-blind, placebo-controlled, randomized clinical trial	Decreased cravings and withdrawal symptoms in both groups, with no significant difference between Bupropion and placebo.
Levin et al. (2013)	N = 103 participants with CUD and MDD	VEN-XR (up to 375 mg/day; n = 51) OR Placebo (n = 52)	A 12-week, double-blind, placebo-controlled	Abstinence was lower in the VEN-XR group compared to the placebo (11.8% versus 36.5%). Mood improvements were associated with a reduction of cannabis use in the placebo group but not VEN-XR.
Weinstein et al. (2014)	N = 52 participants with CUD	Escitalopram (10 mg/day; n = 26) AND 9 weekly CBT and MET group sessions OR Placebo (n = 26) AND 9 weekly CBT and MET group sessions	A 9-week double-blind, placebo-controlled treatment study with 14 weeks follow-up	Three participants in the escitalopram group abstained from cannabis compared to seven in the placebo group. No significant difference in reduction of withdrawal symptoms in either group.
McRae-Clark et al. (2016)	N = 76 participants with CUD	Vilazodone (40 mg/day; n = 41) OR Placebo (n = 35)	An 8-week double-blind, randomized, controlled pilot trial	Participants in both groups reported reduced cannabis use with no significant differences between Vilazodone and placebo treatment.
Transdermal Nicotine Patch (2 Studies, N = 139 participants)				
Hill et al. (2013)	N = 12 participants with CUD and nicotine dependence	TNP (21mg/day × 6 weeks, 14 mg/day × 2 weeks, and 7 mg/day × 2 weeks) AND CBT and NRT OR TNP (14 mg/day × 8 weeks and 7 mg/day × 2 weeks) AND CBT and NRT	A 10-week prospective pilot study	Cannabis use did not significantly decrease during study (10 ± 5.3 inhalations at baseline versus 8.00 ± 5.3 inhalations at end).
Gilbert et al. (2020)	N = 127 participants with CUD	TNP (n = 63) or Placebo patch (n = 64)	Case-control, placebo-controlled study over 15 days	The use of TNP was associated with higher cannabis withdrawal symptoms. Cannabis cravings were reduced in the TNP group compared to placebo post-treatment.
N-Acetylcysteine (4 Studies, N = 525 participants)				
Gray et al. (2010)	N = 18 adolescent participants with CUD	N-acetylcysteine (1,200 mg, 2×/day)	A 4-week open-label pilot study	Cannabis use and craving decreased at the end of treatment.
Gray et al. (2012)	N = 116 participants CUD	N-acetylcysteine (1,200 mg, 2×/day; n = 58) OR placebo (n = 58)	An 8-week double-blind, randomized placebo-controlled trial	Abstinence from cannabis was 50% in N-acetylcysteine treated compared to 25% in placebo group (p = 0.05).

Study	Sample	Intervention	Study design	Results
Roten et al. (2013)	N = 89 participants with CUD	N-acetylcysteine (1,200 mg, 2×/day; n = 45) OR placebo (n = 44)	An 8-week, randomized, placebo-controlled trial	Both groups showed significant decreases in MCQ scores but no significant differences between groups were observed.
Gray et al. (2017)	N = 302 participants, with CUD	N-acetylcysteine (1,200 mg, 2×/day) OR placebo	A 12-week double blind randomized placebo-controlled trial	22.3% of the NAC group abstained from cannabis use compared to 22.4% in the placebo group. The results were not statistically significant ($p = 0.98$).
Mood stabilizers (1 Study, N = 38 participants)				
Johnston et al. (2014)	N = 38 participants with CUD	Lithium (500 mg/day; n = 16) OR placebo (n = 22)	A 3-month double-blind, placebo-controlled parallel-group randomized controlled trial	Cannabis use for both groups deceased. No significant differences between groups.
Anticonvulsants (3 Studies, N = 141 participants)				
Levin et al. (2004)	N = 25 participants with CUD	Divalproex Sodium (1,000 mg/day; n = 13) OR placebo (n = 12)	A 12-week double-blind, placebo-controlled crossover pilot study	Significant reduction in frequency and amount of use, as well as cravings for cannabis in both groups. No statistically significant differences between groups.
Mason et al. (2012)	N = 50 participants with CUD	Gabapentin (1,800 mg/day; n = 25) OR placebo (n = 25)	A 12-week, randomized, double-blind, placebo-controlled trial	Gabapentin significantly decreasing Cannabis use ($p = 0.004$) and significantly lowered withdrawal symptoms ($p < 0.001$) compared to results of the placebo group.
Miranda et al. (2017)	N = 66 youth with CUD	Topiramate (n = 40) OR placebo (n = 26) with MET	A 6-week double-blind, randomized, placebo-controlled pilot study	Topiramate significantly reduced the quantity of cannabis use but did not impact abstinence rates, compared to placebo with MET.
Anxiolytics (2 Studies, N = 217 participants)				
McRae-Clark et al. (2009)	N = 60 participants with CUD	Buspirone (60 mg/day; n = 23) OR placebo (n = 27)	A 12-week double-blind, placebo-controlled trial	Buspirone treatment showed higher cannabis abstinence rates compared to placebo participants verified through UDSs ($p = 0.071$).
McRae-Clark et al. (2015)	N = 157 participants with CUD	Buspirone (60 mg/day; n = 88) OR placebo (n = 87) with MET	A 12-week double-blind, randomized, placebo-controlled trial	Participants in both groups showed reduced cannabis cravings with no significant differences between groups.
Opioid Antagonists (2 Studies, N = 63 participants)				
Haney et al. (2015)	N = 51 participants with CUD	Naltrexone (50 mg/day; n = 23) OR placebo (n = 28)	A 4–6-week outpatient randomized controlled trial	Participants in the placebo group were significantly more likely to self-administer active cannabis compared to the Naltrexone group.

Table 24.2 *(cont.)*

Study	Sample	Treatment	Study Design	Results
Notzon et al. (2018)	N = 12 participants with CUD	Long-acting Naltrexone (380 mg IM at week 1 and week 5)	An 8-week open-label pilot study	Cannabis use frequency significantly decreased compared to baseline ($p = 0.001$).
Neuropeptides (1 Study, N = 16 participants)				
Sherman et al. (2017)	N = 16 participants with CUD	Oxytocin with MET (n = 8) OR Placebo with MET (n = 8)	A 4-week randomized, placebo-controlled trial	Participants receiving oxytocin showed decreased cannabis use and increased MET sessions attended compared to placebo.
Fatty Acid Amide Hydrolase (FAAH) Inhibitors (1 Study, N = 80 participants)				
D'Souza et al. (2019)	N = 80 participants with CUD	PF-04457845 (4 mg/day; n = 46) OR placebo (n = 24)	A double-blind, placebo-controlled parallel group Phase II trial	Use of PF-04457845, a novel FAAH inhibitor, reduced cannabis use and withdrawal symptoms compared to placebo.
Second-Generation Antipsychotics (1 Study, N = 12 participants)				
Cooper et al. (2013)	N = 12 participants with CUD	Quetiapine (200 mg/day) OR placebo	A 30-day double-blind, placebo-controlled trial	Quetiapine group saw decreased cannabis withdrawal symptoms, but increased cannabis cravings and self-administration compared to placebo.
Combination Study: Antidepressant and Skeletal Muscle Relaxant (1 Study, N = 21 participants)				
Haney et al. (2010)	Study 1: N = 10 participants with CUD Study 2: N = 11 participants with CUD	Study 1: Mirtazapine (60 mg/day) AND Baclofen (90 mg/day) OR placebo Study 2: Baclofen (30 mg/day) AND Mirtazapine (30 mg/day) OR placebo	Multi-phasic inpatient controlled Study (Study 1: 16 days, Study 2: 8 days)	Study 1: The combination of Mirtazapine and Baclofen decreased craving for tobacco and cannabis but also decreased cognitive performance. Study 2: There were no effects of lower dose of Baclofen and Mirtazapine on withdrawal symptoms and did not decrease rates of cannabis relapse.

Abbreviations: CUD, cannabis use disorder; mg, milligrams; MDD, major depressive disorder; CWS, cannabis withdrawal scale; MET, motivational enhancement therapy; CBT, cognitive behavioural therapy; PBO, placebo; VEN-XR, venlafaxine-extended release; RCT, randomized controlled trial; TNP, transdermal nicotine patch; NRT, nicotine replacement therapy; NAC, N-acetylcysteine; MCQ, marijuana craving questionnaire; IM, intramuscular; UDS, urine drug screen; FAAH, fatty acid amide hydrolase.

(e.g., replacement strategies) such as dronabinol (Levin et al., 2011, 2016), nabilone (Haney et al., 2013), and nabiximols (Allsop et al., 2014; Lintzeris et al., 2019; Trigo et al., 2018); transdermal nicotine patch (Gilbert et al., 2020; Hill et al., 2013); antidepressants such as escitalopram (Weinstein et al., 2014), mirtazapine (Haney et al., 2010), vilazodone (McRae-Clark et al., 2016), nefazodone (Carpenter et al., 2009), venlafaxine (Levin et al., 2013), and bupropion (Carpenter et al., 2009; Penetar et al., 2012); the mood-stabilizer lithium carbonate (Johnston et al., 2014); anticonvulsant drugs such as gabapentin (Mason et al., 2012), topiramate (Miranda et al., 2017), and divalproex sodium (Levin et al., 2004); the anti-oxidant/nutraceutical N-acetylcysteine (Gray et al., 2010, 2012, 2017; Roten et al., 2013); buspirone (McRae-Clark et al., 2009, 2015), baclofen (Haney et al., 2010); oral (Haney et al., 2015) and injectable (Notzon et al., 2018) naltrexone; atomoxetine (McRae-Clark et al., 2010); baclofen (Haney et al., 2010); the neuroactive peptide hormone oxytocin (Sherman et al., 2017); and the second-generation antipsychotic drug quetiapine (Cooper et al., 2013). Most of these off-label experimental studies and clinical trials have had mixed results (see Table 24.2).

Interestingly, non-approved, investigational medications such as the fatty acid amide hydrolase (FAAH) inhibitor PF-04457845 (D'Souza et al., 2019) have shown promise as a pharmacotherapy for CUD with robust reductions in cannabis use. Given that schizophrenia is associated with endogenous endocannabinoid deficiency (Borgan et al., 2021), treatment with FAAH inhibitors, which increase endogenous levels of anandamide, may be useful for the management of CUD in psychotic patients (D'Souza et al., 2019). However, these medications have not been formally tested in people with schizophrenia or psychotic disorders. One practical concern in psychotic patients with CUD is that many of these off-label medications (e.g., cannabinoids, venlafaxine, atomoxetine) could exacerbate pre-existing psychosis. Taken together, it is clear that current medication treatment strategies for CUD in people with or without psychosis are far from satisfactory and require further study.

24.5 Behavioural Interventions for Psychosis and CUD

Several psychosocial interventions have been studied, based on the premise that what benefits substance users more generally may, with some enhancements, also benefit substance users with psychosis. Significant differences exist across these interventions in terms of intensity, duration, theoretical model used, mode and location of administration, the target group to which they have been applied, and the way that they have been evaluated. These differences make comparison between studies difficult, and also limit the generalizability of findings across groups and settings (Drake et al., 2008). We address these studies under several categories (see Table 24.3).

24.5.1 Motivational Interviewing (MI)

A single study examined the effects of MI plus treatment as usual (TAU) in the treatment of CUD among individuals with psychosis in a single centre clinical trial (Bonsack et al., 2011). In this study, 62 participants were randomized to receive four-to-six 60-minute individual sessions of either MI+TAU or TAU alone. Participants in the MI+TAU group were also offered a further two-to-four booster sessions of MI up to six months post-study inclusion, that were tailored to the needs of each participant. MI sessions were adapted using an integrated, dual diagnosis approach, which emphasized the effects of cannabis use on symptoms of psychosis. Further, to account for potential cognitive impairment in psychosis, MI interviews were structured around a decisional balance grid, which involved the use of simple verbal and visual materials and repetition strategies. Results demonstrated a significant reduction in amount of cannabis used per week and increased readiness to change cannabis use at six months follow-up for the MI+TAU group compared to TAU alone, though differences between groups were not maintained at 12 months.

24.5.2 Studies Integrating Cognitive Behavioural Therapies (CBTs) with Other Modalities

Four studies investigated the use of combination MI plus CBT (MI+CBT) in participants with comorbid psychosis and CUD, with mixed results. A study by Barrowclough et al. (2001) demonstrated positive results in a randomized controlled trial comparing routine psychiatric care alone, with a programme of routine psychiatric care augmented with a comprehensive package of MI, CBT, and family/caregiver

Table 24.3 Behavioural interventions for cannabis use disorder in psychosis (N = 15 studies; N = 1,365 participants)

Study	Sample	Treatment	Study Design	Results
Motivational Interviewing (MI) (1 Study; N = 62 participants)				
Bonsack et al. (2011)	N = 62 participants with CUD and psychosis	MI (n = 30) OR TAU (n = 32)	A single-centre randomized controlled clinical trial	Participants in the MI group saw a significant reduction in amount of cannabis use per week and confidence to change cannabis use, compared to TAU. Differences between groups were not maintained at 12-month follow-up.
Cognitive Behavioural Therapy (CBT) + Other Behavioural Treatment Modalities (4 Studies; N = 329 participants)				
Barrowclough et al. (2001)	N = 33 participants with schizophrenia or schizoaffective disorder and SUD	Routine care OR integrated care (MI, CBT, and family or caregiver intervention)	A randomized, single-blind controlled study	The integrated care group saw a reduction in positive symptoms and an increase in the percentage of days of abstinence from drugs or alcohol over a 12-month period.
James et al. (2004)	N = 63 participants with a SUD and a psychotic disorder	Treatment Group (MET, RP, & harm reduction; n = 32) OR Control group (n = 31, standard community mental health care)	A 6-week, randomized controlled trial	A significant reduction in use and dependence severity was observed in the treatment group compared to control.
Baker et al. (2006)	N = 130 participants with psychosis and a SUD (alcohol, cannabis, and/or amphetamines)	CBT AND MI (10 weeks; n = 65) OR TAU (n = 65)	A 12-month randomized controlled trial	Short-term improvement in cannabis use frequency at 12 months. Results not maintained beyond follow-up.
Hjorthøj et al. (2013)	N = 103 participants with CUD and psychosis	CapOpus+TAU (CBT and MI; n = 52) OR TAU Alone (n = 51)	A 6-month randomized controlled trial	CapOpus+TAU group saw a reduction in amount of cannabis use, but not frequency compared to TAU alone.
Studies in Early Psychosis (5 Studies; N = 328 participants)				
Kavanagh et al. (2004)	N = 25 participants with early onset psychosis and SUD	Standard care (Pharmacotherapy; n = 12) OR treatment (MET; n = 13)	A 12-month randomized, single-blind, controlled study	All participants in the treatment group reported less substance use at 6 months, compared with 7/12 in the standard care group.
Edwards et al. (2006)	N = 47 participants with first episode psychosis and CUD	Treatment condition (CAP: MI, RP & Harm Reduction; n = 23) OR control condition (PE; n = 24).	A single-blind randomized controlled trial	There were no significant differences between the CAP and PE groups on cannabis use.
Bucci et al. (2010)	N = 58 participants aged 12–25 with FEP or UHR for psychosis who used cannabis weekly	CBT, RP, AND MI (8 weeks)	A 12-month naturalistic study	Participants saw a clinically significant reduction in number of cannabis use occasions per week at 12 months follow-up.

Study	Sample	Intervention	Study design	Results
Madigan et al. (2013)	N = 88 participants with early onset psychosis and CUD	GPI (CBT & MI) OR TAU	A 1-year, multi-site, randomized controlled trial	GPI group saw no significant improvements in psychotic symptoms or cannabis use, compared to TAU.
Barrowclough et al. (2014)	N = 110 participants with first-episode psychosis and CUD	1:1:1 randomization CBT AND MI (12 sessions) OR CBT AND MI (24 sessions) OR Standard care (control)	A single-blind randomized controlled trial for up to 24 weeks	No improvements in cannabis use (frequency or amount) or psychotic symptoms was observed in either treatment group compared to the standard care condition.
Contingency Management (CM) (4 Studies; N = 615 participants)				
Sigmon et al. (2000)	N = 18 male participants with SMI and regular cannabis use	CM for cannabis negative UDS OR control	A 25-week randomized, controlled abstinence study	The number of cannabis negative UDS was significantly higher in the incentivized compensation group compared to control.
Sigmon and Higgins (2006)	N = 7 participants with SMI who used cannabis weekly	Voucher-based CM	A 20-week CM study	The participants achieved greater cannabis abstinence during the incentive CM than during the baseline conditions.
Rabin et al. (2018)	N = 39 participants with Schizophrenia. 19 with CUD, 20 controls	CM	A 28-day cannabis abstinence study	Abstinence rates of 42.1% (8/19) in patients and 55% (11/19) in controls ($p = 0.53$) were observed. Increased cannabis withdrawal in both patients and controls supported abstinence.
Sheridan Rains et al. (2019)	N = 551 participants with first-episode psychosis and CUD	CM+PE (n = 272) OR PE (Control group; n = 259)	A two-armed, single-blind, multi-centre, randomized controlled trial	No significant differences in cannabis use or psychiatric hospitalizations between CM +TAU group, compared to control.
Cognitive Enhancement Therapy (CET) (1 Study; N = 31 participants)				
Eack et al. (2015)	N = 31 participants with schizophrenia and SUD (alcohol and/or cannabis)	CET OR TAU	An 18-month, small scale, randomized controlled feasibility study	No significant differences between groups in cannabis use measures were observed.

Abbreviations: CUD, cannabis use disorder; UDS, urine drug screen; NRT, transdermal patch nicotine replacement therapy; CBT, cognitive behavioural therapy; RP, relapse prevention; ND, no dose; MET, motivational enhancement therapy; MI, motivational interviewing; SUD, substance use disorder; CAP, cannabis and psychosis therapy; PE, psychoeducation; SMI, severe mental illness; AUD, alcohol use disorder; CM, contingency management; TAU, treatment as usual; GPI, group-based psychological intervention; UHR, ultra-high risk; FEP, first episode psychosis; CET, cognitive enhancement therapy.

psychoeducational interventions in substance users with schizophrenia. This intervention was delivered at participants' homes over a nine-month period and required the involvement of family or caregivers to ensure consistency of the interventions. Findings suggested that integrated comprehensive care may generate significant improvements in general functioning, reduce positive symptoms, and lead to an increase in the number of days abstinent from drugs and alcohol. Cannabis was the illicit substance most used by participants in this study. In a follow-up study of this cohort, the participants were assessed at 18 months following study conclusion. Participants in the MI+CBT group maintained improvements in functioning and had a greater percentage of days abstinent relative to baseline than did the control group (Haddock et al., 2003).

A study by Baker et al. (2006) in Australia investigated the use of combination MI+CBT in a community sample of participants with chronic psychosis and substance use disorders (alcohol, cannabis, and/ or amphetamines) in a 12-month randomized controlled trial. One hundred and thirty participants were randomized (1:1) to either MI+CBT (10 weekly, 1-hour sessions) or TAU alone. They were assessed on substance use and psychiatric outcomes at baseline, 15 weeks, 8 months, and 12 months. Participants in the MI+CBT group showed short-term improvements in cannabis use and general functioning at 12 months, though results were not maintained beyond this timepoint (Baker et al., 2006). Moreover, another Australian study observed positive results across several domains in a group-based intervention aimed at reducing substance use and improving mental health among cannabis users with chronic psychosis (James et al., 2004). The intervention was tailored to each participant's motivation for drug use and readiness to change, and encompassed aspects of psychoeducational, MI, cognitive-behavioural/relapse-prevention, and harm reduction approaches. The intervention was performed using a manualized six-week programme. A total of 68 participants were enrolled and randomly allocated to routine psychiatric care or routine care plus the group intervention. Significant improvements were observed within the intervention group on psychopathology, chlorpromazine equivalent doses of antipsychotic medication, and reductions in cannabis and polydrug use.

Finally, a study of the combination MI+CBT was conducted with positive results (Hjorthøj et al., 2013).

One hundred and three participants with psychosis and CUD were randomized to receive either six months of the CapOpus intervention (MI+CBT) or TAU (primarily targeted psychotic symptoms). At baseline, monthly joint use was 46.4 across all participants. In the CapOpus group, consumption reduced significantly to 27.3 joints monthly (95% CI = 12.6–41.9) compared to 48.2 monthly in the TAU condition (95% CI = 31.8–64.6) (p = 0.06). Frequency of cannabis use (days of use per month) did not change significantly, with no significant differences between groups (Hjorthøj et al., 2013).

24.5.3 Early Psychosis

Several studies have studied behavioural interventions for substance use in early psychosis. Kavanagh et al. (2004) evaluated a motivational enhancement therapy (MET) approach for addressing substance use among people with recent onset psychosis. Twenty-five in-patients aged 18–35 years with early psychosis and current misuse of non-opioid drugs were allocated randomly to Standard Care (SC) or SC plus Start Over and Survive (SOS). SOS is an intervention based on the principles of MI and relapse-prevention, including psychoeducation and harm-reduction. The intervention was manualized and comprised of three hours of individual treatment over six-to-nine sessions, which was usually completed within 7–10 days. Participant's goals for change were selected in consultation with therapists and included both reduced use and abstinence from substance use. Substance use and related problems were assessed at baseline, 6 weeks and at 3, 6, and 12 months. Final assessments were undertaken blind to the condition to which the participant was allocated. Participants who received the treatment intervention reported less substance use than controls, and this effect was maintained at 12 months follow-up.

In a separate study, Edwards et al. (2006) developed a cannabis-focused intervention for young people with first-episode psychosis. The intervention encompassed MI, goal-setting, relapse-prevention, and psychoeducation about the possible effects of cannabis on psychosis. It was delivered to 23 participants in weekly sessions by trained clinicians over a 3-month period, with each session lasting between 20–60 minutes. The control group (n = 24) was provided with standard care plus psychoeducation only. No significant differences were found between the treatment and control groups at the end of treatment and at six-month follow-up in terms of drug use, psychopathology, and functioning. However, both the treatment and the control group had significantly reduced their cannabis use over this time. The authors concluded that, as neither intervention was found to be superior, relatively simple, general interventions should be considered initially to reduce cannabis use among people with first-episode psychosis. Additionally, in a separate controlled trial in cannabis users (N = 110) with early psychosis, the combination of MI and CBT, either as a 12- or 24-week treatment period versus standard care did not find any differences across the three groups on cannabis use or psychiatric symptom outcomes (Barrowclough et al., 2014).

In a 12-month naturalistic study, Bucci et al. (2010) studied a sample of 58 young adults with first-episode psychosis, or those at ultra-high risk of developing psychosis. All participants received MI +CBT and relapse prevention (RP) for a period of two-to-eight weeks, depending on severity of cannabis use at baseline. The intervention was associated with significant reductions in frequency of cannabis use per day, though global functioning scores were lower at 12 month follow-up for users of cannabis, compared to non-users.

Finally, a study investigating the effects of MI +CBT by Madigan et al. (2013) examined early psychosis participants with CUD in a multi-site trial. A total of 88 participants were randomized (2:1) to either the 12-week group-based psychological intervention (MI+CBT) or TAU. No evidence to indicate an effect of the intervention on domains of cannabis use, global functioning, or attitude to treatment was observed. Notably, participants in the group-based intervention indicated a significant increase in quality-of-life compared to the TAU group, maintained at one-year follow-up.

Thus, the evidence to support the use of MI+CBT in first-episode psychosis patients is mixed and requires further study.

24.5.4 Contingency Management (CM)

CM promotes short-term behavioural change using positive or negative contingencies. There is evidence for the efficacy of CM interventions for people with problematic cannabis use and serious mental illness (Sigmon et al., 2000; Sigmon and Higgins, 2006). In an initial feasibility study in 18 subjects with

schizophrenia or other serious mental illness and cannabis use disorder (CUD) by Sigmon et al. (2000) in Vermont, USA, escalating monetary payments ($25–$100) were associated with an increased number of drug-free urine samples. Subsequently, using a within-subjects design in seven people with schizophrenia and CUD, voucher-based incentives for drug-free urine samples (up to $930 over 12 weeks) were superior to non-contingent payments ($10/urine, irrespective of outcome) over 4 week baseline periods (Sigmon and Higgins, 2006). More recently, in Toronto, Canada, Rabin et al. (2018) employed a 28-day cannabis abstinence paradigm with CM in CUD subjects with and without schizophrenia, using a single contingent $300 payment for cannabis abstinence biochemically-confirmed using quantitative urine toxicology at study endpoint. All participants received brief (<15 minute) behavioural support using MI to engage them in treatment, as well as coping skills therapy to manage cannabis craving and withdrawal symptoms. There were high rates of cannabis abstinence (~43%) in 19 cannabis-dependent schizophrenia outpatients, comparable to the outcomes found in 20 non-psychiatric controls with CUD (~55%; $p = 0.74$).

Finally, Sheridan Rains et al. (2019) conducted a large multi-site controlled trial of CM in cannabis users with early psychosis (the CIRCLE study). Participants were randomized via a secure web-based service 1:1 to either an experimental arm, involving 12 weeks of CM plus a 6-session psychoeducation package, or a control arm, comprising the psychoeducation package only. The total potential voucher reward in the CM intervention was £240. The primary outcome was time to admission to an acute mental health service. Five hundred and fifty-one participants were recruited, and primary outcome data were obtained for 272 (98%) in the CM group and 259 (95%) in the control group. However, there was no statistically significant difference in time to acute psychiatric care (HR = 1.03, 95% CI = 0.76–1.40) between groups. By 18 months, 90 (33%) of the participants in the CM group and 85 (30%) of the control group had been admitted at least once to an acute psychiatric service. Among those who had experienced an acute psychiatric admission, the median time to admission was 196 days in the CM group and 245 days in the control group (p = NS). These results suggest that CM does not prevent psychiatric admission or reduce cannabis use in patients with early psychosis.

Collectively, these studies suggest the potential of CM interventions to promote cannabis use reductions and abstinence in psychotic cannabis users, but further studies are needed.

24.5.5 Cognitive Enhancement Therapy (CET)

A preliminary study of CET in participants with psychosis was conducted by Eack et al. (2015) in a sample of 31 individuals with an SUD (alcohol and/or cannabis) and schizophrenia. In this 18-month, randomized controlled, feasibility study, participants were allocated to either 18-months of cognitive enhancement therapy (CET; n = 22) or TAU (n = 9). The CET intervention involved cognitive remediation that combined facets of computer-based training in attention, memory, and problem-solving with group-based social cognition strategies. Intent-to-treat analyses demonstrated that, compared to the control group (TAU), participants who received CET were significantly less likely to use alcohol (OR = 0.22, 95% CI = 0.05–0.90, p = 0.036), but not cannabis (OR = 1.89, 95% CI = 0.02–142.99], p = 0.77). Further CET studies are required to understand its potential as an intervention for cannabis use in this population.

24.5.6 Non-psychosis Behavioural Studies

There have been several studies of interventions for CUD in non-psychiatric samples. CBT, MI, RP, CM, and MET have been used to address CUD, with mostly positive outcomes (Table 24.4). A single study examined RP versus control for CUD in non-psychiatric populations (Stephens et al., 1994). The same authors conducted a more recent study comparing MI to RP to a delayed treatment control (Stephens et al., 2000). Five studies have been conducted to understand the effects of CBT in CUD among non-psychiatric populations: Copeland et al. (2001) compared one versus six sessions of CBT versus control in a three-armed randomized controlled trial. Rooke et al. (2013) studied web-based CBT intervention compared to controls. Another study examined the combination of CBT + MI versus control (Gates et al., 2012), and a further study examined the effects of CBT compared to multidisciplinary family therapy (MDFT) on cannabis use (Hendriks et al., 2011). Finally, a recent study by Sinadinovic et al. (2020) compared guided web-based treatment planning versus waitlist control. The results of these studies are summarized in Table 24.4.

Other studies have been conducted with MET alone, or in combination with CBT compared to controls (Hoch et al., 2012; Stephens et al., 2004). Moreover, studies combining MET, CBT, and CM for treatment of CUD have also been performed (Budney et al., 2006; Carroll et al., 2006; Kadden et al., 2007; Litt et al., 2020) (see Table 24.4).

24.6 Other Treatment Modalities

Neuromodulation has emerged as a potential treatment option for CUD, including repetitive transcranial magnetic stimulation (rTMS) (Coles et al., 2018; Mahoney et al., 2020), where an electromagnetic coil placed against the scalp produces pulses in rapid succession to targeted brain regions. Most studies have targeted the dorsolateral prefrontal cortex (DLPFC) to modulate cortical excitability and strengthen cognitive control (Bellamoli et al., 2014; Dunlop et al., 2017). High-frequency rTMS has shown promise in reducing drug craving (Diana et al., 2017; Zhang et al., 2019) and use, for several SUDs including CUD (Bellamoli et al., 2014; Coles et al., 2018; Feil and Zangen, 2010; Gorelick et al., 2014; Hanlon et al., 2018; Mahoney et al., 2020; Salling and Martinez, 2016; Zhang et al., 2019). Several factors differ between studies including number of rTMS sessions, site of stimulation, presence of a sham control, whether left, right, or bilaterally administered, sample size, and presence of comorbid psychiatric illnesses. However, a consensus exists that targeting the DLPFC is most effective, given its important role in inhibitory control of reward circuits, including mesocorticolimbic dopamine systems (Ikeda et al., 2019; Moretti et al., 2020). Moreover, given this area is important in executive and inhibitory control, and commonly impaired among people with SUDs, most studies apply high-frequency rTMS (e.g., 10, 20 Hz) to the DLPFC to decrease craving. Recently, our group at CAMH in Toronto, Canada has used high-frequency (20 Hz), sham-controlled rTMS to bilateral DLPFC for 20 sessions over 4 weeks to reduce cannabis use (Cohen's d = 0.55) and improve positive symptoms of schizophrenia in 19 people with schizophrenia and concurrent CUD (Kozak et al., 2021). This finding suggests the promise of neuromodulation paradigms to treat CUD in schizophrenia.

Table 24.4 Behavioural interventions for cannabis use disorder in non-psychiatric samples (N = 13 studies, N = 2,715 participants)

Study	Sample	Treatment	Study Design	Results
Stephens et al. (1994)	N = 212 adult participants with CUD	Relapse Prevention OR Control (SSG)	A 12-month randomized controlled trial	A significant reduction in frequency of cannabis use and related problems was found, with no significant differences between groups.
Stephens et al. (2000)	N = 291 treatment-seeking adults with CUD	MI (Brief, 2 sessions; n = 88) OR RP (14 sessions; n = 117) OR DTC (n = 86)	A 16-month randomized controlled trial	Significant reductions in cannabis use, dependence symptoms, and negative consequences of cannabis use in both treatment groups compared to DTC, with no significant differences between treatments.
Copeland et al. (2001)	N = 229 adult participants with CUD	CBT (1 session) OR CBT (6 sessions) OR DTC	A 12-month randomized controlled trial	Participants in treatment groups (CBT 1 and 6 sessions) reported increased rates of abstinence and less self-reported cannabis-related problems compared to DTC. Participants who received 6 sessions of CBT reported less overall cannabis consumption compared to single session CBT and DTC.
(Marijuana Treatment Project Research Group, 2004)	N = 450 adult participants with CUD	MET (2 sessions; n = 146) OR MET+CBT (9 sessions; n = 156) OR DTC (n = 148)	A 15 month multisite, randomized controlled trial	Individuals in the MET+CBT condition (9 sessions) saw significant reductions in cannabis use, compared to MET alone and the DTC.
Budney et al. (2006)	N = 90 treatment-seeking adults with CUD	CBT (n = 30) OR CM (abstinence-based vouchers; n = 30) OR CBT+CM (n = 30)	A 12-month randomized controlled trial	Results indicated that CM using abstinence-based vouchers were effective in maintaining cannabis abstinence over extended periods of time. CBT did not significantly contribute to abstinence, though it enhanced post-treatment maintenance of cannabis cessation.
Carroll et al. (2006)	N = 136 young adults with CUD	MET+CBT+CM OR MET+CBT OR IDC+CM OR IDC alone	A 4 arm, 6-month randomized controlled trial	A significant main effect of CM on cannabis-free UDS was found. MET+CBT+CM was significantly more effective at reducing cannabis use compared to other treatment groups. Participants who received this treatment maintained reduced frequency and amount of cannabis use at 6-month follow-up.

Table 24.4 (*cont.*)

Study	Sample	Treatment	Study Design	Results
Kadden et al. (2007)	N = 240 adult participants with CUD	MET+CBT+CM OR MET+CBT OR CM alone OR Control condition (case management only)	A 12-month randomized controlled trial	Both treatment groups involving CM saw superior improvements in cannabis abstinence compared to treatments without CM and control. The CM alone group saw the highest abstinence rates of all groups post-treatment. The MET+CBT+CM group showed highest maintained abstinence rates at 1 year follow-up.
Hendriks et al. (2011)	N = 109 adolescent participants with CUD	MDFT OR CBT	A 12 month randomized controlled trial	Participants in both treatment groups saw clinically significant reductions in cannabis use, maintained at follow-up. No significant differences between groups were observed.
Gates et al. (2012)	N = 110 participants with CUD	MI+CBT OR DTC	A 12-week randomized controlled trial	Participants in the treatment group reported significant reductions in symptoms of cannabis dependence and significantly higher levels of cannabis abstinence at 12 weeks compared to the DTC.
Hoch et al. (2012)	N = 122 adult participants with CUD	Treatment Group (MET+CBT +PST; n = 90) OR DTC (n = 32)	A 6 month randomized controlled trial	Cannabis abstinence was achieved in 49% of participants allocated to the treatment group compared to 13% in the DTC group. Further, individuals in the treatment group demonstrated a significant reduction in cannabis use amount, frequency, and overall addiction severity compared to DTC, maintained at 6-month follow-up.
Rooke et al. (2013)	N = 225 adult participants with CUD	Web-based CBT intervention OR Control (6 educational modules)	A 6-week randomized controlled trial	Experimental group reported significantly fewer days of cannabis during the past month, significantly fewer days of smoking, and significantly fewer symptoms of cannabis abuse compared to control participants.
Litt et al. (2020)	N = 198 participants with CUD	MET+CBT+CM OR IATP+CM OR MET+CBT OR IATP	A 14-month randomized controlled trial	IATP conditions saw significantly greater abstinence rates (with and without CM) compared to MET+CBT (with and without CM) group. The addition of CM to the MET+CBT group led to greater abstinence rates than MET+CBT alone.

Table 24.4 (*cont.*)

Study	Sample	Treatment	Study Design	Results
Sinadinovic et al. (2020)	N = 303 adult participants with CUD	Web-based Hybrid Intervention (CBT+PE; n = 151) OR WLC (n = 152)	A double blinded randomized controlled trial with a parallel group design	No significant differences between treatment group and WLC group were observed.

Abbreviations: CUD, cannabis use disorder; SSG, social support group; RP, relapse prevention; CBT, cognitive behavioural therapy; DTC, delayed treatment control; IDC, individual drug counselling; CM, contingency management; MET, motivational enhancement therapy; PST, problem-solving training; WLC, waitlist control; IAPT, individualized assessment and treatment programme; MDFT, multidimensional family therapy.

Finally, in Montreal, Canada, Tatar et al. (2021) have proposed the use of smart-phone and web-based interventions for early psychosis patients with problematic cannabis use, given that these young patients are difficult to treat but tend to favour technology-based assessment and treatment. Further work using digital technologies is warranted to assist cannabis users with psychotic disorders reduce their cannabis use.

24.7 Conclusion and Suggestions for Future Research

While there are some promising behavioural, pharmacological, and novel treatments which have been investigated for treating CUD in schizophrenia and psychosis, none have been validated in large, randomized, definitive controlled studies. It is also challenging to note that no such treatments have been approved for treatment of CUD in the general population. Engaging and retaining patients with psychosis and CUD is very difficult, and will likely require multi-site investigations, using randomized, controlled clinical trials and intensive subject retention strategies including contingency management. Moreover, increases in legalized recreational cannabis use are likely to lead to higher rates of problematic cannabis use in psychotic patients. Thus, a better understanding of the biobehavioural mechanisms that contribute to cannabis addiction in schizophrenia and psychosis may lead to unique treatment approaches using target engagement and validation strategies (e.g., rTMS, CBT). This has the potential to address this devastating co-morbidity in this highly marginalized and difficult to treat population of people with psychosis and CUD.

Funding

This work was supported in part by a National Institute of Drug Abuse (NIDA) grant R21-DA-043949 to Dr George.

Acknowledgements

The helpful and constructive comments on the manuscript by Rachel A. Rabin, Ph.D. (McGill University) is gratefully acknowledged.

References

Abdel-Baki, A., Thibault, D., Medrano, S., et al. (2020). Long-acting antipsychotic medication as first-line treatment of first-episode psychosis with comorbid substance use disorder. *Early Interv Psychiatry*, 14, 69–79.

Adamson, S., Kay-Lambkin, F., Baker, A., et al. (2010). An improved brief measure of cannabis misuse: The cannabis use disorders identification test – revised (CUDIT-R). *Drug Alcohol Depend*, 110, 137–143.

Allsop, D., Copeland, J., Linteris, N., et al. (2014). Nabiximols as an agonist replacement therapy during cannabis withdrawal: A randomized clinical trial. *JAMA Psychiatry*, 71, 281–291.

Arsalan, A., Iqbal, Z., Tariq, M., et al. (2019). Association of smoked cannabis with treatment resistance in schizophrenia. *Psychiatry Res*, 278, 242–247.

Baker, A., Bucci,, S., Lewin, T. J., et al. (2006). Cognitive-behavioural therapy for substance use disorders in people with psychotic disorders: Randomised controlled trial. *Br J Psychiatry*, **188**, 439–448.

Barrowclough, C., Haddock, G., Tarrier, N., et al. (2001). Randomized controlled trial of motivational interviewing, cognitive behavior therapy, and family intervention for patients with comorbid schizophrenia and substance use disorders. *Am J Psychiatry*, **158**, 1706–1713.

Barrowclough, C., Marshall, M., Gregg, L., et al. (2014). A phase-specific psychological therapy for people with problematic cannabis use following a first episode of psychosis: A randomized controlled trial. *Psychol Med*, **44**, 2749–2761.

Bellamoli, E., Manganotti, P., Schwartz, R. P., et al. (2014). rTMS in the treatment of drug addiction: An update about human studies. *Behav Neurol*, **2014**, 815215.

Bersani, G., Orlandi, V., Kotzalidis, G. D., et al. (2002). Cannabis and schizophrenia: Impact on onset, course, psychopathology and outcomes. *Eur Arch Psychiatry Clin Neurosci*, **252**, 86–92.

Bloomfield, M. A., Morgan, C. J., Kapur, S., et al. (2014). The link between dopamine function and apathy in cannabis users: An [18F]-DOPA PET imaging study. *Psychopharmacology (Berl)*, **231**, 2251–2259.

Bonsack, C., Gibellini Manetti, S., Favrod, J., et al. (2011) Motivational intervention to reduce cannabis use in young people with psychosis: A randomized controlled trial. *Psychother Psychosom*, **80**, 287–297.

Borgan, F., Kokkinou, M., and Howes, O. (2021). The cannabinoid CB$_1$ receptor in schizophrenia. *Biol*

Psychiatry Cogn Neurosci Neuroimaging, **6**, 646–659.

Brunette, M. F., Dawson, R., O'Keefe, C. D., et al. (2011). A randomized trial of clozapine vs. other antipsychotics for cannabis use disorder in patients with schizophrenia. *J Dual Diagnosis*, **7**, 50–63.

Bucci, S., Baker, A., Halpin, S. A., et al. (2010). Intervention for cannabis use in young people at ultra high risk for psychosis and in early psychosis. *Mental Health Subst Use*, **3**, 66–73.

Budney, A. J., Moore, B. A., Rocha, H. L., et al. (2006). Clinical trial of abstinence-based vouchers and cognitive-behavioral therapy for cannabis dependence. *J Consult Clin Psychol*, **74**, 307–316.

Carpenter, K. M., McDowell, D., Brooks, D. J., et al. (2009). A preliminary trial: Double-blind comparison of nefazodone, bupropion-SR, and placebo in the treatment of cannabis dependence. *Am J Addict*, **18**, 53–64.

Carroll, K. M., Easton, C. J., Nich, C., et al. (2006). The use of contingency management and motivational/skills-building therapy to treat young adults with marijuana dependence. *J Consult Clin Psychol*, **74**, 955–966.

Coles, A. S., Knezevic, D., George, T. P., et al. (2021). Long-acting injectable antipsychotic treatment in schizophrenia and co-occurring substance use disorders. *Front Psychiatry*, **12**, 808002.

Coles, A. S., Kozak, K., and George, T. P. (2018). A review of brain stimulation for treatment of substance use disorders. *Am J Addict*, **27**, 71–91.

Coles, A. S., Sasiadek, J., and George, T. P. (2019) Pharmacotherapies for co-occurring substance use and bipolar disorders: A systematic review. *Bipolar Dis*, **21**, 595–610.

Compton, M. T., Furman, A. C., and Kaslow, N. J. (2004). Lower negative symptom scores among cannabis-dependent patients with schizophrenia-spectrum disorders: Preliminary evidence from an African American first-episode sample. *Schizophr Res*, **71**, 61–64.

Cooper, Z. D., Foltin, R. W., Hart, C. L., et al. (2013). A human laboratory study investigating the effects of quetiapine on marijuana withdrawal and relapse in daily marijuana smokers. *Addict Biol*, **18**, 993–1002.

Copeland, J., Swift, W., Roffman, R., et al. (2001). A randomized controlled trial of brief cognitive-behavioral interventions for cannabis use disorder. *J Subst Abuse Treat*, **21**, 55–64; discussion 65–66.

D'Souza, D. C., Abi-Saab, W. M., Madonick, S., et al. (2005). Delta-9-tetrahydrocannabinol effects in schizophrenia: Implications for cognition, psychosis, and addiction. *Biol Psychiatry*, **57**, 594–608.

D'Souza, D. C., Cortes-Briones, J., Creatura, G., et al. (2019). Efficacy and safety of a fatty acid amide hydrolase inhibitor (PF-04457845) in the treatment of cannabis withdrawal and dependence in men: A double-blind, placebo-controlled, parallel-group, phase 2a single-site randomized trial. *Lancet Psychiatry*, **6**, 35–45.

Diana, M., Raij, T., Melis, M., et al. (2017). Rehabilitating the addicted brain with transcranial magnetic stimulation. *Nat Rev Neurosci*, **18**, 685–693.

Drake, R. E., and Mueser, K. T. (2001). Managing comorbid schizophrenia and substance abuse. *Curr Psychiat Rep*, **3**, 418–422.

Drake, R. E., O'Neal, E. L., and Wallach, M. A. (2008). A systematic review of psychosocial interventions for people with co-occurring severe mental and substance use disorders. *J Subst Abuse Treat*, **34**, 123–138.

Dunlop, K., Hanlon, C. A., and Downar, J. (2017). Noninvasive brain stimulation treatments for addiction and major depression. *Ann NY Acad Sci*, **1394**, 31–54.

Eack, S. M., Hogarty, S. S., Greenwald, D. P., et al. (2015). Cognitive enhancement therapy in substance misusing schizophrenia: Results of an 18-month feasibility trial. *Schizophr Res*, **161**, 478–483.

Edwards, J., Elkins, K., Hinton, M., et al. (2006). Randomized controlled trial of a cannabis-focused intervention for young people with first-episode psychosis. *Acta Psychiatr Scand*, **114**, 109–117.

Feil, J., and Zangen, A. (2010). Brain stimulation in the study and treatment of addiction. *Neurosci Biobehav Rev*, **34**, 559–574.

Gates, P. J., Norberg, M. M., Copeland, J., et al. (2012). Randomized controlled trial of a novel cannabis use intervention delivered by telephone. *Addiction*, **107**, 2149–2158.

George, T. P., Hill, K. P., and Vaccarino, F. J. (2018). Cannabis legalization and psychiatric disorders: Caveat H-emptor. *Can J Psychiatry*, **63**, 447–450.

Gilbert, D. G., Rabinovich, N. E., and McDaniel, J. T. (2020). Nicotine patch for cannabis withdrawal symptom relief: A randomized controlled trial. *Psychopharmacology (Berl)*, **237**, 1507–1519.

Gorelick, D. A., Zangen, A., and George, M. S. (2014). Transcranial magnetic stimulation in the treatment of substance addiction. *Ann NY Acad Sci*, **1327**, 79–93.

Gray, K. M., Carpenter, M. J., Baker, N. L., et al. (2012). A double-blind, randomized controlled trial of

N-acetylcysteine in cannabis-dependent adolescents. *Am J Psychiatry*, **169**, 805–812.

Gray, K. M., Sonne, S. C., McClure, E. A., et al. (2017). A randomized placebo-controlled trial of N-acetylcysteine for cannabis use disorder in adults. *Drug Alcohol Depend*, **177**, 249–257.

Gray, K. M., Watson, N. L., Carpenter, M. J., et al. (2010). N-acetylcysteine (NAC) in young marijuana users: An open-label pilot study. *Am J Addict*, **19**, 187–189.

Green, A. I. (2007). Treatment of schizophrenia and comorbid substance abuse: Pharmacological approaches. *J Clin Psychiatry*, **67**, S31–S35.

Green, A. I., Burgess, E. S., Dawson, R., et al. (2003). Alcohol and cannabis use in schizophrenia: Effects of clozapine vs. risperidone. *Schizophr Res*, **60**, 81–85.

Green, M. F. (2016). Impact of cognitive and social cognitive impairment on functional outcomes in patients with schizophrenia. *J Clin Psychiatry*, **77**, 8–11.

Guillin, O., Abi-Dargham, A., and Laruelle, M. (2007). Neurobiology of dopamine in schizophrenia. *Int Rev Neurobiol*, **78**, 1–39.

Haddock, G., Barrowclough, C., Tarrier, C., et al. (2003). Cognitive-behavioural therapy and motivational intervention for schizophrenia and substance misuse: 18-month outcomes of a randomised controlled trial. *Br J Psychiatry*, **183**, 418–426.

Hajizadeh, M. (2016). Legalizing and regulating marijuana in Canada: Review of potential economic, social, and health impacts. *Int J Health Policy Manag*, **5**, 453–456.

Haney, M., Cooper, Z. D., Bedi, G., et al. (2013). Nabilone decreases marijuana withdrawal and a laboratory measure of marijuana

relapse. *Neuropsychopharmacology*, **38**, 1557–1565.

Haney, M., Hart, C. L., Vosburg, S. K., et al. (2010). Effects of baclofen and mirtazapine on a laboratory model of marijuana withdrawal and relapse. *Psychopharmacology (Berl)*, **211**, 233–244.

Haney, M., Ramesh, D, Glass, A, et al. (2015). Naltrexone maintenance decreases cannabis self-administration and subjective effects in daily cannabis smokers. *Neuropsychopharmacology*, **40**, 2489–2498.

Hanlon, C. A., Dowdle, L. T., and Henderson, J. S. (2018). Modulating neural circuits with transcranial magnetic stimulation: Implications for addiction treatment development. *Pharmacol Rev*, **70**, 661–683.

Hasin, D. S. (2018). U.S. epidemiology of cannabis use and associated problems. *Neuropsychopharmacology*, **43**, 195–212.

Hendriks, V., van der Schee, E., and Blanken, P. (2011). Treatment of adolescents with a cannabis use disorder: Main findings of a randomized controlled trial comparing multidimensional family therapy and cognitive behavioral therapy in The Netherlands. *Drug Alcohol Depend*, **119**, 64–71.

Hill, K. P., Toto, L. H., Lukas, S. E., et al. (2013). Cognitive behavioral therapy and the nicotine transdermal patch for dual nicotine and cannabis dependence: A pilot study. *Am J Addict*, **22**, 233–238.

Hjorthøj, C. R., Orlovska, S., Fohlmann, A., et al. (2013). Psychiatric treatment following participation in the CapOpus randomized trial for patients with comorbid cannabis use disorder and psychosis. *Schizophr Res*, **151**, 191–196.

Hoch, E., Noack, R., Henker, J., et al. (2012). Efficacy of a targeted cognitive-behavioral treatment program for cannabis use disorders (CANDIS). *Eur Neuropsychopharmacol*, **22**, 267–280.

Ikeda, T., Kobayashi, S., and Morimoto, C. (2019). Effects of repetitive transcranial magnetic stimulation on ER stress-related genes and glutamate, gamma-aminobutyric acid and glycine transporter genes in mouse brain. *Biochem Biophys Rep*, **17**, 10–16.

James, W., Preston, N., Koh, G., et al. (2004). A group intervention which assists patients with dual diagnosis reduce their drug use: A randomized controlled trial. *Psychol Med*, **34**, 983–990.

Johnston, J., Lintzeris, N., Allsop, D. J., et al. (2014). Lithium carbonate in the management of cannabis withdrawal: A randomized placebo-controlled trial in an inpatient setting. *Psychopharmacology (Berl)*, **231**, 4623–4636.

Kadden, R. M., Litt, M. D., Kabela-Cormier, E., et al. (2007). Abstinence rates following behavioral treatments for marijuana dependence. *Addict Behav*, **32**, 1220–1236.

Kavanagh, D. J., Young, R., White, A., et al. (2004). A brief motivational intervention for substance misuse in recent-onset psychosis. *Drug Alcohol Rev*, **23**, 151–155.

Kolliakou, A., Castle, D., Sallis, H., et al. (2012). Reasons for cannabis use in first-episode psychosis: Does strength of endorsement change over 12 months? *Eur Psychiatry*, **30**, 152–159.

Koskinen, J., Lohonen, J., Koponen, H., et al. (2010). Rates of cannabis use disorders in clinical samples of patients with schizophrenia: A meta-analysis. *Schizophr Bull*, **36**, 1115–1124.

Kozak, K., Barr, M. S., and George, T. P. (2017). Traits and biomarkers for addiction risk in schizophrenia. *Curr Addict Rep*, **4**, 14–24.

Kozak, K., Lowe, D. J. E., Sanches, M., et al. (2021). Effects of repetitive transcranial magnetic stimulation (rTMS) on cannabis use and cognitive function in achizophrenia. *Brain Stimulation*, under review.

Krebs, P., Norcross, J. C., Nicholson, J. M., et al. (2018). Stages of change and psychotherapy outcomes: A review and meta-analysis. *J Clin Psychol*, **74**, 1964–1979.

Levin, F., Mariani, J., Brooks, D. J., et al. (2011). Dronabinol for the treatment of cannabis dependence: A randomized, double-blind, placebo-controlled trial. *Drug Alcohol Depend*, **116**, 142–150.

Levin, F., Mariani, J, Brooks, D. J., et al. (2013). A randomized, double-blind, placebo-controlled trial of venlafaxine extended-release for co-occurring cannabis dependence and depressive disorders. *Am J Addict*, **108**, 1084–1094.

Levin, F., Mariani, J. J., Pavlicova, M., et al. (2016). Dronabinol and lofexidine for cannabis use disorder: A randomized, double-blind, placebo-controlled trial. *Drug Alcohol Depend*, **159**, 53–60.

Levin, F., McDowell, D., Evans, S. M., et al. (2004). Pharmacotherapy for marijuana dependence: A double-blind, placebo-controlled pilot study of divalproex sodium. *Am J Addict*, **13**, 21–32.

Lintzeris, N., Bhardwaj, A., Mills, L., et al. (2019). Nabiximols for the treatment of cannabis dependence: A randomized clinical trial. *JAMA Intern Med*, **179**, 1242–1253.

Litt, M. D., Kadden, R. M., Tennen, H., et al. (2020). Individualized assessment and treatment program (IATP) for cannabis use disorder: Randomized controlled trial with and without contingency management. *Psychol Addict Behav*, **34**, 40–51.

Longenecker, J. M., Bagby, R. M., McKenzie, K. J., et al. (2021). Cross-cutting symptom domains predict functioning in psychotic disorders. *J Clin Psychiatry*, **82**, 20m13288.

Lowe, D. J. E., Sasiadek, J. D., Coles, A. S., et al. (2019). Cannabis and mental illness: A review. *Eur Arch Psychiat Clin Neurosci*, **269**, 107–120.

Machielsen, M., Beduin, A. S., Dekker, N., et al. (2012). Differences in craving for cannabis between schizophrenia patients using risperidone, olanzapine or clozapine. *J Psychopharmacol*, **26**, 89–95.

Machielsen, M. W. J., Veltman, D. J., van den Brink, W., et al. (2014). The effect of clozapine and risperidone on attentional bias in patients with schizophrenia and a cannabis use disorder: An FMRI study. *J Psychopharmacol*, **28**, 633–642.

Madigan, K., Brennan, D., Lawlor, E., et al. (2013). A multi-center, randomized controlled trial of a group psychological intervention for psychosis with comorbid cannabis dependence over the early course of illness. *Schizophr Res*, **143**, 138–142.

Mahoney, J. J., 3rd, Hanlon, C. A., Marshalek, P. J., et al. (2020). Transcranial magnetic stimulation, deep brain stimulation, and other forms of neuromodulation for substance use disorders: Review of modalities and implications for treatment. *J Neurol Sci*, **418**, 117149.

Marijuana Treatment Project Research Group. (2004). Brief treatments for cannabis dependence: Findings from a randomized multisite trial. *J Consult Clin Psychol*, **72**, 455–466.

Mason, B., Cream, R., Godell, V., et al. (2012). A proof-of-concept randomized controlled study of gabapentin: Effects on cannabis use, withdrawal and executive function deficits in cannabis-dependent adults. *Neuropsychopharmacology*, **37**, 1689–1698.

McLellan, A. T., Kushner, H., Metzger, D., et al. (1992). The fifth edition of the addiction severity index. *J Subst Abus Treat*, **9**, 199–213.

McRae-Clark, A. L., Baker, N. L., Gray, K. M., et al. (2015). Buspirone treatment of cannabis dependence: A randomized, placebo-controlled trial. *Drug Alcohol Depend*, **156**, 29–37.

et al. (2016). Vilazodone for cannabis dependence: A randomized, controlled pilot trial. *Am J Addict*, **25**, 69–75.

McRae-Clark, A., Carter, R. E., Killeen, T. K., et al. (2009). A placebo-controlled trial of buspirone for the treatment of cannabis dependence. *Drug Alcohol Depend*, **105**, 132–138.

et al. (2010). A placebo-controlled trial of atomoxetine in marijuana-dependent individuals with attention deficit hyperactivity disorder. *Am J Addict*, **19**, 481–489.

Miranda, R., Jr., Treloar, H., Blanchard, A., et al. (2017). Topiramate and motivational enhancement therapy for cannabis use among youth: A randomized placebo-controlled pilot study. *Addict Biol*, **22**, 779–790.

Moretti, J., Poh, E. Z., and Rodger, J. (2020). rTMS-induced changes in glutamatergic and dopaminergic systems: Relevance to cocaine and methamphetamine use disorders. *Front Neurosci*, **14**, 137.

Notzon, D. P., Kelly, M. A., Choi, C. J., et al. (2018). Open-label pilot study of injectable naltrexone for cannabis dependence. *Am J Drug Alcohol Abuse*, **44**, 619–627.

Penetar, D. M., Looby, A. R., Ryan, E. T., et al. (2012). Bupropion reduces some of the symptoms of marihuana withdrawal in chronic marihuana users: A pilot study. *Subst Abuse*, **6**, 63–71.

Potvin, S., Stip, E., Lipp, O., et al. (2006). Quetiapine in patients with comorbid schizophrenia-spectrum and substance use disorders: An open-label trial. *Curr Med Res Opin*, **22**, 1277–1285.

Rabin, R. A., Barr, M. S., Herman, Y., et al. (2017). Effects of extended cannabis abstinence on neurocognitive outcomes in cannabis dependent schizophrenia patients versus non-psychiatric controls. *Neuropsychopharmacology*, **42**, 2259–2271.

Rabin, R. A., and George, T. P. (2017). Understanding the link between cannabinoids and psychosis. *Clin Pharmacol Therap*, **101**, 197–199.

Rabin, R. A., Kozak, K., Herman, Y., et al. (2018). A method to achieve short-term cannabis abstinence in cannabis-dependent patients with schizophrenia and non-psychiatric controls. *Schizophr Res*, **194**, 47–54.

Rabin, R. A., Zakzanis, K. K., and George, T. P. (2011). The effects of cannabis use on neurocognition in schizophrenia: A meta-analysis. *Schizophr Res*, **128**, 111–116.

Rooke, S., Copeland, J., Norberg, M., et al. (2013). Effectiveness of a self-guided web-based cannabis treatment program: Randomized controlled trial. *J Med Internet Res*, **15**, e26.

Roten, A. T., Baker, N. L., and Gray, K. M. (2013). Marijuana craving trajectories in an adolescent marijuana cessation pharmacotherapy trial. *Addict Behav*, **38**, 1788–1791.

Salling, M. C., and Martinez, D. (2016). Brain stimulation in addiction. *Neuropsychopharmacology*, **41**, 2798–2809.

Schnell, T., Koethe, D., Krasnianski, A., et al. (2014). Ziprasidone versus clozapine in the treatment of dually diagnosed (DD) patients with schizophrenia and cannabis use disorders: A randomized study. *Am J Addict*, **23**, 308–312.

Schwilke, E. W., Gulberg, R. G., Darwin, W. D., et al. (2011). Differentiating new cannabis use from residual urinary cannabinoid excretion in chronic, daily cannabis users. *Addiction*, **106**, 499–506.

Sheridan Rains, L., Marston, L., Hinton, M., et al. (2019). Clinical and cost-effectiveness of contingency management for cannabis use in early psychosis: The CIRCLE randomised clinical trial. *BMC Med*, **17**, 161.

Sherman, B. J., Baker, N. L., and McRae-Clark, A. L. (2017). Effect of oxytocin pretreatment on cannabis outcomes in a brief motivational intervention. *Psychiatry Res*, **249**, 318–320.

Sigmon, S. C., and Higgins, S. T. (2006). Voucher-based contingent reinforcement of marijuana abstinence among individuals with serious mental illness. *J Subst Abuse Treat*, **30**, 291–295.

Sigmon, S. C., Steingard, S., Badger, G. J., et al. (2000). Contingent reinforcement of marijuana abstinence among individuals with serious mental illness: A feasibility study. *Exp Clin Psychopharmacol*, **8**, 509–517.

Sinadinovic, K., Johansson, M., Johansson, A. S., et al. (2020). Guided web-based treatment program for reducing cannabis use: A randomized controlled trial. *Addict Sci Clin Pract*, **15**, 9.

Slavet, J. D., Stein, L. A. R., Colby, S. M., et al. (2006). The marijuana ladder: Measuring motivation to change marijuana use in incarcerated adolescents. *Drug Alcohol Depend*, **83**, 42–48.

Spencer, C., Castle, D., and Michie, P. T. (2002). Motivations that maintain substance use among individuals with psychotic disorders. *Schizophr Bull*, **28**, 233–247.

Stephens, R. S., Babor, T. F., Kadden, R., et al. (2004). Brief treatments for cannabis dependence: Findings from a randomized multisite trial. *J Consult Clin Psychol*, **72**, 455–466.

Stephens, R. S., Roffman, R. A., and Curtin, L. (2000). Comparison of extended versus brief treatments for marijuana use. *J Consult Clin Psychol*, **68**, 898–908.

Stephens, R. S., Roffman, R. A., and Simpson, E. E. (1994). Treating adult marijuana dependence: A test of the relapse prevention model. *J Consult Clin Psychol*, **62**, 92–99.

Szerman, N., Basurte-Villamor, I., Vega, P., et al. (2020). Once-monthly long-acting injectable aripiprazole for the treatment of patients with schizophrenia and co-occurring substance use disorders: A multicentre, observational study. *Drugs Real World Outcomes*, **7**, 75–83.

Tang, S. M., Ansarian, A., and Courtney, D. B. (2017). Clozapine treatment and cannabis use in adolescents with psychotic disorders: A retrospective cohort chart review. *J Can Acad Child Adolesc Psychiatry*, **26**, 51–58.

Tatar, O., Abdel-Baki, A., Tra, C., et al. (2021). Technology-based psychological interventions for young adults with early psychosis and cannabis use disorder: Qualitative study of patient and clinician perspectives. *JMIR Form Res*, **5**, e26562.

Trigo, J. M., Soliman, A., Quilty, L. C., et al. (2018). Nabiximols combined with motivational enhancement/cognitive behavioral therapy for the treatment of cannabis dependence: A pilot randomized clinical trial. *PLoS ONE*, **13**, e0190768.

Weinstein, A. M., Miller, H., Bluvstein, I., et al. (2014). Treatment of cannabis dependence using escitalopram in combination with cognitive-behavior therapy: A double-blind placebo-controlled study. *Am J Drug Alcohol Abuse*, **40**, 16–22.

Zhang, J. J. Q., Fong, K. N. K., Ouyang, R. G., et al. (2019). Effects of repetitive transcranial magnetic stimulation (rTMS) on craving and substance consumption in patients with substance dependence: A systematic review and meta-analysis. *Addiction*, **114**, 2137–2149.

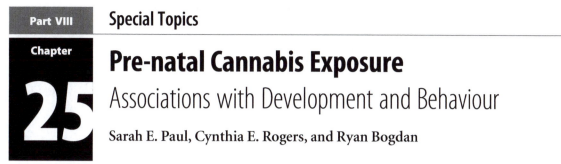

Pre-natal Cannabis Exposure
Associations with Development and Behaviour

Sarah E. Paul, Cynthia E. Rogers, and Ryan Bogdan

25.1 Fact Boxes

Pregnant women are increasingly using cannabis, with rates in the United States doubling from 3.4% to 7% between 2002 and 2017 and daily use increasing three-fold.

The endocannabinoid system is critically involved in implantation and placentation and, during prenatal development, plays crucial roles in neuronal proliferation and differentiation, migration, and synaptogenesis and myelinogenesis.

Pre-natal cannabis exposure, particularly when frequent and continued later in pregnancy, is associated with reductions in birthweight and with pre-term birth.

Offspring exposed to cannabis in utero have elevated rates of externalizing problems, cannabis use, and psychotic-like experiences, with mixed evidence linking exposure to internalizing symptoms and impairments in cognition.

Although more data are needed to better assess the independence of these effects from familial and other confounds, the existing evidence suggests that cannabis use during pregnancy should be discouraged.

Increasingly permissive sociocultural attitudes and laws surrounding cannabis use have been accompanied by a rise in use (Chapter 4; Compton et al., 2016), including among pregnant women. For example, in the United States, past-month cannabis use among pregnant women doubled from 2002/2003 (3.4%) to 2016/2017 (7.0%), with daily use showing an approximately three-fold increase (Volkow et al., 2019). While the reasons for this increase are not fully understood, greater availability following legalization is correlated with greater use during pregnancy (Young-Wolff et al., 2021). Further, women who continue to use cannabis during pregnancy report doing so for health management (e.g., to combat nausea, pain, sleep, anxiety, and stress) and report uncertainty and limited perceptions of potential harm to the baby (Bayrampour et al., 2019). These trends have led to concern because pre-natal cannabis exposure (PCE) may adversely affect the pre-natal environment, neurodevelopment, and health by interfacing with the endocannabinoid system in the placenta and developing foetus. As the tide of public opinion and legislation on cannabis continues to swell toward a sea change of increased permissiveness, it is increasingly important to understand potential consequences following PCE to guide policy. This chapter provides an overview and critical evaluation of existing research examining associations between PCE and outcomes during childhood. First, we highlight the role of the endocannabinoid system in foetal development. Second, we describe observed associations between PCE and neonatal development as well as childhood psychopathology risk and cognition. Finally, we leverage non-human animal experiments to consider putative mechanisms through which PCE may affect these outcomes and conclude by considering challenges to the field and how we may best confront these going forward.

25.2 The Endocannabinoid System and Pre-natal Development

The effects of cannabinoids, including constituents of cannabis such as delta-9-tetrahydrocannabinol (THC), which drives the psychotropic effects of cannabis, arise primarily from their binding to cannabinoid type 1 receptors (CB1Rs) and type 2 receptors (CB2Rs; Chapters 1 and 2). CB1Rs are predominantly expressed in the central nervous system. In addition to their critical roles in long-term synaptic depression and psychiatrically-relevant constructs including reward, anxiety, and stress regulation throughout life (Chapter 2), they also contribute to early neural development. CB1Rs have been detected as early as nine weeks post-conception in humans and in rodent brains at the equivalent of five-to-six weeks in humans (Berrendero et al., 1998; Zurolo et al., 2010). In contrast to ubiquitous distribution in adult brains, CB1Rs during early pre-natal development are preferentially expressed in neural progenitor cells, playing an important regulatory role in neuronal proliferation and differentiation, migration, and, later, synaptogenesis and myelinogenesis (Basavarajappa et al., 2009; Wu et al., 2011). That is, CB1Rs are critically involved in the processes by which neural progenitors multiply, travel to their appropriate locations, find synaptic partners, and by which axons acquire myelin and transmit electrical signals more efficiently. CB2Rs are predominantly expressed in the peripheral nervous system with trace amounts present in brain tissue (Chen et al., 2017); while less is known about the role of CB2Rs, it is conceivable that they may influence neural development through immune processes. Alongside evidence that approximately a third of THC present in maternal plasma traverses the placenta (Hutchings et al., 1989; Yao et al., 2018), it is plausible that PCE, particularly when frequent and heavy, may broadly interfere in proper neuronal maturation and the function of diverse neurotransmitter systems to negatively influence distal child behaviour and cognition. Further, there is also the possibility for indirect effects through influences on maternal behaviour as well as the placenta, which houses CB1Rs and in which cannabinoid signalling plays an important role in key gestational events, including implantation and placentation (Maia et al., 2019). Impairments in these processes may induce adverse neonatal outcomes (e.g., low birthweight), further increasing risk for child behaviour problems and even all-cause mortality (Belbasis et al., 2016; Fan et al., 2013).

25.3 Neonatal Outcomes: Birthweight and Pre-term Birth

Initial evidence from relatively small prospective studies (e.g., the Ottawa Pre-natal Prospective Study [OPPS] and Maternal Health Practices and Child Development study [MHPCD]; Table 25.1) found that PCE is not associated with birthweight (e.g., Cornelius et al., 1995; Fried and O'Connell, 1987), and there was mixed evidence that it may be associated with pre-term birth (e.g., Cornelius et al., 1995; Day et al., 1991; Fried and O'Connell, 1987). However, a sizable and methodologically diverse (e.g., hospital records, prospective studies) literature and meta-analyses have revealed that PCE is associated with reduced birthweight and gestational age at birth (e.g., Baer et al., 2019; Conner et al., 2016; Corsi et al., 2019; El Marroun et al., 2009; Gunn et al., 2016; but see Chabarria et al., 2016; Crume et al., 2018). These associations appear to be driven mainly by frequent maternal use during pregnancy, particularly in later stages (i.e., third trimester; El Marroun et al., 2009; Grzeskowiak et al., 2020; Leemaqz et al., 2016; but see Paul et al., 2021).

What remains unclear is whether PCE may causally induce low birthweight or pre-term birth or whether this relationship is attributable to confounds (e.g., other substance exposure during pregnancy, shared genomic liability). For instance, while several studies have shown that the link between PCE and low birthweight is robust to a multitude of potential confounds (e.g., other pre-natal substance exposures; Crume et al., 2018), a meta-analysis suggests that controlling for pre-natal tobacco exposure reduces this association to trend level and substantially attenuates the association with pre-term birth (Conner et al., 2016). However, causal evidence of a relationship between PCE and low birthweight has emerged from non-human animal experiments showing that daily administration of Δ9-THC or other CB1 agonists at physiologically-plausible levels induces low birthweight (Natale et al., 2020), though these findings have not always been consistent across studies (e.g., Breit et al., 2020). Interestingly, despite evidence linking cannabis use as well as problematic cannabis use to eating behaviour and weight (Alshaarawy and Anthony, 2019), PCE-induced

Table 25.1 Three prospective studies of pre-natal cannabis exposure

Study	Sample Size	Sample Characteristics	Years, Country of Recruitment	Measurement of PCE
Ottawa Pre-natal Prospective Study (OPPS) (Fried, 1995; Fried et al., 1980, 1984).	~700 pregnant women recruited, 190 (140 exposed to substances) offspring followed beyond birth	Predominantly White and middle class	1979–1983 Canada	Interviews each trimester ~15% reported PCE (avg of 6.6 joints/week).
Maternal Health Practices and Child Development Study (MHPCD) (Day et al., 1991; Day and Richardson, 1991)	829 pregnant women recruited, 763 offspring	57% Black, low SES	1982–1985 United States	Interviews at months 4 & 7 and at delivery. ~62% reported PCE (29% $\geq$ 1 joint/day).
Generation R (El Marroun et al., 2009; Jaddoe et al., 2006; Kooijman et al., 2016)	9,778 pregnant women recruited	Population-based sample, predominantly White	2002–2006 Netherlands	Retrospective self-report of PCE before knowledge of pregnancy, prospective report after knowledge. ~3.6% reported PCE.

reductions in birthweight exist independent of effects on maternal feeding behaviour and may instead arise from adverse effects on the placenta and intrauterine foetal growth restriction. Relative to birthweight, pre-term birth has been more seldom examined in animal studies, with existing data providing little evidence of causality (e.g., Campolongo et al., 2007).

The emergence of systematized hospital records has enabled large-scale investigations of PCE and neonatal outcomes. The resulting data (Table 25.2) suggest that PCE, particularly when frequent and continued into later trimesters of pregnancy, is associated with reductions in birthweight and gestational age at birth. Whether these associations are independent of confounding factors remains unclear. Disparities among studies may result from differences in total and cannabis-exposed sample sizes, covariate adjustment, assessment of PCE, or other sample characteristics; more data are needed to better assess independence and causality.

25.4 Psychiatric Risk

25.4.1 Internalizing and Externalizing

Overall, existing evidence supports a relationship between PCE and elevated externalizing problems,

Table 25.2 Level of confidence in the evidence for adverse effects of PCE on neonatal, psychological, and cognitive outcomes

Outcome	Level of Confidence
Neonatal	
Reduced birthweight	Moderate/High
Reduced gestational age at/pre-term birth	Moderate
Psychological	
Internalizing	Low
Externalizing	Moderate
Psychosis/psychotic-like experiences	Low
Cannabis use	Low
Cognitive Deficits	
Broad cognitive ability	Low
Academic achievement	Low
Executive function	Low/Moderate

Note: For many outcomes, evidence is generally stronger for more frequent/heavier cannabis exposure. Low evidence may arise due to the lack of available studies or the accumulation of null results.

while the associations with internalizing symptoms have been weaker and inconsistent. Across samples, PCE has been linked with aggression, impulsivity, and substance use (e.g., Fried et al., 1992; Richardson et al., 2009; but see Bada et al., 2011), particularly when cannabis exposure continues into later stages of pregnancy (Paul et al., 2021). By contrast, few studies have identified associations between PCE and offspring anxiety and depression (El Marroun et al., 2019; Richardson et al., 2009), with some data trending on significance (Paul et al., 2021). In the few studies that have found a significant relationship, the timing of cannabis exposure during pregnancy has not consistently influenced results, with data from MHPCD alternatively showing elevated internalizing symptoms among offspring exposed to cannabis in the first trimester (Goldschmidt et al., 2012) or in the first and third, but not second, trimesters (Gray et al., 2005). Interestingly, some data from animal experiments have revealed that pre-natal cannabinoid exposure elicits anxiogenic-like symptoms in adult offspring (Trezza et al., 2008; but see Manduca et al., 2020). It should be noted that, relative to internalizing problems, externalizing symptoms typically arise earlier and are more readily observable to parents and teachers frequently reporting on such behaviors (Achenbach et al., 1987). These differences may explain, at least in part, disparate findings for internalizing and externalizing problems.

Despite evidence that associations between PCE and externalizing behaviors are robust to potential confounds (e.g., Paul et al., 2021), whether this relationship represents causal influences of PCE remains unclear. For instance, evidence of earlier initiation and increased frequency of cannabis use among offspring exposed to cannabis in utero (e.g., Porath and Fried, 2005; Sonon et al., 2015) may be attributable to inherited propensity to use cannabis and increased environmental access to cannabis rather than independent effects of PCE. Experiments in animals have revealed that exposure to cannabinoids causes increased alcohol drinking, relapse, and conflict behaviour in offspring (Brancato et al., 2020), but animal models of other forms of externalizing behaviors are lacking.

25.4.2 Psychotic-like Experiences

To our knowledge, four studies have explored the relationship between PCE and offspring psychosis proneness, with PCE being linked to psychotic-like experiences in the ABCD study (Fine et al., 2019; Paul et al., 2021) but not in other cohorts (Bolhuis et al., 2018; Zammit et al., 2009). Notably, the association in ABCD was specific to PCE after maternal knowledge of pregnancy and, whereas Zammit et al. (2009) found no evidence that more frequent use was associated with psychotic-like experiences, their sample was underpowered to examine timing effects due to relatively low levels of use (i.e., of the small proportion reporting use, approximately half (n = 37) used less than once per week). Further, although the inclusion of polygenic scores for schizophrenia did not substantially attenuate the association between PCE and psychotic-like experiences in ABCD (Paul et al., 2021), Bolhuis et al. (2018) found that this relationship was not independent of genetic and familial confounds. It is also possible that the null finding reported by Bolhuis et al. (2018) is reflective of the limited data gathered on use past the first trimester, particularly given the ontogeny of the eCB system.

25.4.3 Conclusion

Overall, the state of the evidence linking PCE to behavioural and psychological outcomes in offspring is mixed, though there is more support for associations with externalizing as compared to internalizing symptoms and too few studies of psychotic-like experience to allow strong conclusions. Of note, externalizing symptoms tend to be more observable and arise earlier compared to internalizing problems, so this pattern could possibly reflect the age of the samples and widespread use of caregiver reports. That said, this pattern of results aligns with evidence that PCE may disrupt processes regulating inhibitory control in non-human animals (e.g., Volk and Lewis, 2016). However, given their cross-sectional examination, it is possible that associations with externalizing problems are attributable to genetic susceptibility to cannabis misuse (e.g., during pregnancy) and other externalizing behaviour that is passed to offspring. The temporal disconnection from the pre-natal environment and numerous potentially confounding factors makes it difficult to tease apart independent effects of PCE.

25.5 Cognitive Outcomes: General Cognitive Ability, Executive Function, and Academic Achievement

Measures of general cognitive ability (e.g., IQ) have not been linked with PCE in most studies to date, with data from OPPS showing that offspring exposed to PCE display normative or higher levels of cognitive ability (Fried and Watkinson, 1988; Fried et al., 2003) and data from MHPCD producing some evidence of lower scores on global measures of intelligence (Goldschmidt et al., 2012; Richardson et al., 2009; but see Day et al., 1994). Studies conducted with other samples have not revealed significant associations (e.g., Paul et al., 2021; Rose-Jacobs et al., 2012; Singer et al., 2008), although some data suggest that, relative to children exposed only early in pregnancy or not exposed, those with PCE later in pregnancy show reduced cognitive performance (Paul et al., 2021). Similarly, with respect to executive function deficits, MHPCD and OPPS have documented both impaired (Fried et al., 1992; Leech et al., 1999; Richardson et al., 2002) and enhanced (Fried et al., 1998) levels of sustained attention, as well as normative (e.g., Fried et al., 2003) and enhanced (Fried et al., 1998; Leech et al., 1999) levels of response inhibition. Interestingly, in a small follow-up neuroimaging study of OPPS (n = 31, ages 18–22), those with PCE exhibited normal executive functioning performance alongside increased left posterior brain activity (Smith et al., 2016). This finding was interpreted to reflect a possible compensatory mechanism, wherein those with PCE needed to recruit additional brain regions or further engage typically recruited regions. Performance on other executive functioning tasks in other samples have yielded null results (e.g., Carmody et al., 2011), with the puzzling exception of poorer cognitive flexibility among those exposed to moderate, but not heavy, levels of cannabis in a relatively small sample of 33 exposed and 104 unexposed adolescents (Rose-Jacobs et al., 2011). Finally, the data are also mixed regarding academic achievement, with MHPCD finding that offspring exposed to cannabis exhibit lower overall achievement as well as poorer reading and spelling performance (Goldschmidt et al., 2004, 2012) and studies in other samples finding no evidence of significant associations (e.g., Singer et al., 2008). Although animal models are unable to recapitulate higher order cognitive processes such as intelligence, experiments conducted in animals have revealed that pre-natal exposure to CB1 agonists impairs memory consolidation and retention (Mereu et al., 2003; Silva et al., 2012) as well as performance on mazes and other tests of learning (Antonelli et al., 2005; Gianutsos and Abbatiello, 1972). In rodent studies, passive cannabis vapor exposure in utero has elicited dose-dependent deficits in behavioural flexibility in attentional set-shifting (Weimar et al., 2020). Furthermore, exposure at the equivalent of the third trimester in humans has been shown to impair working memory in rodents (O'Shea and Mallet, 2005), in line with data from MHPCD (Day et al., 1994; Goldschmidt et al., 2008; but see Richardson et al., 2009).

A recent systematic review of 45 studies of PCE and cognitive outcomes concluded that PCE was not associated with clinically significant cognitive deficits (Torres et al., 2020). Out of 1,001 cognitive outcomes, children with PCE exhibited worse performance on only 34 (3.4%) and *better* performance on 9 (0.9%); only 0.3% of the total sample performed below the normal range. Additionally, most studies examined many outcome measures without adjusting for multiple testing, increasing the chance of Type I errors (i.e., false positives). Further, it was common for studies to assess each domain of cognition with a single measure; each idiosyncratic measure may tap into a slight variation of a particular cognitive construct. As documented here and in the systematic review, the sizeable portion of either null or *positive* associations between PCE and cognition both within and across cognitive domains, measures, ages, and samples indicates that this relationship is likely tenuous at best.

25.6 Potential Mechanisms Linking PCE to Childhood Outcomes

If PCE is, in fact, linked to offspring outcomes, how might those associations arise? First, there is the possibility that the observed associations are not independent, but rather are explainable by unmeasured confounders (e.g., other pre-natal substance exposures, genomic liability, pre-conception, and/or paternal cannabis use). Second, PCE may be causally related to the observed outcomes through several non-mutually exclusive biological pathways (e.g., shared genomic and environmental liability). Finally, there is the possibility that PCE may cause individual differences in neonatal development and behaviour. In particular, THC may elicit epigenetic alterations in gene expression; interfere with intrauterine growth and placental function; impede adaptive neuronal development, differentiation, pruning, and related processes; and/or disrupt a range of neurotransmitter systems in the foetus.

A growing body of literature suggests that parental cannabis use, even prior to conception, may contribute to offspring outcomes via epigenetic alterations. Adverse offspring outcomes may result from epigenetic changes induced by direct PCE and/or that are inherited through the germline from pre-conception parental cannabis use. Broadly, epigenetic alterations induced by parental THC exposure have been linked to cross-generational abnormalities in the expression of genes for cannabinoid, dopaminergic, and glutamatergic receptors (Szutorisz et al., 2016; Watson et al., 2015). A genome-wide study in humans discovered that non-specific pre-natal substance exposure was linked to variation in DNA methylation in gestational and adolescent blood samples across genes implicated in neurodevelopment; DNA methylation was further associated with earlier and heavier substance use in adolescence (Cecil et al., 2016). In rodents, paternal THC exposure has resulted in lasting attentional deficits, memory impairments, risk-taking behaviour, increased motivation to self-administer heroin, and alterations in locomotor activity (Holloway et al., 2020; Levin et al., 2019; Szutorisz et al., 2014).

Alongside evidence of lower birthweight among infants exposed to cannabis in utero are data suggesting intrauterine growth restriction (IUGR) and impairments in placental function. Such adverse events may explain not only birthweight reductions but also, in part, later psychopathology and related outcomes among exposed offspring, given an extensive literature linking these neonatal developmental outcomes to risk for later behaviour problems (e.g., Fan et al., 2013). IUGR and deficits in placental function may arise from many factors, with emerging evidence suggesting that THC-induced defects in foetal blood space and reduced glutamatergic receptor expression in the labyrinth zone of the placenta reflect putative mechanisms (Natale et al., 2020). Thus, psychopathology among offspring with PCE may be partially mediated by neonatal events and outcomes, though some data suggest that associations between PCE and externalizing behaviour and psychotic-like experiences, for instance, are robust to the inclusion of birthweight as a covariate (Paul et al., 2021) and highlight the possibility of additional mechanisms (e.g., THC binding in the foetal brain).

PCE may interfere with diverse neurotransmitter systems in the foetus, particularly after CB1Rs are expressed (i.e., after approximately 9 weeks in humans; Zurolo et al., 2010), more directly resulting in adverse childhood outcomes. THC acts as a functional antagonist at CB1Rs (i.e., supplants endogenous endocannabinoid CB1R binding), so PCE may disrupt normal endocannabinoid signalling and, as a result, neuronal maturation and specification, synaptic wiring, and axonal growth and morphology (Tortoriello et al., 2014). PCE may, thus, contribute to cytoarchitectural abnormalities associated with schizophrenia and/or deficits in cognitive control more broadly (Chapters 16 and 21). Abnormalities in glutamatergic signalling have also been identified, with declines in hippocampal glutamate levels disrupting long-term potentiation and negatively impacting offspring cognition (Mereu et al., 2003). Male rodent offspring have displayed reduced social interaction alongside alterations in endocannabinoid-related long-term depression and increased excitability in the medial PFC, perhaps due to reduced endogenous endocannabinoid availability and related reductions in glutamate receptor signalling (Bara et al., 2018).

Finally, PCE has been related to dopaminergic system hyperactivity, which has been implicated in the pathophysiology of schizophrenia and, more generally, in heightened stress responsivity and impaired inhibitory control (Frau et al., 2019; Sagheddu et al., 2021). Specifically, PCE has been associated with mesolimbic dopaminergic hyperactivity as manifested by depolarized resting state membrane potentials, reduced latency to action potential onset, and thus increased excitability and action potential firing (Frau et al., 2019). Offspring have exhibited impulsivity and increased sensitivity to acute THC exposure as a result, both of which may confer risk for diverse psychopathology (Frau et al., 2019). Reduced activity of dopaminergic neurons in the ventral tegmental area (VTA; Sagheddu et al., 2021) in rodent offspring and decreased expression of dopamine D2 receptors in the nucleus accumbens and amygdala in humans (Dinieri et al., 2011; Wang et al., 2004) may represent an adaptive response to a hyperdopaminergic state (Volkow et al., 2007).

These proposed mechanisms likely interact with each other and with other biological and psychological factors. Epigenetic alterations may directly and causally link PCE to offspring psychopathology and/or may constitute a confounding variable arising from pre-conception or paternal cannabis use. Yet, although experiments in non-human animals have the capacity to test for causality, human brains and psychology are substantially more complex than those of animals; mechanistic findings in rodents cannot be cleanly mapped onto humans. As discussed in Section 25.7, researchers of PCE in humans have the challenging task of disentangling effects of exposure from a host of potential confounds.

25.7 Methodological Considerations and Limitations

25.7.1 Measurement

First, we turn to the widespread exclusive use of self-reports. Although MHPCD used deception (i.e., falsely told participants that toxicology screens would be used) to increase self-report accuracy, none of the three primary prospective studies (Table 25.1) collected corroborating toxicology information; this is unfortunately the norm throughout the literature. Sole use of either toxicology or self-report is problematic. Interview and self-report data, unlike toxicology results, allow examination of use patterns over longer periods of time. Toxicology assessments track predominantly recent substance exposure and are further subject to both false positives and negatives (for a recent review, see: Kapur and Aleksa, 2020). However, evidence from recent large-scale investigations and comprehensive reviews suggests that self-report measures tend to underestimate exposure rates, which could result in misclassification of offspring and bias associations downward (e.g., Young-Wolff et al., 2020). Given that the timing of PCE is potentially crucial to consider if there are causal influences due to receptor availability, more frequent interviews and toxicology screens of pregnant mothers are needed to capture PCE chronology.

Second, the potency, frequency, quantity, timing, and mode of cannabis consumption introduce substantial variability to PCE assessment. The more cannabis consumed by the mother and the more potent it is, the higher the THC concentration present in the foetus and the greater the potential deleterious effects. Related to potency is the ratio of THC to the major non-psychoactive component of cannabis, cannabidiol (CBD). Some data suggest that CBD may actually counter intoxicating effects of THC (Chapter 20; Niesink and van Laar, 2013). The average ratio of THC to CBD in confiscated cannabis specimens, however, skyrocketed from ~14 in 1995 to ~80 in 2014 (Chapter 5; ElSohly et al., 2016). It will be important to examine how not only the potency, but also the relative concentrations of these chemicals, may impact associations between PCE and childhood outcomes.

More frequent cannabis consumption also leads to higher THC concentrations and prolonged foetal exposure. Studies that have incorporated frequency and quantity data have indicated that heavier exposure is associated with poorer outcomes. Unfortunately, most of the existing literature does not account for frequency or quantity, and, even when such data are collected, there are no agreed upon definitions of heavy, moderate, or light exposure. Standardized assessment protocols are needed.

Where possible, such assessments must gather information on when during pregnancy cannabis was consumed. Considering that cannabinoid receptors are not expressed until late in the first trimester, studies that examine any cannabis exposure across pregnancy, effectively lumping together exposure across time, may produce results biased toward the null or else confounded by other factors.

Further, all else being equal, whether the cannabis is smoked, vaporized, orally ingested, or otherwise consumed is crucial to consider, but seldom is. Not only can different modes of consumption affect the concentration and rate of THC absorption by the foetus due to differential pharmacokinetic properties (for a review, see Grant et al., 2018), they may also introduce additional chemicals into the mix. Like tobacco smoke, cannabis smoke includes potentially toxic chemical compounds resulting from pyrolysis or incomplete combustion. Compared to tobacco smoke, cannabis smoke exhibits similar or even higher concentrations of possibly teratogenic particulate matter (Graves et al., 2020). Vaporizing and orally ingesting cannabis, by contrast, does not involve combustion. Without accounting for different methods of ingestion, it may not be possible to differentiate the effects of cannabis from the effects attributable to combustion. The inclusion of these aspects of PCE in future research may promote discoveries about the relative risks of various cannabis use behaviors by pregnant women.

25.7.2 Potential Confounds

Another issue is that human studies of PCE are predominantly correlational in nature, and the range of possible confounds is vast. Cannabis use during pregnancy is associated with younger maternal age, lower educational attainment and income, belonging to a minoritized group, being unmarried, being unemployed, having a history of childhood trauma and delinquency, having an unplanned pregnancy, and being exposed to past-year stressful life events (Allen et al., 2020; Brents, 2017; El Marroun et al., 2008). Lower socioeconomic status and past-year stressful life events may directly impact foetal development and/or portend further stresses that may influence childhood outcomes. Women who use cannabis during pregnancy are also more likely to use other substances and have partners who use cannabis or other substances (El Marroun et al., 2008; Ko et al., 2015), and these patterns of substance use may adversely affect offspring.

This non-exhaustive list of potential confounding variables underscores the difficulty in isolating independent effects of PCE, if they exist, in observational work. Most studies to date have controlled for at least some of the more obvious possible confounds, such as co-use of alcohol and tobacco and maternal age. Less commonly assessed, but nonetheless significant, potential confounds include family history of psychopathology and maternal stress exposure. Where included, these covariates are often narrowly construed (Day et al., 2011; Rose-Jacobs et al., 2012).

25.7.3 False Positives and False Negatives

Most studies reviewed here examined more than one outcome. For instance, in investigations of birth outcomes, it is common to simultaneously test birthweight, gestational age, birth length, and head circumference (e.g., Cornelius et al., 1995; Day et al., 1991; Grzeskowiak et al., 2020), frequently in addition to other outcomes. However, very few studies account for the inflated Type I error rate resulting from multiple testing. Type II errors (i.e., false negatives), too, may be especially concerning in this field and even made more likely by the frequent lumping together of exposures across trimesters of pregnancy. Taken together, it is possible that current evidence is contaminated by both false positives and false negatives. It will be important for researchers to correct for multiple testing (e.g., through False Discovery Rate correction), use data reduction techniques, and/or, at the very least, report exact p-values.

25.8 Conclusions, Recommendations, and Future Directions

Overall, the majority of evidence suggests that PCE is associated with reduced birthweight and pre-term birth. A smaller and more mixed literature suggests that PCE may be associated with psychopathology risk in children and in particular externalizing behaviors and psychotic-like experiences. What remains unclear is whether these associations are independent of confounds and whether PCE contributes to these individual differences.

Whether significant associations between PCE and these outcomes are causal and/or arise from shared pre-disposition is difficult to test outside of experimental approaches. However, genetically informed designs may help uncover the extent to which an association is due to shared genetic influence. One study accounted for genomic liability to schizophrenia using a polygenic risk score (PRS) in the association between PCE and psychotic-like experiences (Paul et al., 2021), finding that the inclusion of the PRS did not substantially attenuate this relationship. Other methods, such as sibling crossover designs in which non-twin siblings are discordant for pre-natal exposure, can be leveraged to capture the proportion of variance not attributable to familial confounding (e.g., maternal genetic and other characteristics). That said, such designs have limitations in the context of pregnancy, in that they cannot rule out the possibility of different circumstances leading to cannabis use during one pregnancy and not another.

In addition to family-based designs, additional biological data are needed, as are well-powered studies able to explore the effects of timing of exposure. First, supplementing self-reports with toxicology screens to quantify PCE in prospective studies is crucial. Second, to more fully explore whether and through what pathways PCE may influence offspring, biological (e.g., genetic, neuroimaging, inflammation) data and longitudinal measures of behaviour, cognition, and environmental risk factors are needed. New endeavours (e.g., the HEALthy Brain and Child Development [HBCD] study; https://heal.nih.gov/research/infants-and-children, last accessed 30 October 2022) will incorporate longitudinal neuroimaging, stress exposure, and medical data. These studies aim to target recruitment such that there will be sufficient power to detect PCE-specific effects (e.g., recruiting women who exclusively use cannabis), as well as critically important timing-related influences, and will be positioned to explore mechanistic pathways.

Considering the data presented here, it would be advisable for healthcare providers to caution expectant parents ((of any gender) to be more inclusive of all genders among expectant parents) about plausible risks to foetal and child development. In the spirit of harm reduction, pregnant women should be advised about the likely increased risk associated with combustion. In light of growing cannabis use among pregnant women, rapidly expanding cannabis legalization and accessibility, and declining perceptions of harm, the possibility that even small effects on offspring development may be spread over a sizeable population of infants and children is cause for concern. Thus, until more data are gathered, we recommend against the use of cannabis during pregnancy.

References

Achenbach, T. M., McConaughy, S. H., and Howell, C. T. (1987). Child/adolescent behavioral and emotional problems: Implications of cross-informant correlations for situational specificity. *Psychol Bull*, **101**, 213–232.

Allen, A. M., Jung, A. M., Alexander, A. C., et al. (2020). Cannabis use and stressful life events during the perinatal period: Cross-sectional results from Pregnancy Risk Assessment Monitoring System (PRAMS) data, 2016. *Addiction*, **115**, 1707–1716.

Alshaarawy, O., and Anthony, J. C. (2019). Are cannabis users less likely to gain weight? Results from a national 3-year prospective study. *Int J Epidemiol*, **48**, 1695–1700.

Antonelli, T., Tomasini, M. C., Tattoli, M., et al. (2005). Prenatal exposure to the CB1 receptor agonist WIN 55,212-2 causes learning disruption associated with impaired cortical NMDA receptor function and emotional reactivity changes in rat offspring. *Cereb Cortex*, **15**, 2013–2020.

Bada, H. S., Bann, C. M., Bauer, C. R., et al. (2011). Preadolescent behavior problems after prenatal cocaine exposure: Relationship between teacher and caretaker ratings (Maternal Lifestyle Study). *Neurotoxicol Teratol*, **33**, 78–87.

Baer, R. J., Chambers, C. D., Ryckman, K. K., et al. (2019). Risk of preterm and early term birth by maternal drug use. *J Perinatol*, **39**, 286–294.

Bara, A., Manduca, A., Bernabeu, A., et al. (2018). Sex-dependent effects of in utero cannabinoid exposure on cortical function. *eLife*, **7**, e36234.

Basavarajappa, B. S., Nixon, R. A., and Arancio, O. (2009). Endocannabinoid system: Emerging role from neurodevelopment to neurodegeneration. *Mini Rev Med Chem*, **9**, 448–462.

Bayrampour, H., Zahradnik, M., Lisonkova, S., et al. (2019). Women's perspectives about cannabis use during pregnancy and the postpartum period: An integrative review. *Prev Med*, **119**, 17–23.

Belbasis, L., Savvidou, M. D., Kanu, C., et al. (2016). Birth weight in relation to health and disease in later life: An umbrella review of systematic reviews and meta-analyses. *BMC Med*, **14**, 147.

Berrendero, F., García-Gil, L., Hernández, M. L., et al. (1998). Localization of mRNA expression and activation of signal transduction mechanisms for cannabinoid receptor in rat brain during fetal development. *Development*, **125**, 3179–3188.

Bolhuis, K., Kushner, S. A., Yalniz, S., et al. (2018). Maternal and paternal cannabis use during pregnancy and the risk of psychotic-like experiences in the offspring. *Schizophr Res*, **202**, 322–327.

Brancato, A., Castelli, V., Lavanco, G., et al. (2020). In utero Δ9-tetrahydrocannabinol exposure confers vulnerability towards cognitive impairments and alcohol drinking in the adolescent offspring: Is there a role for neuropeptide Y? *J Psychopharmacol (Oxf)*, **34**, 663–679.

Breit, K. R., Rodriguez, C. G., Lei, A., et al. (2020). Combined vapor exposure to THC and alcohol in pregnant rats: Maternal outcomes and pharmacokinetic effects. *Neurotoxicol Teratol*, **82**, 106930.

Brents, L. K. (2017). Correlates and consequences of prenatal cannabis exposure (PCE): Identifying and characterizing vulnerable maternal populations and determining outcomes for exposed offspring. In: Preedy, V. R. (ed.), *Handbook of Cannabis and Related Pathologies: Biology, Pharmacology, Diagnosis, and Treatment* (pp. 160–170). London: Elsevier Inc.

Campolongo, P., Trezza, V., Cassano, T., et al. (2007). Perinatal exposure to delta-9-tetrahydrocannabinol causes enduring cognitive deficits associated with alteration of cortical gene expression and neurotransmission in rats. *Addict Biol*, **12**, 485–495.

Carmody, D. P., Bennett, D. S., and Lewis, M. (2011). The effects of prenatal cocaine exposure and gender on inhibitory control and attention. *Neurotoxicol Teratol*, **33**, 61–68.

Cecil, C. A. M., Walton, E., Smith, R. G., et al. (2016). DNA methylation and substance-use risk: A prospective, genome-wide study spanning gestation to adolescence. *Transl Psychiatry*, **6**, e976.

Chabarria, K. C., Racusin, D. A., Antony, K. M., et al. (2016). Marijuana use and its effects in pregnancy. *Am J Obstet Gynecol*, **215**, 506.e1–506.e7.

Chen, D. J., Gao, M., Gao, F. F., et al. (2017). Brain cannabinoid receptor 2: Expression, function and modulation. *Acta Pharmacol Sin*, **38**, 312–316.

Compton, W. M., Han, B., Jones, C. M., et al. (2016). Marijuana use and use disorders in adults in the USA, 2002–14: Analysis of annual cross-sectional surveys. *Lancet Psychiatry*, **3**, 954–964.

Conner, S. N., Bedell, V., Lipsey, K., et al. (2016). Maternal marijuana use and adverse neonatal outcomes: A systematic review and meta-analysis. *Obstet Gynecol*, **128**, 713–723.

Cornelius, M. D., Taylor, P. M., Geva, D., et al. (1995). Prenatal tobacco and marijuana use among adolescents: Effects on offspring gestational age, growth, and morphology. *Pediatrics*, **95**, 738–743.

Corsi, D. J., Walsh, L., Weiss, D., et al. (2019). Association between self-reported prenatal cannabis use and maternal, perinatal, and neonatal outcomes. *JAMA*, **322**, 145–152.

Crume, T. L., Juhl, A. L., Brooks-Russell, A., et al. (2018). Cannabis use during the perinatal period in a state with legalized recreational and medical marijuana: The association between maternal characteristics, breastfeeding patterns, and neonatal outcomes. *J Pediatr*, **197**, 90–96.

Day, N. L., Leech, S. L., and Goldschmidt, L. (2011). The effects of prenatal marijuana exposure on delinquent behaviors are mediated by measures of neurocognitive functioning. *Neurotoxicol Teratol*, **33**, 129–136.

Day, N. L., and Richardson, G. A. (1991). Prenatal marijuana use: Epidemiology, methodologic issues, and infant outcome. *Clin Perinatol*, **18**, 77–91.

Day, N. L., Richardson, G. A., Goldschmidt, L., et al. (1994). Effect of prenatal marijuana exposure on the cognitive development of offspring at age three. *Neurotoxicol Teratol*, **16**, 169–175.

Day, N. L., Sambamoorthi, U., Taylor, P., et al. (1991). Prenatal marijuana use and neonatal outcome. *Neurotoxicol Teratol*, **13**, 329–334.

Dinieri, J. A., Wang, X., Szutorisz, H., et al. (2011). Maternal cannabis use alters ventral striatal dopamine D2 gene regulation in the offspring. *Biol Psychiatry*, **70**, 763–769.

El Marroun, H., Bolhuis, K., Franken, I. H. A., et al. (2019). Preconception and prenatal cannabis use and the risk of behavioural and emotional problems in the offspring; a multi-informant prospective longitudinal study. *Int J Epidemiol*, **48**, 287–296.

El Marroun, H., Tiemeier, H., Jaddoe, V. W. V., et al. (2008). Demographic, emotional and social determinants of cannabis use in early pregnancy: The Generation R study. *Drug Alcohol Depend*, **98**, 218–226.

El Marroun, H., Tiemeier, H., Steegers, E. A., et al. (2009). Intrauterine cannabis exposure affects fetal growth trajectories: The Generation R study. *J Am Acad Child Adolesc Psychiatry*, **48**, 1173–1181.

ElSohly, M. A., Mehmedic, Z., Foster, S., et al. (2016). Changes in cannabis potency over the last 2 decades (1995–2014): Analysis of current data in the United States. *Biol Psychiatry*, **79**, 613–619.

Fan, R. G., Portuguez, M. W., and Nunes, M. L. (2013). Cognition, behavior and social competence of preterm low birth weight children at school age. *Clinics*, **68**, 915–921.

Fine, J. D., Moreau, A. L., Karcher, N. R., et al. (2019). Association of prenatal cannabis exposure with psychosis proneness among children in the Adolescent Brain Cognitive Development (ABCD) study. *JAMA Psychiatry*, **76**, 762.

Frau, R., Miczan, V., Traccis, F., et al. (2019). Prenatal THC exposure produces a hyperdopaminergic phenotype rescued by pregnenolone. *Nat Neurosci*, **22**, 1975–1985.

Fried, P. A. (1995). The Ottawa Prenatal Prospective Study (OPPS): Methodological issues and findings – it's easy to throw the baby out with the bath water. *Life Sci*, **56**, 2159–2168.

Fried, P. A., and O'Connell, C. M. (1987). A comparison of the effects of prenatal exposure to tobacco, alcohol, cannabis and caffeine on birth size and subsequent growth. *Neurotoxicol Teratol*, **9**, 79–85.

Fried, P. A., and Watkinson, B. (1988). 12- and 24-month neurobehavioural follow-up of children prenatally exposed to marihuana, cigarettes and alcohol. *Neurotoxicol Teratol*, **10**, 305–313.

Fried, P. A., Watkinson, B., Grant, A., et al. (1980). Changing patterns of soft drug use prior to and during pregnancy: A prospective study. *Drug Alcohol Depend*, **6**, 323–343.

Fried, P. A., Watkinson, B., and Gray, R. (1992). A follow-up study of attentional behavior in 6-year-old children exposed prenatally to marihuana, cigarettes, and alcohol. *Neurotoxicol Teratol*, **14**, 299–311.

(1998). Differential effects on cognitive functioning in 9- to 12-year olds prenatally exposed to cigarettes and marihuana. *Neurotoxicol Teratol*, **20**, 293–306.

(2003). Differential effects on cognitive functioning in 13- to 16-year-olds prenatally exposed to cigarettes and marihuana. *Neurotoxicol Teratol*, **25**, 427–436.

Fried, P. A., Watkinson, B., and Willan, A. (1984). Marijuana use during pregnancy and decreased length of gestation. *Am J Obstet Gynecol*, **150**, 23–27.

Gianutsos, G., and Abbatiello, E. R. (1972). The effect of pre-natal cannabis sativa on maze learning ability in the rat. *Psychopharmacologia*, **27**, 117–122.

Goldschmidt, L., Richardson, G. A., Cornelius, M. D., et al. (2004). Prenatal marijuana and alcohol exposure and academic achievement at age 10. *Neurotoxicol Teratol*, **26**, 521–532.

Goldschmidt, L., Richardson, G. A., Willford, J., et al. (2008). Prenatal marijuana exposure and intelligence test performance at age 6. *J Am Acad Child Adolesc Psychiatry*, **47**, 254–263.

Goldschmidt, L., Richardson, G. A., Willford, J. A., et al. (2012). School achievement in 14-year-old youths prenatally exposed to marijuana. *Neurotoxicol Teratol*, **34**, 161–167.

Grant, K. S., Petroff, R., Isoherranen, N., et al. (2018). Cannabis use during pregnancy: Pharmacokinetics and effects on child development. *Pharmacol Ther*, **182**, 133–151.

Graves, B. M., Johnson, T. J., Nishida, R. T., et al. (2020). Comprehensive characterization of mainstream marijuana and tobacco smoke. *Sci Rep*, **10**, 1–12.

Gray, K. A., Day, N. L., Leech, S., et al. (2005). Prenatal marijuana exposure: Effect on child depressive symptoms at ten years of age. *Neurotoxicol Teratol*, **27**, 439–448.

Grzeskowiak, L. E., Grieger, J. A., Andraweera, P., et al. (2020). The deleterious effects of cannabis during pregnancy on neonatal outcomes. *Med J Aust*, **212**, 519–524.

Gunn, J. K. L., Rosales, C. B., Center, K. E., et al. (2016). Prenatal exposure to cannabis and maternal and child health outcomes: A systematic review and meta-analysis. *BMJ Open*, **6**, e009986.

Holloway, Z. R., Hawkey, A. B., Torres, A. K., et al. (2020). Paternal cannabis extract exposure in rats: Preconception timing effects on

neurodevelopmental behavior in offspring. *NeuroToxicology*, **81**, 180–188.

Hutchings, D. E., Martin, B. R., Gamagaris, Z., et al. (1989). Plasma concentrations of delta-9-tetrahydrocannabinol in dams and fetuses following acute or multiple prenatal dosing in rats. *Life Sci*, **44**, 697–701.

Jaddoe, V. W. V., Mackenbach, J. P., Moll, H. A., et al. (2006). The Generation R study: Design and cohort profile. *Eur J Epidemiol*, **21**, 475–484.

Kapur, B. M., and Aleksa, K. (2020). What the lab can and cannot do: clinical interpretation of drug testing results. *Crit Rev Clin Lab Sci*, **57**, 548–585.

Ko, J. Y., Farr, S. L., Tong, V. T., et al. (2015). Prevalence and patterns of marijuana use among pregnant and nonpregnant women of reproductive age. *Am J Obstet Gynecol*, **213**, 201.e1–201.e10.

Kooijman, M. N., Kruithof, C. J., van Duijn, C. M., et al. (2016). The Generation R study: Design and cohort update 2017. *Eur J Epidemiol*, **31**, 1243–1264.

Leech, S. L., Richardson, G. A., Goldschmidt, L., et al. (1999). Prenatal substance exposure: Effects on attention and impulsivity of 6-year-olds. *Neurotoxicol Teratol*, **21**, 109–118.

Leemaqz, S. Y., Dekker, G. A., McCowan, L. M., et al. (2016). Maternal marijuana use has independent effects on risk for spontaneous preterm birth but not other common late pregnancy complications. *Reprod Toxicol*, **62**, 77–86.

Levin, E. D., Hawkey, A. B., Hall, B. J., et al. (2019). Paternal THC exposure in rats causes long-lasting neurobehavioral effects in the offspring. *Neurotoxicol Teratol*, **74**, 106806.

Maia, J., Midão, L., Cunha, S. C., et al. (2019). Effects of cannabis tetrahydrocannabinol on

endocannabinoid homeostasis in human placenta. *Arch Toxicol*, **93**, 649–658.

Manduca, A., Servadio, M., Melancia, F., et al. (2020). Sex-specific behavioural deficits induced at early life by prenatal exposure to the cannabinoid receptor agonist WIN55, 212-2 depend on mGlu5 receptor signalling. *Br J Pharmacol*, **177**, 449–463.

Mereu, G., Fà, M., Ferraro, L., et al. (2003). Prenatal exposure to a cannabinoid agonist produces memory deficits linked to dysfunction in hippocampal long-term potentiation and glutamate release. *Proc Natl Acad Sci USA*, **100**, 4915–4920.

Natale, B. V., Gustin, K. N., Lee, K., et al. (2020). Δ9-tetrahydrocannabinol exposure during rat pregnancy leads to symmetrical fetal growth restriction and labyrinth-specific vascular defects in the placenta. *Sci Rep*, **10**, 1–15.

Niesink, R. J. M., and van Laar, M. W. (2013). Does cannabidiol protect against adverse psychological effects of THC? *Front Psychiatry*, **4**, 130.

O'Shea, M., and Mallet, P. E. (2005). Impaired learning in adulthood following neonatal Δ9-THC exposure. *Behav Pharmacol*, **16**, 455–461.

Paul, S. E., Hatoum, A. S., Fine, J. D., et al. (2021). Associations between prenatal cannabis exposure and childhood outcomes: Results from the ABCD study. *JAMA Psychiatry*, **78**, 64.

Porath, A. J., and Fried, P. A. (2005). Effects of prenatal cigarette and marijuana exposure on drug use among offspring. *Neurotoxicol Teratol*, **27**, 267–277.

Richardson, G. A., Goldschmidt, L., and Willford, J. (2009). Continued effects of prenatal cocaine use: Preschool development. *Neurotoxicol Teratol*, **31**, 325–333.

Richardson, G. A., Ryan, C., Willford, J., et al. (2002). Prenatal alcohol and marijuana exposure: Effects on neuropsychological outcomes at 10 years. *Neurotoxicol Teratol*, **24**, 309–320.

Rose-Jacobs, R., Augustyn, M., Beeghly, M., et al. (2012). Intrauterine substance exposures and Wechsler Individual Achievement Test-II scores at 11 years of age. *Vulnerable Child Youth Stud*, **7**, 186–197.

Rose-Jacobs, R., Soenksen, S., Appugliese, D. P., et al. (2011). Early adolescent executive functioning, intrauterine exposures and own drug use. *Neurotoxicol Teratol*, **33**, 379–392.

Sagheddu, C., Traccis, F., Serra, V., et al. (2021). Mesolimbic dopamine dysregulation as a signature of information processing deficits imposed by prenatal THC exposure. *Prog Neuropsychopharmacol Biol Psychiatry*, **105**, 110128.

Silva, L., Zhao, N., Popp, S., et al. (2012). Prenatal tetrahydrocannabinol (THC) alters cognitive function and amphetamine response from weaning to adulthood in the rat. *Neurotoxicol Teratol*, **34**, 63–71.

Singer, L. T., Nelson, S., Short, E., et al. (2008). Prenatal cocaine exposure: Drug and environmental effects at 9 years. *J Pediatr*, **153**, 105–111.

Smith, A. M., Mioduszewski, O., Hatchard, T., et al. (2016). Prenatal marijuana exposure impacts executive functioning into young adulthood: An fMRI study. *Neurotoxicol Teratol*, **58**, 53–59.

Sonon, K. E., Richardson, G. A., Cornelius, J. R., et al. (2015). Prenatal marijuana exposure predicts marijuana use in young adulthood. *Neurotoxicol Teratol*, **47**, 10–15.

Szutorisz, H., DiNieri, J. A., Sweet, E., et al. (2014). Parental THC exposure leads to compulsive heroin-seeking and altered striatal synaptic plasticity in the subsequent generation.

Neuropsychopharmacology, **39**, 1315–1323.

Szutorisz, H., Egervári, G., Sperry, J., et al. (2016). Cross-generational THC exposure alters the developmental sensitivity of ventral and dorsal striatal gene expression in male and female offspring. *Neurotoxicol Teratol*, **58**, 107–114.

Torres, C. A., Medina-Kirchner, C., O'Malley, K. Y., et al. (2020). Totality of the evidence suggests prenatal cannabis exposure does not lead to cognitive impairments: A systematic and critical review. *Front Psychol*, **11**, 816.

Tortoriello, G., Morris, C. V., Alpar, A., et al. (2014). Miswiring the brain: Δ9-tetrahydrocannabinol disrupts cortical development by inducing an SCG10/stathmin-2 degradation pathway. *EMBO J*, **33**, 668–685.

Trezza, V., Cuomo, V., and Vanderschuren, L. J. M. J. (2008). Cannabis and the developing brain: Insights from behavior. *Eur J Pharmacol*, **585**, 441–452.

Volk, D. W., and Lewis, D. A. (2016). The role of endocannabinoid signaling in cortical inhibitory neuron dysfunction in schizophrenia. *Biol Psychiatry*, **79**, 595–603.

Volkow, N. D., Fowler, J. S., Wang, G. J., et al. (2007). Dopamine in drug abuse and addiction: Results of imaging studies and treatment implications. *Arch Neurol*, **64**, 1575–1579.

Volkow, N. D., Han, B., Compton, W. M., et al. (2019). Self-reported medical and nonmedical cannabis use among pregnant women in the United States. *JAMA*, **322**, 167–169.

Wang, X., Dow-Edwards, D., Anderson, V., et al. (2004). In utero marijuana exposure associated with abnormal amygdala dopamine D2 gene expression in the human fetus. *Biol Psychiatry*, **56**, 909–915.

Watson, C. T., Szutorisz, H., Garg, P., et al. (2015). Genome-wide DNA

methylation profiling reveals epigenetic changes in the rat nucleus accumbens associated with cross-generational effects of adolescent THC exposure. *Neuropsychopharmacology*, **40**, 2993–3005.

Weimar, H. V., Wright, H. R., Warrick, C. R., et al. (2020). Long-term effects of maternal cannabis vapor exposure on emotional reactivity, social behavior, and behavioral flexibility in offspring. *Neuropharmacology*, **179**, 108288.

Wu, C.-S., Jew, C. P., and Lu, H.-C. (2011). Lasting impacts of prenatal cannabis exposure and the role of endogenous cannabinoids in the developing brain. *Future Neurol*, **6**, 459–480.

Yao, J. L., He, Q. Z., Liu, M., et al. (2018). Effects of Δ(9)-tetrahydrocannabinol (THC) on human amniotic epithelial cell proliferation and migration. *Toxicology*, **394**, 19–26.

Young-Wolff, K. C., Adams, S. R., Padon, A., et al. (2021). Association of cannabis retailer proximity and density with cannabis use among pregnant women in Northern California after legalization of cannabis for recreational use. *JAMA Netw Open*, **4**, e210694.

Young-Wolff, K. C., Sarovar, V., Tucker, L. Y., et al. (2020). Validity of self-reported cannabis use among pregnant females in Northern California. *J Addict Med*, **14**, 287–292.

Zammit, S., Thomas, K., Thompson, A., et al. (2009). Maternal tobacco, cannabis and alcohol use during pregnancy and risk of adolescent psychotic symptoms in offspring. *Br J Psychiatry*, **195**, 294–300.

Zurolo, E., Iyer, A. M., Spliet, W. G. M., et al. (2010). CB1 and CB2 cannabinoid receptor expression during development and in epileptogenic developmental pathologies. *Neuroscience*, **170**, 28–41.

Cannabis Use and Violence

Giulia Trotta, Paolo Marino, Victoria Rodriguez, Robin M. Murray, and Evangelos Vassos

26.1 Introduction

There is a strong worldwide trend toward liberalizing policy toward cannabis use and commercializing its sale (Murray and Hall, 2020). According to the World Drug Report 2021, habitual cannabis users were estimated at 192 million worldwide, making cannabis the most widely used illicit substance (World Drug Report, 2021). Even if only a minority of users suffer adverse effects, given the high number of people smoking cannabis, its use has become a health concern. In particular, increasing concern has been expressed regarding the spread of high-potency cannabis (i.e., concentration of tetrahydrocannabinol >10%), especially within the young, and much attention has focused on the now well-established evidence that prolonged heavy use increases the likelihood of psychosis (Di Forti et al., 2019).

The question of whether the use of cannabis is associated with violence has gained attention more recently. A meta-analysis in patients with severe mental illnesses found a moderate association between cannabis use and violence (Dellazizzo et al., 2019). Schizophrenia and other psychoses are associated with violence and violent offending, but it seems that most of the excess risk is mediated by comorbidity with substance abuse (Fazel et al., 2009). Absolute rates of violent crime over 5–10 years are typically below 5% in individuals with mental illness but increase to more than 10% in those with substance misuse (Bujarski et al., 2016).

This chapter aims to elucidate whether, and to what extent, cannabis use is associated with violent events. This may provide a better insight on the pathogenic mechanisms involved and have the potential for guiding future preventive strategies.

26.2 Measurement of Cannabis Use

According to the 2021 European Monitoring Centre for Drugs and Drug Addiction (EMCDDA) report, at present the most widely available type of cannabis used across Europe has an average 20–28% of THC content, which is twice as much as traditional herbal cannabis (European Monitoring Centre for Drugs and Drug Addiction, 2021). Many products available on the market have high-THC content. Consequentially, cannabis users are currently exposed to much higher doses of THC than previously, which raises concerns for a higher risk of dependence and mental health problems. The following are some of the results cited in the 2021 EMCDDA report:

- A 2015–2020 survey of 26 European countries estimates that cannabis use in the 15–34 age group category averages 15.4% (ranging from 3.4% in Hungary to 21.8% in France). Narrowing the age-range up to 24-years of age resulted in a rate of 19.2% (9.1 million) in the last year and 10.3% (4.9 million) in the last month.
- Of school children, 2.4% reported having smoked cannabis for the first time at age 13 or younger (ESPAD, 2019).
- In 2019, around 111,000 individuals started treatment for problematic use of cannabis in Europe, comprising 35% of all drug-related treatment demands. Fifty-one percent of first-time entrants to treatment reported daily cannabis use in the last month.

Another report (Aebi and Tiago, 2020) showed that individuals in prison, compared with the general population, report higher rates of drug use and drug-related problems. Although the link between drugs and crime is not simple (Stuart and Rich, 2018), it is known that problematic drug use increases the rates of offending and increases the likelihood of spending time in prison, especially recurrent short periods of imprisonment. A recent review of 12 European countries showed an average 61% of lifetime prevalence of illicit drug use on entry to prison, with cannabis being the most frequently reported substance (van de Baan et al., 2022).

Many instruments are currently used to assess cannabis consumption and related problems. Although most have good reliability, there is no gold standard tool yet (López-Pelayo et al., 2015). In fact, there are different definitions of cannabis consumption, depending on different frequency patterns and, consequently, it is not easy to assess comprehensively all those patterns in relation to violence.

26.3 Measurement of Violence

According to the Global Study on Homicide, 464,000 people died from violent crimes in 2017, making violence one of the leading causes of deaths worldwide (United Nation Office on Drugs and Crime, 2019).

Violence is defined as 'the intentional use of physical force or power, threatened or actual, against oneself, another person, or against a group or community, that either results in or has a highly likelihood of resulting in injury, death, psychological harm, mal development or deprivation' (Krug et al., 2002, p. 5).

A 'typology of violence' has been developed based on the World Health Organization's definition, that includes different categories and types of violent acts to have a better understanding of the phenomenon and the contexts in which it occurs (*Prevention of Violence: Public Health Priority*, WHO, 2016). It also helps to link the different categories and types allowing a holistic approach to intervention.

Three categories of violence have been identified:

- *Self-directed violence* refers to violent acts that individuals inflict upon themselves and includes self-abuse/mutilation and suicidal behaviors.
- *Inter-personal violence* refers to violent acts inflicted on another individual and its sub-groups are family and intimate partner violence and community violence, depending on the relationship between victims and perpetrators.
- *Collective violence* refers to an instrumental use of violent acts for achieving specific purposes such as political, economic, and social.

The types of violence are identified depending on the nature of the acts, as follows:

- *Physical violence*: The intentional use of physical force, used with the potential for causing harm, injury, disability, or death. It includes pushing, grabbing, biting, choking, shaking, slapping, punching, hitting, burning, use of a weapon, use of restraint or one's body against another person and others.
- *Sexual violence*: A sexual act attempted or committed against someone who has not freely given consent, or who is unable to consent or refuse. This includes forced, drug/alcohol-facilitated, or unwanted penetration, sexual touching, or non-contact acts of a sexual nature.
- *Psychological violence* (or emotional or mental abuse): verbal and non-verbal communication aimed at harming another individual mentally or emotionally, or to exert control over another person.
- *Neglect*: When a caregiver fails to fulfil needs for which an individual is unable to care for themselves, depriving them of adequate care. Neglect includes the failure to provide supervision, nourishment, or medical care.

According to the summary provided here, narrowed for the purpose of this chapter, the difficulty to assess such a complex phenomenon is evident. In fact, when assessing violence, different types of data are needed but those do not necessarily fulfil different purposes comprehensively in terms of (a) describing the impact of violence, (b) understanding which factor increases the risk for violent perpetration and victimization, and (c) evaluating the effects of specific prevention programmes. It is also difficult to assess different categories and types of violence based on data provided from databases and/or collected by different evaluation or risk assessment. It is a heterogeneous phenomenon not easy to be harmonized, as different studies may provide either self-reported data and/or criminal records.

26.3.1 Cannabis Association with Being the Perpetrator of Violence

Cannabis use and violence often co-occur during adolescence and early adulthood, and it is difficult to disentangle the direction of the association. A higher prevalence of cannabis use in relation to violent behaviors was found both among a large nationally representative sample of high school students (Blitstein et al., 2005) and a Brazilian cohort of adolescents (Silva et al., 2014). However, it could be hypothesized that (i) substance use causes violence, (ii) violence causes substance use, and (iii) the relationship is bidirectional. Lim and Lui (2016) tried to clarify this complex relationship investigating the cross-lagged effects for perpetration and cannabis use. Cannabis use significantly predicted the risk of violence perpetration in adolescence and early adulthood but not later in life. It must be noted that also perpetration was significantly associated with subsequent cannabis use.

An association between adolescent former and current cannabis use and a variety of emotional and behavioural problems has been well established by cross-sectional studies (Moore et al., 2007). These findings were confirmed by a prospective population study which investigated the longitudinal associations between externalizing and internalizing psychopathology and cannabis, showing that cannabis use often precedes criminal offences, especially among males (Miettunen et al., 2014). Moreover, a Norwegian population-based study followed up adolescents and young adults from 13 to 27 years of age, examining the association between cannabis use and subsequent criminal charges (Pedersen and Skardhamar, 2010). After adjusting for relevant confounding factors, such as alcohol and other illegal substances, the relationship remained robust. Nevertheless, the increased risk of later registered crime was mainly due to drug-specific charges while no association was found for other types of violence, such as for criminal gain.

The co-occurrence of substance use and intimate partner violence perpetration has been studied extensively, but findings are contradictory for cannabis. Data from the National Epidemiologic Survey on Alcohol and Related Conditions showed increased odds of intimate partner violence perpetration for all types of substances, including cannabis (Afifi et al., 2012). There was no evidence of gender-specific associations and interactions between partner violence perpetration and individual cannabis use within a large forensic sample (Crane et al., 2014); on the contrary, cannabis seemed to play a role in moderating the association between problematic alcohol use and intimate partner violence. Similarly, another study found no increased risk of intimate partner violence perpetration by cannabis users compared to users of other substances, such as alcohol.

The effect of cannabis use on partner violence has been examined in non-European populations. A longitudinal study examined predictors of intimate partner violence perpetration among Latinos, indicating important gender differences for young adults (Grest et al., 2018). However, this probably reflected more culture-related factors such as acculturation and

traditional gender role attitude rather than cannabis consumption. Indeed, cannabis was not a statistically significant predictor of intimate partner violence perpetration. Another study investigated the association between trajectories of cannabis use from adolescence into young adulthood and violence among ethnic minorities such as African Americans and Puerto Ricans (Brook et al., 2014). Cannabis use, regardless of different developmental progressions, such as increasing chronic use, moderate use, and former use, was associated with a greater risk of violent behaviour using weapons compared to non-users.

In summary, a review of the relevant literature suggests that cannabis users are at increased risk of carrying out inter-personal violence, including severe types of violence such as aggravated assault, sexual aggression, fighting, and robbery.

26.3.2 Cannabis Association with Being the Victim of Violence

Several studies have examined the association between cannabis use and risk of being a victim of violence. An association between substance use and intimate partner violence victimization has been reported, and the relationship seems to be even stronger among those who were treated for substance abuse. Among different substances, robust findings were found for cannabis and intimate partner violence victimization, indicating that cannabis use is important for understanding the risk of experiencing violence.

Although cross-sectional studies reveal an association between women's cannabis use and experiencing physical violence from an intimate partner, the temporal ordering of these variables is not clearly established. However, a longitudinal examination of the association provided evidence that women who use cannabis are at increased risk of experiencing subsequent partner violence (Testa et al., 2003). In addition, another longitudinal study investigated whether cannabis use predicted intimate partner violence among newly married couples (Smith et al., 2014). Consistent with the literature, both cannabis use and intimate partner violence tended to decline during marriage and no association was demonstrated.

Since most studies have been focused on intimate partner violence, data is lacking on non-partner violent assault. However, there is evidence on the association between cannabis use and subsequent victimization also in this context. A study examined the cannabis use–violence relationship across the life course investigating how early cannabis use longitudinally affects the risk of victimization in subsequent life stages (Lim and Lui, 2016). Early cannabis use was significantly related to victimization in adolescence and early adulthood with an increasing magnitude of the effect during these transitions.

Only a few studies reported a dose–response relationship, suggesting a greater risk of violence after heavy cannabis use. For example, Amaro et al. (1990) showed an increasing association in the odds of being a victim of violence in those with frequent cannabis use. Moreover, in a South African study, frequent cannabis users reported higher rates of exposure to single or multiple types of violent acts compared to infrequent and non-users (Morojele and Brook, 2006).

26.3.3 Cannabis and Risk of Violence among Psychiatric Patients

Nowadays, it is well known that psychiatric patients have an increased risk of violence either in being perpetrators or victims (Stuart, 2003). A recent meta-analysis of 12 studies investigating the risk of violence in patients with severe mental illness who use cannabis (Dellazizzo et al., 2020) showed a moderate association between cannabis use and violence (OR = 3.02, CI = 2.01–4.54), which was stronger when considering cannabis misuse (OR = 5.8, CI = 3.27–10.28). The authors conclude that there is no single explanation for this association. Cannabis may determine poorer clinical outcome, leading to a higher risk of relapse, persistent positive symptoms, poor adherence, and treatment resistance which, in addition to the substance use itself, are potential risk factors for violent behaviour. Individuals with severe mental disorders represent an at-risk group, considering their higher rate of cannabis use compared to the general population.

26.4 Possible Mechanisms Underlying the Association between Cannabis and Violence

The associations between cannabis use and violence could be explained by different potential mechanisms, such as the neurobiological effect of the substance

after acute use, and importantly during abstinence and withdrawal, and social factors, for example the violent/criminal lifestyles of cannabis users. Chronic cannabis consumption may lead, in a dose–response manner, to overall and domain-specific cognitive impairments (e.g., attention, executive function, inhibition, and problem-solving). Indeed, prolonged and heavy cannabis use can negatively affect brain circuitry, inducing alterations in brain regions rich in CB-1 receptors, such as the amygdala and the anterior cingulate cortex, and affecting not only cognitive functions, but also affective and emotional regulation (e.g., anger and hostility) (Bloomfield et al., 2019). Poor cognition and defective emotional processing could then be associated with an increased risk of aggressive behaviour.

Abstinence and withdrawal have also been suggested as mechanisms linking cannabis and violence (Schlienz et al., 2017). Symptoms such as irritability, anxiety, restlessness, and impaired functioning may likewise contribute to subsequent aggressiveness. Most importantly, at a behavioural level, regular cannabis use may increase susceptibility to experience paranoia, and to interpret neutral stimuli as potentially threatening. Additionally, circumstantial factors may play a role in the positive association between cannabis and aggressiveness. As cannabis users tend to be more impulsive and risk-taking, it could be hypothesized that their risky lifestyle may expose them to antisocial and criminal behaviors (Moore and Stuart, 2005).

Cannabis misuse might have stronger effects on cognition and emotions in psychiatric patients rather than the general population. This could lead to severe symptoms such as paranoia, panic, and the feeling of loss of control and depersonalization. Furthermore, it is known that manic and psychotic symptoms get worse in the context of cannabis intoxication (Gibbs et al., 2015). Consequently, violent acts may be mediated by those psychopathological effects of cannabis misuse. Previous research has shown there is no association between aggression and cannabis withdrawal symptoms among people without a history of violent acts (Smith et al., 2013). On the other hand, withdrawal may improve aggressive behaviour among those with a previous history of aggression. Hence, when analysing this association, other non-pharmacological factors must be considered such as personality antisocial traits and peer influences (Moore and Stuart, 2005).

26.5 Limitations of the Available Evidence

We observed large heterogeneity of definitions for violence and methods of assessment for cannabis use in our literature review. This, on one hand, hinders the estimation of a 'global' effect of cannabis on violence and, on the other, indicates that the association between cannabis use and violence exists in different settings and populations.

Secondly, most current studies did not conduct a detailed assessment of cannabis exposure/pattern of use (type of cannabis, dosage, THC and CBD ratio, frequency of use, etc.), which may differentially be associated with violence. Studies that target dose–response analyses are needed. Moreover, very few studies controlled their findings for relevant confounding factors, such as other drug use (i.e., alcohol and stimulants), so sometimes the specific contribution of cannabis use is not clear.

Third, most studies were cross-sectional and retrospective, and it is not possible to be sure that the exposure to cannabis use definitely occurred prior to violence, thus presenting issues related to temporality and causal interference. The violence and cannabis use relationship is very complex and the extant research regarding the directionality of this relationship is inconclusive. The specific longitudinal linkages between cannabis use and later violence have not been researched extensively; thus, more prospective, longitudinal studies are required to disentangle the direction of the association and conclude any causal relations.

26.6 Conclusion

The available research suggests an association between cannabis use and risk of being a perpetrator and a victim of violence. Therefore, from a social perspective, cannabis use may be a useful preventive intervention target, particularly among at-risk groups such as psychiatric patients, to mitigate the risk. At a clinical level, this review of the available literature supports the need for a comprehensive assessment of cannabis use. However, further research is needed to overcome limitations in the current studies on cannabis use and violence and answer the unresolved questions as to the direction of the association and the potential mechanisms involved.

References

Aebi, M. F., and Tiago, M. M. (2020). Prisons and prisoners in Europe in pandemic times: An evaluation of the short-term impact of the COVID-19 on prison populations. *Universite de Lausanne* (Junio): 1–17.

Afifi, T. O., Henriksen, C. A., Asmundson, G. J. G., et al. (2012). Victimization and perpetration of intimate partner violence and substance use disorders in a nationally representative sample. *J Nervous Mental Dis*, **200**, 684–691.

Amaro, H., Fried, L. E., Cabral, H., et al. (1990). Violence during pregnancy and substance use. *Am J Public Health*, **80**, 575–579.

van de Baan, F. C., Montanari, L., Royuela, L., et al. (2022). Prevalence of illicit drug use before imprisonment in Europe: Results from a comprehensive literature review. *Drugs Educ Prevent Policy*, **29**, 1–12.

Blitstein, J. L., Murray, D. M., Lytle, L. A., et al. (2005). Predictors of violent behavior in an early adolescent cohort: Similarities and differences across genders. *Health Educ Behav*, **32**, 175–194.

Bloomfield, M. A. P., Hindocha, C., Green, S. F., et al. (2019). The neuropsychopharmacology of cannabis: A review of human imaging studies. *Pharmacol Ther*, **195**, 132–161.

Brook, J. S., Lee, J. Y., Finch, S. J., et al. (2014). Developmental trajectories of marijuana use from adolescence to adulthood: Relationship with using weapons including guns. *Aggress Behav*, **40**, 229–237.

Bujarski, S. J., McDaniel, C. E., Lewis, S. F., et al. (2016). Past-month marijuana use is associated with self-reported violence among trauma-exposed adolescents.

J Child Adolesc Subst Abuse, **26**, 111–118.

Crane, C. A., Oberleitner, L. M. S., Devine, S., et al. (2014). Substance use disorders and intimate partner violence perpetration among male and female offenders. *Psychol Violence*, **4**, 322–333.

Dellazizzo, L., Potvin, S., Beaudoin, M., et al. (2019). Cannabis use and violence in patients with severe mental illnesses: A meta-analytical investigation. *Psychiatry Res*, **274**, 42–48.

Dellazizzo, L., Potvin, S., Dou, B. Y., et al. (2020). Association between the use of cannabis and physical violence in youths: A meta-analytical investigation. *Am J Psychiatry*, **177**, 619–626.

Di Forti M., Quattrone D., Freeman T. P., et al. (2019). The contribution of cannabis use to variation in the incidence of psychotic disorder across Europe (EU-GEI): A multicentre case-control study. *The Lancet Psychiatry* **6**, 427–436.

ESPAD. (2019). *Results from the European School Survey Project on Alcohol and Other Drugs.* Available at: https://europa.eu/! Xy37DU. Last accessed 23 November 2021.

European Monitoring Centre for Drugs and Drug Addiction. (2021). *European Drug Report Trends and Developments.* Lisbon: EMCDDA.

Fazel, S., Gulati, G., Linsell, L., et al. (2009). Schizophrenia and violence: Systematic review and meta-analysis. *PLoS Med*, **6**, e1000120.

Gibbs, M., Winsper, C., Marwaha, S., et al. (2015). Cannabis use and mania symptoms: A systematic review and meta-analysis. *J Affect Disord*, **171**, 39–47.

Grest, C. V., Amaro, H., and Unger, J. (2018). Longitudinal predictors of intimate partner violence perpetration and victimization in Latino emerging adults. *J Youth Adolesc*, **47**, 560–574.

Krug, E. G., Dahlberg, L. L., Mercy, J. A., et al. (2002). *World Report on Violence and Health.* Geneva: World Health Organization.

Lim, J. Y., and Lui, C. K. (2016). Longitudinal associations between substance use and violence in adolescence through adulthood. *J Social Work Pract Addict*, **16**, 72–92.

López-Pelayo, H., Batalla, A., Balcells, M. M., et al. (2015). Assessment of cannabis use disorders: A systematic review of screening and diagnostic instruments. *Psychol Med*, **45**, 1121–1133.

Miettunen, J., Murray, G. K., Jones, P. B., et al. (2014). Longitudinal associations between childhood and adulthood externalizing and internalizing psychopathology and adolescent substance use. *Psychol Med*, **44**, 1727–1738.

Moore, T. H., Zammit, S., Lingford-Hughes, A., et al. (2007). Cannabis use and risk of psychotic or affective mental health outcomes: A systematic review. *Lancet*, **370**, 319–328.

Moore, T. M., and Stuart, G. L. (2005). A review of the literature on marijuana and interpersonal violence. *Aggress Violent Behav*, **10**, 171–192.

Morojele, N. K., and Brook, J. S. (2006). Substance use and multiple victimisation among adolescents in South Africa. *Addict Behav*, **31**, 1163–1176.

Murray, R. M., and Hall, W. (2020). Will legalization and commercialization of cannabis use increase the incidence and prevalence of psychosis? *JAMA Psychiatry*, **77**, 777–778.

Pedersen, W., and Skardhamar, T. (2010). Cannabis and crime: Findings from a longitudinal study. *Addiction*, **105**, 109–118.

Schlienz, N. J., Budney, A. J., Lee, D. C., et al. (2017). Cannabis withdrawal: A review of neurobiological mechanisms and sex differences. *Curr Addict Rep*, **4**, 75–81.

Silva, R. J. D. S., Soares, N. M. M., and Cabral De Oliveira, A. C. (2014). Factors associated with violent behavior among adolescents in northeastern Brazil. *Sci World J*, **2014**, 863918.

Smith, P. H., Homish, G. G., Leonard, K. E., et al. (2013). Marijuana withdrawal and aggression among a representative sample of U.S. marijuana users. *Drug Alcohol Depend*, **132**, 63–68.

Smith, P. H., Homish, G. G., Lorraine Collins, R., et al. (2014). Couples' marijuana use is inversely related to their intimate partner violence over the first 9 years of marriage. *Psychol Addict Behav*, **28**, 734–742.

Stuart, A., and Rich, J. D. J. (eds.) (2018). *Drug Use in Prisoners: Epidemiology, Implications, and Policy Responses.* Oxford: Oxford University Press.

Stuart, H. (2003). Violence and mental illness: An overview. *World Psychiatry*, **2**, 121.

Testa, M., Livingston, J. A., and Leonard, K. E. (2003). Women's substance use and experiences of intimate partner violence: A longitudinal investigation among a community sample. *Addict Behav*, **28**, 1649–1664.

United Nation Office on Drugs and Crime. (2019). *UNODC World Drug Report 2019.* Available at: https://wdr.unodc.org/wdr2019/index.html. Last accessed 3 November 2022.

World Drug Report. (2021). *UNODC World Drug Report 2021.* Available at: www.unodc.org/unodc/en/data-and-analysis/wdr2021.html. Last accessed 23 November 2021.

World Health Organization. (2016). *Prevention of Violence: Public Health Priority.* Available at: https://apps.who.int/iris/handle/10665/179463. Last accessed 24 November 2021.

Cannabis Withdrawal

27

Jane Metrik and Kayleigh N. McCarty

27.1 Introduction

The cannabis withdrawal syndrome is a diagnosis and a criterion of cannabis use disorder (CUD) in the American Psychiatric Association's (2013) *Diagnostic and Statistical Manual of Mental Disorders, DSM-5* and cannabis dependence in the International Classification of Diseases and Related Health Problems, ICD-10 and ICD-11 (World Health Organization, 2018). Withdrawal occurs when a drug is abruptly discontinued following prolonged exposure, which is indicative of neurological adaptation to the drug (Koob and Volkow, 2016). Cessation of heavy chronic regular use is associated with a cannabis withdrawal syndrome observed in humans and in a variety of animal species (Budney et al., 2003; Haney, 2005; Schlienz and Vandrey, 2019). A substantial amount of scientific evidence from pre-clinical, clinical, and epidemiological studies support reliability, validity, and clinical significance of cannabis withdrawal syndrome (Agrawal et al., 2008; Budney, 2006; Budney et al., 2006; Compton et al., 2009; Haney and Spealman, 2008; Hasin et al., 2008; Lynskey and Agrawal, 2007). Because physiological withdrawal symptoms resulting from cannabis use tend to be milder relative to opiates or benzodiazepines (National Academies of Sciences, Engineering, and Medicine, 2017), cannabis withdrawal symptoms were not previously considered clinically significant according to DSM-IV (American Psychiatric Association, 1994). With more clear evidence of clinical significance of cannabis withdrawal syndrome (Budney et al., 2003, 2008) much of the controversy that historically surrounded cannabis' addiction potential has been resolved.

27.2 Symptoms and Clinical Course

The DSM-5 symptoms that comprise cannabis withdrawal syndrome include irritability/anger/ aggression, nervousness/anxiety, sleep difficulty, decreased appetite or weight loss, restlessness, depressed mood, and physical symptoms such as abdominal pain, shakiness/tremors, sweating, fever, chills, and headaches (American Psychiatric Association, 2013). To meet criteria for cannabis withdrawal, individuals must endorse at least three of these symptoms that are causing distress and impairment, and these symptoms must occur following cessation of heavy and prolonged cannabis use. The symptoms of muscle tension, shakiness, chills, sweating, and nausea/stomach pain are less common (Budney et al., 2003; Haney et al., 1999, 2004). Symptoms of cannabis withdrawal typically develop within 24–72 hours after cessation of cannabis use (Budney et al., 2003). Peak magnitude of symptoms occurs two-to-five days post-cessation (Budney et al., 2003; Haney et al., 1999). Most symptoms resolve after two-to-three weeks of abstinence and return to baseline levels before cannabis use (Budney et al., 2003; Kouri and Pope, 2000).

Withdrawal is alleviated by administration of tetrahydrocannabinol (THC) (Haney et al., 1999, 2004) suggesting that THC plays an essential role in the development of cannabis use disorder and expression of withdrawal (Cooper and Haney, 2008). Of note, potency (% THC) of most cannabis strains has increased substantially (Chandra et al., 2019; ElSohly et al., 2016), with current cannabis containing $\geq 20\%$ THC. Widely available high-potency products (~80% THC) are implicated in increasing CUD rates and may be implicated in cannabis withdrawal expression (Meier, 2017). Relative to low potency cannabis, use of high potency cannabis was associated with more severe symptoms of CUD, which may include withdrawal (Freeman et al., 2019). Synthetic cannabinoids, which have higher cannabinoid receptor affinity and efficacy than THC, pose a greater risk for dependence and withdrawal severity than cannabis. Among daily users of synthetic cannabinoids, abrupt cessation has been associated with withdrawal symptoms that are more severe and protracted, relative to those following discontinuation of THC. Seizures, cardiovascular (e.g., tachycardia, chest pain), and respiratory symptoms have been reported along with more moderate withdrawal symptoms (e.g., anxiety, insomnia, headaches, nausea) common among cannabis users (Cooper, 2016). In fact, patients seeking synthetic cannabinoid treatment often require inpatient detoxification (Macfarlane and Christie, 2015). As greater potency of THC is implicated in more severe cannabis withdrawal symptoms, synthetic cannabinoid withdrawal severity appears to also correlate with greater frequency and quantity of the drug consumed (Cooper, 2016).

Sleep difficulty is one of the most endorsed symptoms of cannabis withdrawal. Sleep disturbance persists for at least 45 days following cannabis cessation and may take longer than other cannabis withdrawal symptoms to resolve (Budney et al., 2003). Trouble falling asleep is often considered to be among the more distressing symptoms of cannabis withdrawal (Allsop et al., 2011). In particular, disturbing dreams are often the most intensely experienced aspect of sleep problems (Allsop et al., 2011). Not surprisingly, several studies suggest that withdrawal-related sleep problems are cited as a primary reason for cannabis relapse (Arendt et al., 2007; Budney et al., 2008; Levin et al., 2010; Wiesbeck et al., 1996). While pharmacologically cannabis exacerbates objective sleep behaviors including decreased REM and slow wave sleep, it has also been found to improve self-reported sleep onset (Bolla et al., 2008; Garcia and Salloum, 2015; Gates et al., 2016; Nicholson et al., 2004; Pacek et al., 2017). Thus, sleep disturbance motivates cannabis use maintenance and is often endorsed as a salient reason for use (Reinarman et al., 2011; Schofield et al., 2006; Tringale and Jensen, 2011). In fact, cannabis-related sleep motives and withdrawal-related sleep disruptions may be an important underlying reason for why cannabis users may be ambivalent about quitting use. Furthermore, using cannabis specifically as a means of managing sleep problems was found to be the dominant mechanism explicating the relations between co-occurring mood disorders with cannabis use, cannabis-related problems, and cannabis use disorder (Metrik et al., 2016). In addition, cannabis users are more likely to report difficulty sleeping than those who do not use cannabis (Freeman et al.,

2010; Glozier et al., 2010; Mednick et al., 2010; Wong et al., 2009).

Sleep disturbance, restlessness, change in appetite/weight, and mood disturbance are common symptoms across all drugs of abuse (Schlienz and Vandrey, 2019). However, cannabis and tobacco withdrawal share the most similarities in terms of the presenting symptoms and time course (Budney et al., 2008; Vandrey et al., 2005, 2008). Withdrawal from each of these substances can include symptoms of anger/aggression, anxiety/nervousness, depressed mood, irritability, restlessness, and sleep difficulty. Cannabis withdrawal and tobacco withdrawal also affect both appetite and weight. Cannabis withdrawal decreases appetite and weight, whereas tobacco withdrawal increases appetite and weight (Vandrey et al., 2005). Regarding time course, the onset of cannabis withdrawal symptoms is most similar to that of stimulant withdrawal symptoms, and in general develops slower than symptoms of tobacco, alcohol, or opioid withdrawal. Peak cannabis withdrawal effects and the duration of these effects are similar to the time course of effects present with other substances, and tobacco in particular (Hughes et al., 1994). Unlike withdrawal from some other substances, cannabis withdrawal does not pose serious medical or psychiatric risk and typically does not require medical attention (American Psychiatric Association, 2013; Budney and Hughes, 2006).

27.3 Clinical Significance

Symptoms of cannabis withdrawal have been documented across a wide range of populations, including treatment-seeking and non-treatment-seeking samples, and settings including inpatient, outpatient, and research laboratories (Schlienz and Vandrey, 2019). According to the *DSM-5*, diagnosable withdrawal syndrome must result in significant impairment or distress (American Psychiatric Association, 2013). Collateral reports from friends and family of participants abstaining from cannabis noted an increase in several symptoms, including aggression, irritability, and nervousness after discontinuing cannabis use (Budney et al., 2001, 2003). In those abstinent from cannabis, withdrawal symptom severity is also positively associated with functional impairment (i.e., interference with normal daily activities; Allsop et al., 2012). In addition, cannabis withdrawal symptoms are negatively reinforcing, such that a desire to relieve the distress caused by withdrawal symptoms is commonly endorsed as a reason for resuming cannabis use after a period of abstinence (Copersino et al., 2010; Levin et al., 2010). Alternatively, individuals may use other substances, such as alcohol or tobacco, to relieve discomfort associated with cannabis withdrawal (Budney et al., 2008). The presence of withdrawal symptoms may also be associated with poorer treatment outcomes in those seeking treatment for CUD (Budney et al., 2019a).

A substantial number of cannabis users endorse attempts to cease or reduce cannabis use, with individuals seeking treatment for CUD averaging more than six attempts at quitting (Budney et al., 2007a). This substantive experience with quitting, and by extension with cannabis withdrawal that motivates resumed use, contributes to the development of salient learned associations surrounding cannabis cessation. In a study of cannabis cognitions about the expected outcomes of reducing or stopping cannabis use, anticipation of mood disturbance (i.e., irritability, anxiety, depression symptoms of cannabis withdrawal) was identified as a unique dimension of cannabis cessation expectancies. Stronger expectancies of worsening mood states upon cannabis cessation were observed among more frequent users and those endorsing greater craving after overnight deprivation (Metrik et al., 2017). In other studies, the majority of non-treatment-seeking adult cannabis users indicated that cannabis withdrawal directly contributed to the decision to resume cannabis use during a quit attempt or was the motivating factor for use of other substances including alcohol, tobacco, and sedatives (Budney et al., 2000, 2004, 2006).

Cannabis use disorder is highly comorbid with a number of psychiatric conditions, including psychotic disorders and mood and anxiety disorders (Hasin et al., 2016). In fact, prevalence of CUD among individuals with schizophrenia is substantially higher (~ 25%) relative to that in the general population (see Chapter 24). Negative affective states, as well as sleep disturbance, commonly experienced during cannabis withdrawal can mask as symptoms of depression and anxiety upon clinical presentation. Therefore, symptoms of psychiatric disorders and cannabis withdrawal may be difficult to differentiate among individuals with CUD or heavy cannabis users with co-occurring psychiatric diagnoses. While possible increase in psychiatric symptoms may be of clinical concern to patients with dual diagnosis attempting

cannabis cessation, sustained cannabis abstinence does not necessarily change the severity of psychotic symptoms in patients with schizophrenia and in fact may be associated with less severe depressive symptoms over time (Rabin et al., 2018). Nevertheless, cannabis treatment engagement and retention of patients with psychotic disorders is very difficult (see Chapter 24), and more research on cannabis withdrawal is needed in this population.

Furthermore, relief of anxiety and depression are the most common reasons for cannabis use among medical cannabis patients (Bonn-Miller et al., 2014; Kosiba et al., 2019; Metrik et al., 2018; Walsh et al., 2017) and among individuals who use cannabis recreationally (Osborn et al., 2015). In addition, medical cannabis users are more likely to endorse daily use than those who use recreationally (Kosiba et al., 2019; Lin et al., 2016; Metrik et al., 2018). Thus, individuals using cannabis medicinally may be at greater risk for developing symptoms of cannabis withdrawal due to frequent use patterns. In fact, daily cannabis quantity is found to be positively associated with withdrawal severity (Budney et al., 1999). Together these studies suggest that aversive psychological and mood states experienced during cannabis withdrawal may motivate cannabis use as an emotion regulatory strategy to reduce or manage these symptoms. Unsuccessful cessation efforts can further heighten symptoms of depression and anxiety, particularly among individuals with affective vulnerability or comorbid psychiatric disorders. Clinically, distinction between mood disturbance attributable to cannabis withdrawal versus psychiatric comorbidity has great utility because careful assessment of cannabis withdrawal syndrome may facilitate evidence-based therapeutic intervention specific to the presenting disorder.

27.4 Neurobiological Mechanisms of Cannabis Withdrawal

Pre-clinical research implicates the cannabinoid receptor type 1 (CB1), a G-coupled receptor that facilitates the psychoactive, intoxicating, and rewarding or positive effects of cannabis (Pertwee, 2005), in the expression of cannabis withdrawal (Ledent et al., 1999; Lichtman and Martin, 2002). CB1 receptor density and function is reduced with chronic cannabis exposure, with greater downregulation in cortical regions. On the other hand, prolonged abstinence in cannabis-dependent animals results in rapid recovery of CB1 receptor density and function, with faster stabilization in sub-cortical regions (D'Souza et al., 2016). Molecular genetic studies with the CB1 knockout mice, in which the CB1 receptor has been deleted or knocked out, demonstrate that these mice fail to exhibit withdrawal precipitated by the SR 141716A selective CB1 receptor antagonist (Lichtman and Martin, 2006). CB1 agonists have been shown to relieve withdrawal resulting from abrupt discontinuation of THC administration in animals and in humans (Schlienz et al., 2017).

In humans, imaging studies suggest that daily cannabis use is associated with a downregulation in CB1 receptor, possibly contributing to increased tolerance and eventually the development of withdrawal following abstinence from cannabis (Hirhoven et al., 2012). In fact, lower CB1 receptor density was associated with greater severity of cannabis withdrawal when symptoms were at their peak (on the second day of abstinence) (D'Souza et al., 2016). Similar to animal models, data from human studies suggest that CB1 receptor downregulation rapidly reverses with cannabis cessation and stabilizes to normal levels after 28 days of abstinence (D'Souza et al., 2016; Hirhoven et al., 2012). Taken together these studies indicate that cannabis withdrawal is a result of CB1 receptor downregulation attributed to repeated exposure to CB1 receptor agonists (e.g., THC).

27.5 Individual Differences in Cannabis Withdrawal

Only a sub-set of regular cannabis users develop symptoms of cannabis withdrawal. Survey studies suggest that approximately 30% of daily or near-daily cannabis users experience cannabis withdrawal (Wiesbeck et al., 1996; Young et al., 2002), though this estimate increases among individuals enrolled in CUD treatment studies or human laboratory studies (50–95%; Budney et al., 1998; Copeland et al., 2001; Crowley et al., 1998; Mikulich et al., 2001; Stephens et al., 2002). Individual differences may explain why some cannabis users are at greater risk for developing cannabis withdrawal.

27.6 Demographics

Sex differences in cannabis withdrawal symptoms have been examined in several studies. Women are more likely to report symptoms of cannabis withdrawal than men among those seeking treatment for CUD (Herrmann et al., 2015) and non-treatment seekers (Copersino et al., 2010). Specifically, women are more likely to report greater physiological symptoms of withdrawal relative to men (Cooper and Haney, 2014; Copersino et al., 2010). Pre-clinical studies indicate similar patterns. Female Sprague-Dawley rats exhibited reduced locomotor activity in response to cannabis withdrawal (Harte-Hargrove and Dow-Edwards, 2012; Marusich et al., 2014).

Very few studies have examined the effects of race and ethnicity on the experience of cannabis withdrawal symptoms. One study suggested that there may not be racial differences between the likelihood of reporting a cannabis withdrawal symptom, but race may influence the type of symptom endorsed. Specifically, Copersino et al. (2010) found that white individuals were more likely to endorse increased anxiety, difficulty sleeping, craving for cannabis, and decrease in appetite in response to cannabis cessation relative to Black/African American respondents. Of note, this study also described racial differences in pattern of cannabis use, with Black/African American participants reporting a younger age at first cannabis use and a shorter duration of lifetime cannabis use, suggesting that observed differences in withdrawal may be due to differences in cannabis use patterns rather than racial differences. Levin et al. (2010) found no significant differences in reported withdrawal symptoms between White and Black/African American individuals.

Studies have documented the presence of cannabis withdrawal symptoms in adolescent treatment-seeking samples (Vandrey et al., 2005). Notably, Vandrey et al. (2005) indicated that the prevalence of cannabis withdrawal symptoms in adolescents was lower than that observed in a similar study of treatment-seeking adults, suggesting that symptoms of cannabis withdrawal are more common and severe among adults (Budney et al., 1999). This finding aligns with the results from a human laboratory study that directly compared acute effects of cannabis administration in adolescents versus adults (Mokrysz et al., 2016). Adolescents reported blunted intoxication, were less cognitively impaired, but endorsed increased cannabis craving, suggesting decreased sensitivity to negative effects in youth relative to adults. On the other hand, in another study comparing cannabis withdrawal symptoms among adolescents and young adults (ages 16–36), there were no significant effects of age on cannabis withdrawal symptoms (Preuss et al., 2010). Similarly, adult-only studies have also found no effect of age on cannabis withdrawal symptoms (Allsop et al., 2011; Levin et al., 2010). However, age may influence the types of symptoms endorsed. One study suggested that older adults may be more likely to endorse increased sex drive and increased anxiety during cannabis withdrawal relative to younger adults (Copersino et al., 2010).

27.7 Cannabis Use History

Increased frequency of cannabis use is associated with a greater likelihood of experiencing withdrawal. In non-treatment seeking adults, using cannabis at least once weekly was associated with greater severity of withdrawal symptoms (Levin et al., 2010). Similar patterns are observed in frequent cannabis users, with a positive association between past month cannabis use quantity and number of withdrawal symptoms endorsed (Gorelick et al., 2012). Another study in non-treatment seeking adults failed to find a significant association between cannabis use quantity and severity of withdrawal symptoms (Allsop et al., 2011). Similarly, studies on treatment-seeking adolescents have failed to support an association between the amount of cannabis consumed in the previous month and cannabis withdrawal symptoms, suggesting that persistence of use may alone contribute to withdrawal symptoms (Milin et al., 2008). Alternatively, it is possible that future investigations with samples of users consuming high potency cannabis products may in fact link severity of cannabis withdrawal with higher THC quantity (Freeman et al., 2019).

27.8 Psychological Traits and Psychiatric Conditions

Substance use disorders often co-occur with other psychiatric conditions, including psychotic disorders, mood disorders, anxiety disorders, or trauma- or stress-related disorders (Grant et al., 2016; Hasin et al., 2016). Substance users with co-occurring mental health disorders are more likely to endorse symptoms of withdrawal (Ahmadi et al., 2008; Livne et al., 2019; Weinberger et al., 2010). Individuals with schizophrenia are particularly likely to experience cannabis withdrawal, with about 75% of chronic cannabis users with this diagnosis reporting numerous symptoms of withdrawal during a quit attempt (Boggs et al., 2013). Furthermore, withdrawal symptoms are often more severe among those with co-occurring psychiatric conditions (American Psychiatric Association, 2013). Limited research has focused on the effects of co-occurring psychiatric problems on cannabis withdrawal specifically. Cannabis withdrawal is more common among those seeking treatment for substance use disorders, regardless of substance type (Chauchard et al., 2014; Hesse and Thylstrup, 2013; Vorspan et al., 2010). Symptoms of cannabis withdrawal are also more common among those seeking treatment for other mental health conditions (Boggs et al., 2013; Dawes et al., 2011). Notably, a study on treatment seeking adolescents reported no significant associations between cannabis withdrawal and co-occurring psychiatric disorders (Greene and Kelly, 2014). In addition, among a sample of non-treatment seeking adults, cannabis withdrawal symptoms were more prevalent among individuals with a psychiatric diagnosis, but this difference was observed only for one week after cannabis cessation (Schuster et al., 2017). In a sample of young adults and adolescents with co-occurring DSM-IV cannabis dependence and major depression, 92% of individuals meeting criteria for cannabis dependence endorsed cannabis withdrawal (Cornelius et al., 2008). Cannabis withdrawal may also be more likely among those with personality disorder diagnoses (Livne et al., 2019).

27.9 Genetics and Heritability

Studies suggest that genetics may influence one's likelihood of experiencing cannabis withdrawal. Twin studies have suggested that cannabis withdrawal is moderately heritable, with approximately 50% of variation in withdrawal accounted for by genetic influences (Verweij et al., 2013). Of note, the genetic influences on cannabis withdrawal were nearly the same (99%) as those contributing to the diagnoses of DSM-IV cannabis abuse or cannabis dependence. Linkage analyses have identified chromosomal regions associated with the cannabis withdrawal symptom of 'nervous, tense, restless, or irritable' (Ehlers et al., 2010b). Experiencing nervousness during cannabis withdrawal has also been found to be one of the most heritable cannabis use disorder symptoms along with craving (Ehlers et al., 2010a).

Previous work suggests that variations in the *CNR1* gene that encodes the CB1 receptor and variation in the fatty acid amide hydrolase enzyme (*FAAH*) gene are implicated in reducing negative affect due to cannabis withdrawal (Haughey et al., 2008; Schacht et al., 2009). Single nucleotide polymorphisms in the *CNR1* gene may also play a role in the experience of cannabis withdrawal during periods of abstinence (Haughey et al., 2008). Haughey et al. (2008) found that variation in the *CNR1* gene was associated with withdrawal symptom severity in daily cannabis smokers. Schacht et al. (2009) studied variation in the *FAAH* gene in daily cannabis users in relation to cannabis' acute effects on abstinence-related intermediate phenotypes, such as craving, withdrawal, and subjective effects. Results from this study suggest that variation in the *FAAH* gene was also associated with withdrawal symptom severity. Other studies have posited an important environmental role in the development of cannabis withdrawal. A longitudinal study of children suggested that early childhood maltreatment led to the development of symptoms of cannabis abuse and dependence including withdrawal in adolescence (Oshri et al., 2011).

27.10 Treatment of Cannabis Withdrawal

27.10.1 Behavioural Interventions

Cannabis withdrawal symptoms may cause significant distress and are known to contribute to relapse among adults and adolescents seeking treatment for CUD (Budney et al., 2004; Cornelius et al., 2008). Cannabis cessation attempts among daily users interested in quitting are frequent and short-lived, with few achieving sustained abstinence (Budney et al., 2019b). The presence of cannabis withdrawal symptoms in the clinical course of CUD underscores the importance of implementing behavioural treatments that specifically incorporate skills training aimed at minimizing the clinical impact of withdrawal on resumed use.

Efficacious psychotherapeutic approaches for CUD include motivational-enhancement therapy (MET), cognitive-behavioural therapy (CBT), and abstinence-based contingency-management (CM) (Budney et al., 2007; Dutra et al., 2008; Metrik and Ramesh, 2018). A combination of MET, CBT, and/or abstinence-based CM appears to be the most potent behavioural intervention for adults and adolescents

with CUD (Davis et al., 2015; Dennis et al., 2004). However, only the minority of cannabis users demonstrate desired outcomes with CUD treatment, with relapse rates as high as they are for other substance use disorders (Budney et al., 2019b).

Contingency management is based on frequent monitoring of the target behaviour (e.g., abstinence) and the provision of tangible incentives (e.g., prizes or cash vouchers) for target behaviour (Budney et al., 2006; Prendergast et al., 2006). A number of randomized-controlled trials (RCTs) utilizing a combination of manualized MET/CBT (9–14 weekly individual sessions) and weekly CM monetary-based reinforcement of cannabis-negative urine specimens have demonstrated increased abstinence at the end of treatment and up to 12 months (Budney et al., 2000, 2006; Carroll et al., 2006; Kadden et al., 2007; Stanger et al., 2009). As a stand-alone treatment, CM produces equivalent outcomes to MET/CBT/CM during treatment and comparable outcomes to CBT at follow-up but appears to be less efficacious than the combined CBT+CM intervention post-treatment with respect to cannabis abstinence (Budney et al., 2006; Kadden et al., 2007).

Cognitive-behavioural conceptualization of substance use disorder is that of learned behaviour that develops over time when particular emotional states or cues associated with substance use produce cravings often followed by substance use. Individuals with substance use disorder use substances to cope with cravings or problems; therefore, acquisition of alternative coping skills is essential in CBT-based treatment approaches (Monti et al., 2001). Furthermore, behavioural treatments focused on coping skills for mood and stress management (Buckner et al., 2014) are specifically indicated for individuals planning to stop using cannabis who may be at risk for experiencing cannabis withdrawal. Negative affective states (i.e., increased anxiety, irritability, depressed mood) as well as sleep difficulty experienced during cannabis withdrawal motivate resumed cannabis use for coping reasons (Buckner and Zvolensky, 2014; Johnson et al., 2010; Simons et al., 2005) to decrease distress (Bonn-Miller et al., 2010; Potter et al., 2011). This type of short-term relief of negative affect from cannabis withdrawal (Metrik et al., 2011) is negatively reinforcing (Baker et al., 2004) and is responsible for CUD maintenance and progression in CUD severity (Bonn-Miller and Zvolensky, 2009; Farris et al., 2016; Metrik et al.,

2016). Therefore, behavioural interventions focused on increasing an individual's tolerance for emotional distress, increasing mindfulness (Potter et al., 2011; Segal et al., 2004), and decreasing avoidance of distress via specific strategies such as coping with cannabis urges are indicated for treatment goals centred on abstinence from cannabis. Cognitive-behavioural relapse prevention (Steinberg et al., 2005) or mindfulness-based relapse prevention (Bowen et al., 2011) emphasize coping with craving and negative affect skills training interventions and are successful in terms of long-term abstinence outcomes (Bowen et al., 2014).

27.10.2 Pharmacological Interventions

At the present time there are no Food and Drug Administration-approved pharmacotherapies for CUD. Because cannabis withdrawal symptoms abate with re-administration of cannabis (i.e., relapse to problematic use), much of the focus of pharmacotherapy development for CUD has been on alleviating symptoms of withdrawal (Hart, 2005). The pharmacotherapy development literature related to CUD has been previously summarized in considerable detail (Balter et al., 2014; Benyamina et al., 2008; Budney et al., 2010; Metrik and Ramesh, 2018; Ramesh and Haney, 2015; Vandrey and Haney, 2009); however, recent clinical efficacy data reviewed later in this chapter support a number of promising pharmacological medication compounds for further testing. Most of the research on CUD pharmacotherapeutic approaches is limited to small-scale laboratory models and small open-label trials with a specific focus on symptomatic treatment of cannabis withdrawal.

Medications investigated in clinical laboratory settings include cannabinoid substitutes (partial agonists of the CB1 receptor), such as dronabinol (synthetic encapsulated delta-9-tetrahydrocannabinol, THC) and nabilone. Studies incorporating this type of an agonist approach assess effects of treatment with dronabinol on withdrawal in heavy cannabis smokers. Human laboratory studies with dronabinol (50–60 mg/day) significantly decreased cravings, anxiety, chills, and sleep problems but did not affect self-administration (Haney et al., 2004, 2008). The findings of these studies were extended to an outpatient setting that showed that oral THC (10 or 30 mg, 3 times a day for 15 days) attenuated cannabis withdrawal symptoms such as aggression, craving,

troubled sleep, and irritability (Budney et al., 2007a, 2007b). An RCT in 156 participants examining dronabinol (40 mg/day) (Levin et al., 2011) found that all participants reduced cannabis use over time, irrespective of treatment, and there was no significant difference between treatment groups in the proportion of participants who achieved two weeks of abstinence at the end of the medication phase. However, the dronabinol group had higher treatment retention (77%) compared to placebo (61%) and, consistent with laboratory studies, withdrawal symptoms were significantly lower in the dronabinol group than placebo. Nabilone, a cannabinoid agonist with better bioavailability and a more reliable dose–response function than dronabinol (Bedi et al., 2013), significantly reversed withdrawal-induced irritability and disruptions in sleep and food intake as well as cannabinoid self-administration (6, 8 mg/day, for 8 days) (Haney et al., 2013). Positive findings on improvement in cannabis withdrawal symptoms from this human laboratory study suggest that nabilone is a promising candidate for investigation in a clinical trial for CUD treatment and relapse prevention.

An RCT in 51 treatment-seeking cannabis users found nabiximols (Sativex®; 1:1 ratio of THC (86.4 mg) and cannabidiol (80 mg)) attenuated cannabis withdrawal symptoms and improved patient retention in treatment (Allsop et al., 2015). Long-term reductions in cannabis use were not observed in this study; however, another RCT utilizing the same dose of nabiximols showed reduced cannabis use following 12 weeks of medication treatment (Lintzeris et al., 2019). Overall, nabiximols trials yielded mixed findings with respect to treatment of cannabis withdrawal including non-significant results (Trigo et al., 2018). An RCT testing cannabidiol (CBD), a non-psychoactive component of THC (and also present in nabiximols), in 82 individuals with CUD found that both 400 mg and 800 mg CBD were more effective than placebo at reducing cannabis use during four weeks of treatment; however, only the 800 mg dose significantly reduced cannabis withdrawal symptoms (Freeman et al., 2020).

Non-cannabinoid pharmacological agents including anticonvulsant gabapentin, oxytocin, and n-acetylcysteine also yielded promising findings. Gabapentin (1,200 mg/day for 12 weeks) significantly attenuated withdrawal severity and reduced cannabis use as compared to placebo (Mason et al., 2012). Although study retention was low in this proof-of-concept clinical trial, further research on gabapentin is indicated. The hormone, oxytocin, administered in conjunction with MET behavioural treatment in an RCT with 16 people reduced cannabis use at the end of treatment; however, no data on withdrawal symptoms were reported (Sherman et al., 2017). Glutamatergic modulator n-acetylcysteine showed initial promise in reducing cannabis-positive urine drug tests in an RCT with cannabis-dependent adolescents (Gray et al., 2012) but a larger study with 302 adults did not replicate this finding (Gray et al., 2017), and neither study published data on the medication's effect on withdrawal symptoms.

Inhibition of fatty acid amide hydrolase (FAAH) enzyme that degrades the endocannabinoid anandamide has shown efficacy in an RCT with 46 men with cannabis dependence. Specifically, relative to placebo, FAAH-inhibitor treatment (4 mg per day for 3 weeks following precipitated cannabis withdrawal during a 5-day hospital stay) reduced symptoms of cannabis withdrawal and lowered cannabis use at the end of treatment (D'Souza et al., 2019). Importantly, subjective improvements in withdrawal-induced sleep disturbance and objective changes in sleep architecture were observed during cannabis abstinence in the FAAH-inhibitor treatment condition. Unlike THC-substitution therapy, FAAH inhibitors do not have abuse liability and offer long-acting, safe, and highly efficacious treatment option for CUD. Multisite clinical trial is now underway to establish efficacy of the FAAH inhibitor in a larger more diverse sample.

In summary, the most promising cannabis withdrawal pharmacotherapy to date are preparations containing THC such as nabilone and FAAH-inhibitor that were shown to reduce a broad range of withdrawal symptoms associated with cannabis abstinence in users with CUD and in cannabis self-administration. Nabiximols have also shown promise in clinical trials in reducing cannabis withdrawal symptoms but not in promoting long-term abstinence. High dose of CBD has demonstrated efficacy in terms of reducing cannabis withdrawal and cannabis use during treatment. Ultimately, integrating pharmacotherapy treatment with behavioural interventions to alleviate withdrawal symptoms particularly in initial stages of CUD treatment should improve treatment outcomes and reduce relapse risk.

27.11 Conclusion

Cannabis withdrawal is a clinically significant syndrome commonly marked by mood and sleep disturbance symptoms as well as appetite decline or weight loss and restlessness. Withdrawal symptoms develop within 24–72 hours, peak within 2–5 days, and mostly resolve within 2–3 weeks following cannabis cessation. Cannabis withdrawal affects approximately a third of daily users but over half of individuals who seek CUD treatment. Although not life-threatening, cannabis withdrawal must be thoroughly assessed and treated because its psychological and physiological symptoms cause significant distress and pose high risk for relapse. Repeated cessation attempts and resumed use are negatively reinforcing, presenting major challenges to individuals trying to abstain from problematic cannabis use. Behavioural interventions aimed at mitigating cannabis withdrawal symptoms have limited efficacy, and there are no current medications available for treatment of cannabis withdrawal syndrome or CUD. A number of pharmacotherapy development studies and clinical trials are currently underway and appear promising. Additional research needs to elucidate the impact of cannabis withdrawal in vulnerable populations, particularly those with co-occurring psychotic disorders. Furthermore, increasing potency and availability of a variety of cannabis products with much higher concentration of THC (e.g., edibles, concentrates) may disproportionally place vulnerable cannabis users at risk for developing CUD and at risk for cannabis withdrawal syndrome of greater severity.

References

Agrawal, A., Pergadia, M. L., Saccone, S. F., et al. (2008). An autosomal linkage scan for cannabis use disorders in the nicotine addiction genetics project. *Arch Gen Psychiatry*, **65**, 713–721.

Ahmadi, J., Kampman, K., Dackis, C., et al. (2008). Cocaine withdrawal symptoms identify 'type B' cocaine-dependent patients. *Am J Addict*, **17**, 60–64.

Allsop, D. J., Copeland, J., Norberg, M. M., et al. (2012). Quantifying the clinical significance of cannabis withdrawal. *PLoS ONE*, **7**, 1–12.

Allsop, D. J., Lintzeris, N., Copeland, J., et al. (2015). Cannabinoid replacement therapy (CRT): Nabiximols (Sativex) as a novel treatment for cannabis withdrawal. *Clin Pharmacol Therap*, **97**, 571–574.

Allsop, D. J., Norberg, M. M., Copeland, J., et al. (2011). The cannabis withdrawal scale development: Patterns and predictors of cannabis withdrawal and distress. *Drug Alcohol Depend*, **119**, 123–129.

American Psychiatric Association. (1994). *Diagnostic and Statistical Manual of Mental Disorders (DSM-IV)*. Washington, DC: American Psychiatric Association.

(2013). *Diagnostic and Statistical Manual of Mental Disorders (5th Ed.)*. Arlington, VA: American Psychiatric Publishing.

Arendt, M., Rosenberg, R., Foldager, L., et al. (2007). Withdrawal symptoms do not predict relapse among subjects treated for cannabis dependence. *Am J Addict*, **16**, 461–467.

Baker, T. B., Piper, M. E., McCarthy, D. E., et al. (2004). Addiction motivation reformulated: An affective processing model of negative reinforcement. *Psychol Rev*, **111**, 33–51.

Balter, R. E., Cooper, Z. D., and Haney, M. (2014). Novel pharmacologic approaches to treating cannabis use disorder. *Curr Addict Rep*, **1**, 137–143.

Bedi, G., Cooper, Z. D., and Haney, M. (2013). Subjective, cognitive and cardiovascular dose-effect profile of nabilone and dronabinol in marijuana smokers. *Addict Biol*, **18**, 872–881.

Benyamina, A., Lecacheux, M., Blecha, L., et al. (2008). Pharmacotherapy and psychotherapy in cannabis withdrawal and dependence. *Expert Rev Neurother*, **8**, 479–491.

Boggs, D. L., Kelly, D. L., Liu, F., et al. (2013). Cannabis withdrawal in chronic cannabis users with schizophrenia. *J Psychiatric Res*, **47**, 240–245.

Bolla, K. I., Lesage, S. R., Gamaldo, C. E., et al. (2008). Sleep disturbance in heavy marijuana users. *Sleep*, **31**, 901–908.

Bonn-Miller, M. O., Boden, M. T., Bucossi, M. M., et al. (2014). Self-reported cannabis use characteristics, patterns and helpfulness among medical cannabis users. *Am J Drug Alcohol Abuse*, **40**, 23–30.

Bonn-Miller, M. O., Vujanovic, A., Twohig, M. P., et al. (2010). Posttraumatic stress symptom severity and marijuana use coping motives: A test of the mediating role of non-judgmental acceptance within a trauma-exposed community sample. *Mindfulness*, **1**, 98–106.

Bonn-Miller, M. O., and Zvolensky, M. J. (2009). An evaluation of the nature of marijuana use and its motives among young adult active users. *Am J Addict*, **18**, 409–416.

Bowen, S., Chawla, N., and Marlatt, G. A. (2011). *Mindfulness-based Relapse Prevention for Addictive Behaviors: A Clinician's Guide*. New York: Guilford Press.

Bowen, S., Witkiewitz, K., Clifasefi, S. L., et al. (2014). Relative efficacy of mindfulness-based relapse prevention, standard relapse prevention, and treatment as usual for substance use disorders: A randomized clinical trial. *JAMA Psychiatry*, **71**, 547–556.

Buckner, J. D., and Zvolensky, M. J. (2014). Cannabis and related impairment: The unique roles of cannabis use to cope with social anxiety and social avoidance. *Am J Addict*, **23**, 598–603.

Buckner, J. D., Zvolensky, M. J., Schmidt, N. B., et al. (2014). Integrated cognitive behavioral therapy for cannabis use and anxiety disorders: Rationale and development. *Addict Behav*, **39**, 495–496.

Budney, A. J. (2006). Are specific dependence criteria necessary for different substances: How can research on cannabis inform this issue? *Addiction*, **101**, 125–133.

Budney, A. J., Borodovsky, J.T. and Knapp, A. A. (2019a). Clinical manifestations of cannabis use disorder. In Montoya, I. D., and Weiss, S. R. B. (eds.) *Cannabis Use Disorders* (pp. 85–91). Cham: Springer International Publishing.

Budney, A. J., Higgins, S. T., Radanovich, K. J., et al. (2000). Adding voucher-based incentives to coping skills and motivational enhancement improves outcomes during treatment for marijuana dependence. *J Consult Clin Psychol*, **68**, 1051–1061.

Budney, A. J., and Hughes, J. R. (2006). The cannabis withdrawal syndrome. *Curr Opin Psychiatry*, **19**, 233–238.

Budney, A. J., Hughes, J. R., Moore, M. A., et al. (2001). Marijuana abstinence effects in marijuana smokers maintained in their home environment. *Arch Gen Psychiatry*, **58**, 917–924.

Budney, A. J., Moore, B. A., Rocha, L. A., et al. (2006). Clinical trial of abstinence-based vouchers and cognitive-behavioral therapy for cannabis dependence. *J Consult Clin Psychol*, **74**, 307–316.

Budney, A. J., Moore, B. A., and Vandrey, R. (2004). Review of the validity and significance of cannabis withdrawal syndrome. *Am J Psychiatry*, **161**, 1967–1977.

Budney, A. J., Moore, B. A., Vandrey, R. G., et al. (2003). The time course and significance of cannabis withdrawal. *J Abnormal Psychol*, **112**, 393–402.

Budney, A. J., Novy, P. L., and Hughes, J. R. (1999). Marijuana withdrawal among adults seeking treatment for marijuana dependence. *Addiction*, **94**, 1311–1322.

Budney, A. J., Radonovich, K. J., Higgins, S. T., et al. (1998). Adults seeking treatment for marijuana dependence: A comparison with cocaine-dependent treatment seekers. *Exp Clin Psychopharmacol*, **6**, 419–426.

Budney, A. J., Roffman, R., Stephens, R. S., et al. (2007a). Marijuana dependence and its treatment. *Addict Sci Clin Pract*, 4, 4–16.

Budney, A. J., Sofis, M. J., and Borodovsky, J. T. (2019b). An update on cannabis use disorder with comment on the impact of policy related to therapeutic and recreational cannabis use. *Eur Arch Psychiatry Clin Neurosci*, **269**, 73–86.

Budney, A. J., Vandrey, R. G., Hughes, J. R., et al. (2007b). Oral delta-9-tetrahydrocannabinol suppresses cannabis withdrawal symptoms. *Drug Alcohol Depend*, 86, 22–29.

(2008). Comparison of cannabis and tobacco withdrawal: Severity and contribution to relapse. *J Subst Abuse Treat*, **35**, 362–368.

Budney, A. J., Vandrey, R. G., and Stanger, C. (2010). Intervenções farmacológica e psicossocial para os distúrbios por uso da cannabis. *Revista Brasileira de Psiquiatria*, **32**, 546–555.

Carroll, K. M., Easton, E. J., Nich, C., et al. (2006). The use of contingency management and motivational/skills-building therapy to treat young adults with marijuana dependence. *J Consult Clin Psychol*, **74**, 955–966.

Chandra, S., Radwan, M. M., Majumdar, C. G., et al. (2019). New trends in cannabis potency in USA and Europe during the last decade (2008–2017). *Eur Arch Psychiatry Clin Neurosci*, **269**, 5–15.

Chauchard, E., Goncharov, O., Krupitsky, E., et al. (2014). Cannabis withdrawal in patients with and without opioid dependence. *Subst Abuse*, **35**, 230–234.

Compton, W. M., Saha, T. D., Conway, K. P., et al. (2009). The role of cannabis use within a dimensional approach to cannabis use disorders. *Drug Alcohol Depend*, **100**, 221–227.

Cooper, Z. D. (2016). Adverse effects of synthetic cannabinoids: Management of acute toxicity and withdrawal. *Curr Psychiatry Rep*, **18**, 52.

Cooper, Z. D., and Haney, M. (2008). Cannabis reinforcement and dependence: Role of the cannabinoid CB1 receptor: Cannabis dependence. *Addict Biol*, **13**, 188–195.

(2014). Investigation of sex-dependent effects of cannabis in daily cannabis smokers. *Drug Alcohol Depend*, **136**, 85–91.

Copeland, J., Swift, W., and Rees, V. (2001). Clinical profile of participants in a brief intervention program for cannabis use disorder. *J Subst Abuse Treat*, 20, 45–52.

Copersino, M. L., Boyd, S. J., Tashkin, D. P., et al. (2010). Sociodemographic characteristics of cannabis smokers and the experience of cannabis withdrawal. *Am J Drug Alcohol Abuse*, 36, 311–319.

Cornelius, J. R., Chung, T., Martin, C., et al. (2008). Cannabis withdrawal is common among treatment-seeking adolescents with cannabis dependence and major depression, and is associated with rapid relapse to dependence. *Addict Behav*, 33, 1500–1505.

Crowley, T. J., Macdonald, M. J., Whitmore, E. A., et al. (1998). Cannabis dependence, withdrawal, and reinforcing effects among adolescents with conduct disorder symptoms and substance use disorders. *Drug Alcohol Depend*, 50, 27–37.

D'Souza, D. C., Cortes-Briones, J., Creatura, G., et al. (2019). Efficacy and safety of a fatty acid amide hydrolase inhibitor (PF-04457845) in the treatment of cannabis withdrawal and dependence in men: A double-blind, placebo-controlled, parallel group, phase 2a single-site

randomised controlled trial. *Lancet Psychiatry*, **6**, 35–45.

D'Souza, D. C., Cortes-Briones, J. A., Ranganathan, M., et al. (2016). Rapid changes in cannabinoid 1 receptor availability in cannabis-dependent male subjects after abstinence from cannabis. *Biol Psychiatry Cogn Neurosci Neuroimaging*, **1**, 60–67.

Davis, M. L., Powers, M. B., Handelsman, P., et al. (2015). Behavioral therapies for treatment-seeking cannabis users: A meta-analysis of randomized controlled trials. *Eval Health Prof*, **38**, 94–114.

Dawes, G. M., Sitharthan, T., Conigrave, K. M., et al. (2011). Patients admitted for inpatient cannabis detoxification: Withdrawal symptoms and impacts of common comorbidities. *J Subst Use*, **16**, 392–405.

Dennis, M. L., Funk, R., Harrington Godley, S., et al. (2004). Cross-validation of the alcohol and cannabis use measures in the Global Appraisal of Individual Needs (GAIN) and Timeline Followback (TLFB; Form 90) among adolescents in substance abuse treatment. *Addiction*, **99**, 120–128.

Dutra, L., Stathopoulou, G., Basden, S. L., et al. (2008). A meta-analytic review of psychosocial interventions for substance use disorders. *Am J Psychiatry*, **165**, 179–187.

Ehlers, C. L., Gizer, I. R., Vieten, C., et al. (2010a). Cannabis dependence in the San Francisco Family Study: Age of onset of use, DSM-IV symptoms, withdrawal, and heritability. *Addict Behav*, **35**, 102–110.

(2010b). Linkage analyses of cannabis dependence, craving, and withdrawal in the San Francisco family study. *Am J Med Genet B Neuropsychiatr Genet*, **153B**, 802–811.

ElSohly, M. A., Mehmedic, Z., Foster, S., et al. (2016). Changes in cannabis potency over the last 2 decades (1995–2014): Analysis of current data in the United States. *Biol Psychiatry*, **79**, 613–619.

Farris, S. G., Metrik, J., Bonn-Miller, M. O., et al. (2016). Anxiety sensitivity and distress intolerance as predictors of cannabis dependence symptoms, problems, and craving: The mediating role of coping motives. *J Stud Alcohol Drugs*, **77**, 889–897.

Freeman, D., Brugha, T., Meltzer, H., et al. (2010). Persecutory ideation and insomnia: Findings from the second British National Survey of Psychiatric Morbidity. *J Psychiatr Res*, **44**, 1021–1026.

Freeman, T. P., Groshkova, T., Cunningham, A., et al. (2019). Increasing potency and price of cannabis in Europe, 2006–16: Cannabis in Europe. *Addiction*, **114**, 1015–1023.

Freeman, T. P., Hindocha, C., Baio, G., et al. (2020). Cannabidiol for the treatment of cannabis use disorder: A phase 2a, double-blind, placebo-controlled, randomised, adaptive Bayesian trial. *Lancet Psychiatry*, **7**, 865–874.

Garcia, A. N., and Salloum, I. M. (2015). Polysomnographic sleep disturbances in nicotine, caffeine, alcohol, cocaine, opioid, and cannabis use: A focused review. *Am J Addict*, **24**, 590–598.

Gates, P., Albertella, L., and Copeland, J. (2016). Cannabis withdrawal and sleep: A systematic review of human studies. *Subst Abuse*, **37**, 255–269.

Glozier, N., Martiniuk, A., Patton, G., et al. (2010). Short sleep duration in prevalent and persistent psychological distress in young adults: The DRIVE study. *Sleep*, **33**, 1139–1145.

Gorelick, D. A., Levin, K. H., Copersino, M. L., et al. (2012).

Diagnostic criteria for cannabis withdrawal syndrome. *Drug Alcohol Depend*, **123**, 141–147.

Grant, B. F., Goldstein, R. B., Saha, T. D., et al. (2016). Epidemiology of *DSM-5* drug use disorder: Results from the National Epidemiologic Survey on Alcohol and Related Conditions–III. *JAMA Psychiatry*, **73**, 39.

Gray, K. M., Carpenter, M. J., Baker, N. L., et al. (2012). A double-blind randomized controlled trial of N-acetylcysteine in cannabis-dependent adolescents. *Am J Psychiatry*, **169**, 805–812.

Gray, K. M., Sonne, S. C., McClure, E. A., et al. (2017). A randomized placebo-controlled trial of N-acetylcysteine for cannabis use disorder in adults. *Drug Alcohol Depend*, **177**, 249–257.

Greene, M. C., and Kelly, J. F. (2014). The prevalence of cannabis withdrawal and its influence on adolescents' treatment response and outcomes: A 12-month prospective investigation. *J Addict Med*, **8**, 359–367.

Haney, M. (2005). The marijuana withdrawal syndrome: Diagnosis and treatment. *Curr Psychiatry Rep*, **7**, 360–366.

Haney, M., Cooper, Z. D., Bedi, G., et al. (2013). Nabilone decreases marijuana withdrawal and a laboratory measure of marijuana relapse. *Neuropsychopharmacology*, **38**, 1557–1565.

Haney, M., Hart, C. L., Vosburg, S. K., et al. (2004). Marijuana withdrawal in humans: Effects of oral THC or divalproex. *Neuropsychopharmacology*, **29**, 158–170.

(2008). Effects of THC and lofexidine in a human laboratory model of marijuana withdrawal and relapse. *Psychopharmacology*, **197**, 157–168.

Haney, M., and Spealman, R. (2008). Controversies in translational

research: Drug self-administration. *Psychopharmacology*, **199**, 403–419.

Haney, M., Ward, A. S., Comer, S. D., et al. (1999). Abstinence symptoms following oral THC administration to humans. *Psychopharmacology*, **141**, 385–394.

Hart, C. L. (2005). Increasing treatment options for cannabis dependence: A review of potential pharmacotherapies. *Drug Alcohol Depend*, **80**, 147–159.

Harte-Hargrove, L. C., and Dow-Edwards, D. L. (2012). Withdrawal from THC during adolescence: Sex differences in locomotor activity and anxiety. *Behav Brain Res*, **231**, 48–59.

Hasin, D. S., Kerridge, B. T., Saha, T. D., et al. (2016). Prevalence and correlates of DSM-5 cannabis use disorder, 2012–2013: Findings from the national epidemiologic survey on alcohol and related conditions-III. *Am J Psychiatry*, **173**, 588–599.

Hasin, D. S., Keyes, K. M., Alderson, D., et al. (2008). Cannabis withdrawal in the United States: Results from NESARC. *J Clin Psychiatry*, **69**, 1354–1363.

Haughey, H. M., Marshall, E., Schacht, J. P., et al. (2008). Marijuana withdrawal and craving: Influence of the cannabinoid receptor 1 (CNR1) and fatty acid amide hydrolase (FAAH) genes. *Addiction*, **103**, 1678–1686.

Herrmann, E. S., Weerts, E. M., and Vandrey, R. (2015). Sex differences in cannabis withdrawal symptoms among treatment-seeking cannabis users. *Exp Clin Psychopharmacol*, **23**, 415–421.

Hesse, M., and Thylstrup, B. (2013). Time-course of the DSM-5 cannabis withdrawal symptoms in poly-substance abusers. *BMC Psychiatry*, **13**, 1–11.

Hirhoven, J., Goodwin, R. S., Li, C.-T., et al. (2012). Reversible and regionally selective downregulation of brain cannabinoid CB1 receptors in chronic daily cannabis smokers. *Mol Psychiatry*, **17**, 642–649.

Hughes, J. R., Higgins, S. T., and Bickel, W. K. (1994). Nicotine withdrawal versus other drug withdrawal syndromes: Similarities and dissimilarities. *Addiction*, **89**, 1461–1470.

Johnson, K., Mullin, J. L., Marshall, E. C., et al. (2010). Exploring the mediational role of coping motives for marijuana use in terms of the relation between anxiety sensitivity and marijuana dependence. *Am J Addict*, **19**, 277–282.

Kadden, R. M., Litt, M. D., Kabela-Cormier, E., et al. (2007). Abstinence rates following behavioral treatments for marijuana dependence. *Addict Behav*, **32**, 1220–1236.

Koob, G. F., and Volkow, N. D. (2016). Neurobiology of addiction: A neurocircuitry analysis. *Lancet Psychiatry*, **3**, 760–773.

Kosiba, J. D., Maisto, S. A., and Ditre, J. W. (2019). Patient-reported use of medical cannabis for pain, anxiety, and depression symptoms: Systematic review and meta-analysis. *Soc Sci Med*, **233**, 181–192.

Kouri, E. M., and Pope Jr., H. G. (2000). Abstinence symptoms during withdrawal from chronic marijuana use. *Exp Clin Psychopharmacol*, **8**, 483–492.

Ledent, C., Valverde, O., Cossu, G., et al. (1999). Unresponsiveness to cannabinoids and reduced addictive effects of opiates in CB1 receptor knockout mice. *Science*, **283**, 401–404.

Levin, F. R., Mariani, J. J., Brooks, D. J., et al. (2011). Dronabinol for the treatment of cannabis dependence: A randomized, double-blind, placebo-controlled trial. *Drug Alcohol Depend*, **116**, 142–150.

Levin, K. H., Copersino, M. L., Heishman, S. J., et al. (2010). Cannabis withdrawal symptoms in non-treatment-seeking adult cannabis smokers. *Drug Alcohol Depend*, **111**, 120–127.

Lichtman, A. H., and Martin, B. R. (2002). Marijuana withdrawal syndrome in the animal model. *J Clin Pharmacol*, **42**, 20S–27S.

(2006). Understanding the phamacology and physiology of cannabis dependence. In *Cannabis Dependence: Its Nature, Consequences, and Treatment* (pp. 37–57). Cambridge: Cambridge University Press.

Lin, L. A., Ilgen, M. A., Jannausch, M., et al. (2016). Comparing adults who use cannabis medically with those who use recreationally: Results from a national sample. *Addict Behav*, **61**, 99–103.

Lintzeris, N., Bhardwaj, A., Mills, L., et al. (2019). Nabiximols for the treatment of cannabis dependence: A randomized clinical trial. *JAMA Intern Med*, **179**, 1242–1253.

Livne, O., Shmulewitz, D., Lev-Ran, S., et al. (2019). DSM-5 cannabis withdrawal syndrome: Demographic and clinical correlates in U.S. adults. *Drug Alcohol Depend*, **195**, 170–177.

Lynskey, M. T., and Agrawal, A. (2007). Psychometric properties of DSM assessments of illicit drug abuse and dependence: Results from the National Epidemiologic Survey on Alcohol and Related Conditions (NESARC). *Psychol Med*, **37**, 1345–1355.

Macfarlane, V., and Christie, G. (2015). Synthetic cannabinoid withdrawal: A new demand on detoxification services: Synthetic cannabinoid detoxification. *Drug Alcohol Rev*, **34**, 147–153.

Marusich, J. A., Lefever, T. W., Antonazzo, K. R., et al. (2014). Evaluation of sex differences in cannabinoid dependence. *Drug Alcohol Depend*, **137**, 20–28.

Mason, B. J., Crean, R., Goodell, V., et al. (2012). A proof-of-concept randomized controlled study of gabapentin: Effects on cannabis use, withdrawal and executive function deficits in cannabis-dependent adults. *Neuropsychopharmacology*, **37**, 1689–1698.

Mednick, S. C., Christakis, N. A., and Fowler, J. H. (2010). The spread of sleep loss influences drug use in adolescent social networks. *PLoS ONE*, **5**, e9775.

Meier, M. H. (2017). Associations between butane hash oil use and cannabis-related problems. *Drug Alcohol Depend*, **179**, 25–31.

Metrik, J., Bassett, S. S., Aston, E. R., et al. (2018). Medicinal versus recreational cannabis use among returning veterans. *Transl Issues Psychol Sci*, **4**, 6–20.

Metrik, J., Farris, S. G., Aston, E. R., et al. (2017). Development and initial validation of a marijuana cessation expectancies questionnaire. *Drug Alcohol Depend*, **177**, 163–170.

Metrik, J., Jackson, K., Bassett, S. S., et al. (2016). The mediating roles of coping, sleep, and anxiety motives in cannabis use and problems among returning veterans with PTSD and MDD. *Psychol Addict Behav*, **30**, 743–754.

Metrik, J., Kahler, C. W., McGeary, J. E., et al. (2011). Acute effects of marijuana smoking on negative and positive affect. *J Cogn Psychother*, **25**, 10.1891/0889-8391.25.1.31.

Metrik, J., and Ramesh, D. (2018). Cannabis use disorder. In MacKillop, J., Kenna, G. A., Leggio, L., et al. (eds.) *Integrating Psychological and Pharmacological Treatments for Addictive Disorders: An Evidence-Based*

Guide (pp. 150–171). New York: Routledge.

Mikulich, S. K., Hall, S. K., Whitmore, E. A., et al. (2001). Concordance between DSM-III-R and DSM-IV diagnoses of substance use disorders in adolescents. *Drug Alcohol Depend*, **61**, 237–248.

Milin, R., Manion, I., Dare, G., et al. (2008). Prospective assessment of cannabis withdrawal in adolescents with cannabis dependence: A pilot study. *J Am Acad Child Adolesc Psychiatry*, **47**, 174–179.

Mokrysz, C., Freeman, T. P., Korkki, S., et al. (2016). Are adolescents more vulnerable to the harmful effects of cannabis than adults? A placebo-controlled study in human males. *Transl Psychiatry*, **6**, 1–10.

Monti, P. M., Colby, S. M., and O'Leary, T. A. (eds.) (2001). *Adolescents, Alcohol, and Substance Abuse: Reaching Teens through Brief Interventions*. New York: Guilford Press.

National Academies of Sciences, Engineering, and Medicine. (2017). *The Health Effects of Cannabis and Cannabinoids: The Current State of Evidence and Recommendations for Research*. Washington, DC: The National Academies Press.

Nicholson, A. N., Turner, C., Stone, B. M., et al. (2004). Effect of Delta-9-tetrahydrocannabinol and cannabidiol on nocturnal sleep and early-morning behavior in young adults. *J Clin Psychopharmacol*, **24**, 305–313.

Osborn, L. A., Lauritsen, K. J., Cross, N., et al. (2015). Self-medication of somatic and psychiatric conditions using botanical marijuana. *J Psychoactive Drugs*, **47**, 345–350.

Oshri, A., Rogosch, F. A., Burnette, M. L., et al. (2011). Developmental pathways to adolescent cannabis abuse and dependence: Child maltreatment, emerging

personality, and internalizing versus externalizing psychopathology. *Psychol Addict Behav*, **25**, 634–644.

Pacek, L. R., Herrmann, E. S., Smith, M. T., et al. (2017). Sleep continuity, architecture and quality among treatment-seeking cannabis users: An in-home, unattended polysomnographic study. *Exp Clin Psychopharmacol*, **25**, 295–302.

Pertwee, R. G. (2005). Pharmacological actions of cannabinoids. *Hbk Exp Pharmacol*, **168**, 1–51.

Potter, C. M., Vujanovic, A. A., Marshall-Berenz, E. C., et al. (2011). Posttraumatic stress and marijuana use coping motives: The mediating role of distress tolerance. *J Anxiety Disord*, **25**, 437–443.

Prendergast, M., Podus, D., Finney, J., et al. (2006). Contingency management for treatment of substance use disorders: A meta-analysis. *Addiction*, **101**, 1546–1560.

Preuss, U. W., Watzke, A. B., Zimmermann, J., et al. (2010). Cannabis withdrawal severity and short-term course among cannabis-dependent adolescent and young adult inpatients. *Drug Alcohol Depend*, **106**, 133–141.

Rabin, R. A., Kozak, K., Zakzanis, K. K., et al. (2018). Effects of extended cannabis abstinence on clinical symptoms in cannabis dependent schizophrenia patients versus non-psychiatric controls. *Schizophr Res*, **194**, 55–61.

Ramesh, D., and Haney, M. (2015). Treatment of cannabis use disorders. In el-Guebaly, N., Carrà, G., and Galanter, M. (eds.) *Textbook of Addiction Treatment: International Perspectives* (pp. 367–380). Milan: Springer Milan.

Reinarman, C., Nunberg, H., Lanthier, F., et al. (2011). Who are medical marijuana patients? Population characteristics from nine

California assessment clinics. *J Psychoactive Drugs*, **43**, 128–135.

Schacht, J. P., Selling, R. E., and Hutchison, K. E. (2009). Intermediate cannabis dependence phenotypes and the FAAH C385A variant: An exploratory analysis. *Psychopharmacology*, **203**, 511–517.

Schlienz, N. J., Budney, A. J., Lee, D. C., et al. (2017). Cannabis withdrawal: A review of neurobiological mechanisms and sex differences. *Curr Addict Rep*, **4**, 75–81.

Schlienz, N. J., and Vandrey, R. (2019). Cannabis withdrawal. In Montoya, I. D., and Weiss, S. R. B. (eds.) *Cannabis Use Disorders* (pp. 93–102). Cham: Springer International Publishing.

Schofield, D., Tennant, C., Nash, L., et al. (2006). Reasons for cannabis use in psychosis. *Aust NZ J Psychiatry*, **40**, 570–574.

Schuster, R. M., Fontaine, M., Nip, E., et al. (2017). Prolonged cannabis withdrawal in young adults with lifetime psychiatric illness. *Prevent Med*, **104**, 40–45.

Segal, Z. V., Teasdale, J. D., and Williams, J. M. G. (2004). Mindfulness-based cognitive therapy: Theoretical rationale and empirical status. In Hayes, S. C., Follette, V. M., and Linehan, M. M. (eds.) *Mindfulness and Acceptance: Expanding the Cognitive-Behavioral Tradition* (pp. 45–65). New York: Guilford Press.

Sherman, B. J., Baker, N. L., and McRae-Clark, A. L. (2017). Effect of oxytocin pretreatment on cannabis outcomes in a brief motivational intervention. *Psychiatry Res*, **249**, 318–320.

Simons, J. S., Gaher, R. M., Correia, C. J., et al. (2005). An affective-motivational model of marijuana and alcohol problems among college students. *Psychol Addict Behav*, **19**, 326–334.

Stanger, C., Budney, A. J., Kamon, J. L., et al. (2009). A randomized trial of contingency management for adolescent marijuana abuse and dependence. *Drug Alcohol Depend*, **105**, 240–247.

Steinberg, K. L., Roffman, R. A., Carroll, K. M., et al. (2005). *Brief Counseling for Marijuana Dependence: A Manual for Treating Adults*. Baltimore, MD: Center for Substance Abuse Treatment, Substance Abuse and Mental Health Services Administration.

Stephens, R. S., Babor, T. F., Kadden, R., et al. (2002). The marijuana treatment project: Rationale, design, and participant characteristics. *Addiction*, 97, 109S–124S.

Trigo, J. M., Soliman, A., Quilty, L. C., et al. (2018). Nabiximols combined with motivational enhancement/cognitive behavioral therapy for the treatment of cannabis dependence: A pilot randomized clinical trial. *PLoS ONE*, **13**, e0190768–e0190768.

Tringale, R., and Jensen, C. (2011). Cannabis and Insomnia: Patients commonly report that use of cannabis reduces the time it takes them to fall asleep: Whether or not insomnia was the complaint with which they presented. *O'Shaughnessy's*, Autumn, 31–32.

Vandrey, R. G., Budney, A. J., Hughes, J. R., et al. (2008). A within-subject comparison of withdrawal symptoms during abstinence from cannabis, tobacco, and both substances. *Drug Alcohol Depend*, **92**, 48–54.

Vandrey, R., Budney, A. J., Kamon, J. L., et al. (2005). Cannabis withdrawal in adolescent treatment seekers. *Drug Alcohol Depend*, **78**, 205–210.

Vandrey, R., and Haney, M. (2009). Pharmacotherapy for cannabis dependence: How close are we? *CNS Drugs*, **23**, 543–553.

Verweij, K .J. H., Agrawal, A., Nat, N. O., et al. (2013). A genetic perspective on the proposed inclusion of cannabis withdrawal in DSM-5. *Psychol Med*, **43**, 1713–1722.

Vorspan, F., Guillem, E., Bloch, V., et al. (2010). Self-reported sleep disturbances during cannabis withdrawal in cannabis-dependent outpatients with and without opioid dependence. *Sleep Med*, **11**, 499–500.

Walsh, Z., Gonzalez, R., Crosby, K., et al. (2017). Medical cannabis and mental health: A guided systematic review. *Clin Psychol Rev*, **51**, 15–29.

Weinberger, A. H., Desai, R. A., and McKee, S. A. (2010). Nicotine withdrawal in US smokers with current mood, anxiety, alcohol use, and substance use disorders. *Drug Alcohol Depend*, **108**, 7–12.

Wiesbeck, G. A., Schuckit, M. A., Kalmijn, J. A., et al. (1996). An evaluation of the history of a marijuana withdrawal syndrome in a large population. *Addiction*, **91**, 1469–1478.

Wong, M. M., Brower, K. J., and Zucker, R. A. (2009). Childhood sleep problems, early onset of substance use and behavioral problems in adolescence. *Sleep Med*, **10**, 787–796.

World Health Organization. (2018). *International Classification of Diseases for Mortality and Morbidity Statistics (11th Revision)*. Geneva: World Health Organization.

Young, S. E., Corley, R. P., Stallings, M. C., et al. (2002). Substance use, abuse and dependence in adolescence: Prevalence, symptom profiles and correlates. *Drug Alcohol Depend*, **68**, 309–322.

Chapter

28

Cannabis and Addiction

H. Valerie Curran, Will Lawn, and Tom P. Freeman

28.1 Introduction

Cannabis is now the main reason for first time entry into drug treatment services within the European Union (Schettino and Hoch, 2015). Globally, there are more people in treatment for cannabis addiction than addiction to any other drug, including opiates (UNODC, 2017). At the same time, most of the estimated 192 million last-year cannabis users (UNODC, 2020) worldwide (nearly 4% of the population) use infrequently without developing problems. Approximately 22 million people are currently addicted to cannabis, which is roughly equivalent to the number addicted to opiates, and substantially larger than the number addicted to psychostimulants (Degenhardt et al., 2018). The estimated chance of becoming addicted to cannabis after lifetime exposure is between 9% and 34% (Anthony et al., 1994; Leung et al., 2020; Lopez-Quintero et al., 2011a; Marel et al., 2019), which is slightly lower than for alcohol (15–38%) and substantially lower than for opioids (23–47%) or psychostimulants (17–50%) (Anthony et al., 1994; Lopez-Quintero et al., 2011b; Marel et al., 2019). For past year users in the United States, 30% met criteria for cannabis use disorder (CUD) (Hasin et al., 2016). In comparison, that figure was 17.5% for alcohol and 80% for tobacco.

Estimates of prevalence depend on definitions of addiction. For example, the Fifth Edition of the *Diagnostic and Statistical Manual of Mental Disorders* (*DSM-5*) (American Psychiatric Association, 2013) amalgamated previous categories of substance abuse (considered as milder problems) and dependence (considered as more severe problems) with a single diagnosis of 'substance use disorder' (SUD) that can vary in severity. Cannabis use disorder (CUD) is defined as: A problematic pattern of cannabis use leading to clinically significant impairment or distress, as manifested by at least two of the following symptoms: craving cannabis; lack of control over amount used; unsuccessful attempts to cut down; much time devoted to obtaining, using, or recovering from the drug; reduction in other activities; use despite problems caused; failure to fulfil other obligations; use in situations in which it is physically hazardous; tolerance to the drug; and withdrawal symptoms upon cessation. Mild CUD is diagnosed when two or three of these symptoms are present, moderate CUD with four or five symptoms, and severe CUD with six or more symptoms. Addiction is considered by some to be approximately equivalent to severe substance use disorder (Heilig et al., 2021).

The International Classification of Diseases 11th revision (ICD-11) includes the diagnosis of cannabis dependence, which is defined as 'a disorder of regulation of cannabis use arising from repeated or continuous use of cannabis' (WHO, 2018). Similar to the DSM-5 diagnosis of CUD, ICD-11 cannabis dependence is characterized by a strong internal drive to use cannabis, which is manifested by an impaired ability to control use, increasing priority over other activities, and persistent use despite harm or negative consequences. These experiences are often accompanied by a subjective sensation of urge or craving to use cannabis. Physiological features of dependence may also be present, including tolerance to the effects of cannabis and withdrawal symptoms following cessation. The linguistic quagmire of terms like addiction, dependence, and CUD is also evident in the language used to describe the extent of cannabis use. 'Heavy use' can refer to once a month or once a day or repeated consumption throughout each day. Unlike standard units of alcohol, the field of cannabis use lacks agreed metrics for quantifying use (Freeman and Lorenzetti, 2020). Cannabis can vary enormously in potency, cannabinoid profile, and route of administration. Heterogeneity in measures of cannabis use and what constitutes heavy use also impact the lack of agreed-upon outcomes for the treatment of cannabis addiction (Loflin et al., 2020).

Cannabis addiction develops as a consequence of chronic neuroadaptations over time to repeated cannabis use (Ferland and Hurd, 2020). These neuroadaptations lead to withdrawal symptoms when cannabis use is markedly reduced or stopped, and a specific cannabis withdrawal syndrome has been identified (see Chapter 27). Of over 140 cannabinoids identified in cannabis plants, delta-9-tetrahydrocannabinol (THC) underpins the main euphoric and 'stoned' effects, as well as its amnestic and attentional effects (Ramaekers et al., 2021). In contrast, cannabidiol (CBD) may moderate some effects of THC (Freeman et al., 2019). Estimates of prevalence of problematic use have varied as the THC content of street cannabis has risen markedly over the past two decades, whereas its cannabidiol (CBD) content has stayed constant or slightly decreased (see also Chapter 5) (Freeman et al., 2021). In Europe and Australia, high-potency cannabis containing 15% THC or more and less than 0.1% CBD currently dominates the recreational drug market. Use of cannabis with higher concentrations of THC is associated with an increased risk of cannabis addiction (Freeman and Winstock, 2015; Hines et al., 2020). The marked changes over time in THC content may limit the relevance of older, longitudinal cohort studies (e.g., the New Zealand birth cohort study) to understanding the risk of addiction and other outcomes of people who use cannabis today. Increases in THC concentrations have implications for the burden of disease associated with cannabis addiction. For example, rising THC over time has been associated with a faster progression of cannabis addiction symptom onset (Arterberry et al., 2019) and an increase in the number of people entering treatment for cannabis addiction (Freeman et al., 2018).

28.2 Neurobiology

As detailed in Chapters 1 and 2, the brain's natural endogenous endocannabinoid (eCB) system comprises cannabinoid receptors (CB1R and CB2R) and endogenous ligands (anandamide and 2-arachidonoylglycerol – 2-AG) and associated enzymes responsible for their degradation (e.g., Fatty Acid Amide Hydrolase – FAAH). THC is a partial agonist of the CB1R (Pertwee, 2008) and this underpins its subjective effects (Huestis et al., 2001). CB1Rs are abundantly expressed in brain regions relevant to addiction which mediate the neural processes underlying reward, emotional regulation, cognition, and inhibitory control (Curran et al., 2016). Positron emission tomography (PET) imaging of daily cannabis users have revealed considerable deficiencies in CB1R levels compared to controls, particularly in cortical regions, that correlate with both years of cannabis use and severity of withdrawal symptoms, and which rapidly normalize during abstinence from cannabis (D'Souza et al., 2016; and see Chapter 16).

Unlike psychostimulant addiction, alterations to dopamine D2/3 receptor densities in heavy cannabis users have not been found (Albrecht et al., 2013; Urban et al., 2012), although dopamine synthesis capacity may be compromised (Bloomfield et al., 2014). A number of magnetic resonance imaging (MRI) studies have aimed to detect morphological and functional differences between addicted and non-addicted cannabis users, with some evidence for differences. Smaller and altered shapes of hippocampi have been reported in those addicted to cannabis (Chye et al., 2019; Lorenzetti et al., 2020). Furthermore, in prospective studies, cannabis cue-induced brain activity (Vingerhoets et al., 2016) and working memory network function (Cousijn et al., 2014) predicted addiction severity.

28.3 Vulnerability and Resilience to Cannabis Addiction

As only a minority of cannabis users develop addiction, many other factors play an important role in determining an individual's vulnerability. In turn the interaction of these various factors underpins the very significant individual differences observed in the effects of cannabis use (see Box 28.1). Cannabis addiction often co-occurs with addictions to other drugs. Concurrent tobacco use has been identified as a risk factor in several studies (Hindocha et al., 2015; Hines et al., 2016). Males typically have an earlier opportunity to use cannabis, a greater risk of addiction, and a faster progression from first use to addiction. This is consistent with normative data from European treatment services: the mean age of first treatment is 25 years; of first cannabis use is 17 years; and 84% of treated individuals are male (EMCDDA, 2021). Interestingly, a three-year prospective study of daily users found that variables related directly to cannabis use did not predict transition to addiction; more important were current environmental factors such as living alone and negative life events (such as having

Box 28.1   Risk factors for cannabis addiction

Risk factor	Notes
Frequency of use	Greater frequency of use ↑ addiction severity
Amount of cannabis	Larger amounts of cannabis in joints, pipes and vaporizers ↑ addiction severity
Potency of cannabis	Use of high-potency cannabis ↑ addiction severity Average THC level ↑ population level cannabis treatment admissions
Urinary THC metabolites	Greater levels of urinary carboxy-THC ↑ addiction severity
Gender	Being male ↑ addiction risk
Age	Younger age of onset or being an adolescent ↑ addiction risk
Mental health problems	Depression, anxiety, attention-deficit, and post-traumatic stress disorders ↑ addiction risk
Socioeconomic status/financial income	Low socioeconomic status and smaller family income ↑ addiction risk
Parental death	Parental death in childhood ↑ addiction risk
Tobacco	Cannabis users who use tobacco with cannabis or use tobacco leaf 'blunts' ↑ addiction severity
Illicit drugs	Use of other illicit drugs ↑ addiction risk
Personality traits	Impulsivity and novelty seeking ↑ addiction severity Behavioural inhibition ↓ addiction severity
Motives for use	Using cannabis in order to 'cope' ↑ addiction severity
Recent life events	Recent negative events occurring ↑ addiction severity

had a major financial crisis) (van der Pol et al., 2013b). On the contrary, other studies have shown that those who use cannabis more frequently (Coffey and Patton, 2016; Curran et al., 2019), in larger quantities (Cuttler and Spradlin, 2017), and those who use higher potency cannabis (Freeman and Winstock, 2015; Hines et al., 2020), are more likely to be addicted. A separate prospective study of cannabis users highlighted parental death, use of other illicit drugs, and recent negative life events as significant predictors of future cannabis addiction (von Sydow et al., 2002). Personality traits including impulsivity, novelty-seeking, and behavioural inhibition have also been associated with cannabis problems (Papinczak et al., 2019; von Sydow et al., 2002).

Vulnerability and Genetic Factors: A meta-analysis of 24 twin studies (Verweij et al., 2017) suggested that genetic influences account for around 55% of the vulnerability to cannabis addiction, with shared environmental factors and non-shared environmental factors accounting for much lower proportions

(17.5% and 27.5%, respectively). There is some evidence of genetic variants associated with cannabis use disorder from genome-wide association studies, which show some specificity but were also associated with genetic liability to cannabis use and other mental health disorders such as ADHD, depression, and schizophrenia (Johnson et al., 2020) (for a review of genetic factors see Chapter 30).

Vulnerability and Comorbidities: Like other addictions, cannabis addiction often occurs along with other mental health problems. Epidemiological evidence indicates a possible association between regular cannabis use and the development of anxiety (Chapter 11) and depression (Chapter 12). However, the evidence is more mixed and less consistent than that for an association between cannabis use and psychosis (see Chapters 14 and 16). One study compared the mental health of individuals who were dependent on cannabis (according to DSM-IV criteria) with that of non-dependent cannabis users who had similar patterns and levels of cannabis use.

301

Only the dependent users had comorbid depression and anxiety problems (van der Pol et al., 2013a). Depression and anxiety disorders are not only cross-sectionally associated with addiction but are also predictive of whether individuals transition from use to severe CUD (Flórez-Salamanca et al., 2013). An Australian study reported that anxiety disorders are more common in those with cannabis addiction (41%) than those who use cannabis without addiction (21%), and far greater than those who do not use cannabis (11%) (Teesson et al., 2012). In the United States, mood disorders, anxiety disorders, post-traumatic stress disorder, and personality disorders are all significantly associated with past year CUD with odds ratios of 3–5 (Hasin et al., 2016).

28.4 Age-dependent Vulnerability: Adolescence and Adulthood

Adolescence is a critical period for brain development in which there is an overall decrease in cortical grey matter alongside an increase in white matter (Giedd et al., 1999) and a time when crucial psychological, social, and personal changes occur (Blakemore and Choudhury, 2006). The endocannabinoid (eCB) system continues to mature during adolescence, with fluctuations in CB1R expression and anandamide and 2-AG levels, and it modulates the development of other neural networks (Galve-Roperh et al., 2009). As exogenous cannabinoids affect the functioning of the eCB system, it is plausible that prolonged use during adolescence disrupts the neurodevelopmental maturational processes during this period (Lubman et al., 2007). Thus, the human brain may be more vulnerable to cannabis at the time when use of the drug often begins (for full discussion of pubertal exposure to cannabis and the brain, see Chapters 7 and 8), including the risk of transitioning to addiction.

In Europe, the prevalence of cannabis dependence for 14–17 year-olds is 1.8% and it is 0.3% for 18–64 year-olds (Wittchen et al., 2011). Indeed, it has been reliably shown that adolescents who use cannabis are considerably more likely to develop cannabis addiction than adults who use cannabis (Chen et al., 2005, 2009; Han et al., 2019; Millar et al., 2021; Volkow et al., 2021). A recent study showed the odds of having cannabis addiction in people who use cannabis are decreased by 11% for each year of delayed cannabis onset (Millar et al., 2021). The effect size reflecting adolescent vulnerability to cannabis

addiction varies. One recent study reported that, in the years proximal to initiation, those aged 12–15 are roughly twice as likely to develop addiction than those aged 18–25 (Han et al., 2019), while another reported a 13-times greater risk for 13–15 year-olds in comparison to those aged 21 and over (Chen et al., 2005). Considering all studies together, an approximate estimate is that those under 18 are three times more likely to develop cannabis addiction in comparison to people over 18.

It is not yet known why adolescents are at a greater risk to cannabis addiction. The transitional state of the eCB system (Galve-Roperh et al., 2009), the putatively greater reward sensitivity, and weaker self-control mechanisms likely contribute. Alternatively, the differential acute effects of cannabis in adolescents and adults could contribute to adolescent vulnerability to addiction. In an early study, we directly compared the acute effects of cannabis on adolescents (16–17 year-olds) with adults (24–28 year-olds) using a randomized, placebo-controlled design (Mokrysz et al., 2016). On active cannabis, adolescents felt less stoned, reported fewer psychotomimetic symptoms, were more impulsive on a response inhibition task, and wanted more cannabis than adults. This profile of adolescent resilience to acute cannabis effects may contribute to escalated use.

To further explore this, in a project called CANN-TEEN we compared the performance of 24 adolescents with 24 adults (matched for days per week cannabis use and pre-morbid IQ) on measures sensitive to acute cannabis effects on three separate occasions after they inhaled three separate types of cannabis: cannabis with 0.107 mg/kg THC ('THC') (8 mg THC for a 75 kg person) or THC plus 0.320 mg/kg CBD ('THC+CBD') (24 mg CBD for a 75 kg person), or placebo cannabis ('PLA'). We found no adolescent sensitivity/vulnerability in subjective effect, verbal memory, or psychotomimetic effect (Lawn et al, 2023). The same study also assessed reward sensitivity on the Monetary Incentive Delay (MID) task during fMRI Adolescents showed no increased vulnerability compared with adults and CBD did not significantly moderate the effects of THC (Skumlien et al, 2022a). Using the same MID task with 125 adolescent and adult cannabis users and well matched non-using controls to explore chronic effects, we again found that reward anticipation and feedback processing appear spared in adolescent and adult cannabis users (Skumlien et al, 2022b).

However, significantly more adolescent than adult cannabis users had severe CUD (Lawn et al, 2022). Longitudinal data from this project, and from the exciting ABC project, should clarify vulnerability factors in adolescents' varied usage and experiences of the effects of strains of cannabis.

28.5 Treatments for Cannabis Use Disorder

As with most addictions, only a minority of problematic cannabis users will actively seek treatment. It is estimated that 85% of people with cannabis addiction do not seek treatment (Hasin et al., 2016). This partly reflects the significant social stigma which remains associated with addiction as well as the normalization of cannabis use in some sections of society. It is important that comorbidities are assessed and treated appropriately alongside the cannabis addiction itself. However, there is little evidence that standard interventions are effective when individuals specifically have a psychotic disorder (Lees et al., 2021).

28.5.1 Psychosocial Treatments

As detailed in Box 28.2, psychosocial treatments are currently the mainstay for individuals with cannabis addiction who present to drug services. These include Cognitive Behavioural Therapy (CBT), Motivational Enhancement Therapy (MET), and Contingency Management (CM). These therapies can reduce the frequency of cannabis use and symptoms of addiction and can be delivered in combination (Gates et al., 2016; Lees et al., 2021). Meta-analysis of all psychosocial treatments combined versus control have found effect sizes of Cohen's d = 0.8 (Dutra et al., 2008) and Hedges' g = 0.4 (Davis et al., 2015). Psychotherapies are appropriate for use with adolescents and involvement of their family can enhance therapeutic outcomes. Combinations of CBT, MET, and CM can be particularly effective, with CM adding significantly to the longevity of abstinence periods. At short-term follow-up (four months), combined MET and CBT double abstinence rates; however, after nine months interventions usually have no discernible effect (Gates et al., 2016). There is accumulating evidence that delivering interventions digitally may be especially helpful in reducing barriers to entering treatment (Budney et al., 2019).

28.5.2 Pharmacological Treatments

A recent systematic review concluded that there are no effective pharmacological treatments for cannabis addiction judged by patients achieving abstinence at treatment end (Nielsen et al., 2019). The most frequently studied interventions included in that review were substitution cannabinoid treatments. These generally involved synthetic THC (dronabinol) or a combination of THC with CBD in a 1:1 ratio (nabiximols) in combination with psychotherapy. Overall, the evidence in that review suggested that, while substitution treatments typically reduce withdrawal symptoms, there was no consistent evidence for their effectiveness in reducing cannabis use. However, a more recent and larger trial found evidence for reduced frequency of cannabis use following 12-weeks of nabiximols treatment compared to placebo (Lintzeris et al., 2019). Furthermore, a frequentist network meta-analysis

Box 28.2 Psychosocial treatments for cannabis addiction	
Therapy	**Description**
Cognitive behavioural therapy (CBT) & relapse prevention (RP)	Aims to improve patients' awareness of high-risk situations and thought processes that increase the likelihood of cannabis use. Teaches patients how to deal with and cope with these triggers, thus minimizing relapse. Non-drug rewarding behaviors are used to replace cannabis use.
Motivational enhancement therapy (MET)	Uses a collaborative approach between therapist and patient to elicit 'change talk', resolve ambivalence, and enhance motivation to reduce or abstain from cannabis. Therapists employ open questions, affirmations, reflections, and positive summaries. The spirit of MET is non-judgmental and aims to evoke change from within the patient.
Contingency management (CM)	Patients are paid in money or vouchers when they demonstrate successful abstinence from cannabis.

Box 28.3 Promising pharmacological treatments for cannabis addiction

Drug	Putative mechanism	Trial results
Cannabidiol	Inhibitor of FAAH; CB1R allosteric modulation; GRP55 agonist; Serotonin-1a receptor partial agonist	400 and 800 mg CBD reduced urinary carboxy-THC and days abstinent compared to placebo at the end of 4 weeks of treatment (Freeman et al., 2020).
Nabilone	CB1R agonist	No difference reported between nabilone and placebo (Hill et al., 2017), but frequentist network meta-analysis suggests there may be a positive impact of nabilone (Bahji et al., 2021).
Topiramate	GABA agonist, glutamate antagonist	Topiramate decreased number of grams smoked per day of use, but abstinence rates were similar. Drop-out was higher in topiramate group (Miranda et al., 2017).
FAAH inhibitor	Inhibition of FAAH and increase of anandamide	Reduced cannabis withdrawal and reduced cannabis use in the FAAH inhibitor group compared to placebo (D'Souza et al., 2019).
Nabiximols (THC and CBD)	CB1R agonist	In one study, nabiximols reduced withdrawal symptoms compared to placebo, but did not affect cannabis use (Allsop et al., 2014), in another it reduced cannabis use compared to placebo (Lintzeris et al., 2019).
Dronabinol	CB1R agonist	Treatment retention was higher and withdrawal symptoms lower on dronabinol than placebo, but cannabis use was similar (Levin et al., 2011).
Gabapentin	GABA analogue	Gabapentin reduced grams of cannabis per week and urinary THC metabolites compared to placebo (Mason et al., 2012).
N-acetylcysteine	Glutamate agonist	N-acetylcysteine increased odds of a negative urine test for cannabis use compared to placebo in adolescents, but this was not replicated in a larger sample (Gray et al., 2017).

suggested that nabilone, a synthetic cannabinoid that mimics the effects of THC, as well as topiramate, an anticonvulsant also used for alcohol use disorder, reduced cannabis use relative to placebo (Bahji et al., 2021). Gabapentin and n-acetylcysteine have also shown promise in some, but not all, studies (Lees et al., 2021). These are summarized in Box 28.3.

Since the Cochrane review (Nielsen et al., 2019) two trials which use treatments that act on the eCB system in different ways have been reported. One approach has been to use fatty acid amide hydrolase (FAAH) inhibitors which might potentiate eCB signalling by inhibiting the enzyme that degrades the endocannabinoid anandamide. One study administered a FAAH inhibitor (PF-04457845; N = 46) or placebo (N = 24) during five-to-eight days of enforced abstinence from cannabis in hospital followed by three weeks of outpatient treatment (D'Souza et al.,

2019). Relative to placebo, treatment with PF-04457845 reduced symptoms of cannabis withdrawal on the first two days of treatment. At four weeks treatment, the FAAH inhibitor was associated with lowered self-reported cannabis use and lower urinary carboxy-THC (THC-COOH) concentrations. A large Phase III trial is now underway. A second trial administered CBD for four weeks at daily doses of 0, 200, 400, and 800 mg alongside six sessions of MET (Freeman et al., 2020). This RCT used an adaptive Bayesian design, which resulted in the 200 mg dose being eliminated from the trial an early stage due to lack of efficacy. At final analysis, both the 400 and 800 mg doses reduced cannabis use at 4 weeks (THC-COOH concentrations and days abstinent from cannabis). These non-substitution treatments have the potential to treat CUD through eCB mechanisms which avoid the potential risks associated with THC treatments.

28.6 Natural Progression of People with Cannabis Addiction

A systematic review reported that, over one year, 17% of people with cannabis addiction remitted (Calabria et al., 2010). In a German study of the natural progression of cannabis use over four years, 15% of people with cannabis addiction and 25–40% of heavy users without addiction had stopped using (von Sydow et al., 2001). Users often make multiple brief quit attempts and transition between periods of abstinence, reduced use, and normal use; sustained abstinence is difficult to achieve. However, across an entire lifetime, like in other addictions, the majority of people with cannabis addiction (97%) will remit (Lopez-Quintero et al., 2011a). Indeed, in a sample of people with cannabis addiction, half of them will remit after six years, which is much faster than for alcohol (14 years) and tobacco (26 years).

28.7 Medicinal Use of Cannabis and Addiction

Benefits of cannabis and cannabinoids have received scant research attention compared with that given to their harms. Recreational users of the drug clearly use it for its perceived benefits and not for its harms.

Cannabis has been legalized for medical use in an ever-increasing number of countries. A growing body of scientific evidence supports the use of medical cannabis for a range of therapeutic indications and prescriptions are mainly for daily dosing. In parallel with these developments, concerns have been expressed by many prescribers that increased use will lead to patients developing cannabis addiction. Cannabis addiction has been widely researched in non-medical users, and these findings have often been projected onto patients using medical cannabis (Schlag et al., 2021). However, studies exploring medical cannabis dependence are scarce and the appropriate methodology to measure this construct is only now in development. How, and to what extent, do concerns about problems of dependence in non-medical cannabis users apply to prescribed medical users? The main issues related to medical cannabis and CUD include the importance of dose, potency, cannabinoid content, pharmacokinetics and route of administration, frequency of use, as well as set and setting. Medical and non-medical cannabis users differ in significant ways, although a minority will use for both purposes. There are many questions about the potential for medical cannabis use to lead to CUD but the answers will not simply be found by extrapolating findings from the non-medical cannabis literature. It is, therefore, imperative to address these questions empirically in order to minimize harms of medical cannabis use.

In a recent publication, we draw out a set of recommendations for increasing the safety of medical cannabis prescribing so that risks of CUD are minimized (Schlag et al., 2021). These include:

- minimizing THC dose and maximizing CBD content;
- ensuring supply of GMP product;
- following guidelines for safer use;
- monitoring of use and dose over time;
- personalizing prescriptions; and
- balancing patient need with the potential for harm.

New research designs should be considered for assessing potential medical benefits of cannabis in differing clinical disorders rather than wait years for costly randomized controlled trials. Real world evidence can additionally be useful in having greater applicability to actual day-to-day clinical practice and outcomes.

28.8 How Will Legalization Affect Cannabis Addiction?

Based on the history of alcohol and tobacco, as cannabis prices fall, an increase in frequent, heavy cannabis use and cannabis addiction are expected (Hall and Lynskey, 2020; and see Chapter 6) Indeed, there is some evidence of this occurring in adolescents, but not adults, from jurisdictions where recreational cannabis has been legalized (Cerdá et al., 2020). Large-scale studies in the United States have reported inconsistent findings regarding the association between medical cannabis legalization and rates of adult cannabis addiction (Leung et al., 2018). Given the nascent recreational markets in the United States, Canada, and Uruguay, and their varied approaches, we will have to wait a number of years before successfully judging the impact on rates of addiction.

28.9 Conclusion

One priority for cannabis research should be extending the evidence base to understand how individual differences (including age, gender, cannabis use history, culture, co-occurring mental health issues, genetic and epigenetic factors) influence the effects of cannabis. Another is to elucidate effects of different usage patterns and types of cannabinoids ingested, facilitated by standardized metrics and terminology. Measuring and reporting dose using the 5 mg Standard THC Unit (Freeman and Lorenzetti, 2020) is now a requirement for research funded by the National Institute of Drug Abuse, the National institute of Mental Health, and other National Institute of Health funders. Amongst other reasons, this requirement is intended to help researchers capture reductions in cannabis use more accurately when investigating treatments for cannabis addiction (Volkow, 2021).

How patterns of cannabis use will change as the medicalization and legalization of cannabis proliferates across many parts of the globe is not known. But even a small percentage increase in the current 192 million recreational users worldwide will mean a considerable surge in absolute numbers. Drug policy should promote harm reduction by providing a more regulated and safe market where low potency products are provided, prices are regulated, harm reduction advice is available to adolescents as well as older users, and advertising in legal cannabis jurisdictions is prohibited or, at least, strictly controlled. These actions would help to prevent many cases of cannabis addiction. For those with cannabis addiction, the stigma of seeking treatment needs to be reduced. This may include increasing the accessibility of successful online approaches to CUD that can be delivered in the individual's own home.

References

Albrecht, D. S., Skosnik, P. D., Vollmer, J. M., et al. (2013). Striatal D2/D3 receptor availability is inversely correlated with cannabis consumption in chronic marijuana users. *Drug Alcohol Depend*, **128**, 52–57.

Allsop, D. J., Copeland, J., Lintzeris, N., et al. (2014). Nabiximols as an agonist replacement therapy during cannabis withdrawal: A randomized clinical trial. *JAMA Psychiatry*, **71**, 281–291.

American Psychiatric Association. (2013). DSM-5 diagnostic classification. In *Diagnostic and Statistical Manual of Mental Disorders*. Washington, DC: American Psychiatric Association.

Anthony, J. C., Warner, L. A., and Kessler, R. C. (1994). Comparative epidemiology of dependence on tobacco, alcohol, controlled substances, and inhalants: Basic findings from the National Comorbidity Survey. *Exp Clin Psychopharmacol*, **2**, 244–268.

Arterberry, B. J., Padovano, H. T., Foster, K. T., et al. (2019). Higher average potency across the United States is associated with progression to first cannabis use disorder symptom. *Drug Alcohol Depend*, **195**, 186–192.

Bahji, A., Meyyappan, A. C., Hawken, E. R., et al. (2021). Pharmacotherapies for cannabis use disorder: A systematic review and network meta-analysis. *Int J Drug Policy*, **97**, 103295.

Blakemore, S. J., and Choudhury, S. (2006). Development of the adolescent brain: Implications for executive function and social cognition. *J Child Psychol Psychiatry*, **47**, 296–312.

Bloomfield, M. A. P., Morgan, C. J., Egerton, A., et al. (2014). Dopaminergic function in cannabis users and its relationship to cannabis-induced psychotic symptoms. *Biol psychiatry*, **75**, 470–478.

Budney, A. J., Sofis, M. J., and Borodovsky, J. T. (2019). An update on cannabis use disorder with comment on the impact of policy related to therapeutic and recreational cannabis use. *Eur Arch Psychiatry Clin Neurosci*, **269**, 73–86.

Calabria, B., Degenhardt, L., Briegleb, C., et al. (2010). Systematic review of prospective studies investigating 'remission' from amphetamine, cannabis, cocaine or opioid dependence. *Addict Behav*, **35**, 741–749.

Cerdá, M., Mauro, C., Hamilton, A., et al. (2020). Association between recreational marijuana legalization in the United States and changes in marijuana use and cannabis use disorder from 2008 to 2016. *JAMA Psychiatry*, **77**, 165–171.

Chen, C. Y., O'Brien, M. S., and Anthony, J. C. (2005). Who becomes cannabis dependent soon after onset of use? Epidemiological evidence from the United States: 2000–2001. *Drug Alcohol Depend*, **79**, 11–22.

Chen, C. Y., Storr, C. L., and Anthony, J. C. (2009). Early-onset drug use and risk for drug dependence problems. *Addict Behav*, **34**, 319–322.

Chye, Y., Lorenzetti, V., Suo, C., et al. (2019). Alteration to hippocampal volume and shape confined to cannabis dependence: A multi-site study. *Addict Biol*, **24**, 822–834.

Coffey, C., and Patton, G. C. (2016). Cannabis use in adolescence and young adulthood: A review of findings from the Victorian Adolescent Health Cohort Study. *Can J Psychiatry*, **61**, 318–327.

Cousijn, J., Wiers, R. W., Ridderinkhof, K. R., et al. (2014). Effect of baseline cannabis use and working-memory network function on changes in cannabis use in heavy cannabis users:

A prospective fMRI study. *Hum Brain Mapp*, **35**, 2470–2482.

Curran, H. V., Freeman, T. P., Mokrysz, C., et al. (2016). Keep off the grass? Cannabis, cognition and addiction. *Nat Rev Neurosci*, **17**, 293–306.

Curran, H. V., Hindocha, C., Morgan, C. J. A., et al. (2019). Which biological and self-report measures of cannabis use predict cannabis dependency and acute psychotic-like effects? *Psychol Med*, **49**, 1574–1580.

Cuttler, C., and Spradlin, A. (2017). Measuring cannabis consumption: Psychometric properties of the daily sessions, frequency, age of onset, and quantity of cannabis use inventory (DFAQ-CU). *PLoS ONE*, **12**, e0178194.

D'Souza, D. C., Cortes-Briones, J., Creatura, G., et al. (2019). Efficacy and safety of a fatty acid amide hydrolase inhibitor (PF-04457845) in the treatment of cannabis withdrawal and dependence in men: A double-blind, placebo-controlled, parallel group, phase 2a single-site randomised controlled trial. *Lancet Psychiatry*, **6**, 35–45.

D'Souza, D. C., Cortes-Briones, J. A., Ranganathan, M., et al. (2016). Rapid changes in cannabinoid 1 receptor availability in cannabis-dependent male subjects after abstinence from cannabis. *Biol Psychiatry Cogn Neurosci Neuroimaging*, **1**, 60–67.

Davis, M. L., Powers, M. B., Handelsman, P., et al. (2015). Behavioral therapies for treatment-seeking cannabis users: A meta-analysis of randomized controlled trials. *Eval Health Prof*, **38**, 94–114.

Degenhardt, L., Charlson, F., Ferrari, A., et al. (2018). The global burden of disease attributable to alcohol and drug use in 195 countries and territories, 1990–2016: A systematic analysis

for the Global Burden of Disease Study 2016. *Lancet Psychiatry*, **5**, 987–1012.

Dutra, L., Stathopoulou, G., Basden, S. L., et al. (2008). A meta-analytic review of psychosocial interventions for substance use disorders. *Am J Psychiatry*, **165**, 179–187.

EMCDDA. (2021). *European Drug Report*. Luxembourg: Publications Office of the European Union.

Ferland, J.-M. N., and Hurd, Y. L. (2020). Deconstructing the neurobiology of cannabis use disorder. *Nat Neurosci*, **23**, 600–610.

Flórez-Salamanca, L., Secades-Villa, R., Hasin, D. S., et al. (2013). Probability and predictors of transition from abuse to dependence on alcohol, cannabis, and cocaine: Results from the national epidemiologic survey on alcohol and related conditions. *Am J Drug Alcohol Abuse*, **39**, 168–179.

Freeman, A. M., Petrilli, K., Lees, R., et al. (2019). How does cannabidiol (CBD) influence the acute effects of delta-9-tetrahydrocannabinol (THC) in humans? A systematic review. *Neurosci Biobehav Rev*, **107**, 696–712.

Freeman, T. P., Craft, S., Wilson, J., et al. (2021). Changes in delta-9-tetrahydrocannabinol (THC) and cannabidiol (CBD) concentrations in cannabis over time: Systematic review and meta-analysis. *Addiction*, **116**, 1000–1010.

Freeman, T. P., Hindocha, C., Baio, G., et al. (2020). Cannabidiol for the treatment of cannabis use disorder: A phase 2a, double-blind, placebo-controlled, randomised, adaptive Bayesian trial. *Lancet Psychiatry*, **7**(10), pp. 865–874.

Freeman, T. P., and Lorenzetti, V. (2020). 'Standard THC units': A proposal to standardize dose across all cannabis products and

methods of administration. *Addiction*, **115**, 1207–1216.

Freeman, T. P., van der Pol, P., Kuijpers, W., et al. (2018). Changes in cannabis potency and first-time admissions to drug treatment: A 16-year study in the Netherlands. *Psychol Med*, **48**, 2346–2352.

Freeman, T. P., and Winstock, A. R. (2015). Examining the profile of high-potency cannabis and its association with severity of cannabis dependence. *Psychol Med*, **45**, 3181–3189.

Galve-Roperh, I., Palazuelos, J., Aguado, T., et al. (2009). The endocannabinoid system and the regulation of neural development: Potential implications in psychiatric disorders. *Eur Arch Psychiatry Clin Neurosci*, **259**, 371–382.

Gates, P. J., Sabioni, P., Copeland, J., et al. (2016). Psychosocial interventions for cannabis use disorder. *Cochrane Database Syst Rev*, **2016**, CD005336.

Giedd, J. N., Blumenthal, J., Jeffries, N. O., et al. (1999). Brain development during childhood and adolescence: A longitudinal MRI study. *Nat Neurosci*, **2**, 861–863.

Gray, K. M., Sonne, S. C., McClure, E. A., et al. (2017). A randomized placebo-controlled trial of N-acetylcysteine for cannabis use disorder in adults. *Drug Alcohol Depend*, **177**, 249–257.

Hall, W., and Lynskey, M. (2020). Assessing the public health impacts of legalizing recreational cannabis use: The US experience. *World Psychiatry*, **19**, 179–186.

Han, B., Compton, W. M., Blanco, C., et al. (2019). Time since first cannabis use and 12-month prevalence of cannabis use disorder among youth and emerging adults in the United States. *Addiction*, **114**, 698–707.

Hasin, D. S., Kerridge, B. T., Saha, T. D., et al. (2016). Prevalence and correlates of DSM-5 cannabis use disorder, 2012–2013: Findings from the National Epidemiologic Survey on Alcohol and Related Conditions–III. *Am J Psychiatry*, **173**, 588–599.

Heilig, M., MacKillop, J., Martinez, D., et al. (2021). Addiction as a brain disease revised: Why it still matters, and the need for consilience. *Neuropsychopharmacology*, **46**, 1715–1723.

Hill, K. P., Palastro, M. D., Gruber, S. A., et al. (2017). Nabilone pharmacotherapy for cannabis dependence: A randomized, controlled pilot study. *Am J Addict*, **26**, 795–801.

Hindocha, C., Shaban, N. D. C., Freeman, T. P., et al. (2015). Associations between cigarette smoking and cannabis dependence: A longitudinal study of young cannabis users in the United Kingdom. *Drug Alcohol Depend*, **148**, 165–171.

Hines, L. A., Freeman, T. P., Gage, S. H., et al. (2020). Association of high-potency cannabis use with mental health and substance use in adolescence. *JAMA Psychiatry*, **77**, 1044–1051.

Hines, L. A., Morley, K. I., Strang, J., et al. (2016). Onset of opportunity to use cannabis and progression from opportunity to dependence: Are influences consistent across transitions? *Drug Alcohol Depend*, **160**, 57–64.

Huestis, M. A., Gorelick, D. A., Heishman, S. J., et al. (2001). Blockade of effects of smoked marijuana by the CB1-selective cannabinoid receptor antagonist SR141716. *Arch Gen Psychiatry*, **58**, 322–328.

Johnson, E. C., Demontis, D., Thorgeirsson, T. E., et al. (2020). A large-scale genome-wide association study meta-analysis of cannabis use disorder. *Lancet Psychiatry*, **7**, 1032–1045.

Lawn W, Mokrysz C, Lees R et al. (2022). The CannTeen Study: Cannabis use disorder, depression, anxiety, and psychotic-like symptoms in adolescent and adult cannabis users and age-matched controls. *J Psychopharmacol*. **36**, 1350–1361.

Lees, R., Hines, L. A., D'Souza, D. C., et al. (2021). Psychosocial and pharmacological treatments for cannabis use disorder and mental health comorbidities: A narrative review. *Psychol Med*, **51**, 353–364.

Leung, J., Chan, G. C. K., Hides, L., et al. (2020). What is the prevalence and risk of cannabis use disorders among people who use cannabis? A systematic review and meta-analysis. *Addict Behav*, **109**, 106479.

Leung, J., Chiu, C. Y. V., Stjepanović, D., et al. (2018). Has the legalisation of medical and recreational cannabis use in the USA affected the prevalence of cannabis use and cannabis use disorders? *Curr Addict Rep*, **5**, 403–417.

Levin, F. R., Mariani, J. J., Brooks, D. J., et al. (2011). Dronabinol for the treatment of cannabis dependence: A randomized, double-blind, placebo-controlled trial. *Drug Alcohol Depend*, **116**, 142–150.

Lintzeris, N., Bhardwaj, A., Mills, L., et al. (2019). Nabiximols for the treatment of cannabis dependence: A randomized clinical trial. *JAMA Intern Med*, **179**, 1242–1253.

Loflin, M. J. E., Kiluk, B. D., Huestis, M. A., et al. (2020). The state of clinical outcome assessments for cannabis use disorder clinical trials: A review and research agenda. *Drug Alcohol Depend*, **212**, 107993.

Lopez-Quintero, C., Hasin, D. S., de los Cobos, J. P., et al. (2011a). Probability and predictors of remission from life-time nicotine, alcohol, cannabis or cocaine dependence: Results from the national epidemiologic survey on alcohol and related conditions. *Addiction*, **106**, 657–669.

Lopez-Quintero, C., Pérez de los Cobos, J., Hasin, D. S., et al. (2011b). Probability and predictors of transition from first use to dependence on nicotine, alcohol, cannabis, and cocaine: Results of the National Epidemiologic Survey on Alcohol and Related Conditions (NESARC). *Drug Alcohol Depend*, **115**, 120–130.

Lorenzetti, V., Chye, Y., Suo, C., et al. (2020). Neuroanatomical alterations in people with high and low cannabis dependence. *Aust NZ J Psychiatry*, **54**, 68–75.

Lubman, D. I., Yücel, M., and Hall, W. D. (2007). Substance use and the adolescent brain: A toxic combination? *J Psychopharmacol*, **21**, 792–794.

Marel, C., Sunderland, M., Mills, K. L., et al. (2019). Conditional probabilities of substance use disorders and associated risk factors: Progression from first use to use disorder on alcohol, cannabis, stimulants, sedatives and opioids. *Drug Alcohol Depend*, **194**, 136–142.

Mason, B. J., Crean, R., Goodell, V., et al. (2012). A proof-of-concept randomized controlled study of gabapentin: Effects on cannabis use, withdrawal and executive function deficits in cannabis-dependent adults. *Neuropsychopharmacology*, **37**, 1689–1698.

Millar, S. R., Mongan, D., Smyth, B. P., et al. (2021). Relationships between age at first substance use and persistence of cannabis use and cannabis use disorder. *BMC Public Health*, **21**, 1–11.

Miranda Jr, R., Treloar, H., Blanchard, A., et al. (2017). Topiramate and motivational enhancement therapy for cannabis use among youth: A randomized placebo-controlled pilot study. *Addict Biol*, 22, 779–790.

Mokrysz, C., Freeman, T. P., Korkki, S., et al. (2016). Are adolescents more vulnerable to the harmful effects of cannabis than adults? A placebo-controlled study in human males. *Transl Psychiatry*, 6, e961–e961.

Nielsen, S., Gowing, L., Sabioni, P., et al. (2019). Pharmacotherapies for cannabis dependence. *Cochrane Database Syst Rev*, 1, CD008940.

Papinczak, Z. E., Connor, J. P., Feeney, G. F. X., et al. (2019). Testing the biosocial cognitive model of substance use in cannabis users referred to treatment. *Drug Alcohol Depend*, 194, 216–224.

Pertwee, R. G. (2008). The diverse CB1 and CB2 receptor pharmacology of three plant cannabinoids: Δ9-tetrahydrocannabinol, cannabidiol and Δ9-tetrahydrocannabivarin. *Br J Pharmacol*, 153, 199–215.

van der Pol, P., Liebregts, N., de Graaf, R., et al. (2013a). Mental health differences between frequent cannabis users with and without dependence and the general population. *Addiction*, 108, 1459–1469.

(2013b). Predicting the transition from frequent cannabis use to cannabis dependence: A three-year prospective study. *Drug Alcohol Depend*, 133, 352–359.

Ramaekers, J. G., Mason, N. L., Kloft, L., et al. (2021). The why behind the high: Determinants of neurocognition during acute cannabis exposure. *Nat Rev Neurosci*, 22, 439–454.

Schettino, J., and Hoch, E. (2015). *Treatment of Cannabis-related Disorders in Europe*. Luxembourg: Publications Office of the European Union.

Schlag, A. K., Hindocha, C., Zafar, R., et al. (2021). Cannabis based medicines and cannabis dependence: A critical review of issues and evidence. *J Psychopharmacol*, 35, 773–785.

Skumlien M., Freeman, T. P, Hall, R. et al. (2022a). The effects of acute cannabis with and without cannabidiol on neural reward anticipation in adults and adolescents, Biological Psychiatry: Cognitive Neuroscience and Neuroimaging (2022), doi.org/10.1016/j.bpsc.2022.10.004.

Skumlien M., Mokrysz, C., Freeman, T. P. et al. (2022b). Neural responses to reward anticipation and feedback in adult and adolescent cannabis users and controls. *Neuropsychopharmacology*. 47, 1976–1983.

von Sydow, K., Lieb, R., Pfister, H., et al. (2001). The natural course of cannabis use, abuse and dependence over four years: A longitudinal community study of adolescents and young adults. *Drug Alcohol Depend*, 64, 347–361.

(2002). What predicts incident use of cannabis and progression to abuse and dependence? A 4-year prospective examination of risk factors in a community sample of adolescents and young adults. *Drug Alcohol Depend*, 68, 49–64.

Teesson, M., Slade, T., Swift, W., et al. (2012). Prevalence, correlates and comorbidity of DSM-IV cannabis use and cannabis use disorders in Australia. *Aust NZ J Psychiatry*, 46, 1182–1192.

UNODC. (2017). *World Drug Report*. Geneva: United Nations.

(2020). *World Drug Report*. Geneva: United Nations.

Urban, N. B. L., Slifstein, M., Thompson, J. L., et al. (2012). Dopamine release in chronic cannabis users: A [11c] raclopride positron emission tomography study. *Biol Psychiatry*, 71, 677–683.

Verweij, K. J. H., Abdellaoui, A., Nivard, M. G., et al. (2017). Genetic association between schizophrenia and cannabis use. *Drug Alcohol Depend*, 171, 117–121.

Vingerhoets, W. A. M., Koenders, L., van den Brink, W., et al. (2016). Cue-induced striatal activity in frequent cannabis users independently predicts cannabis problem severity three years later. *J Psychopharmacol*, 30, 152–158.

Volkow, N. (2021). *Establishing 5 mg of THC as the Standard Unit for Research*. Available at: www.drugabuse.gov/about-nida/noras-blog/2021/05/establishing-5mg-thc-standard-unit-research. Last accessed 31 October 2022.

Volkow, N. D., Han, B., Einstein, E. B., et al. (2021). Prevalence of substance use disorders by time since first substance use among young people in the US. *JAMA Pediatr*, 175, 640–643.

WHO. (2018). *International Classification of Diseases for Mortality and Morbidity Statistics (11th Revision)*. Geneva: World Health Organization.

Wittchen, H. U., Jacobi, F., Rehm, J., et al. (2011). The size and burden of mental disorders and other disorders of the brain in Europe 2010. *Eur Neuropsychopharmacol*, 21, 655–679.

Chapter

29

Tobacco Use among Individuals with Cannabis Use

Insights into Co-use and Why It Matters for People with Psychosis

Rachel A. Rabin, Erin A. McClure, and Tony P. George

29.1 Introduction

A prominent but underappreciated concern for individuals using cannabis is the co-use of other substances, especially tobacco and its primary psychoactive ingredient, nicotine. Interestingly, cannabis and tobacco co-use is more common than using cannabis alone. Data from adults in the United States (US) indicate that the rate of past month co-use is more than double the rate of using solely cannabis (5.2% versus 2.3%) (Schauer et al., 2015). With respect to the last 12-months, 22% of US adults report cannabis and tobacco co-use (Gravely et al., 2020), with other countries showing even higher rates. For example, in Canada this statistic reaches 25% (Statistics Canada, 2020), while in the United Kingdom and Australia co-use is 77.2% (Hindocha et al., 2016) and 86% (Gravely et al., 2020), respectively, underscoring that co-use is a global phenomenon. Notably, in many countries, cannabis and tobacco are frequently mixed together in the same preparation and, in some cases, users may be unaware of tobacco exposure, tempering co-use statistics (Schauer et al., 2017).

Cannabis and tobacco co-use can refer to sequential use or simultaneous use. The former refers to using each substance on separate occasions often with no temporal proximity or relationship in use. However, one exception is the practice of 'chasing', which refers to smoking tobacco immediately following cannabis. In contrast, simultaneous use implies consumption of these substances at the same time (i.e., co-administration). The main route of simultaneous administration is through smoking. Tobacco can be added to joints, a process referred to as 'mulling', where up to one half of a cigarette can be added to a joint. Alternatively, cigars can be hollowed out and replaced by cannabis: known as a 'blunt'. While processes of simultaneous use may result in relatively low quantities of tobacco compared to tobacco-only consumption, research suggests that

these practices can yield comparable rates of tobacco exposure to that of light and moderate cigarette smokers (Belanger et al., 2013). A similar pattern is seen with sequential co-use, in that individuals who report smoking both cannabis and tobacco cigarettes consumed more cigarettes compared to those smoking cigarettes alone (Flatz et al., 2013). Given that inhalation is the predominant route of administration of both drugs, this may be another factor driving continued co-use [see Agrawal and Lynskey (2009) for a review]. Importantly, methods of co-use administration can vary by country (Smith et al., 2020a), culture (Kelly, 2005), and age (Chadi et al., 2019; Trivers et al., 2018; Wang et al., 2016).

Cannabis legalization has contributed to an increase in the development and marketing of new methods and tools that facilitate co-use. Electronic cigarettes (e-cigarettes) and other methods of vaping, which may be used to deliver cannabis and/or nicotine, are becoming increasingly popular, especially among youth (Giroud et al., 2015; Trivers et al., 2018). These devices heat liquid or solid preparations of the substance to allow the user to inhale the psychoactive compounds (e.g., THC and/or nicotine) in a non-combustible form. The attractiveness of vaping stems from the perception that it may be a healthier, safer alternative to smoking (Ambrose et al., 2014; Lee et al., 2016). However, emerging data confirms that these delivery systems are far from being-free. Vapours from e-cigarettes contain alarming concentrations of heavy metals and carcinogenic substances (Rubinstein et al., 2018), and vaping can intensify the exposure to psychoactive ingredients (Mehmedic et al., 2010), which ironically can lead to the initiation of cigarette smoking behaviors (Lowe, 2019). Vaping is also more discrete than other forms of smoking (no smell), which may explain their appeal to minors as well as their use in places where smoking is restricted (Morean et al., 2015).

Over the last several decades there has been a substantial effort focused on reducing tobacco use worldwide (WHO, 2003). However, despite declining rates of tobacco-only use (G. B. D. Tobacco Collaborators, 2017), rates of daily cannabis and tobacco co-use are rising (Goodwin et al., 2018), suggesting persistence of tobacco use among cannabis users. Accordingly, cannabis use may be propelling the use of tobacco and preventing successful tobacco quit attempts (Rabin and George, 2015). Evidence of the reverse has also been observed. Tobacco use reinforces cannabis use and is a clinical marker for greater cannabis relapse and poorer treatment outcomes (Haney et al., 2013). Currently, there are no approved medications for cannabis use disorders (CUD), and behavioural treatments yield only modest abstinence rates that decline once treatment is discontinued (Brezing and Levin, 2018; Gates et al., 2016; and see Chapter 24). Conceivably, among co-users, treatment for CUD can be augmented if co-occurring tobacco use is considered and potentially addressed through treatment, highlighting the need to better understand cannabis use in the context of tobacco use. Therefore, this chapter reviews the evidence for: (1) mechanisms driving the high rates of tobacco use among cannabis users; (2) the interactive effects of co-use on the brain, clinical outcomes, and physical health; and (3) the implications for treating cannabis and tobacco co-use, particularly in people with schizophrenia and other psychotic disorders.

29.2 Mechanisms Underlying Co-use

29.2.1 Synergistic Effects

There is considerable overlap between the human endocannabinoid system and cholinergic systems, the neurobiological systems in the brain implicated with cannabis use and tobacco use, respectively (Adermark, 2011; and see Chapters 1 and 2). Independently, both substances promote the release of mesolimbic dopamine, contributing to the reinforcing properties of each drug (Cheer et al., 2004; Grenhoff et al., 1986). One theory proposed to explain the high rates of tobacco use among cannabis users is that adding tobacco to cannabis can potentiate and prolong the euphoric and rewarding effects of cannabis (Tullis et al., 2003). Evidence suggests that when tobacco is added to cannabis in the right

proportions, extraction of THC can be increased by up to 50% (Van der Kooy et al., 2009). In line with this, in a sample of co-users, Penetar et al. (2005) demonstrated that pre-treatment with a transdermal nicotine patch increased subjective cannabis ratings of 'stimulated' and 'high' on a visual analogue scale, compared to placebo (Penetar et al., 2005). In a qualitative study, participants commonly reported using a tobacco cigarette following cannabis as a means of increasing the euphoric effects of cannabis, a practice that was referred to as 'boosting' (Lee et al., 2010). Another study of college student co-users found that 65% had smoked both substances in the same hour, with 31% reporting that they smoked tobacco to prolong the effects of cannabis (Ramo et al., 2013). These results are in line with a large online survey (N = 432 adults) that concluded that nicotine may enhance the rewarding effects of cannabis for some, but not all users (Akbar et al., 2019).

Findings from studies conducted in animals provide further support for an 'enhancing' effect of nicotine on cannabis. For example, a recent pre-clinical study found that chronic nicotine exposure increased sensitivity to the rewarding effects of low doses of THC in mice regardless of whether delivered by electronic cigarette or cigarette smoking (Ponzoni et al., 2019), suggesting that the method of administration of nicotine/tobacco may be irrelevant. Collectively, these studies demonstrate enhanced effects of cannabis when co-used with tobacco, which may contribute to the development of CUD. Thus, it is not surprising that, among cannabis users, tobacco use is associated with a greater number of cannabis dependence symptoms (Ream et al., 2008) and may mediate the transition of cannabis use to CUD (Hindocha et al., 2015).

However, not all studies support a synergistic effects of tobacco on cannabis use. Using a double-blind, 2 (active cannabis, placebo cannabis) × 2 (active tobacco, placebo tobacco) crossover design in non-dependent cannabis and tobacco co-users, Hindocha et al. (2017b) observed that tobacco did not influence the rewarding effects of cannabis. Similarly, another study that employed a mixed-methods approach found that participants did not perceive a synergistic effect with co-use (Berg et al., 2018). Thus, the synergistic relationship between cannabis and tobacco may be complex, with factors such as dose, timing, method of administration, previous cannabis/tobacco history, and insight moderating the reinforcing effects of co-use. In addition, common genetic influences associated with cannabis and tobacco use may also play a role in increasing the reinforcing and synergistic effects associated with co-use (Agrawal et al., 2010).

29.2.2 Compensatory Effects

29.2.2.1 Withdrawal

A cannabis withdrawal syndrome occurs in ~90% of individuals with CUD and may include cravings, anxiety, depression, changes in appetite and sleep, as well as irritability (Budney and Hughes, 2006; and see Chapter 27). Its onset typically occurs 24 hours after the last use of cannabis, peaks 2–6 days later, and can last up to 14 days (Budney et al., 2003). The persistence of these symptoms may contribute to the development of CUD and difficulty quitting cannabis (Budney et al., 2003). Accumulating research suggests that tobacco may be consumed as a means to counteract cannabis withdrawal symptoms. For example, Levin et al. (2010) assessed a large sample (N = 469) of adult cannabis smokers who had made a quit attempt. Almost half of the study participants (~48%) reported using tobacco to relieve a cannabis withdrawal symptom, and 37.7% of participants reported increasing their tobacco use during a quit attempt (Levin et al., 2010). Consistent with these findings, a cannabis abstinence study conducted in patients with schizophrenia who co-used cannabis and tobacco observed that compensatory increases in tobacco use were most pronounced in the first seven days of abstinence but returned to baseline levels by day 28 of abstinence (Rabin et al., 2018). It is unknown whether these patients are substituting cannabis for tobacco purposefully in an attempt to assist with their cessation or inadvertently. Interestingly, the same pattern of increased tobacco use during cannabis abstinence was not observed in a comparison group of non-psychiatric controls (Rabin et al., 2018). Furthermore, in a cross-sectional study in patients with schizophrenia, former and never cannabis smokers had elevated rates of tobacco use compared to current cannabis users (Rabin et al., 2014). In a more recent study, Gilbert et al. (2020) examined the effects of experimental administration of nicotine on cannabis withdrawal symptoms. Participants with CUD were randomized to receive either a low dose (7 mg) nicotine patch or placebo patch over 15 days

of cannabis abstinence (Gilbert et al., 2020). Results showed that the nicotine patch, relative to placebo, selectively attenuated negative affect starting seven days post-patch-initiation, which continued throughout the duration of cannabis abstinence. Interestingly, this reduction in negative affect occurred irrespective of current smoking status (i.e., in individuals who were non-smokers and light tobacco smokers). Future studies are needed to further examine the potential effects of tobacco/nicotine and how these substances can be safely administered to cannabis treatment-seekers to attenuate withdrawal symptoms and bolster rates of cannabis abstinence.

29.2.2.2 Cognition

In general, acute cannabis and tobacco use exert contrasting effects on cognitive function. While cannabis administration is associated with impairments in attention, memory, and executive function (Curran et al., 2016; D'Souza et al., 2004), tobacco administration improves these processes (Heishman et al., 2010). Thus, among cannabis users, co-use of tobacco may be a strategy to offset cannabis-induced cognitive difficulties; a phenomenon that has been demonstrated by several (but not all) studies. One study compared verbal memory and learning performance between cannabis and tobacco co-users and tobacco users with a minimal history of cannabis use, under a tobacco satiated condition and following 24-hours of tobacco abstinence. During the abstinence condition, cannabis users had worse performance relative to tobacco-only participants; however, during the smoking *ad libitum* condition, differences were no longer present between the two groups. In addition, functional magnetic resonance imaging showed that nicotine withdrawal increased task-related activation in the frontocortical region and was associated with decreased frontoparietal connectivity during high working memory load tasks. These findings suggest that, among cannabis users, cannabis-induced deficits in verbal memory and learning performance and its associated impairment in neural activation may be masked under conditions of tobacco satiation (Jacobsen et al., 2007), supporting compensatory actions of cannabis and tobacco. In another study, Schuster et al. (2015) examined whether episodic memory performance of young adults who used cannabis regularly varied with respect to level of past year tobacco exposure. Findings revealed that, while cannabis use was associated with worse memory scores in cannabis users who smoked cigarettes sporadically in the previous year, this relationship was absent in cannabis users who consistently smoked cigarettes (Schuster et al., 2015).

Using ecological momentary assessment, a subsequent study by this group reported similar findings, indicating that, when cannabis and tobacco were combined, working memory performance was better than when cannabis was used alone (Schuster et al., 2016). Partially supporting these findings, an experimental study that compared administration of cannabis and tobacco alone versus co-administration demonstrated that tobacco may counteract the cognitive impairing effects of cannabis, but only on selective aspects of memory – namely delayed recall – but not for immediate or verbal recall (Hindocha et al., 2017a). Whether tobacco's masking effect on cannabis-induced cognitive dysfunction extends to cognitive functions other than memory and learning has been examined in only one published study. Using a randomized double-blind design, Francis et al. (2022) investigated the effects of acute nicotine administration (6 mg) on sensory gating, the process of filtering out unnecessary stimuli from the environment, in cannabis users with no history of tobacco use (Francis et al., 2022). Relative to placebo, acute nicotine administration did not affect sensory gating; however, this study included non-smokers, who may have a differential cognitive response to nicotine relative to smokers (Wignall and de Wit, 2011). Taken together, there is strong evidence to support the compensatory effects of cannabis and tobacco on cognitive function, which may in part reinforce co-using behaviors. Future studies exploring the effects of co-use on a broader range of cognitive domains (e.g., executive function, attention) are warranted, especially in people with schizophrenia and other psychotic disorders, who have amongst the highest rates of tobacco and cannabis co-use (Koskinen et al., 2010; de Leon and Diaz, 2005).

29.3 Consequences of Co-use

29.3.1 Brain Morphology

While the independent effects of tobacco use (Peng et al., 2018; Sutherland et al., 2016; Zhang et al., 2011) and cannabis use (Lorenzetti et al., 2019) on brain structure are well studied, only two studies to date have investigated their combined effects, notably in small samples (<22 co-users) (Filbey et al., 2015; Wetherill et al., 2015). Both of these studies examined grey matter volume differences across four groups of participants: cannabis- and tobacco-only users, co-users, and non-substance users. Filbey et al. (2015) performed a region-of-interest analysis using FreeSurfer-generated volumes of the hippocampus, given its role in memory and learning performance (Squire and Zola-Morgan, 1991). The investigators reported that individuals who used cannabis only and co-used cannabis with tobacco had smaller hippocampal volumes compared to tobacco-only users and non-using controls (Filbey et al., 2015). In the other study, Wetherill et al. (2015) used a whole-brain voxel-wise approach to determine group differences in grey matter volume. In contrast to the findings of Filbey et al.'s (2015) study, no group effects in hippocampal volume were observed (Wetherill et al., 2015). However, a significant group effect was observed in the left putamen, thalamus, right precentral gyrus, and left cerebellum. Compared to non-substance users, all other groups exhibited larger grey matter volumes in the left putamen. Cannabis-only users also had larger grey matter volume than non-substance users in the right precentral gyrus. Cannabis-only users and co-users had smaller grey matter thalamic volume compared to non-substance users. Lastly, tobacco-only users and co-users had smaller cerebellar grey matter volume than non-substance users. Given the paucity of data, more studies employing larger samples are necessary to draw conclusions as to whether individuals with co-use exhibit different structural patterns compared to single substance users and non-substance users. Further, these studies should aim to determine the clinical correlates of morphological abnormalities in co-users given that studies in other addictive samples have reported that lower grey matter volume in the hippocampus, cerebellum, and putamen is associated with greater drug consumption, worse cognitive function, and more difficulty maintaining abstinence, respectively (Qian et al., 2019; Rabin et al., 2020, 2021). Hence, if co-use is associated with greater brain atrophy compared to atrophy associated with either substance alone, then it follows that the clinical effects that are mediated via grey matter volume may be worse than that of either substance alone (see Figure 29.1).

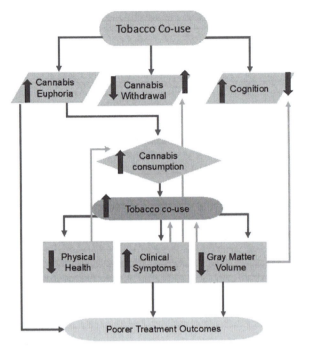

Figure 29.1 This diagram illustrates how tobacco co-use reinforces use of cannabis and tobacco and ultimately hampers successful treatment outcomes (i.e., abstinence). Mechanisms such as increased euphoric effects of cannabis, attenuation of cannabis withdrawal, and compensatory cognitive improvements, contribute to the high rates of tobacco co-use among cannabis users, which in turn can lead to greater cannabis consumption and increased tobacco co-use. Secondary pathways (in light grey) serve to further reinforce co-using behaviors.

29.3.2 Brain Function

Investigating reward sensitivity and neural activity to rewarding stimuli in individuals with substance use disorders (SUDs) compared to healthy controls can provide important insights into how drug users process salient cues. Only recently have researchers started to investigate whether neural activity differs between cannabis- and tobacco-only users and co-users. Karoly et al. (2015) used a monetary incentive delay task to probe reward sensitivity indexed by neural activation in the nucleus accumbens, a key structure in the brain reward system. Findings showed that the tobacco-only group had lower activation in the nucleus accumbens during reward anticipation compared to cannabis and tobacco co-users and non-substance users. No group differences emerged between the cannabis-only group and the other groups. In contrast, a subsequent study employing a similar task reported that cannabis use was associated with decreased neural response in the nucleus accumbens, during reward anticipation; an effect that was not modulated by previous or concurrent tobacco use (Martz et al., 2016).

Using a cue-reactivity paradigm, Kuhns et al. (2020) examined neural activity in response to cannabis cues in a sample of cannabis- and tobacco-only users, co-users, and non-substance using controls (Kuhns et al., 2020). The cannabis-only group demonstrated heightened cannabis cue-induced activity in the amygdala compared with non-substance using controls; an effect not seen in co-users. Unexpectedly, tobacco-only users had heightened cue reactivity in the amygdala and striatum compared to co-users and non-substance using controls, suggesting that tobacco use does play an important role in cannabis cue reactivity, but less so for co-users. While only a handful of studies have been conducted using fMRI, reward related neural activity appears to be most compromised in tobacco-only users compared to cannabis-only users and co-users. This pattern of results may suggest that functional impairments in brain activity may be a trait characteristic that is unique to tobacco-only users; however, this is only speculative given the limited number of studies conducted.

29.3.3 Clinical Outcomes

The relationship between psychopathology and substance use is well established (Boyle and Offord, 1991). What is less known is whether mental health outcomes differ between cannabis and tobacco co-users versus single substance users. In a sample of cannabis treatment-seekers, Moore and Budney reported that co-users had greater psychiatric severity compared to cannabis-only users as measured by the Brief Symptom Inventory (Derogatis, 1993); however, this study did not include a tobacco-only comparison group limiting interpretation of the findings (Moore and Budney, 2001). Consistent with these results, a recent study using data from a nationally representative sample in Great Britain found that rates of depression were highest among co-users (32%), were comparable across cannabis-only (18.3%) and tobacco-only (20.3%) users, and lowest in non-using controls (12.3%); a similar pattern of results was reported for symptoms of anxiety (Hindocha et al., 2021). Another study found that tobacco-only users had the highest level of anxiety, while co-users reported more anxiety than cannabis-only users and non-substance-users (Bonn-Miller et al., 2010).

To date, only one study has reported on the association of cannabis and tobacco co-use patterns and psychiatric diagnoses (other than SUDs). Peters et al. (2014) analysed data from a sample of the National Epidemiologic Survey on Alcohol and Related Conditions (NESARC) that included adults with concurrent CUD and nicotine dependence, CUD only, and nicotine dependence only (Peters et al., 2014). Co-use was associated with a higher prevalence of bipolar disorder and personality disorders compared to cannabis- and tobacco-only users while, compared to tobacco-only, co-use was also associated with higher rates of anxiety disorders, which may serve to further complicate co-use treatment (Rabin, 2020). With respect to substance use and SUDs, co-users tend to have greater rates of alcohol use and other drugs of abuse compared to tobacco-only users (Ramo et al., 2012). Lastly, cannabis and tobacco co-use is associated with an increased likelihood of heavier cannabis use and for meeting diagnostic criteria for both CUD and nicotine dependence (Peters et al., 2012; Ream et al., 2008; Rubinstein et al., 2014). Overall, these studies suggest additive or interactive effects of cannabis and tobacco co-use on psychiatric symptoms and diagnoses as compared to single substance use. This may in turn contribute to greater cannabis and tobacco co-use in an attempt to alleviate these symptoms (i.e., a bidirectional relationship; see Figure 29.1) (Quello et al., 2005). Furthermore, given that anxiety and depression are the most commonly experienced symptoms during cannabis withdrawal (Livne et al., 2019), the clinical effects associated with co-use may exacerbate cannabis withdrawal symptoms culminating in greater compensatory use of tobacco (Figure 29.1).

29.3.4 Physical Health

While the therapeutic potential of cannabis to treat a broad range of medical conditions has been the subject of many studies, results regarding its efficacy remain inconclusive (Cohen et al., 2019). Thus, while many are aiming to improve their physical health with cannabis, ironically, cannabis may exert effects that are detrimental to one's health. For one, a recent study demonstrated that medical cannabis legalization was positively associated with tobacco co-use such that there was a higher proportion of co-users in states where medical marijuana was legal compared to states where it was illegal, suggesting that medical cannabis use may inadvertently increase tobacco use (Wang et al., 2016).

Research investigating the effects of co-use on respiratory disease documents an increased risk of developing chronic obstructive pulmonary disease compared to smoking cannabis alone (Tan et al., 2009), with another study reporting a link between co-use and cardiovascular disease biomarkers (Meier and Hatsukami, 2016). Similarly, adult co-users had both poorer smoking-specific health problems (e.g., emphysema, airway disease) and poorer general health compared to adults who used cannabis-only (Rooke et al., 2013). Recent data have also demonstrated that co-users have significantly higher urinary concentrations of several combustion by-products (e.g., acrylonitrile, acrylamine, and polycyclic aromatic hydrocarbons) compared to tobacco-only users (Smith et al., 2020b), suggesting potential additive toxicant exposure among co-users. Furthermore, although marketed as a safer alternative to smoking, there is growing evidence that electronic delivery systems are associated with worrisome health risks. For example, there has been a steady climb in the number of cases of e-cigarette or vaping product use-associated lung injury (EVALI) (Moritz et al., 2019), with the majority (>80%) of these patients reporting co-use (Perrine et al., 2019). In contrast, a large study did not find an association between co-use and physical health problems (Peters et al., 2014). However, it is important to note that large effect sizes of disease markers may only be apparent in samples that include older adults, when health problems are more likely to emerge (Mehra et al., 2006). Research has not fully uncovered the full breadth of physical health consequences associated with co-using behaviors. As new methods for co-use appear on the market, it will be necessary to collect long-term data before declaring such products as safer alternatives to smoking.

29.4 Treatment Implications for Co-users

As detailed in Chapter 24, there are currently are no approved medications for CUD and behavioural treatments yield only modest abstinence rates that decline once treatment is discontinued (Brezing and Levin, 2018; Gates et al., 2016). In contrast, there are several approved medications for tobacco use with evidence that combination therapy can be quite effective (Stead et al., 2016). Despite the high rates of co-use, tobacco and cannabis use are rarely co-treated. In light of the synergistic and compensatory effects associated with co-use (as outlined previously), treating both substances may present additional challenges as compared to treating one substance alone. To this end, a recent systematic review and meta-analysis that evaluated the impact of interventions that were designed to address cannabis, tobacco, co-use, and/or poly-substance use among cannabis and tobacco co-users found that single and multi-substance interventions addressing cannabis and/or tobacco have not shown a clear effect on either substance (Walsh et al., 2020).

In order to develop effective treatment approaches for co-use, it is important to understand how tobacco use may influence cannabis treatment outcomes. Preliminary evidence from a laboratory study suggested that tobacco co-use among cannabis users increased the likelihood of cannabis relapse compared to non-tobacco smokers (Haney et al., 2013). Moreover, a clinical study reported that treatment-seeking cannabis users who co-used tobacco had a significantly lower percentage of cannabis-negative urines and relapsed more quickly compared to former tobacco users (Moore and Budney, 2001). These and other studies (de Dios et al., 2009; Gray et al., 2017; McClure et al., 2014) suggest that tobacco co-use may significantly hamper cannabis treatment outcomes (i.e., achieving sustained cannabis abstinence).

From the evidence reviewed in this chapter, it is clear that the relationship between cannabis and tobacco use is complex and thus, it follows that there is currently no gold standard for treating co-use. Importantly, cannabis and tobacco co-use may serve to compromise treatment outcomes for one or both substances. In Figure 29.1, we depict the mechanisms that may underlie high rates of tobacco co-use among cannabis users (increased euphoric effects of cannabis, attenuation of cannabis withdrawal, and compensatory cognitive improvements), which in turn may increase cannabis consumption and thereby increase tobacco co-use. Over time, these mechanisms may strengthen to further reinforce co-use, ultimately making reductions and abstinence even more challenging.

Traditionally, interventions for comorbid substance use have been poorly developed and it remains to be determined whether treatment for cannabis and tobacco co-use may benefit from an integrated approach. A caveat of the latter is that the co-users must want to quit both substances (McClure et al., 2019); nevertheless, this approach is surely beneficial from a financial and resource perspective (Kalman et al., 2010). Indeed, more research is necessary to elucidate the potential reasons for poor outcomes among co-users, and to do this researchers and clinicians must incorporate better metrics to index co-use (Hindocha et al., 2021).

29.5 Conclusion

Clearly, cannabis and tobacco use are inter-related. The high prevalence of co-use and their associated neural, clinical, and physical consequences underscore the need to better understand mechanisms underlying co-use. Moreover, co-users are a heterogeneous population (e.g., diverse age range, presence of psychopathology) with variable and dynamic practices of co-use, which will likely continue to diversify as more products and delivery devices enter the market; factors which serve to further complicate understanding and treating co-use. Encouragingly, research does indeed suggest that treating cannabis and tobacco co-use is feasible, albeit effective interventions for these individuals will *not* be a 'one size fits all' approach. Given that cannabis-tobacco co-use is prevalent globally, the development of effective interventions for cannabis and tobacco co-use should be deemed a public health priority, especially among populations with high rates of co-use, such as individuals with schizophrenia and other psychoses.

Funding

This review was funded by grants from the Fonds de Recherche du Québec – Santé (FRQS) and the Canada First Research Excellence Fund awarded to McGill University for the Healthy Brains for Healthy Lives to Dr Rabin, and funds from the Astrid H. Flaska and CAMH Foundations and the National Institute of Drug Abuse (NIDA) grant R21-DA-043949 to Dr George.

References

Adermark, L. (2011). Modulation of endocannabinoid-mediated long-lasting disinhibition of striatal output by cholinergic interneurons. *Neuropharmacology*, **61**, 1314–1320.

Agrawal, A., and Lynskey, M. T. (2009). Tobacco and cannabis co-occurrence: Does route of administration matter? *Drug Alcohol Depend*, **99**, 240–247.

Agrawal, A., Silberg, J. L., Lynskey, M. T., et al. (2010). Mechanisms underlying the lifetime co-occurrence of tobacco and cannabis use in adolescent and young adult twins. *Drug Alcohol Depend*, **108**, 49–55.

Akbar, S. A., Tomko, R. L., Salazar, C. A., et al. (2019). Tobacco and cannabis co-use and interrelatedness among adults. *Addict Behav*, **90**, 354–361.

Ambrose, B. K., Rostron, B. L., Johnson, S. E., et al. (2014). Perceptions of the relative harm of cigarettes and e-cigarettes among U.S. youth. *Am J Prev Med*, **47**, S53–S60.

Belanger, R. E., Marclay, F., Berchtold, A., et al. (2013). To what extent does adding tobacco to cannabis expose young users to nicotine? *Nicotine Tob Res*, **15**, 1832–1838.

Berg, C. J., Payne, J., Henriksen, L., et al. (2018). Reasons for marijuana and tobacco co-use among young adults: A mixed methods scale development study. *Subst Use Misuse*, **53**, 357–369.

Bonn-Miller, M. O., Zvolensky, M. J., and Johnson, K. A. (2010). Uni-morbid and co-occurring marijuana and tobacco use: Examination of concurrent associations with negative mood states. *J Addict Dis*, **29**, 68–77.

Boyle, M. H., and Offord, D. R. (1991). Psychiatric disorder and substance use in adolescence. *Can J Psychiatry*, **36**, 699–705.

Brezing, C. A., and Levin, F. R. (2018). The current state of pharmacological treatments for cannabis use disorder and withdrawal. *Neuropsychopharmacology*, **43**, 173–194.

Budney, A. J., and Hughes, J. R. (2006). The cannabis withdrawal syndrome. *Curr Opin Psychiatry*, **19**, 233–238.

Budney, A. J., Moore, B. A., Vandrey, R. G., et al. (2003). The time course and significance of cannabis withdrawal. *J Abnorm Psychol*, **112**, 393–402.

Chadi, N., Schroeder, R., Jensen, J. W., et al. (2019). Association between electronic cigarette use and marijuana use among adolescents and young adults: A systematic review and meta-analysis. *JAMA Pediatr*, **173**, e192574.

Cheer, J. F., Wassum, K. M., Heien, M. L., et al. (2004). Cannabinoids enhance subsecond dopamine release in the nucleus accumbens of awake rats. *J Neurosci*, **24**, 4393–4400.

Cohen, K., Weizman, A., and Weinstein, A. (2019). Positive and negative effects of cannabis and cannabinoids on health. *Clin Pharmacol Ther*, **105**, 1139–1147.

Curran, H. V., Freeman, T. P., Mokrysz, C., et al. (2016). Keep off the grass? Cannabis, cognition and addiction. *Nat Rev Neurosci*, **17**, 293–306.

D'Souza, D. C., Perry, E., MacDougall, L., et al. (2004). The psychotomimetic effects of intravenous delta-9-tetrahydrocannabinol in healthy individuals: Implications for psychosis. *Neuropsychopharmacology*, **29**, 1558–1572.

Derogatis, L. R. (1993). *Brief Symptom Inventory: Administration, Scoring and Procedures Manual*. Minneapolis, MN: Systems Inc.

de Dios, M. A., Vaughan, E. L., Stanton, C. A., et al. (2009). Adolescent tobacco use and substance abuse treatment outcomes. *J Subst Abuse Treat*, **37**, 17–24.

Filbey, F. M., McQueeny, T., Kadamangudi, S., et al. (2015). Combined effects of marijuana and nicotine on memory performance and hippocampal volume. *Behav Brain Res*, **293**, 46–53.

Flatz, A., Belanger, R. E., Berchtold, A., et al. (2013). Assessing tobacco dependence among cannabis users smoking cigarettes. *Nicotine Tob Res*, **15**, 557–561.

Francis, A. M., Parks, A., Choueiry, J., et al. (2022). Sensory gating in tobacco-naive cannabis users is unaffected by acute nicotine administration. *Psychopharmacology*, **239**, 1279–1288.

G. B. D. Tobacco Collaborators. (2017). Smoking prevalence and attributable disease burden in 195 countries and territories, 1990–2015: A systematic analysis from the Global Burden of Disease Study 2015. *Lancet*, **389**, 1885–1906.

Gates, P. J., Sabioni, P., Copeland, J., et al. (2016). Psychosocial interventions for cannabis use disorder. *Cochrane Database Syst Rev*, **5**, CD005336.

Gilbert, D. G., Rabinovich, N. E., and McDaniel, J. T. (2020). Nicotine patch for cannabis withdrawal symptom relief: A randomized controlled trial. *Psychopharmacology (Berl)*, **237**, 1507–1519.

Giroud, C., de Cesare, M., Berthet, A., et al. (2015). E-cigarettes: A review of new trends in cannabis use. *Int J Environ Res Public Health*, **12**, 9988–10008.

Goodwin, R. D., Pacek, L. R., Copeland, J., et al. (2018). Trends in daily cannabis use among cigarette smokers: United States, 2002–2014. *Am J Public Health*, **108**, 137–142.

Gravely, S., Driezen, P., Smith, D. M., et al. (2020). International differences in patterns of cannabis use among adult cigarette smokers: Findings from the 2018 ITC Four Country Smoking and Vaping Survey. *Int J Drug Policy*, **79**, 102754.

Gray, K. M., Sonne, S. C., McClure, E. A., et al. (2017). A randomized placebo-controlled trial of N-acetylcysteine for cannabis use disorder in adults. *Drug Alcohol Depend*, **177**, 249–257.

Grenhoff, J., Aston-Jones, G., and Svensson, T. H. (1986). Nicotinic effects on the firing pattern of midbrain dopamine neurons. *Acta Physiol Scand*, **128**, 351–358.

Haney, M., Bedi, G., Cooper, Z. D., et al. (2013). Predictors of marijuana relapse in the human laboratory: Robust impact of tobacco cigarette smoking status. *Biol Psychiatry*, **73**, 242–248.

Heishman, S. J., Kleykamp, B. A., and Singleton, E. G. (2010). Meta-analysis of the acute effects of nicotine and smoking on human performance. *Psychopharmacology (Berl)*, **210**, 453–469.

Hindocha, C., Brose, L. S., Walsh, H., et al. (2021). Cannabis use and co-use in tobacco smokers and non-smokers: Prevalence and associations with mental health in a cross-sectional, nationally representative sample of adults in Great Britain, 2020. *Addiction*, **116**, 2209–2219.

Hindocha, C., Freeman, T. P., Ferris, J. A., et al. (2016). No smoke without tobacco: A global overview of cannabis and tobacco routes of administration and their association with intention to quit. *Front Psychiatry*, **7**, 104.

Hindocha, C., Freeman, T. P., Xia, J. X., et al. (2017a). Acute memory and psychotomimetic effects of cannabis and tobacco both 'joint' and individually: A placebo-controlled trial. *Psychol Med*, **47**, 2708–2719.

Hindocha, C., Lawn, W., Freeman, T. P., et al. (2017b). Individual and combined effects of cannabis and tobacco on drug reward processing in non-dependent users. *Psychopharmacology (Berl)*, **234**, 3153–3163.

Hindocha, C., Shaban, N. D., Freeman, T. P., et al. (2015). Associations between cigarette smoking and cannabis dependence: A longitudinal study of young cannabis users in the United Kingdom. *Drug Alcohol Depend*, **148**, 165–171.

Jacobsen, L. K., Pugh, K. R., Constable, R. T., et al. (2007). Functional correlates of verbal memory deficits emerging during nicotine withdrawal in abstinent adolescent cannabis users. *Biol Psychiatry*, **61**, 31–40.

Kalman, D., Kim, S., Digirolamo, G., et al. (2010). Addressing tobacco use disorder in smokers in early remission from alcohol dependence: The case for integrating smoking cessation services in substance use disorder treatment programs. *Clin Psychol Rev*, **30**, 12–24.

Karoly, H. C., Bryan, A. D., Weiland, B. J., et al. (2015). Does incentive-elicited nucleus accumbens activation differ by substance of abuse? An examination with adolescents. *Dev Cogn Neurosci*, **16**, 5–15.

Kelly, B. C. (2005). Bongs and blunts: Notes from a suburban marijuana subculture. *J Ethn Subst Abuse*, **4**, 81–97.

Koskinen, J., Lohonen, J., Koponen, H., et al. (2010). Rate of cannabis use disorders in clinical samples of patients with schizophrenia: A meta-analysis. *Schizophr Bull*, **36**, 1115.

Kuhns, L., Kroon, E., Filbey, F., et al. (2020). Unraveling the role of cigarette use in neural cannabis cue reactivity in heavy cannabis users. *Addict Biol*, **26**, e12941.

Lee, D. C., Crosier, B. S., Borodovsky, J. T., et al. (2016). Online survey characterizing vaporizer use among cannabis users. *Drug Alcohol Depend*, **159**, 227–233.

Lee, J. P., Battle, R. S., Lipton, R., et al. (2010). 'Smoking': Use of cigarettes, cigars and blunts among Southeast Asian American youth and young adults. *Health Educ Res*, **25**, 83–96.

de Leon, J., and Diaz, F. J. (2005). A meta-analysis of worldwide studies demonstrates an association between schizophrenia and tobacco smoking behaviors. *Schizophr Res*, **76**, 135–157.

Levin, K. H., Copersino, M. L., Heishman, S. J., et al. (2010). Cannabis withdrawal symptoms in non-treatment-seeking adult cannabis smokers. *Drug Alcohol Depend*, **111**, 120–127.

Livne, O., Shmulewitz, D., Lev-Ran, S., et al. (2019). DSM-5 cannabis withdrawal syndrome: Demographic and clinical correlates in U.S. adults. *Drug Alcohol Depend*, **195**, 170–177.

Lorenzetti, V., Chye, Y., Silva, P., et al. (2019). Does regular cannabis use affect neuroanatomy? An updated systematic review and meta-analysis of structural neuroimaging studies. *Eur Arch Psychiatry Clin Neurosci*, **269**, 59–71.

Lowe, D. J. E., Coles, A. S., George, T. P., et al. (2019). E-cigarettes. In Danovitch, I., and Mooney, L. J. (eds.) *The Assessment and Treatment of Addiction: Best Practices and New Frontiers*, 1st ed. (pp. 43–56). New York: Elsevier.

Martz, M. E., Trucco, E. M., Cope, L. M., et al. (2016). Association of marijuana use with blunted nucleus accumbens response to reward anticipation. *JAMA Psychiatry*, **73**, 838–844.

McClure, E. A., Baker, N. L., and Gray, K. M. (2014). Cigarette smoking during an N-acetylcysteine-assisted cannabis cessation trial in adolescents. *Am J Drug Alcohol Abuse*, **40**, 285–291.

McClure, E. A., Tomko, R. L., Salazar, C. A., et al. (2019). Tobacco and cannabis co-use: Drug substitution, quit interest, and cessation preferences. *Exp Clin Psychopharmacol*, **27**, 265–275.

Mehmedic, Z., Chandra, S., Slade, D., et al. (2010). Potency trends of delta9-THC and other cannabinoids in confiscated cannabis preparations from 1993 to 2008. *J Forensic Sci*, **55**, 1209–1217.

Mehra, R., Moore, B. A., Crothers, K., et al. (2006). The association between marijuana smoking and lung cancer: A systematic review. *Arch Intern Med*, **166**, 1359–1367.

Meier, E., and Hatsukami, D. K. (2016). A review of the additive health

risk of cannabis and tobacco co-use. *Drug Alcohol Depend*, **166**, 6–12.

Moore, B. A., and Budney, A. J. (2001). Tobacco smoking in marijuana-dependent outpatients. *J Subst Abuse*, **13**, 583–596.

Morean, M. E., Kong, G., Camenga, D. R., et al. (2015). High school students' use of electronic cigarettes to vaporize cannabis. *Pediatrics*, **136**, 611–616.

Moritz, E. D., Zapata, L. B., Lekiachvili, A., et al. (2019). Update: Characteristics of patients in a national outbreak of E-cigarette, or vaping, product use-associated lung injuries – United States, October 2019. *MMWR Morb Mortal Wkly Rep*, **68**, 985–989.

Penetar, D. M., Kouri, E. M., Gross, M. M., et al. (2005). Transdermal nicotine alters some of marihuana's effects in male and female volunteers. *Drug Alcohol Depend*, **79**, 211–223.

Peng, P., Li, M., Liu, H., et al. (2018). Brain structure alterations in respect to tobacco consumption and nicotine dependence: A comparative voxel-based morphometry study. *Front Neuroanat*, **12**, 43.

Perrine, C. G., Pickens, C. M., Boehmer, T. K., et al. (2019). Characteristics of a multistate outbreak of lung injury associated with E-cigarette use, or vaping – United States, 2019. *MMWR Morb Mortal Wkly Rep*, **68**, 860–864.

Peters, E. N., Budney, A. J., and Carroll, K. M. (2012). Clinical correlates of co-occurring cannabis and tobacco use: A systematic review. *Addiction*, **107**, 1404–1417.

Peters, E. N., Schwartz, R. P., Wang, S., et al. (2014). Psychiatric, psychosocial, and physical health correlates of co-occurring cannabis use disorders and nicotine dependence. *Drug Alcohol Depend*, **134**, 228–234.

Ponzoni, L., Moretti, M., Braida, D., et al. (2019). Increased sensitivity to Delta(9)-THC-induced rewarding effects after seven-week exposure to electronic and tobacco cigarettes in mice. *Eur Neuropsychopharmacol*, **29**, 566–576.

Qian, W., Huang, P., Shen, Z., et al. (2019). Brain gray matter volume and functional connectivity are associated with smoking cessation outcomes. *Front Hum Neurosci*, **13**, 361.

Quello, S. B., Brady, K. T., and Sonne, S. C. (2005). Mood disorders and substance use disorder: A complex comorbidity. *Sci Pract Perspect*, **3**, 13–21.

Rabin, R. A. (2020). Commentary on Walsh et al. (2020): Tobacco and cannabis co-use- considerations for treatment. *Addiction*, **115**, 1815–1816.

Rabin, R. A., Dermody, S. S., and George, T. P. (2018). Changes in tobacco consumption in cannabis dependent patients with schizophrenia versus non-psychiatric controls during 28-days of cannabis abstinence. *Drug Alcohol Depend*, **185**, 181–188.

Rabin, R. A., and George, T. P. (2015). A review of co-morbid tobacco and cannabis use disorders: Possible mechanisms to explain high rates of co-use. *Am J Addict*, **24**, 105–116.

Rabin, R. A., Giddens, J. L., and George, T. P. (2014). Relationship between tobacco and cannabis use status in outpatients with schizophrenia. *Am J Addict*, **23**, 170–175.

Rabin, R. A., Mackey, S., Parvaz, M. A., et al. (2020). Common and gender-specific associations with cocaine use on gray matter volume: Data from the ENIGMA addiction working group. *Hum Brain Mapp*, **43**, 543–554.

Rabin, R. A., Parvaz, M. A., Alia-Klein, N., et al. (2021). Emotion recognition in individuals with cocaine use disorder: The role of abstinence length and the social brain network. *Psychopharmacology (Berl)*, **239**, 1019–1033.

Ramo, D. E., Liu, H., and Prochaska, J. J. (2012). Tobacco and marijuana use among adolescents and young adults: A systematic review of their co-use. *Clin Psychol Rev*, **32**, 105–121.

Ramo, D. E., Liu, H., and Prochaska, J. (2013). Validity and reliability of the nicotine and marijuana interaction expectancy (NAMIE) questionnaire. *Drug Alcohol Depend*, **131**, 166–170.

Ream, G. L., Benoit, E., Johnson, B. D., et al. (2008). Smoking tobacco along with marijuana increases symptoms of cannabis dependence. *Drug Alcohol Depend*, **95**, 199–208.

Rooke, S. E., Norberg, M. M., Copeland, J., et al. (2013). Health outcomes associated with long-term regular cannabis and tobacco smoking. *Addict Behav*, **38**, 2207–2213.

Rubinstein, M. L., Delucchi, K., Benowitz, N. L., et al. (2018). Adolescent exposure to toxic volatile organic chemicals from E-cigarettes. *Pediatrics*, **141**, e20173557.

Rubinstein, M. L., Rait, M. A., and Prochaska, J. J. (2014). Frequent marijuana use is associated with greater nicotine addiction in adolescent smokers. *Drug Alcohol Depend*, **141**, 159–162.

Schauer, G. L., Berg, C. J., Kegler, M. C., et al. (2015). Assessing the overlap between tobacco and marijuana: Trends in patterns of co-use of tobacco and marijuana in adults from 2003–2012. *Addict Behav*, **49**, 26–32.

Schauer, G. L., Rosenberry, Z. R., and Peters, E. N. (2017). Marijuana and tobacco co-administration in blunts, spliffs, and mulled cigarettes: A systematic literature review. *Addict Behav*, **64**, 200–211.

Schuster, R. M., Crane, N. A., Mermelstein, R., et al. (2015). Tobacco may mask poorer episodic memory among young adult cannabis users. *Neuropsychology*, **29**, 759–766.

Schuster, R. M., Mermelstein, R. J., and Hedeker, D. (2016). Ecological momentary assessment of working memory under conditions of simultaneous marijuana and tobacco use. *Addiction*, **111**, 1466–1476.

Smith, D. M., Miller, C., O'Connor, R. J., et al. (2020a). Modes of delivery in concurrent nicotine and cannabis use ('co-use') among youth: Findings from the International Tobacco Control (ITC) Survey. *Subst Abus*, **42**, 1–9.

Smith, D. M., O'Connor R, J., Wei, B., et al. (2020b). Nicotine and toxicant exposure among concurrent users (co-users) of tobacco and cannabis. *Nicotine Tob Res*, **22**, 1354–1363.

Squire, L. R., and Zola-Morgan, S. (1991). The medial temporal lobe memory system. *Science*, **253**, 1380–1386.

Statistics Canada. (2020). *Canadian Cannabis Survey 2020: Summary*. Ottawa: Statistics Canada.

Stead, L. F., Koilpillai, P., Fanshawe, T. R., et al. (2016). Combined pharmacotherapy and behavioural interventions for smoking cessation. *Cochrane Database Syst Rev*, **3**, CD008286.

Sutherland, M. T., Riedel, M. C., Flannery, J. S., et al. (2016). Chronic cigarette smoking is linked with structural alterations in brain regions showing acute nicotinic drug-induced functional modulations. *Behav Brain Funct*, **12**, 16.

Tan, W. C., Lo, C., Jong, A., et al. (2009). Marijuana and chronic obstructive lung disease: A population-based study. *CMAJ*, **180**, 814–820.

Trivers, K. F., Phillips, E., Gentzke, A. S., et al. (2018). Prevalence of cannabis use in electronic cigarettes among US youth. *JAMA Pediatr*, **172**, 1097–1099.

Tullis, L. M., Dupont, R., Frost-Pineda, K., et al. (2003). Marijuana and tobacco: A major connection? *J Addict Dis*, **22**, 51–62.

Van der Kooy, F., Pomahacova, B., and Verpoorte, R. (2009). Cannabis smoke condensate II: Influence of tobacco on tetrahydrocannabinol levels. *Inhal Toxicol*, **21**, 87–90.

Walsh, H., McNeill, A., Purssell, E., et al. (2020). A systematic review and Bayesian meta-analysis of interventions which target or assess co-use of tobacco and cannabis in single- or multi-substance interventions. *Addiction*, **115**, 1800–1814.

Wang, J. B., Ramo, D. E., Lisha, N. E., et al. (2016). Medical marijuana legalization and cigarette and marijuana co-use in adolescents and adults. *Drug Alcohol Depend*, **166**, 32–38.

Wetherill, R. R., Jagannathan, K., Hager, N., et al. (2015). Cannabis, cigarettes, and their co-occurring use: Disentangling differences in gray matter volume. *Int J Neuropsychopharmacol*, **18**, pyv061.

WHO. (2003). *Framework Convention on Tobacco Control*. Geneva: World Health Organization.

Wignall, N. D., and de Wit, H. (2011). Effects of nicotine on attention and inhibitory control in healthy nonsmokers. *Exp Clin Psychopharmacol*, **19**, 183–191.

Zhang, X., Salmeron, B. J., Ross, T. J., et al. (2011). Factors underlying prefrontal and insula structural alterations in smokers. *Neuroimage*, **54**, 42–48.

Cannabis Addiction Genetics

Suhas Ganesh and Arpana Agrawal

30.1 Introduction

While there has been some controversy about the addictive potential of cannabis, about 6% of the US adult general population meet criteria for DSM-5 Cannabis Use Disorder (CUD) during their lifetime (Hasin et al., 2015). The rates of CUD are much higher among lifetime cannabis users, as ~ one in five (19.5%) develop CUD (Hasin, 2018). Chapters 27 and 28 outline the criteria that comprise CUD, including the more recent demonstration that CUD includes a distinct withdrawal syndrome. Here we examine the role of a major contributor to the likelihood that a cannabis user will develop CUD – genetics. We will provide evidence for the heritability of CUD from twin and genomic studies, outline major genome-wide association findings, compare genetic influences on cannabis use and CUD, outline the role of genetics in CUD comorbidities and brain development, characterize gene–environment inter-play, and briefly discuss the implications of this genetic underpinning.

30.2 Twin Studies

30.2.1 Heritability

Early family studies documented that rates of CUD were elevated in individuals with a family history of alcohol and other forms of drug dependence (Bierut et al., 1998). Twin studies – which rely on comparisons of the trait correlation within identical (monozygotic) and fraternal (dizygotic) pairs – suggest that about 50–60% of the variability in cannabis use and CUD is attributable to the additive effects of segregating loci (Verweij et al., 2010). There is no evidence from twin studies that non-additive effects of these loci contribute to the heritability of cannabis use or CUD. The remainder of the variability in cannabis use and CUD has been largely credited to two types of environmental factors. Based on a meta-analysis, about 25% of the variance in starting to use cannabis

is due to those environmental factors that are shared by members of a twin pair, with the remaining 25% being due to environmental factors that make members of twin pairs different from each other. The role of twin-shared environment is slightly lower for CUD – about 15–20%, with a corresponding modestly higher contribution of twin-specific environment. In contrast, cannabis availability (i.e., how easy it is to access cannabis at a certain age) is influenced by twin-shared environment to a greater degree and its heritability is modest (h2 ~ 20%; twin-shared ~ 40%) (Gillespie et al., 2007). Evidence for different heritabilities and the changing role of genetics and environment in men and women is limited, however, there is a hint of a more prominent role of genetic factors for CUD (59% versus 51%) in women when compared to men (see Box 30.1).

30.2.2 Developmental Change

For most substances, and especially those that are socially tolerated at some level, heritability tends to increase in more permissive environments, like those that emerge in early adulthood. Longitudinal studies suggest that the heritability of cannabis use follows a similar pattern, with one study suggesting that, while cannabis use is primarily (80%) due to twin-shared environment prior to age 14, heritable factors begin to exert a modest influence until age 21 at which point they gain prominence (~50%) and then subsequently decline, then increase, and eventually stabilize (Kendler et al., 2008). Another study compared two American states – Minnesota and Colorado – as a comparison of the effect of legalization of recreational cannabis on shifts in heritable variation between adolescence and adulthood. In both states, baseline use at age 16.5 years was heritable to a similar degree (42–50%) but the rate of change in Minnesota (where recreational cannabis is not currently legal) was due to genetic factors (82%) while genetic factors were

---

Box 30.1 Heritability of cannabis use and CUD

- Heritability of cannabis use and CUD in twin studies are estimated to be ~50–60%, mostly attributable to additive effects of genetic variation.
- In cannabis use, both shared and non-shared environment explain ~25% of variance in the trait.
- In CUD in contrast, the role of non-shared environment is higher than shared environment.
- Heritable influences on cannabis use emerge during late adolescence and young adulthood.
- Heritable influences also play a part in determining age at exposure, opportunity and access to cannabis.

---

attenuated (22%) in favour of twin-shared environment (55%) in Colorado. In the Minnesota sample, where extensive longitudinal data were available, cannabis use began to decline in the late 20s, with variability in this pattern attributable to genetic influences. As the authors note, the observation of lower heritability in the Colorado data (where recreational cannabis is legal) is inconsistent with prior studies that show heightened genetic influence in the context of greater permissiveness. While the authors caution sampling error, it is also possible that increasing cannabis accessibility in the context of legalization is better measured by environmental factors shared by twins regardless of zygosity (e.g., distance to a retailer, family values regarding drug use) than by differences in genetic susceptibility, although this is merely speculative.

30.2.3 Genetic Correlation between Cannabis Availability, Use and CUD; Exposure Opportunity

Much like other drugs of abuse, the development of CUD is contingent on an individual accessing the drug, experimenting with it, and repeatedly using it. Genetic liability plays a role in age at exposure opportunity (earliest age when an individual may have been able to access cannabis; h2 ~ 65%) and availability (ease of access; h2 ~ 18%), although the latter is primarily due to twin-shared environment (34%) (Gillespie et al., 2007; Hines et al., 2018). About 45% of the genetic factors influencing frequency of cannabis use are shared with those that also make an individual more likely to have an earlier age at which they were exposed to cannabis. This estimate is lower for availability and only 3% of the variability in starting to use cannabis is due to the effect of genetic factors affecting availability of the drug, although nearly all of the twin-shared environmental effect on starting to use cannabis is related to availability. In contrast, genes influencing cannabis

initiation and those implicated in later cannabis problems are highly correlated, at least in twin studies (as high as 80–90% overlapping genetic factors for cannabis use and problems) (e.g., Agrawal et al., 2012).

Twin studies suggest that, despite developmental shifts, the role of genetic factors on using and misusing cannabis is unequivocal. The remainder of this chapter focuses on the search for the genetic variants that undergird this heritability.

30.3 Genomic Studies

The earliest genomic studies identified regions of the genome that were more likely to be inherited by individuals with CUD and, therefore, assumed to be tightly linked to causal genes (e.g., chromosome 4; Agrawal et al., 2008). Subsequently, genes in these regions as well as other genes that were nominated for their role in reward-related pathways (e.g., the *DRD2* gene that encodes a dopamine receptor) or in endocannabinoid signalling pathways (e.g., the gene encoding the cannabinoid receptor 1, *CNR1*) were examined. These 'candidate' gene approaches provided mixed findings. In addition to being limited by relatively small sample sizes that hindered statistical power, they were also penalized by a high false discovery rate that may have arisen from the inherent process underlying the nomination of these genes and, even further, the selective nature of the variants studied within each gene (Agrawal and Lynskey, 2009). Given the many caveats associated with such candidate variants, we focus our attention instead on the hypothesis-free method of interrogating all of the commonly occurring genetic polymorphisms in the genome using genome-wide association studies (GWASs) which have, thus far, provided limited support for candidate genes for cannabis use and misuse (Verweij et al., 2012).

While there have been numerous smaller GWAS, two large GWAS that meta-analysed data across tens of thousands of individuals have produced insights into the genomic contributions to cannabis use and CUD. In the first GWAS of nearly 185,000 individuals, eight single nucleotide polymorphisms (SNPs) – single base pair changes found commonly along the genome – were found to be associated with lifetime cannabis use (Pasman et al., 2018). The threshold for statistical significance in GWASs is high (p-values $\leq 5 \times 10^{-8}$) and, even though these SNP variants were highly significantly associated with cannabis use when compared to other similar variants, each individual variant contributed a very small effect (e.g., beta coefficients = 0.04–0.07). When examined at a gene-wise level, 35 genes were found to be influential for cannabis use, and the most notable signal from both variant and gene analyses was in *CADM2*, a gene that encodes the Cell Adhesion Molecule 2. This brain-expressed gene has been implicated in numerous GWAS of psychologically relevant traits (Morris et al., 2019), including alcohol use and risk-taking which have historically been genetically linked to cannabis use. Genetically bred obese mice lacking the *CADM2* gene in the hypothalamus tend to have lower body fat and improvements in their insulin response, suggesting its role in energy homeostasis (Yan et al., 2018). Another intriguing finding was in *NCAM1* (Neural Cell Adhesion Molecule 1) which is located in the same gene cluster as the *DRD2* dopamine D2 receptor encoding gene. Several other genes were identified by integrating the GWAS data with gene expression data from post-mortem brain tissue, – and genes previously linked to neuropsychiatric disorders, obesity, and cognition were implicated, albeit with very modest effects on liability to cannabis use.

The largest GWAS for CUD included nearly 21,000 cases with CUD diagnosis and over 363,000 control individuals (Johnson et al., 2020). Two genome-wide significant signals were identified, one in the gene encoding *FOXP2*, a gene with a long-standing relationship to speech as well as development of brain regions that regulate reward response, and another that potentially regulates expression of the gene encoding the nicotinic acetylcholine receptor alpha 2 (*CHRNA2*) which has been implicated in tobacco smoking and schizophrenia. The association with *CHRNA2* persisted even after accounting for smoking and schizophrenia. Both genes are robustly expressed in the brain but, similar to results for cannabis use and nearly all other psychiatric traits, the contribution of each individual variant was exceedingly modest (OR = 0.89–1.11). When the GWASs of cannabis use and CUD were evaluated for signals across the entire genome and not only those that were significant, a genome-wide heritability (or SNP-h2) of ~11% was recovered for both cannabis use and CUD, notably lower than projections from twin studies, as has been the case for most psychiatric traits. Consistent with twin studies, the genome-wide liability to cannabis use and CUD was correlated (rG $\sim$ 0.5). This missing heritability, or the difference between twin-h2 and SNP-h2, often declines as the sample sizes for GWASs increase but could also be influenced by biases in twin studies that inflate h2 (e.g., assortative mating) and those in GWASs that render the SNP-h2 less comprehensive (e.g., GWASs cannot account for the effects of very uncommonly occurring genetic differences in the genome).

Despite the moderate genetic correlation between cannabis use and CUD, their genetic relationship with other traits and disorders varies. Both cannabis use and CUD are genetically correlated with tobacco smoking, alcohol consumption, and alcohol use disorder, as well as other forms of drug use. They also demonstrate positive genetic correlations with general risk-taking, major depression, and schizophrenia. However, notable differences exist for other traits. While educational attainment (measured as number of years of schooling) is genetically correlated with lower liability to CUD, it is associated with higher liability to cannabis use. Similarly, CUD is correlated with higher genetic liability to body mass index (BMI) and related cardio-metabolic traits (Johnson et al., 2020), as well as risk for COVID-19 hospitalization (Hatoum et al., 2021), but associations with cannabis use genetics are either negative or not significant. Notably, CUD polygenic risk is associated with small reductions in white matter volume in children, while cannabis use polygenic risk appears to be related to increased (albeit non-significant) white matter volume. These distinctions suggest that, despite some similar genes influencing both cannabis use and CUD, genetic liability to cannabis use that is distinct from risk for developing CUD might represent a more adaptive aspect of behaviour. For instance, one might posit that individuals who are genetically predisposed to experimenting with cannabis but are resilient to progression to CUD might also bear a correlated pre-disposition to mechanisms that support more years of schooling and lower gains in BMI.

Box 30.2 Genomic Studies

- The largest GWAS to date has identified 35 genes associated with lifetime cannabis use, with the strongest signals in *CADM2* and *NCAM1* genes.
- The largest GWAS in CUD has identified significant associations in *FOXP2* and *CHRNA2* genes.
- Cannabis use and CUD are mutually genetically correlated and also with tobacco and alcohol use disorders, major depression, and schizophrenia.
- Educational attainment, BMI, and white matter volume demonstrate divergent directions of association for cannabis use (positively or not-significantly) and CUD (negatively).

Prior studies contrasting alcohol use with alcohol use disorder have produced similar – and even more stark – distinctions that implicated the role of socio-economic status (SES) in impeding progression from typical drinking to disordered drinking. Alcohol frequency (i.e., how often a person drinks) appears to be genetically correlated with increased SES and educational attainment, while alcohol quantity (i.e., how much they drink) is a genetic correlate of lower SES and education, and only the latter is genetically related to risk for drinking problems (Marees et al., 2020). In contrast, the genetics of ever smoking cigarettes and nicotine dependence both relate to lower educational attainment and SES. Cannabis is juxtaposed between these two drugs – while educational attainment is differentially associated with cannabis use and use disorder, genetic liability to both cannabis use and use disorder is associated with lower SES. These analyses speak to the complex relationship between stages of cannabis use and psychosocial and behavioural indices that broadly assess livelihood (e.g., cognition, academic attainment, neighbourhood, income) (see Box 30.2).

30.4 Specificity versus Shared Genetic Vulnerability for Cannabis Use, CUD, and Other Substance Use Disorders (SUD)

Family and twin studies suggest that a majority of genetic influences on CUD are shared with those that affect alcohol, nicotine, and other illicit drug use disorders (Kendler et al., 2003; Merikangas et al., 2009; Tsuang et al., 2001). There is evidence for a single (or at most, two highly correlated) genetic factor influencing all substance use disorders but at least one longitudinal study suggests that the prominence of this general genetic risk factor on CUD diminishes as individuals age from adolescence into early

and middle adulthood (Vrieze et al., 2012). Twin studies remained inconclusive as to whether cannabis-specific genetic factors exist (Palmer et al., 2012; Xian et al., 2008). GWAS have recapitulated much of the support for common genetic variants that operate across all drugs of abuse although most have relied on the earlier GWAS of cannabis use but even when considering the current largest GWAS of CUD, little support for drug-specific loci have emerged (Abdellaoui et al., 2021; Jang et al., 2022; Waldman et al., 2020). This is in contrast to the genetics of alcohol, nicotine, and opioid use disorders, each of which have singled out substance-specific genes (e.g., alcohol dehydrogenase variants for alcohol, nicotinic receptor, and cytochrome P450 variants for nicotine, and variants in the mu-opioid receptor for opioids). Even in the large GWAS of CUD, variants in the gene encoding the endocannabinoid receptors were not genome-wide significant nor have there been significant findings in cytochrome genes that play a role in conversion of the psychoactive component of cannabis – THC – to its metabolites. The lack of cannabis-specific loci may be attributed to a few factors: first, their effects may be significant but so small that very large sample sizes will be required to identify them; second, our assessment of CUD may be too imperfect to capture metabolism relevant signals and further complicated by modified bioavailability during combustion and due to the fat soluble nature of THC; third, the psychoactive effects of THC do occur via targeting of numerous and diffuse neurotransmitter pathways, thus overemphasizing general versus specific genetic liability; and, fourth, it is likely that CUD rarely occurs in isolation from other forms of substance misuse (e.g., commonly co-occurs with alcohol and nicotine problems) and, therefore, even in its true state, is more likely to capture the genetics of comorbid SUD.

30.4.1 Gateway Hypothesis

The frequent co-morbidity of cannabis use, and CUD, with other SUDs, with cannabis onset preceding the onset of other SUDs noted in epidemiological studies, led to the 'gateway hypothesis' in addiction (Secades-Villa et al., 2015) see Box 30.3. According to this hypothesis, cannabis acts as a gateway drug to the use of other illicit substances with an implicit suggestion of a *causal hypothesis* of the effect of cannabis exposure by altering the response to other substances of abuse (Kandel and Kandel, 2015). Multiple alternative explanations have also been proposed to explain the observed association between cannabis use and CUD, and other SUDs viz.

1. *common genetic liability* – shared genetic vulnerability for cannabis use, CUD and other SUDs;
2. *common confounding liability* – shared vulnerability to externalizing and/or internalizing psychopathology which in turn increase the risk for both cannabis use, CUD and other SUDs; and
3. *common environmental risk* factors for cannabis use, CUD, and other SUDs.

These hypotheses are not mutually exclusive, and the prevailing evidence supports more than one of these possibilities to explain the observed correlation between cannabis use, CUD, and other SUDs.

While twin and genomic studies provide ample support for *common genetic liability*, demonstrating causation for multi-factorial behaviours such as drug use is complicated in naturalistic settings. Monozygotic twins discordant for an exposure such as cannabis use and CUD provide a valuable model to tease apart the causal effects of an exposure (e.g., early cannabis use) on another phenotype, such as other SUDs. Monozygotic twins share all of their segregating genes and, therefore, differences in behaviour within pairs of such twins cannot be due to genetic factors. In pairs of twins where one uses cannabis (particularly at an early age) while the other does not, we can examine whether other illicit drug use is more common in cannabis users even when they are compared to their genetically identical co-twin. Such studies have consistently shown that the twin with cannabis use and specifically early onset cannabis use has higher odds for the use as well as developing a use disorder for alcohol and other substances, even in countries where cannabis is legally tolerated (Agrawal et al., 2004; Lessem et al., 2006; Lynskey

et al., 2003, 2006; Vink et al., 2020). These results provide support to the gateway hypothesis suggesting a causal impact of cannabis use on other SUDs. However, the discordant twin model fails to account for potential confounders that are unique to the twin who uses cannabis, including peer providers of cannabis and other drugs, or social milieu that encourage all forms of drug use. Therefore, it is difficult to conclude whether this excess risk for illicit drug use in cannabis users is due to biochemical or psychosocial mechanisms.

Genomic studies also provide opportunities to study causation. Currently, the GWAS of cannabis use and use disorder, as well as of other illicit drugs, are somewhat underpowered to test such genetic causal mechanisms. Other support for the causal hypothesis is derived from animal models which have shown that exposing adolescent rodents to THC enhances later self-administration of other drugs (e.g., opioids, cocaine) (Ellgren et al., 2007; Scherma et al., 2020).

Externalizing psychopathology, such as Attention Deficit Hyperactivity Disorder (ADHD), is frequently comorbid with cannabis use and CUD as well as other SUDs and shared genetic liability has been suggested for these syndromes (Vilar-Ribó et al., 2021). GWAS studies of cannabis use (Pasman et al., 2018) and CUD (Demontis et al., 2019; Johnson et al., 2020) have consistently noted a robust genetic association with ADHD. Thus, the liability to ADHD may in part explain the observed co-morbidity of cannabis use and CUD with other SUDs (Wimberley et al., 2020). However, a recent GWAS of externalizing behaviours suggests that the shared genetic liability between cannabis, other drug use, and ADHD may generalize to a broad range of impulsive, disinhibited, and developmentally precocious behaviours (Linnér et al., 2020). The literature surrounding the genetic underpinnings of correlations between cannabis use, CUD, and internalizing disorders, such as depression and anxiety, also supports the correlated liabilities hypothesis, but there is emerging evidence that early or excessive cannabis use may exert some causal influence on depression and suicidal thoughts and behaviours, over and above these correlated vulnerabilities (Agrawal et al., 2017).

In summary, *common genetic liability* for cannabis use, CUD, and other SUDs has been consistently demonstrated in genome-wide genetic studies. While discordant-twin studies lend some support for the

---

Box 30.3 Genetics of cannabis use, CUD, and other SUDs

- Both twin and genomic studies support shared genetic risk for cannabis use, CUD, and other SUDs.
- Genomic studies of cannabis use and CUD have thus far not identified signals that specifically implicate genes in the endocannabinoid system or enzymes involved in cannabinoid metabolism.
- Evidence supports common confounding risk for externalizing and internalizing psychopathology underlying cannabis use, CUD, and other SUDs.
- Gateway hypothesis suggests that cannabis use may alter the response to other substances and thus propensity for developing other SUDs.
- Twin and genomic studies provide mixed and inconclusive evidence in support of the gateway hypothesis.

Box 30.4 Cannabis and psychosis: From genetics to causation

- Epidemiological studies suggest a causal influence of cannabis use on psychosis.
- Genome-wide genetic studies alternately suggest operation of reverse causal mechanisms or common confounding liability.
- Mendelian randomization studies in GWAS of cannabis use suggest a bidirectional causal influence with greater support for schizophrenia genetic risk pre-disposing to cannabis use.
- Similar analysis in CUD also supports in part the influence of genetic confounding and reverse causal influences.

---

causal hypothesis, these are yet to be fully investigated in large scale genetic association studies that can assess causality bi-directionally (Vink et al., 2020). *Common confounding liability* to externalizing psychopathology has also been frequently demonstrated in GWAS studies of cannabis use and CUD, suggesting that these mechanisms are not mutually exclusive and often operate in conjunction with *shared/unique environmental risk* factors to manifest in cannabis use and CUD with comorbid SUD.

30.4.2 Genetics and Mental Health Comorbidity of Cannabis Use and CUD

Chapters 11–14 have covered the comorbid presentations of psychosis and depression/anxiety with cannabis use and CUD. Here we outline what genetic studies have to say about these relationships (see Box 30.4).

30.5 Cannabis Use, CUD, and Psychosis

The co-morbidity of psychosis with cannabis use and CUD has been frequently reported in epidemiological studies leading to a causal hypothesis to explain the observed association between cannabis exposure and psychosis. However, recent advances in psychiatric genomics have shed light on potential genetic confounding and reverse causal mechanisms that may in-part explain the observed comorbidity. 'Genetic confounding' refers to a scenario where the common

underlying genetic factors increase the risk for both cannabis use and CUD as well as psychosis, while 'reverse causality' refers to a scenario where the liability for psychosis may operate through certain mechanisms to increase the risk for cannabis use and CUD. We provide a summary of the literature on the genetic factors that explain the comorbidity of cannabis use and CUD with psychosis, with a focus on recent genome-wide genetic studies. Interested readers are referred to a recent viewpoint on genetically informed methods to clarify the cannabis–psychosis association (Gillespie and Kendler, 2021) (see Box 30.4).

30.5.1 Psychosis and 'Lifetime Cannabis Use'

Mendelian Randomization (MR) has been used to disentangle the direction of causal relationship between schizophrenia and cannabis use using summary data from their respective GWASs. Gage et al. (2017) noted evidence for bidirectional causal effects but a stronger causal influence for schizophrenia genetic risk on cannabis use. Vaucher et al. (2018) noted a causal influence of genetic risk for cannabis use on schizophrenia. More recently, Pasman et al. (2018), in one of the largest GWAS of lifetime cannabis use, noted that liability to schizophrenia increases the risk of lifetime cannabis use. In summary, these studies, while not accounting for frequency or severity of use, nor potency, lend support to the reverse causal hypothesis. They contradict non-genetic studies showing elevated risk for first-episode psychosis in those who use high-potency cannabis but whether genetic confounding also plays a role in these studies should be evaluated (Di Forti et al., 2015).

30.5.2 Psychosis and CUD

In one of the largest GWAS to date in CUD (Johnson et al., 2020), the authors noted that schizophrenia and CUD were positively genetically correlated suggesting a shared underlying genetic risk (confounding). While these authors did not perform a two-sample MR, they did not note a causal effect of liability for CUD on any of the correlated traits including schizophrenia. The genetic relationship between CUD and psychosis has also been examined with polygenic risk scores (PRS). Calculated from large discovery GWAS, PRS represent a person-level summary score of the additive genetic risk – comprised of several genetic variants that individually confer small increase in risk – for a complex phenotype. In one study, schizophrenia PRS did not predict CUD in controls or in subjects with psychiatric disorders other than schizophrenia in a Danish sample (Hjorthoj et al., 2021) arguing against shared genetic liability, but other PRS studies have documented genetic overlap (e.g., Power et al., 2014). As larger GWAS studies in CUD emerge, MR studies will be better able to throw light on the direction of causal relationship between regular/frequent cannabis use and psychosis. One study that examined additive and joint effects of polygenic liability to schizophrenia and multiple environmental risk factors noted that regular cannabis use and schizophrenia PRS additively increase the risk for schizophrenia (Guloksuz et al., 2019). Most recently, using the current largest GWAS of CUD, the authors did not find a significant causal effect CUD on schizophrenia. They concluded that common underlying genetic risk factors increased the risk for both CUD and schizophrenia rather than genetic risk for CUD having a causal effect on schizophrenia (Johnson et al., 2021).

In summary, genetically informed studies are challenging the previously assumed solely causal relationship between cannabis use, CUD, and schizophrenia with the uncovering of confounding and reverse causal effects to explain the relationship. However, larger studies of cannabis use and CUD will be needed to clarify the extent to which each of these mechanisms contribute to the observed relationship.

30.5.3 Genetics of Cannabis Use and CUD in Depression, Anxiety, and Suicide

As reviewed in-depth in Chapters 12–14, cannabis use, specifically in adolescence, has been associated with incidences of depression, anxiety, and suicidality (Gobbi et al., 2019). Causal, confounding, and reverse causal mechanisms that were discussed in the context of cannabis and psychosis are also relevant in the context of depression, anxiety, and suicidal ideations and attempts, albeit to a variable extent. By modelling the comorbidity of depression and CUD in a large sample of (n = 2,410) mono- and di-zygotic twins, Smolkina et al. (2017) noted a causal influence of CUD on depression rather than the two syndromes sharing correlated (confounding) liabilities. Another large twin study that included 13,896 twins found evidence for increased odds of major depression and suicidal ideation in monozygotic twins with frequent use of cannabis even after accounting for potential confounding variables. These findings provide support for a causal role of frequent cannabis use in depression and suicidal ideation beyond predisposing factors (Agrawal et al., 2017). Based on GWASs, cannabis use and CUD are positively genetically correlated with depressive symptoms and major depressive disorder (MDD) (Demontis et al., 2019; Johnson et al., 2020; Pasman et al., 2018). Further, polygenic risk for cannabis use is significantly associated with MDD and self-harm (Hodgson et al., 2020). While both cannabis use and CUD were positively correlated with MDD, the magnitude of the genetic correlation was significantly higher for CUD compared to cannabis use (Johnson et al., 2020). This study also noted that polygenic risk for CUD was significantly associated with anxiety, phobic, and dissociative disorders, in addition to MDD and related mood disorders (Johnson et al., 2020). Future studies in larger samples will be able to enumerate the extent of causal, reverse-causal, or confounding genetic relationships between these phenotypes.

30.5.4 Genetics of Cannabis Use and CUD in Cognition, School Performance, and Neurodevelopment

Since cannabis use typically begins in adolescence and features of CUD typically set in by young adulthood, the effects of cannabis use and CUD on cognition, scholastic performance, and educational attainment have been a topic of significant interest. The acute and lasting effects of cannabis on cognition have been reviewed in Chapter 9. Here we provide a summary of the genetic relationship between cannabis use and CUD with cognition and educational attainment. Twin studies suggest the role of twin-shared environment in the relationship between cannabis use and cognition, as well as education (e.g., Verweij et al., 2013). However, as noted before, while the genomic liability to cannabis use is positively correlated, the liability to CUD is negatively correlated with this educational attainment (Johnson et al., 2020). A part of this association could be explained by the positive association noted between CUD-PRS and human intelligence (Demontis et al., 2019). Furthermore, few of the genes identified to be associated with lifetime cannabis use, namely *CNNM2* and *CCDC101*, have previously been associated with intelligence and cognitive performance (Pasman et al., 2018). Unlike CUD, lifetime cannabis use has been found to be associated with higher fluid intelligence in phenotype association studies. This divergence is possibly explained by confounders including social factors, or personality factors that may increase the chance of initial exposure to cannabis but protect against progression to misuse.

In addition to psychosis, mood disorders, and scholastic outcomes, the genetic liability for cannabis use and CUD have been shown to overlap with liability for other neurodevelopmental processes. Similar to psychosis, the intersections of cannabis use and CUD with genetic diathesis for neurodevelopment can be understood from the following broad perspectives: (1) The genetic liability for or the genes implicated in cannabis use and CUD may have important functions relevant to other neurodevelopmental processes; (2) Genetic diathesis for neurodevelopmental disorders can pre-dispose individuals to cannabis use and CUD; and (3) Cannabis use and CUD can act as an environmental provocateur that moderates the genetic diathesis for other neurodevelopmental disorders to result in atypical neurodevelopmental outcomes. In Section 30.5.5 we briefly review each of these scenarios.

As noted in Section 30.3, early linkage and candidate gene association studies of CUD examined several candidate genes in the endocannabinoid system as well as those relevant to neuronal function (Agrawal and Lynskey, 2009), but these results were poorly replicated. Among the loci identified in the recent cannabis use GWAS, several genes such as *CADM2 and NCAM1* have critical neurodevelopmental functions (Pasman et al., 2018). Similarly, one of the two loci identified in GWAS of CUD with genome-wide significance threshold mapped to a region that regulates the expression of *FOXP2* gene in the brain, a gene identified to be critical for synaptic plasticity and language development (Johnson et al., 2020). In the same study, the authors noted that PRS for CUD was significantly associated with white matter volume in cannabis-naïve children, even after accounting for any other substance use or pre-natal exposure. On average, children in the higher quartile of CUD-PRS were noted to have 1% lower white matter volume compared to the lowest quartile. These results highlight the effect of genetic liability to CUD on neuronal development even prior to onset of cannabis use.

The genetic relationship between impulsivity, Attention Deficit Hyperactivity Disorder (ADHD), and SUDs has been extensively investigated (Wimberley et al., 2020). In a two-sample MR analysis, the liability for ADHD has been demonstrated to exert a causal effect on lifetime cannabis use (Soler Artigas et al., 2020). Furthermore, ADHD-PRS have also been shown to predict CUD in a Danish study (Hjorthoj et al., 2021). These results support the role of liability to a neurodevelopmental phenotype such as ADHD on development of cannabis use and CUD.

Lastly, cannabis use in early adolescence has been demonstrated to interact with schizophrenia genetic risk, measured as PRS, to result in lower cortical thickness in a large cohort of adolescents (French et al., 2015) (see Box 30.5).

30.5.5 Gene–Environment Inter-play

Twin-specific environmental factors are responsible for a substantial amount of variability in cannabis use and CUD (20–50%). Several environmental factors have been studied in the context of substance use and misuse – notably peer deviance, low parental monitoring, and childhood trauma. While these environments independently increase susceptibility to SUDs, there is also support for their inter-play with genetic risk. Across different studies, the heritability of substance use increases with increasing permissiveness of the environment. In other words, genetic factors appear to gain prominence in the context of

> **Box 30.5** Cannabis, brain development, and mental health
>
> - Genetic risk for cannabis use and CUD is positively correlated with the risk for depression, anxiety, and suicidal attempt.
> - Twin studies suggest that a mix of correlated and causal pathways may link cannabis use, CUD, and depression.
> - Educational attainment is positively genetically correlated with cannabis use, but negatively with CUD.
> - Genes implicated in cannabis use (*CADM2, NCAM1*) and CUD (*FOXP2*) have pleotropic influences on neurodevelopment.
> - Brain development shared genetic underpinnings with liability to CUD but not cannabis use.

drug-use promoting environments, which have been variously indexed by greater peer deviance and peer drug use, lower parental supervision, less religiosity, greater urbanicity, and access to drugs (Agrawal et al., 2010; Dick et al., 2007, 2009). While most of these environments are particularly risk-conferring during childhood and adolescence, the role of trauma appears to be enduring, although childhood exposure has typically been considered most severe (Meyers et al., 2018; Sartor et al., 2015; Werner et al., 2016).

Relatively few twin studies have systematically examined the impact of gene–environment inter-play underlying cannabis use and CUD specifically. Many studies that have examined this phenomenon have mostly relied on candidate genes in the dopaminergic or the serotonergic system (Milaniak et al., 2015). The interaction of polygenic risk for cannabis use and CUD with psychosocial vulnerabilities is being investigated. One such study found that PRS for cannabis use moderated cannabis use and CUD symptom-count only in a sub-group exposed to trauma but not in the trauma un-exposed sub-group (Meyers et al., 2019) but did not find a moderating effect of religiosity. Another study found that, while PRS for cannabis use and peer cannabis use were independently associated with longitudinal trajectories of cannabis use, they did not interact to modify risk (Johnson et al., 2019). As PRS become more informative, the ability to detect genetic effects that are specific to certain environments will significantly improve. The identification of environments that provide resilience against genetic vulnerability and genotypes that confer plasticity in environmental response will be critical if future prevention and intervention efforts are to derive knowledge from genomic studies.

30.6 Conclusion

Twin and genomic studies have clearly documented that, much like other substance use and psychiatrically relevant traits, cannabis use and CUD are polygenic and multi-factorial traits. Recent studies of cannabis-naïve youth also suggest that subtle pre-existing variability in brain structure may precede onset of cannabis use. A portion of the comorbidity between CUD and psychosocial (e.g., educational attainment), psychiatric (e.g., psychosis, suicide), and health-related (e.g., cognition, body mass index) traits is attributable to shared genetic pathways. Interestingly, despite extensive prior literature linking cannabis use and CUD to genes engaged in endocannabinoid signalling pathways, loci in these genes were not identified. This may speak to the extremely small effects that are typical for such highly heterogeneous and polygenic traits, and the lower sample size of CUD GWAS relative to other psychiatric disorders. It is plausible that, as has been noted for other psychiatric disorders, increasing sample size will produce loci in these genes, or those in other genes that exert regulatory effects on endocannabinoid signalling. Yet, the novel loci that are being identified, such as those in *FOXP2*, indicate genetic pathways that are more generally related to risky behaviours. Despite these discoveries, polygenic risk scores (PRS) for cannabis use and CUD are currently only responsible for a very modest proportion of attributable risk, <1% and, therefore, while of interest in scientific studies, are of limited clinical utility. Importantly, genetic susceptibility for CUD should be viewed within the context of environmental factors. Particularly for traits such as cannabis use and CUD that are routinely subjected to environmental variability (e.g., policy-level, potency), genetic contributions may vary within these environmental contexts.

Acknowledgement

Dr Agrawal receives funding from the National Institutes of Health. She is grateful for a career development grant from the National Institute on Drug Abuse (NIDA: K02DA032573) which has supported her genetic studies of cannabis use and CUD. Dr Ganesh is supported by a NARSAD young investigator grant from the Brain and Behavior Research Foundation.

References

Abdellaoui, A., Smit, D. J. A., van den Brink, W., et al. (2021). Genomic relationships across psychiatric disorders including substance use disorders. *Drug Alcohol Depend*, **220**, 108535.

Agrawal, A., Balasubramanian, S., Smith, E. K., et al. (2010). Peer substance involvement modifies genetic influences on regular substance involvement in young women. *Addiction*, **105**, 1844–1853.

Agrawal, A., and Lynskey, M. T. (2009). Candidate genes for cannabis use disorders: Findings, challenges and directions. *Addiction*, **104**, 518–532.

Agrawal, A., Neale, M. C., Prescott, C. A., et al. (2004). A twin study of early cannabis use and subsequent use and abuse/dependence of other illicit drugs. *Psychol Med*, **34**, 1227–1237.

Agrawal, A., Nelson, E. C., Bucholz, K. K., et al. (2017). Major depressive disorder, suicidal thoughts and behaviours, and cannabis involvement in discordant twins: A retrospective cohort study. *Lancet Psychiatry*, **4**, 706–714.

Agrawal, A., Pergadia, M. L., Saccone, S. F., et al. (2008). An autosomal linkage scan for cannabis use disorders in the nicotine addiction genetics project. *Arch Gen Psychiatry*, **65**, 713–721.

Agrawal, A., Verweij, K. J., Gillespie, N. A., et al. (2012). The genetics of addiction-a translational perspective. *Transl Psychiatry*, **2**, e140.

Bierut, L. J., Dinwiddie, S. H., Begleiter, H., et al. (1998). Familial transmission of substance dependence: Alcohol, marijuana, cocaine, and habitual smoking: A report from the Collaborative Study on the Genetics of Alcoholism. *Arch Gen Psychiatry*, **55**, 982–988.

Demontis, D., Rajagopal, V. M., Thorgeirsson, T. E., et al. (2019).

Genome-wide association study implicates CHRNA2 in cannabis use disorder. *Nat Neurosci*, **22**, 1066–1074.

Di Forti, M., Marconi, A., Carra, E., et al. (2015). Proportion of patients in south London with first-episode psychosis attributable to use of high potency cannabis: A case-control study. *Lancet Psychiatry*, **2**, 233–238.

Dick, D. M., Bernard, M., Aliev, F., et al. (2009). The role of socioregional factors in moderating genetic influences on early adolescent behavior problems and alcohol use. *Alcohol Clin Exp Res*, **33**, 1739–1748.

Dick, D. M., Viken, R., Purcell, S., et al. (2007). Parental monitoring moderates the importance of genetic and environmental influences on adolescent smoking. *J Abnorm Psychol*, **116**, 213–218.

Ellgren, M., Spano, S. M., and Hurd, Y. L. (2007). Adolescent cannabis exposure alters opiate intake and opioid limbic neuronal populations in adult rats. *Neuropsychopharmacology*, **32**, 607–615.

French, L., Gray, C., Leonard, G., et al. (2015). Early cannabis use, polygenic risk score for schizophrenia and brain maturation in adolescence. *JAMA Psychiatry*, **72**, 1002–1011.

Gage, S. H., Jones, H. J., Burgess, S., et al. (2017). Assessing causality in associations between cannabis use and schizophrenia risk: A two-sample Mendelian randomization study. *Psychol Med*, **47**, 971–980.

Gillespie, N. A., and Kendler, K. S. (2021). Use of genetically informed methods to clarify the nature of the association between cannabis use and risk for schizophrenia. *JAMA Psychiatry*, **78**, 467–468.

Gillespie, N. A., Kendler, K. S., Prescott, C. A., et al. (2007). Longitudinal modeling of genetic and environmental influences on

self-reported availability of psychoactive substances: Alcohol, cigarettes, marijuana, cocaine and stimulants. *Psychol Med*, **37**, 947–959.

Gobbi, G., Atkin, T., Zytynski, T., et al. (2019). Association of cannabis use in adolescence and risk of depression, anxiety, and suicidality in young adulthood: A systematic review and meta-analysis. *JAMA Psychiatry*, **76**, 426–434.

Guloksuz, S., Pries, L. K., Delespaul, P., et al. (2019). Examining the independent and joint effects of molecular genetic liability and environmental exposures in schizophrenia: Results from the EUGEI study. *World Psychiatry*, **18**, 173–182.

Hasin, D. S. (2018). US epidemiology of cannabis use and associated problems. *Neuropsychopharmacology*, **43**, 195–212.

Hasin, D. S., Saha, T. D., Kerridge, B. T., et al. (2015). Prevalence of marijuana use disorders in the United States between 2001–2002 and 2012–2013. *JAMA Psychiatry*, **72**, 1235–1242.

Hatoum, A. S., Morrison, C. L., Colbert, S. M. C., et al. (2021). Genetic liability to cannabis use disorder and COVID-19 hospitalization. *Biol Psychiatry Glob Open Sci*, **1**, 317–323.

Hines, L. A., Morley, K. I., Rijsdijk, F., et al. (2018). Overlap of heritable influences between cannabis use disorder, frequency of use and opportunity to use cannabis: Trivariate twin modelling and implications for genetic design. *Psychol Med*, **48**, 2786–2793.

Hjorthoj, C., Uddin, M. J., Wimberley, T., et al. (2021). No evidence of associations between genetic liability for schizophrenia and development of cannabis use disorder. *Psychol Med*, **51**, 479–484.

Hodgson, K., Coleman, J. R. I., Hagenaars, S. P., et al. (2020).

Cannabis use, depression and self-harm: Phenotypic and genetic relationships. *Addiction*, 115, 482–492.

Jang, S. K., Saunders, G., Liu, M., et al. (2022). Genetic correlation, pleiotropy, and causal associations between substance use and psychiatric disorder. *Psychol Med*, 52, 968–978.

Johnson, E. C., Demontis, D., Thorgeirsson, T. E., et al. (2020). A large-scale genome-wide association study meta-analysis of cannabis use disorder. *Lancet Psychiatry*, 7, 1032–1045.

Johnson, E. C., Hatoum, A. S., Deak, J. D., et al. (2021). The relationship between cannabis and schizophrenia: A genetically informed perspective. *Addiction*, 116, 3227–3234.

Johnson, E. C., Tillman, R., Aliev, F., et al. (2019). Exploring the relationship between polygenic risk for cannabis use, peer cannabis use and the longitudinal course of cannabis involvement. *Addiction*, 114, 687–697.

Kandel, D., and Kandel, E. (2015). The gateway hypothesis of substance abuse: Developmental, biological and societal perspectives. *Acta Paediatr*, 104, 130–137.

Kendler, K. S., Jacobson, K. C., Prescott, C. A., et al. (2003). Specificity of genetic and environmental risk factors for use and abuse/dependence of cannabis, cocaine, hallucinogens, sedatives, stimulants, and opiates in male twins. *Am J Psychiatry*, 160, 687–695.

Kendler, K. S., Schmitt, E., Aggen, S. H., et al. (2008). Genetic and environmental influences on alcohol, caffeine, cannabis, and nicotine use from early adolescence to middle adulthood. *Arch Gen Psychiatry*, 65, 674–682.

Lessem, J. M., Hopfer, C. J., Haberstick, B. C., et al. (2006). Relationship between adolescent marijuana use and young adult illicit drug use. *Behav Genet*, 36, 498–506.

Linnér, R. K., Mallard, T. T., Barr, P. B., et al. (2020). Multivariate genomic analysis of 1.5 million people identifies genes related to addiction, antisocial behavior, and health. *bioRxiv*, 2020.10.16.342501.

Lynskey, M. T., Heath, A. C., Bucholz, K. K., et al. (2003). Escalation of drug use in early-onset cannabis users vs co-twin controls. *JAMA*, 289, 427–433.

Lynskey, M. T., Vink, J. M., and Boomsma, D. I. (2006). Early onset cannabis use and progression to other drug use in a sample of Dutch twins. *Behav Genet*, 36, 195–200.

Marees, A. T., Smit, D. J. A., Ong, J. S., et al. (2020). Potential influence of socioeconomic status on genetic correlations between alcohol consumption measures and mental health. *Psychol Med*, 50, 484–498.

Merikangas, K. R., Li, J. J., Stipelman, B., et al. (2009). The familial aggregation of cannabis use disorders. *Addiction*, 104, 622–629.

Meyers, J. L., Salvatore, J. E., Aliev, F., et al. (2019). Psychosocial moderation of polygenic risk for cannabis involvement: The role of trauma exposure and frequency of religious service attendance. *Transl Psychiatry*, 9, 269.

Meyers, J. L., Sartor, C. E., Werner, K. B., et al. (2018). Childhood interpersonal violence and adult alcohol, cannabis, and tobacco use disorders: variation by race/ethnicity? *Psychol Med*, 48, 1540–1550.

Milaniak, I., Watson, B., and Jaffee, S. R. (2015). Gene–environment interplay and substance use: A review of recent findings. *Curr Addict Rep*, 2, 364–371.

Morris, J., Bailey, M. E. S., Baldassarre, D., et al. (2019). Genetic variation in CADM2 as a link between psychological traits and obesity. *Sci Rep*, 9, 7339.

Palmer, R. H., Button, T. M., Rhee, S. H., et al. (2012). Genetic etiology of the common liability to drug dependence: Evidence of common and specific mechanisms for DSM-IV dependence symptoms. *Drug Alcohol Depend*, 123, S24–S32.

Pasman, J. A., Verweij, K. J. H., Gerring, Z., et al. (2018). GWAS of lifetime cannabis use reveals new risk loci, genetic overlap with psychiatric traits, and a causal influence of schizophrenia. *Nat Neurosci*, 21, 1161–1170.

Power, R. A., Verweij, K. J., Zuhair, M., et al. (2014). Genetic predisposition to schizophrenia associated with increased use of cannabis. *Mol Psychiatry*, 19, 1201–1204.

Sartor, C. E., Agrawal, A., Grant, J. D., et al. (2015). Differences between African-American and European-American women in the association of childhood sexual abuse with initiation of marijuana use and progression to problem use. *J Stud Alcohol Drugs*, 76, 569–577.

Scherma, M., Qvist, J. S., Asok, A., et al. (2020). Cannabinoid exposure in rat adolescence reprograms the initial behavioral, molecular, and epigenetic response to cocaine. *Proc Natl Acad Sci USA*, 117, 9991–10002.

Secades-Villa, R., Garcia-Rodriguez, O., Jin, C. J., et al. (2015). Probability and predictors of the cannabis gateway effect: A national study. *Int J Drug Policy*, 26, 135–142.

Smolkina, M., Morley, K. I., Rijsdijk, F., et al. (2017). Cannabis and depression: A twin model approach to co-morbidity. *Behav Genet*, 47, 394–404.

Soler Artigas, M., Sanchez-Mora, C., Rovira, P., et al. (2020). Attention-deficit/hyperactivity disorder and

331

lifetime cannabis use: Genetic overlap and causality. *Mol Psychiatry*, **25**, 2493–2503.

Tsuang, M. T., Bar, J. L., Harley, R. M., et al. (2001). The Harvard twin study of substance abuse: What we have learned. *Harv Rev Psychiatry*, **9**, 267–279.

Vaucher, J., Keating, B. J., Lasserre, A. M., et al. (2018). Cannabis use and risk of schizophrenia: A Mendelian randomization study. *Mol Psychiatry*, **23**, 1287–1292.

Verweij, K. J., Huizink, A. C., Agrawal, A., et al. (2013). Is the relationship between early-onset cannabis use and educational attainment causal or due to common liability? *Drug Alcohol Depend*, **133**, 580–586.

Verweij, K. J., Zietsch, B. P., Liu, J. Z., et al. (2012). No association of candidate genes with cannabis use in a large sample of Australian twin families. *Addict Biol*, **17**, 687–690.

Verweij, K. J., Zietsch, B. P., Lynskey, M. T., et al. (2010). Genetic and environmental influences on cannabis use initiation and problematic use: A meta-analysis of twin studies. *Addiction*, **105**, 417–430.

Vilar-Ribó, L., Sánchez-Mora, C., Rovira, P., et al. (2021). Genetic overlap and causality between substance use disorder and attention-deficit and hyperactivity disorder. *Am J Med Genet B Neuropsychiatr Genet*, **186**, 140–150.

Vink, J. M., Veul, L., Abdellaoui, A., et al. (2020). Illicit drug use and the genetic overlap with cannabis use. *Drug Alcohol Depend*, **213**, 108102.

Vrieze, S. I., Hicks, B. M., Iacono, W. G., et al. (2012). Decline in genetic influence on the co-occurrence of alcohol, marijuana, and nicotine dependence symptoms from age 14 to 29. *Am J Psychiatry*, **169**, 1073–1081.

Waldman, I. D., Poore, H. E., Luningham, J. M., et al. (2020). Testing structural models of psychopathology at the genomic level. *World Psychiatry*, **19**, 350–359.

Werner, K. B., McCutcheon, V. V., Agrawal, A., et al. (2016). The association of specific traumatic experiences with cannabis initiation and transition to problem use: Differences between African-American and European-American women. *Drug Alcohol Depend*, **162**, 162–169.

Wimberley, T., Agerbo, E., Horsdal, H. T., et al. (2020). Genetic liability to ADHD and substance use disorders in individuals with ADHD. *Addiction*, **115**, 1368–1377.

Xian, H., Scherrer, J. F., Grant, J. D., et al. (2008). Genetic and environmental contributions to nicotine, alcohol and cannabis dependence in male twins. *Addiction*, **103**, 1391–1398.

Yan, X., Wang, Z., Schmidt, V., et al. (2018). Cadm2 regulates body weight and energy homeostasis in mice. *Mol Metab*, **8**, 180–188.

Chapter

31

Snoozing on Pot: Cannabis and Sleep

Patrick D. Skosnik and Toral S. Surti

31.1 Summary

The average human spends approximately 25 years in the dark. That is to say, roughly a third of an individual's life-span is spent in sleep, underscoring sleep's biological necessity. Research on the importance of sleep has grown substantially in recent years. Healthy sleep serves many critical functions, including proper neurodevelopment, energy conservation, brain waste clearance, modulation of immune responses, neurocognition, mood, memory consolidation, and performance/vigilance. Surprisingly, regardless of its importance, sleep is relatively understudied in psychiatry.

Evidence has emerged in recent years demonstrating that sleep is partially modulated by the brain's endocannabinoid system. Additionally, both acute and chronic cannabis exposure disrupts several aspects of sleep. Therefore, the current chapter will summarize the current state of the literature on cannabinoids and sleep. First, a review of the importance of sleep in mental health will be undertaken. Next, a brief discussion of the neurobiology of sleep and the role of endocannabinoids will be considered. What is known about the effects of acute and chronic cannabinoids on sleep will follow, including recent research on treatments for sleep disturbances during cannabis withdrawal. Lastly, potential future directions in the emerging field of cannabinoids and sleep will be put forward, including the role of cannabinoids and sleep in psychosis.

31.2 Overview of Sleep Structure in Humans and Biological Importance

Sleep is defined as behavioural quiescence with decreased responsiveness to weak stimuli, albeit arousable with robust or salient stimuli. If sleep is limited, there is an increased need for it due to homeostatic drive. This homeostatic control of sleep suggests that its function is vital and, in every known

animal studied (including invertebrates and animals without a central nervous system), these periods of rest are observed (Anafi et al., 2019). Indeed, across species, healthy sleep serves many critical functions, including proper neurodevelopment, energy conservation, brain waste clearance, modulation of immune responses, neurocognition, mood, memory consolidation, and performance/vigilance (Zielinski et al., 2016).

In humans (and in some non-human animals), it is possible to use polysomnography (PSG) to determine the quantity and quality of sleep. PSG uses multiple sensors for physiological measurements, including cardiac activity, breathing, muscle activity, brain activity with electroencephalography (EEG), and eye movements with electrooculography (EOG) throughout a period of expected sleep. Patterns of combinations of brain, muscle, and eye activity have been categorized into different stages of sleep.

Human sleep includes rapid eye movement (REM) and non-REM (NREM) sleep. NREM sleep occurs in three stages, NREM1, NREM2, and NREM3 (NREM3 was previously split into NREM3 and NREM4, but these have now been consolidated according to the American Academy of Sleep Medicine, AASM). As shown in Figure 31.1A (Sleep Hypnogram), adult sleep begins in NREM1, transitions to deeper sleep through NREM2 and then NREM3, and ultimately reaches REM sleep. Each successive stage is more difficult to arouse from. REM sleep, like wakefulness, is a period of high metabolic activity in the brain, though muscle tone is lowest in REM. NREM sleep is a period of low metabolic activity in the brain. NREM1 is light sleep. NREM3 is characterized predominantly by slow wave sleep (SWS), named as such due to the large amplitude, low frequency (0.5–2 Hz) oscillations that characterize it (Figure 31.1B EEG Spectrogram). In normal adult sleep, humans' cycle through four-to-six cycles of NREM/REM sleep over the typical course of a night, so that each sleep cycle

A. Sleep Hypnogram

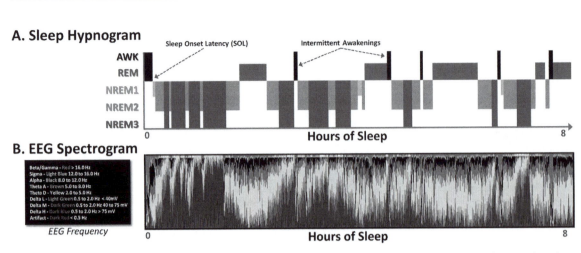

Figure 31.1 (A) A representative hypnogram of healthy human sleep. As can be seen, NREM sleep, particularly NREM3, decreases throughout the sleep cycle while REM sleep increases. (B) A corresponding sleep EEG spectrogram of healthy human sleep. Note the preponderance of high amplitude slow wave (delta) sleep in NREM sleep, low amplitude mixed frequency EEG in other sleep stages, and the predominance of low amplitude beta/gamma frequencies during wake periods. A black and white version of this figure will appear in some formats. For the colour version, please refer to the plate section.

lasts about 60–120 minutes. Typically, these cycles are not identical over the course of the night; early in the night, there is more NREM and SWS predominance, and later there is more time in REM sleep. PSG measures of interest for this review include total sleep time (TST), sleep onset latency (SOL), wake time after sleep onset (WASO), sleep efficiency (SE), minutes spent in each stage, percentage of sleep for each stage, latency to each stage, and number of cycles.

31.3 Sleep and Mental Health Are Intricately Connected

Although humans spend roughly a third of their lives in slumber, and major advances have taken place with respect to the biological necessity of sleep, the role of sleep has been relatively understudied in psychiatry. As aptly expressed by Bassetti et al. (2015), 'Despite these important and exciting new insights, the opportunities of diagnosing and treating sleep–wake disturbances are frequently not adequately addressed or are neglected in neurological and psychiatric practice . . .'. That being said, the role of altered sleep in psychopathology is increasingly being appreciated by clinicians and researchers alike.

For example, sleep disturbances in anxiety and mood disorders have long been recognized, so that sleep disturbances are part of the diagnostic criteria

for these illnesses. The majority of people with generalized anxiety disorder, post-traumatic stress disorder, and major depressive disorder (MDD) have problems with sleep. In MDD, there are characteristic PSG findings including decreased REM latency, increased REM, and decreased SWS (Krystal, 2020). The diagnosis of mania in bipolar disorder requires three of seven symptoms spanning at least one week, one of which is decreased need for sleep (DSM-5).

Germane to the topic of this book, sleep disturbances are very common in schizophrenia (SZ), even though sleep abnormalities are not part of the diagnostic criteria for psychotic disorders (Chouinard et al., 2004; Cohrs, 2008).

Sleep disturbances are not merely a frequent manifestation of psychiatric illnesses; they also influence and contribute to psychiatric symptoms. For example, sleep problems in SZ are associated with worse psychotic symptoms (e.g., hallucinations, delusions, and disorganized thinking and behaviour) (Reeve et al., 2015); greater cognitive impairment (Cazzullo et al., 1977; Manoach et al., 2004, 2016); poorer quality-of-life (Hofstetter et al., 2005; Ritsner et al., 2004; Xiang et al., 2009); and increased risk for future suicide attempts (Li et al., 2016). Insomnia (Robertson et al., 2019) and circadian rhythm disorders (Jones and Benca, 2015; Zanini et al., 2013) are more common in SZ than in healthy populations, and circadian disturbances in those at clinically high risk for developing psychosis are associated with worsened prognosis for psychotic symptoms and functioning (Lunsford-Avery et al., 2017). In addition to frequent (subjective) complaints about sleep, PSG studies have shown objective evidence of sleep disturbances, including decreased TST, decreased sleep efficiency, increased SOL, increased WASO, decreased slow-wave sleep, and disturbances in REM sleep in SZ (Chan et al., 2017). The importance of characterizing sleep in SZ is also underscored by preliminary data which suggests that sleep can disrupt learning in SZ (Surti et al., 2018).

Given the relationship between cannabis and psychosis, the emerging evidence of alterations in sleep in SZ is intriguing, given that (1) the endocannabinoid system may be integrally involved in the neurobiology of sleep, (2) acute and chronic exposure to cannabis has been shown to affect sleep, and (3) endocannabinoid dysfunction has been reported in SZ. The remainder of this chapter will, thus, focus on the role of cannabinoids in sleep.

31.4 Neurobiology of Sleep: Potential Role of Cannabinoids (Pre-clinical Evidence)

31.4.1 Basic Neurobiology of Sleep

Sleep is a highly complex neurobiological process, which involves multiple functionally redundant/parallel neural networks and several neurotransmitter systems (Schwartz and Kilduff, 2015). These networks include nuclei that are either wake- or sleep-promoting, which then interact with areas that modulate circadian rhythms (e.g., the suprachiasmatic nucleus). Wake-promoting networks primarily include monoaminergic and cholinergic systems, particularly in the brainstem ascending reticular activating system (ARAS). For example, stimulation of the ARAS results in low voltage, mixed high-frequency EEG which is a signature of wakefulness (and, to an extent, REM sleep). Excitatory inputs to the ARAS are largely from the lateral hypothalamus via orexin neurons. Sleep-promoting nuclei include the pons, lateral hypothalamus, and brainstem, and they are primarily mediated by the inhibitory neurotransmitter gamma aminobutyric acid (GABA). This may be particularly relevant to the role of cannabinoids in sleep, as central cannabinoid receptors (CB1) are largely involved in the modulation of GABA release throughout the brain (Lu and Mackie, 2016). Lastly, while beyond the scope of this chapter, it should be noted that various other neurotransmitters are implicated in the sleep/wake cycle including adenosine, neuronal nitric oxide, and several neuropeptides (Schwartz and Kilduff, 2015).

31.4.2 Endocannabinoids and Sleep

Evidence has accumulated suggesting that the endocannabinoid system, including the highly ubiquitous CB1 receptor and the endocannabinoid neuromodulators N-arachidonoylethanolamine (anandamide) and 2-arachidonoylglycerol (2-AG), is intricately involved in the normal sleep/wake cycle. For example, Santucci et al. (1996) first demonstrated that the CB1 antagonist/inverse agonist SR141716A decreased the time spent in NREM and REM sleep in rats as assessed with EEG (Santucci et al., 1996). The authors thus postulated that activation of CB1 receptors by endocannabinoids may be part of the normal sleep/wake cycle in mammals. This finding has since been replicated with the CB1 antagonist AM251 (Goonawardena et al., 2015) and AM281 (Pava et al., 2016). Supporting the notion that endocannabinoids are involved in sleep, it has been shown that the fatty acid oleamide, which does not bind to CB1 receptors, may be promoting sleep by enhancing anandamide levels via the inhibition of fatty acid amide hydrolase (FAAH), the enzyme responsible for the metabolism of anandamide (Mechoulam et al., 1997). Subsequently, it was shown that intracerebral ventricular administration of anandamide in rats increased NREM and REM sleep in rats (Murillo-Rodriguez et al., 1998), an effect which was blocked by the co-administration of SR141716A (Murillo-Rodriguez et al., 2001). Moreover, evidence suggests that anandamide exhibits diurnal variation, with increased levels in the hypothalamus during sleep in rodents (Murillo-Rodriguez et al., 2006). This diurnal variation of endocannabinoids has also been shown in assays of peripheral levels of anandamide in humans (Vaughn et al., 2010). Lastly it should be noted that 2-AG may also be involved in sleep modulation, as injection of 2-AG into the lateral hypothalamus increases REM sleep (but not NREM), and this effect was blocked by AM251 (Perez-Morales et al., 2013).

In sum, the findings described in this section provide strong evidence that the endocannabinoids anandamide and 2-AG are sleep-promoting. Activation of the endocannabinoid system is tightly regulated spatially and temporally. While endocannabinoids are produced on demand, rapidly removed/inactivated, and have very local effects, delta-9-tetrahydrocannabinol (THC) by contrast produces more generalized and longer lasting effects (Lu and Mackie, 2016). Furthermore, anandamide and 2-AG are partial agonist and full agonists of cannabinoid receptors, respectively, with a 3- to 4-fold higher affinity for the CB1 versus CB2. By contrast, THC is a partial agonist which binds to CB1 and CB2 with the same affinity. Overall, THC has non-physiological effects that may disrupt normal endocannabinoid functioning. Given this putative role of the endocannabinoid system in the sleep/wake cycle, it would thus follow that the 'non-physiological' activation of CB1 receptors by exogenous cannabinoid agonists (i.e., THC) would disrupt normal sleep mechanisms.

31.4.3 Exocannabinoids and Sleep

Early work on the effect of cannabis extracts on sleep in various pre-clinical models suggest that phytocannabinoids, like THC, alter sleep, with a general trend of increasing NREM while decreasing REM, and tolerance to some of these effects has been observed (for a review, see Kesner and Lovinger, 2020). More recently, it has been shown that the systemic administration of THC decreased REM sleep in rodents (Carley et al., 2002), although, surprisingly, this effect was not blocked by the CB1 antagonist AM251 or the CB2 antagonist AM630 (Calik and Carley, 2017), suggesting the additional possibility of a non-cannabinoid receptor mechanism. Congruent with the abovementioned work with phytocannabinoids, Pava et al. (2016) demonstrated that the potent synthetic CB1 agonist CP47,497 increased NREM and decreased REM sleep, effects that were blocked by the CB1 antagonist AM281 (Pava et al., 2016). Similar to Pava et al. (2016), these results were also observed with the synthetic CB1 agonist WIN55,212 (Goonawardena et al., 2015). Taken together, these

pre-clinical findings on both endo- and exocannabinoids summarized in this section provide the backdrop and mechanistic foundation whereby cannabis exposure may alter normal sleep function in humans.

31.5 Effects of Exocannabinoids (Cannabis and THC) on Human Sleep

31.5.1 Acute Effects

Clinicians are likely very familiar with patients who state they use cannabis as a sleep aid. This clinical experience is corroborated by a study of more than 1,500 individuals utilizing medicinal cannabis from a dispensary that found nearly two-thirds of patients reported decreasing the use of sleep aids after initiation of medical cannabis (Piper et al., 2017). While the common impression of those using cannabis is that it promotes more restful sleep, laboratory sleep studies of people administered cannabis or THC show more nuanced effects.

Acute effects of cannabis on sleep have been examined in small studies, with different doses and different preparations of cannabis and THC. The studies vary in days of drug administration and route of administration, either oral or inhaled. In most studies, cannabis or THC has been given prior to normal sleep onset time. In addition to these differences among studies, the acute effects of cannabis seem to also depend upon whether there is recent regular cannabis use, as will be reviewed in Section 31.5.2. Finally, most studies of the acute effects of cannabis on sleep have been done in a small number of young, healthy male volunteers, so a true understanding of the effects of cannabis on sleep will require larger studies with more diverse participants. These studies have shown themes of an increase in SWS, a possibly related decrease in REM sleep, decreased SOL, and decreased WASO, though not consistently.

Increased SWS has been reported with oral THC (Feinberg et al., 1975; Freemon, 1982; Pivik et al., 1972) and with smoked cannabis (Barratt et al., 1974) in small studies of young healthy people. Barratt et al. (1974) observed that the percentage of sleep that was SWS peaked on the fourth night of marijuana use, and then decreased so that, after the tenth night of administration, the percentage of SWS sleep was lower than baseline, suggesting tolerance to the SWS-inducing effect of cannabis. With high nightly doses of oral THC, however, a decrease in SWS was not seen after 7–10 nights (Feinberg et al., 1975). Not all studies of acute THC administration have resulted in increased SWS (Hosko et al., 1973; Nicholson et al., 2004). In their crossover design study where 8 people were given placebo, 5 mg orobuccal THC/5 mg cannabidiol (CBD), 15 mg THC, or 15 mg THC with 15 mg CBD each on 1 night with challenges separated by 1 week, Nicholson et al. (2004) did not observe increases in SWS with THC alone but, rather, saw decreased SWS only when THC was given with CBD.

Changes in REM with acute THC or cannabis administration have also been found, including a decreased percentage of REM sleep (Feinberg et al., 1975; Pivik et al., 1972) and decreased eye movements, but REM changes have also not been observed consistently (Freemon, 1972; Hosko et al., 1973; Nicholson et al., 2004). Interestingly, some researchers have observed a paradoxical decrease in REM with shortened REM latency (Feinberg et al., 1976), suggesting that the decreased REM latency may not be due to REM rebound effect following REM deficit.

Increases in TST and decreases in WASO and SOL have not been seen as often as one would expect given how often people report using cannabis to ameliorate sleep. Decreased SOL was found with oral THC in otherwise healthy people with insomnia, but there was no significant change in sleep interruptions and no reported change in TST, as measured by researchers observing sleeping participants every 15 minutes (Cousens and DiMascio, 1973). In a study of four young men, TST was higher on the night of oral THC administration and the following night compared to baseline (Pivik et al., 1972). Studies have also found no improvements in TST, SOL, and WASO (Nicholson et al., 2004).

31.5.2 Chronic Effects

Determining the long-term effects of chronic cannabis exposure on sleep is complicated by the possibility that disordered sleep may be a characteristic of people who go on to use cannabis – poor sleep may drive people to use cannabis, or habitual cannabis administration, and poor sleep may share common

underlying neurobiology, including genetics (Winiger et al., 2021). Subjective measures of sleep are less accurate in individuals using cannabis compared to those who are not (McPherson et al., 2021), and insomnia is present in 25% of cannabis users (Pacek et al., 2017). Age of onset of regular cannabis may also predict adult sleep duration/quality. In one study, onset of cannabis use before age 17 years was associated with shorter reported sleep duration compared to those who did not use and those with an age of onset of regular cannabis use after the age of 17 (Winiger et al., 2019). The relationship between the age of initiation of regular cannabis use and sleep duration, however, is more complicated; in the same study, later age of onset was associated with longer sleep duration than those who never used cannabis. Additionally, when 170 cannabis users were compared to 170 non-using volunteers, the association between early cannabis use and sleep problems was only seen in women (McPherson et al., 2021).

Objective measures of sleep in habitual cannabis users also demonstrate sleep abnormalities. In a study of 87 adults who used cannabis regularly, sleep efficiency was <85% in 55% of the sample, 31% had SOL >30 minutes, and half had WASO >30 minutes (Pacek et al., 2017). Comparisons of sleep in cannabis users versus non-users have found decreased SWS (Pranikoff et al., 1973) and an increased percentage of REM sleep in cannabis users (Karacan et al., 1976). Further decreases in SWS and increases in percentage REM sleep are seen with withdrawal after chronic use, as discussed in Section 31.5.3.

31.5.3 Withdrawal Effects

Compared to acute or chronic cannabis exposure, the clinical effects of cannabis withdrawal on sleep, at least for an important sub-group of people, seem the most significant. In people meeting criteria for cannabis withdrawal syndrome, nearly 70% have reported sleep disturbances (Livne et al., 2019). While sleep in cannabis withdrawal differs compared to the sleep during regular cannabis use that preceded withdrawal, it is less clear whether sleep during cannabis withdrawal differs from sleep in healthy people who do not use cannabis. A study of 20 people abstaining for 24–36 hours from their regular cannabis use compared to abstinent age- and sex-matched control volunteers showed no differences in any sleep parameters (Karacan et al., 1976). It may be, however, there is a sub-set of people who, after regular cannabis use, are at particularly high risk for sleep disturbances during withdrawal. Consistent with the idea that a sub-set of people are prone to sleep abnormalities with cannabis withdrawal, people using cannabis who reported sleep problems as symptoms of past cannabis withdrawal had significant differences in sleep compared to healthy abstinent volunteers (Bolla et al., 2008).

Studies have shown that, during withdrawal from regular cannabis use in young adults, TST decreases and SOL increases (Bolla et al., 2010; Feinberg et al., 1975; Freemon, 1982). In one study of seven young men with cannabis withdrawal, the decrease in TST was explained by increased SOL (Feinberg et al., 1975), however, increased WASO during cannabis withdrawal has also been found (Bolla et al., 2010) so that both difficulty falling asleep and increased midnight awakenings may be contributing.

Decreased SWS has also been repeatedly seen during cannabis withdrawal (Bolla et al., 2008; Feinberg et al., 1975). In adults, SWS does not normalize after four weeks of abstinence (D'Souza et al., 2019) and represents a potential therapeutic target for cannabis use disorder. It is possible that recovery of SWS varies with age or other biological factors, as suggested by a study of adolescents who used alcohol and marijuana regularly (Cohen-Zion et al., 2009). Compared to healthy, abstinent adolescents, those using substances had decreased SWS after 2 days of abstinence, but this SWS deficit had recovered by 28 days of abstinence. While it may be that the shorter duration of use in adolescents leads to fewer consequences for sleep in extended abstinence or that the adolescent brain is able to more quickly recover in withdrawal, another possibility is there are distinct long-term effects of cannabis withdrawal on brain health at different stages of the lifespan. Given the continued high rates of cannabis use in adolescents (Albaugh et al., 2021), and increasing use among the elderly (Han et al., 2017), it is worth studying further whether there are distinct effects of cannabis withdrawal on sleep from adolescence to advanced age. Nearly all studies of sleep during cannabis withdrawal (as well as during acute and chronic use of cannabis) have been done in young, healthy adults who are mostly male.

REM is often altered, usually increased (possibly due to REM rebound), in cannabis withdrawal. Withdrawal from oral THC, oral marijuana extract, or cannabis in male cannabis users has resulted in an increased percentage of REM sleep and a decreased REM latency (D'Souza et al., 2019; Feinberg et al., 1975, 1976). This phenomenon has also been observed in a very small (n = 2) sample of female cannabis users (Freemon, 1972). Usually the first sleep cycle has the least REM sleep, but this is not consistently the case during cannabis withdrawal, and REM may take >10 days of abstinence to normalize (Feinberg et al., 1976). These findings of increased REM and earlier REM onset are consistent with REM rebound, an increase in REM to either compensate for a prior deficit in REM sleep or adapt to physiologic stress during wakefulness (Suchecki et al., 2012).

In addition to changes in basic sleep architecture, other features of sleep are probably altered in cannabis withdrawal. Periodic limb movements (PLMs) are jerking movements of the limbs, usually the legs, preceding REM sleep, and when they disrupt sleep in the absence of another sleep disorder, periodic limb movement disorder (PLMD) is diagnosed. PLMs often co-occur with restless leg syndrome and are most common in people over age 65 years, but after young adult heavy cannabis users were abstinent for 2 weeks, PLMs were increased, and associated with both higher cannabis use and longer duration of use (Bolla et al., 2010).

31.6 Treating Cannabis-Related Sleep Disturbances

While there are currently no FDA-approved treatments for cannabis use disorder, there are promising developments in this area utilizing drugs that target the brain's endocannabinoid system. Chronic exposure to exogenous cannabinoids induces down-regulation of CB1 receptors (D'Souza et al., 2016; Hirvonen et al., 2012). This reduction in CB1, coupled with the decrease in THC during cannabis withdrawal, leads to markedly decreased CB1 activity and endocannabinoid dysregulation. Thus, one pharmacological strategy is to administer exogenous CB1 agonists. Dronabinol, an orally administered synthetic THC approved by the FDA for treating weight loss in Acquired Immunodeficiency Syndrome (AIDS) and chemotherapy-induced nausea and vomiting, has improved subjective reports of sleep in cannabis withdrawal in some laboratory studies (Budney et al., 2007; Haney et al., 2004; Vandrey et al., 2013) but not in others (Haney et al., 2008; Hart et al., 2002) and, in one laboratory study, dronabinol increased sleep onset latency (Haney et al., 2008).

A second possible pharmacological strategy is to increase CB1 activity during cannabis withdrawal by inhibiting the degradation of endogenous cannabinoids. As stated in Section 31.4.2, FAAH breaks down the endocannabinoid anandamide, and there is a safe and well tolerated inhibitor of FAAH, termed PF-04457845 (Huggins et al., 2012; Li et al., 2012). In a double-blind randomized placebo-controlled study in men with cannabis use disorder, PF-04457845 decreased cannabis use and symptoms of cannabis withdrawal (D'Souza et al., 2019). Importantly, participants receiving PF-04457845 also had improved sleep, reporting deeper sleep and longer sleep duration than those receiving placebo. PF-04457845 increased NREM3 sleep, as measured (Hart et al., 2002) by PSG, during early withdrawal, normalizing the most characteristic effect of cannabis withdrawal on brain activity during sleep. In post-hoc tests, participants taking the FAAH inhibitor also had less REM sleep after four weeks than those on placebo, suggesting that the increased REM sleep in cannabis withdrawal can also be treated with FAAH inhibition.

Treating sleep disturbances directly may also help to prevent or quit cannabis use. Many people report using cannabis as a sleep aid. Though insomnia is not typically one of the qualifying reasons to use medicinal cannabis, one quarter of adults using medicinal cannabis report sleep is the primary reason they use cannabis (Bonn-Miller et al., 2014). Among adolescents using cannabis and other illicit substances, 69% reported they used cannabis to help sleep (Boys et al., 2001). One predictor of future substance use is the perception from the user that the substance is serving a function (Boys et al., 1999), such as promoting sleep; hence, improving both the subjective experience of sleep and physiologically measured sleep could curtail cannabis use.

Zolpidem is a non-benzodiazepine $GABA_A$ receptor agonist that is FDA-approved for short-term treatment of insomnia and, in small laboratory-based studies, has been shown to improve reported sleep quality and objectively measured sleep efficiency in cannabis withdrawal (Herrmann et al., 2016; Vandrey et al., 2011), but, when given alone, does not target other symptoms of withdrawal or decrease cannabis use (Herrmann et al., 2016). Similarly, quetiapine, a sedating antipsychotic often used to treat insomnia despite a lack of evidence supporting this use (Sateia et al., 2017), has improved sleep in a laboratory study of cannabis withdrawal without improving mood disturbances or cannabis cravings (Cooper et al., 2013). Though these small studies have not shown improvement in cannabis use, it may be that, in a sub-set of patients with cannabis use disorder, treating sleep disturbances does help curb cannabis use.

Cognitive behavioural therapy for insomnia (CBT-I) is the first-line treatment for insomnia (Qaseem et al., 2016; Schutte-Rodin et al., 2008) and includes several components: relaxation training, biofeedback, sleep restriction, sleep hygiene, stimulus control (promoting association between the bed and sleep and cognitive control (finding and changing attitudes that encumber sleep). CBT-I was tested in adolescents who used substances, all of whom used cannabis, and were all offered the intervention of six sessions (Bootzin and Stevens, 2005). Those who completed six sessions compared to non-completers had improved sleep, but the effects on substance use were not easy to determine since all participants had just ended substance abuse treatment before the study. Cognitive therapy could be especially helpful in female cannabis users, who have reported more cognitive distortions about sleep compared to male cannabis users (Pacek et al., 2017).

One problem with CBT-I has been that it is underused and difficult to access (Koffel et al., 2018), given the few trained therapists. Internet-based CBT-I, however, has proven effective for insomnia (Zachariae et al., 2016) as well as for depressive symptoms in people with insomnia (Christensen et al., 2016). Other delivery methods, such as CBT-I mobile apps, are emerging. Though they require further evaluation, one has been piloted in Veterans with cannabis use disorder (Babson et al., 2015).

Other behavioural interventions might also decrease cannabis use by treating sleep disturbances. Exercise is proven to help sleep disturbances (Amiri et al., 2021; Li et al., 2021). In a randomized controlled trial of 6 continuous days of 35-minute sessions of aerobic exercise versus stretching in people with cannabis withdrawal, aerobic exercise improved TST, WASO, and sleep efficiency, as measured by wrist actigraphy, though it did not improve participants' subjective sleep (McCartney et al., 2021). As suggested by a recent meta-analysis demonstrating that exercise improves sleep disturbance, longer interventions may be more effective (Amiri et al., 2021) and should be studied.

31.7 Cannabis, Sleep, and Psychosis

Cannabinoids and their role in sleep may represent a 'convergence zone' contributing to the pathophysiology of psychosis. As discussed in Section 31.3, altered sleep may be a core feature of SZ, which could have downstream effects on symptoms and cognition (e.g., sleep-dependent learning). While speculative, this could be due in part to a dysregulation of the endocannabinoid system in SZ. For example, while results have been mixed, a pattern of altered CB1 and endocannabinoid levels have been observed in psychosis (Borgan et al., 2021; Garani et al., 2021; Ranganathan et al., 2016). These endocannabinoid abnormalities would be expected to disrupt the normal sleep/wake cycle in SZ.

The high rates of cannabis use in SZ populations could also contribute to altered sleep in psychosis, acting synergistically with those intrinsic to SZ or creating them. As discussed in Section 31.3, SZ, like chronic cannabis use and cannabis withdrawal, is associated with decreases in SWS, TST, sleep efficiency, and REM disturbances. It is also possible that cannabis use, sleep disturbances, and psychosis share common aetiologies. Genome-wide association studies have implicated shared genetic risk between SZ and cannabis use disorder (Johnson et al., 2020), SZ and sleep disturbances (O'Connell et al., 2021), and sleep deficits and cannabis use (Winiger et al., 2021).

Lastly, antipsychotic medications can ameliorate sleep disturbances in SZ (Krystal et al., 2008). However, the sleep-promoting effects of different antipsychotics in SZ may be influenced by whether patients are using cannabis or not. Thomas-Brown at al. (2018) found that, while both haloperidol and risperidone treatment during inpatient admission for SZ were associated with improved sleep in patients who were not using cannabis, only risperidone was associated with improved sleep in those who had evidence of recent cannabis use (Thomas-Brown et al., 2018). Hence, the optimal treatments for sleep disturbances in SZ may vary depending on patients' cannabis use patterns.

31.8 Conclusion and Future Directions

To recapitulate, sleep is a vital neurobiological process, and evidence has mounted that the endocannabinoid system plays a key role in the sleep/wake cycle. Acute administration and chronic use of THC and cannabis have been shown to alter sleep in small studies of healthy, young people. Sleep disturbances are also part of cannabis withdrawal syndrome and include increased sleep complaints, decreased SWS, and increased REM. Given that sleep changes with age and differs with sex, future research should include younger and older individuals as well as more women, to determine how generalizable the current findings are, as well as to determine which interventions may be most effective for preventing and treating cannabis use in different populations. Sleep may, thus, provide an in-road to treating cannabis use disorder. Promising interventions worthy of further study include pharmacological manipulation of the endocannabinoid system via FAAH inhibition, CBT-I, and aerobic exercise. Future studies could incorporate a combination of these pharmacologic and behavioural interventions.

Given the link between cannabinoids and psychosis as summarized in the current volume, the role of cannabis-induced sleep alterations in psychosis prone individuals and SZ patients warrants further study. Finally, we need to learn whether cannabis use should influence our treatment of sleep impairments in SZ.

31.9 Fact Boxes

Box 31.1 Biological importance of sleep and role in mental health

- Roughly a third of an individual's life-span is spent in sleep, clearly underscoring sleep's biological necessity.
- Healthy sleep serves many critical functions, including proper neurodevelopment, energy conservation, brain waste clearance, modulation of immune responses, neurocognition, mood, memory consolidation, and performance/vigilance.
- While relatively understudied, sleep plays a key role in various psychiatric illnesses, including anxiety, depression, bipolar disorder, and schizophrenia.

Box 31.2 The endocannabinoid system and sleep (pre-clinical models)

- The endocannabinoid system plays a key role in the sleep–wake cycle.
- CB1 antagonists disrupt sleep.
- The naturally-occurring endocannabinoids anandamide and 2-AG are sleep promoting, increasing both SWS and REM sleep.
- Anandamide exhibits a diurnal variation, which is correlated with sleep.
- Administration of exogenous cannabinoids disrupts sleep, typically by increasing SWS and decreasing REM sleep.

Box 31.3 Cannabis use and sleep in humans

- Acute cannabis or THC administration in humans increases SWS and decreases REM sleep, mirroring finds in pre-clinical models.
- Chronic cannabis use is associated with alterations in various sleep measures including sleep efficiency, sleep onset latency, and awakenings after sleep onset.
- Sleep problems are one of the most reported effects of cannabis withdrawal.
- Objective measures have shown that decreased SWS and increased REM sleep is commonly observed in cannabis withdrawal.
- Promising interventions for treating sleep disturbances in cannabis use disorder include pharmacological manipulation of the endocannabinoid system via FAAH inhibition, CBT-I, and aerobic exercise.

References

Albaugh, M. D., Ottino-Gonzalez, J., Sidwell, A., et al. (2021). Association of cannabis use during adolescence with neurodevelopment. *JAMA Psychiatry*, **78**, 1031–1040.

Amiri, S., Hasani, J., and Satkin, M. (2021). Effect of exercise training on improving sleep disturbances: A systematic review and meta-analysis of randomized control trials. *Sleep Med*, **84**, 205–218.

Anafi, R. C., Kayser, M. S., and Raizen, D. M. (2019). Exploring phylogeny to find the function of sleep. *Nat Rev Neurosci*, **20**, 109–116.

Babson, K. A., Ramo, D. E., Baldini, L., et al. (2015). Mobile app-delivered cognitive behavioral therapy for insomnia: Feasibility and initial efficacy among veterans with cannabis use disorders. *JMIR Res Protoc*, **4**, e87.

Barratt, E. S., Beaver, W., and White, R. (1974). The effects of marijuana on human sleep patterns. *Biol Psychiatry*, **8**, 47–54.

Bassetti, C. L., Ferini-Strambi, L., Brown, S., et al. (2015). Neurology and psychiatry: Waking up to opportunities of sleep: State of the art and clinical/research priorities for the next decade. *Eur J Neurol*, **22**, 1337–1354.

Bolla, K. I., Lesage, S. R., Gamaldo, C. E., et al. (2008). Sleep disturbance in heavy marijuana users. *Sleep*, **31**, 901–908.

(2010). Polysomnogram changes in marijuana users who report sleep disturbances during prior abstinence. *Sleep Med*, **11**, 882–889.

Bonn-Miller, M. O., Boden, M. T., Bucossi, M. M., et al. (2014). Self-reported cannabis use characteristics, patterns and helpfulness among medical cannabis users. *Am J Drug Alcohol Abuse*, **40**, 23–30.

Bootzin, R. R., and Stevens, S. J. (2005). Adolescents, substance abuse, and the treatment of insomnia and daytime sleepiness. *Clin Psychol Rev*, **25**, 629–644.

Borgan, F., Kokkinou, M., and Howes, O. (2021). The cannabinoid CB1 receptor in schizophrenia. *Biol Psychiatry Cogn Neurosci Neuroimaging*, **6**, 646–659.

Boys, A., Marsden, J., Griffiths, P., et al. (1999). Substance use among young people: The relationship between perceived functions and intentions. *Addiction*, **94**, 1043–1050.

Boys, A., Marsden, J., and Strang, J. (2001). Understanding reasons for drug use amongst young people: A functional perspective. *Health Educ Res*, **16**, 457–469.

Budney, A. J., Vandrey, R. G., Hughes, J. R., et al. (2007). Oral delta-9-tetrahydrocannabinol suppresses cannabis withdrawal symptoms. *Drug Alcohol Depend*, **86**, 22–29.

Calik, M. W., and Carley, D. W. (2017). Effects of cannabinoid agonists and antagonists on sleep and breathing in Sprague-Dawley rats. *Sleep*, **40**, zsx112.

Carley, D. W., Paviovic, S., Janelidze, M., et al. (2002). Functional role for cannabinoids in respiratory

stability during sleep. *Sleep*, **25**, 391–398.

Cazzullo, C. L., Fornari, M. G., Maffei, C., et al. (1977). Sleep, psychophysiological functioning and learning processes in schizophrenia. *Act Nerv Super (Praha)*, **19**, 409–417.

Chan, M. S., Chung, K. F., Yung, K. P., et al. (2017). Sleep in schizophrenia: A systematic review and meta-analysis of polysomnographic findings in case-control studies. *Sleep Med Rev*, **32**, 69–84.

Chouinard, S., Poulin, J., Stip, E., et al. (2004). Sleep in untreated patients with schizophrenia: A meta-analysis. *Schizophr Bull*, **30**, 957–967.

Christensen, H., Batterham, P. J., Gosling, J. A., et al. (2016). Effectiveness of an online insomnia program (SHUTi) for prevention of depressive episodes (the GoodNight Study): A randomised controlled trial. *Lancet Psychiatry*, **3**, 333–341.

Cohen-Zion, M., Drummond, S. P., Padula, C. B., et al. (2009). Sleep architecture in adolescent marijuana and alcohol users during acute and extended abstinence. *Addict Behav*, **34**, 976–979.

Cohrs, S. (2008). Sleep disturbances in patients with schizophrenia: Impact and effect of antipsychotics. *CNS Drugs*, **22**, 939–962.

Cooper, Z. D., Foltin, R. W., Hart, C. L., et al. (2013). A human laboratory study investigating the effects of quetiapine on marijuana withdrawal and relapse in daily marijuana smokers. *Addict Biol*, **18**, 993–1002.

Cousens, K., and DiMascio, A. (1973). (-) Delta 9 THC as an hypnotic. An experimental study of three dose levels. *Psychopharmacologia*, **33**, 355–364.

D'Souza, D. C., Cortes-Briones, J., Creatura, G., et al. (2019). Efficacy and safety of a fatty acid amide hydrolase inhibitor (PF-04457845) in the treatment of cannabis withdrawal and dependence in men: A double-blind, placebo-controlled, parallel group, phase 2a single-site randomised controlled trial. *Lancet Psychiatry*, **6**, 35–45.

D'Souza, D. C., Cortes-Briones, J. A., Ranganathan, M., et al. (2016). Rapid changes in CB1 receptor availability in cannabis dependent males after abstinence from cannabis. *Biol Psychiatry Cogn Neurosci Neuroimaging*, **1**, 60–67.

Feinberg, I., Jones, R., Walker, J., et al. (1975). Effects of high dosage delta-9-tetrahydrocannabinol on sleep patterns in man. *Clin Pharmacol Ther*, **17**, 458–466.

et al. (1976). Effects of marijuana extract and tetrahydrocannabinol on electroencephalographic sleep patterns. *Clin Pharmacol Ther*, **19**, 782–794.

Freemon, F. R. (1972). Effects of marihuana on sleeping states. *JAMA*, **220**, 1364–1365.

(1982). The effect of chronically administered delta-9-tetrahydrocannabinol upon the polygraphically monitored sleep of normal volunteers. *Drug Alcohol Depend*, **10**, 345–353.

Garani, R., Watts, J. J., and Mizrahi, R. (2021). Endocannabinoid system in psychotic and mood disorders, a review of human studies. *Prog Neuropsychopharmacol Biol Psychiatry*, **106**, 110096.

Goonawardena, A. V., Plano, A., Robinson, L., et al. (2015). Modulation of food consumption and sleep–wake cycle in mice by the neutral CB1 antagonist ABD459. *Behav Pharmacol*, **26**, 289–303.

Han, B. H., Sherman, S., Mauro, P. M., et al. (2017). Demographic trends among older cannabis users in the

United States, 2006–13. *Addiction*, **112**, 516–525.

Haney, M., Hart, C. L., Vosburg, S. K., et al. (2004). Marijuana withdrawal in humans: Effects of oral THC or divalproex. *Neuropsychopharmacology*, **29**, 158–170.

(2008). Effects of THC and lofexidine in a human laboratory model of marijuana withdrawal and relapse. *Psychopharmacology (Berl)*, **197**, 157–168.

Hart, C. L., Haney, M., Ward, A. S., et al. (2002). Effects of oral THC maintenance on smoked marijuana self-administration. *Drug Alcohol Depend*, **67**, 301–309.

Herrmann, E. S., Cooper, Z. D., Bedi, G., et al. (2016). Effects of zolpidem alone and in combination with nabilone on cannabis withdrawal and a laboratory model of relapse in cannabis users. *Psychopharmacology (Berl)*, **233**, 2469–2478.

Hirvonen, J., Goodwin, R. S., Li, C. T., et al. (2012). Reversible and regionally selective downregulation of brain cannabinoid CB1 receptors in chronic daily cannabis smokers. *Mol Psychiatry*, **17**, 642–649.

Hofstetter, J. R., Lysaker, P. H., and Mayeda, A. R. (2005). Quality of sleep in patients with schizophrenia is associated with quality of life and coping. *BMC Psychiatry*, **5**, 13.

Hosko, M. J., Kochar, M. S., and Wang, R. I. (1973). Effects of orally administered delta-9-tetrahydrocannabinol in man. *Clin Pharmacol Ther*, **14**, 344–352.

Huggins, J. P., Smart, T. S., Langman, S., et al. (2012). An efficient randomised, placebo-controlled clinical trial with the irreversible fatty acid amide hydrolase-1 inhibitor PF-04457845, which modulates endocannabinoids but fails to induce effective analgesia in patients with pain due to osteoarthritis of the knee. *Pain*, **153**, 1837–1846.

Johnson, E. C., Demontis, D., Thorgeirsson, T. E., et al. (2020). A large-scale genome-wide association study meta-analysis of cannabis use disorder. *Lancet Psychiatry*, **7**, 1032–1045.

Jones, S. G., and Benca, R. M. (2015). Circadian disruption in psychiatric disorders. *Sleep Med Clin*, **10**, 481–493.

Karacan, I., Fernandez-Salas, A., Coggins, W. J., et al. (1976). Sleep electroencephalographic-electrooculographic characteristics of chronic marijuana users: Part I. *Ann N Y Acad Sci*, **282**, 348–374.

Kesner, A. J., and Lovinger, D. M. (2020). Cannabinoids, endocannabinoids and sleep. *Front Mol Neurosci*, **13**, 125.

Koffel, E., Bramoweth, A. D., and Ulmer, C. S. (2018). Increasing access to and utilization of cognitive behavioral therapy for insomnia (CBT-I): A narrative review. *J Gen Intern Med*, **33**, 955–962.

Krystal, A. D. (2020). Sleep therapeutics and neuropsychiatric illness. *Neuropsychopharmacology*, **45**, 166–175.

Krystal, A. D., Goforth, H. W., and Roth, T. (2008). Effects of antipsychotic medications on sleep in schizophrenia. *Int Clin Psychopharmacol*, **23**, 150–160.

Li, G. L., Winter, H., Arends, R., et al. (2012). Assessment of the pharmacology and tolerability of PF-04457845, an irreversible inhibitor of fatty acid amide hydrolase-1, in healthy subjects. *Br J Clin Pharmacol*, **73**, 706–716.

Li, S., Li, Z., Wu, Q., et al. (2021). Effect of exercise intervention on primary insomnia: A meta-analysis. *J Sports Med Phys Fitness*, **61**, 857–866.

Li, S. X., Lam, S. P., Zhang, J., et al. (2016). Sleep disturbances and suicide risk in an 8-year longitudinal study of schizophrenia-spectrum disorders. *Sleep*, **39**, 1275–1282.

Livne, O., Shmulewitz, D., Lev-Ran, S., et al. (2019). DSM-5 cannabis withdrawal syndrome: Demographic and clinical correlates in U.S. adults. *Drug Alcohol Depend*, **195**, 170–177.

Lu, H. C., and Mackie, K. (2016). An introduction to the endogenous cannabinoid system. *Biol Psychiatry*, **79**, 516–525.

Lunsford-Avery, J. R., Goncalves, B., Brietzke, E., et al. (2017). Adolescents at clinical-high risk for psychosis: Circadian rhythm disturbances predict worsened prognosis at 1-year follow-up. *Schizophr Res*, **189**, 37–42.

Manoach, D. S., Cain, M. S., Vangel, M. G., et al. (2004). A failure of sleep-dependent procedural learning in chronic, medicated schizophrenia. *Biol Psychiatry*, **56**, 951–956.

Manoach, D. S., Pan, J. Q., Purcell, S. M., et al. (2016). Reduced sleep spindles in schizophrenia: A treatable endophenotype that links risk genes to impaired cognition? *Biol Psychiatry*, **80**, 599–608.

McCartney, D., Isik, A. D., Rooney, K., et al. (2021). The effect of daily aerobic cycling exercise on sleep quality during inpatient cannabis withdrawal: A randomised controlled trial. *J Sleep Res*, **30**, e13211.

McPherson, K. L., Tomasi, D. G., Wang, G. J., et al. (2021). Cannabis affects cerebellar volume and sleep differently in men and women. *Front Psychiatry*, **12**, 643193.

Mechoulam, R., Fride, E., Hanus, L., et al. (1997). Anandamide may mediate sleep induction. *Nature*, **389**, 25–26.

Murillo-Rodriguez, E., Cabeza, R., Mendez-Diaz, M., et al. (2001). Anandamide-induced sleep is blocked by SR141716A, a CB1 receptor antagonist and by U73122, a phospholipase C inhibitor. *Neuroreport*, **12**, 2131–2136.

Murillo-Rodriguez, E., Desarnaud, F., and Prospero-Garcia, O. (2006). Diurnal variation of arachidonoylethanolamine, palmitoylethanolamide and oleoylethanolamide in the brain of the rat. *Life Sci*, **79**, 30–37.

Murillo-Rodriguez, E., Sanchez-Alavez, M., Navarro, L., et al. (1998). Anandamide modulates sleep and memory in rats. *Brain Res*, **812**, 270–274.

Nicholson, A. N., Turner, C., Stone, B. M., et al. (2004). Effect of delta-9-tetrahydrocannabinol and cannabidiol on nocturnal sleep and early-morning behavior in young adults. *J Clin Psychopharmacol*, **24**, 305–313.

O'Connell, K. S., Frei, O., Bahrami, S., et al. (2021). Characterizing the genetic overlap between psychiatric disorders and sleep-related phenotypes. *Biol Psychiatry*, **90**, 621–631.

Pacek, L. R., Herrmann, E. S., Smith, M. T., et al. (2017). Sleep continuity, architecture and quality among treatment-seeking cannabis users: An in-home, unattended polysomnographic study. *Exp Clin Psychopharmacol*, **25**, 295–302.

Pava, M. J., Makriyannis, A., and Lovinger, D. M. (2016). Endocannabinoid signaling regulates sleep stability. *PLoS ONE*, **11**, e0152473.

Perez-Morales, M., de la Herran-Arita, A. K., Mendez-Diaz, M., et al. (2013). 2-AG into the lateral hypothalamus increases REM sleep and cFos expression in melanin concentrating hormone neurons in rats. *Pharmacol Biochem Behav*, **108**, 1–7.

Piper, B. J., Dekeuster, R. M., Beals, M. L., et al. (2017). Substitution of medical cannabis for pharmaceutical agents for pain, anxiety, and sleep. *J Psychopharmacol*, **31**, 569–575.

Pivik, R. T., Zarcone, V., Dement, W. C., et al. (1972). Delta-9-tetrahydrocannabinol and synhexl: Effects on human sleep patterns. *Clin Pharmacol Ther*, **13**, 426–435.

Pranikoff, K., Karacan, I., Larson, E. A., et al. (1973). Effects of marijuana smoking on the sleep EEG. Preliminary studies. *JFMA*, **60**, 28–31.

Qaseem, A., Kansagara, D., Forciea, M. A., et al. (2016). Management of chronic insomnia disorder in adults: A clinical practice guideline from the American College of Physicians. *Ann Intern Med*, **165**, 125–133.

Ranganathan, M., Cortes-Briones, J., Radhakrishnan, R., et al. (2016). Reduced brain cannabinoid receptor availability in schizophrenia. *Biol Psychiatry*, **79**, 997–1005.

Reeve, S., Sheaves, B., and Freeman, D. (2015). The role of sleep dysfunction in the occurrence of delusions and hallucinations: A systematic review. *Clin Psychol Rev*, **42**, 96–115.

Ritsner, M., Kurs, R., Ponizovsky, A., et al. (2004). Perceived quality of life in schizophrenia: Relationships to sleep quality. *Qual Life Res*, **13**, 783–791.

Robertson, I., Cheung, A., and Fan, X. (2019). Insomnia in patients with schizophrenia: Current understanding and treatment options. *Prog Neuropsychopharmacol Biol Psychiatry*, **92**, 235–242.

Santucci, V., Storme, J. J., Soubrie, P., et al. (1996). Arousal-enhancing properties of the CB1 cannabinoid receptor antagonist SR 141716A in rats as assessed by electroencephalographic spectral and sleep–waking cycle analysis. *Life Sci*, **58**, PL103–PL110.

Sateia, M. J., Buysee, D. J., Krystal, A. D., et al. (2017). Clinical practice guideline for the pharmacologic treatment of chronic insomnia in adults: An American Academy of Sleep Medicine Clinical Practice guideline. *J Clin Sleep Med*, **13**, 307–349.

Schutte-Rodin, S., Broch, L., Buysse, D., et al. (2008). Clinical guideline for the evaluation and management of chronic insomnia in adults. *J Clin Sleep Med*, **4**, 487–504.

Schwartz, M. D., and Kilduff, T. S. (2015). The neurobiology of sleep and wakefulness. *Psychiatr Clin North Am*, **38**, 615–644.

Suchecki, D., Tiba, P. A., and Machado, R. B. (2012). REM sleep rebound as an adaptive response to stressful situations. *Front Neurol*, **3**, 41.

Surti, T. S., Skosnik, P. D., Ranganathan, M., et al. (2018). Sleep-dependent perceptual learning in schizophrenia. *57th Annual Meeting of the American College of Neuropsychopharmacology*, December 2018, Hollywood, FL.

Thomas-Brown, P. L., Martin, J. S., Sewell, C. A., et al. (2018). Risperidone provides better improvement of sleep disturbances than haloperidol therapy in schizophrenia patients with cannabis-positive urinalysis. *Front Pharmacol*, **9**, 769.

Vandrey, R., Smith, M. T., McCann, U. D., et al. (2011). Sleep disturbance and the effects of extended-release zolpidem during cannabis withdrawal. *Drug Alcohol Depend*, **117**, 38–44.

Vandrey, R., Stitzer, M. L., Mintzer, M. Z., et al. (2013). The dose effects of short-term dronabinol (oral THC) maintenance in daily cannabis users. *Drug Alcohol Depend*, **128**, 64–70.

Vaughn, L. K., Denning, G., Stuhr, K. L., et al. (2010). Endocannabinoid signalling: Has it got rhythm? *Br J Pharmacol*, **160**, 530–543.

Winiger, E. A., Ellingson, J. M., Morrison, C. L., et al. (2021). Sleep deficits and cannabis use behaviors: An analysis of shared genetics using linkage disequilibrium score regression and polygenic risk prediction. *Sleep*, **44**, zsaa188.

Winiger, E. A., Huggett, S. B., Hatoum, A. S., et al. (2019). Onset of regular cannabis use and adult sleep duration: Genetic variation and the implications of a predictive relationship. *Drug Alcohol Depend*, **204**, 107517.

Xiang, Y. T., Weng, Y. Z., Leung, C. M., et al. (2009). Prevalence and correlates of insomnia and its impact on quality of life in Chinese schizophrenia patients. *Sleep*, **32**, 105–109.

Zachariae, R., Lyby, M. S., Ritterband, L. M., et al. (2016). Efficacy of internet-delivered cognitive-behavioral therapy for insomnia: A systematic review and meta-analysis of randomized controlled trials. *Sleep Med Rev*, **30**, 1–10.

Zanini, M., Castro, J., Coelho, F. M., et al. (2013). Do sleep abnormalities and misaligned sleep/circadian rhythm patterns represent early clinical characteristics for developing psychosis in high risk populations? *Neurosci Biobehav Rev*, **37**, 2631–2637.

Zielinski, M. R., McKenna, J. T., and McCarley, R. W. (2016). Functions and mechanisms of sleep. *AIMS Neurosci*, **3**, 67–104.

Chapter 32

Cannabinoids as Medicines
What the Evidence Says and What It Does Not Say

Marco De Toffol, Elena Dragioti, Andre Ferrer Carvalho, and Marco Solmi

---

Box 32.1 Summary of evidence of psychiatric and medical risks and benefits associated with cannabis

- All sources of evidence, namely observational studies, randomized controlled trials, and Mendelian Randomization studies, consistently indicate that use of cannabis is associated with increased risk of psychosis.
- Observational studies and randomized controlled trials point toward a potentially increased risk of certain psychiatric symptoms – including mania – with use of cannabis.
- Observational studies and randomized controlled trials consistently point toward an association between cannabis use and cognitive impairment, notably in the short-term but with some effects persisting.
- Observational studies report an association between cannabis use and motor vehicle accident risk.
- Interventional studies show that cannabidiol can be effective for epilepsy in children,
- Cannabis-based medicines can be effective in improving muscle spasticity in multiple sclerosis, chronic pain syndromes, and nausea/vomiting in palliative care

---

32.1 Introduction

As covered extensively in other chapters of this book, *Cannabis sativa* is commonly used recreationally, mostly due to the effects of its main psychoactive cannabinoid, delta-9-tetrahydrocannabinol (THC). In the last several years, the properties of a number of cannabinoids have being studied for their utility in medical treatment, often with rather mixed outcomes. One of the complexities for this type of research is that *Cannabis sativa* contains more than 100 cannabinoids, which are characterized by different pharmacological profiles: delineating which chemical is responsible – alone or in concert with others – for particular outcomes, is difficult.

The psychoactive properties and addictive potential of cannabis is ascribed to THC, the main psychoactive constituent. Recent years have seen a steadily increasing THC potency in plant cannabis (Bhattacharyya et al., 2010; and see Chapter 5). As detailed in Chapters 1 and 2, THC acts through CB1 receptor binding, largely present in the brain's neurons and astrocytes, and through CB2 receptors, mainly expressed by immune cells. THC-rich medicinal cannabis is prescribed and is being studied for a variety of different medical conditions, including, but not limited to, pain control and nausea and vomiting during chemotherapy.

Conversely, cannabidiol (CBD) has been proposed as a treatment for cannabis use disorder, as it does not produce the 'high' experienced with THC, and thus it does not carry the same potential for addiction, nor does it have psychosis-inducing effects. CBD has also been used for the treatment of neurological disorders such as certain forms of childhood epilepsy; it is claimed by some researchers to be useful for anxiety (Chapter 12) and sleep disorders (see Chapter 31); and even as a treatment for schizophrenia (see Chapter 20).

As outlined in Tables 32.1 and 32.2, a number of studies have been published reporting on outcomes of exposure to cannabis or cannabinoids or cannabis-based medicines. Observational studies, in particular, have focused on detrimental effects of cannabis use, through use of longitudinal designs and analysis of outcomes not possible to study in randomized controlled trials (RCTs), such as motor vehicle accidents (MVA). Additionally, RCTs have investigated the effects of cannabis-based medicines on a number of medical conditions, and they also report adverse events, such as nausea and anxiety. Finally, Mendelian Randomization (MR) studies have explored adverse outcomes associated with cannabis use disorder, with multiple MR studies focusing on schizophrenia as an outcome of interest.

Table 32.1 Outcomes investigated and relative population of interest and cannabis exposure

Population	Cannabis type exposure	Outcomes
General population (adults)	Cannabis	Cognition
Schizophrenia (adults)	Cannabis use	Cognition
Healthy subjects, psychosis (adults)	Cannabis use	Cognition
General population	Cannabis use	IQ
First-episode psychosis (adolescents, adults)	Cannabis use	Cognition
Non-psychotic users	Cannabis use	Brain alterations
General population (adolescents, adults)	Regular cannabis use	Brain volume
General population (adolescents, adults)	Regular cannabis use	Brain executive and default mode network
Psychosis (adolescents, adults)	Cannabis (smoked)	Antipsychotics adherence
Psychosis	Cannabis use (current, past)	Psychosis relapse
Ultra-high risk of psychosis (adolescents, adults)	Cannabis use	Psychosis (transition to)
General population (adolescents, adults)	Cannabis use	Depression, psychosis symptoms, and suicidal ideation
General population (adolescents, adults)	Cannabis use	Age at onset of schizophrenia and other psychoses
General population (adolescents)	Cannabis use	Psychosis
Healthy subjects	Intravenous, oral, or nasal THC, CBD	Psychiatric symptoms
General population (adolescents, adults)	Cannabis use (normal and heavy)	Depression
General population (adolescents, young adults)	Cannabis	Depression (symptoms or disorder)
General population (adolescents, adults)	Cannabis use	Suicide ideation, attempt, and suicide
General population (adults)	Cannabis use	Mania symptoms
Pregnancy (adults)	Marijuana use	Low birth weight
Pregnancy (adults)	Cannabis use	Decreased birth weight
General population (adolescents, adults)	THC	Car crash death/injuries
Drivers (adults)	Cannabis, testing THC positive	Car crush and car crush culpability
General population (adolescents, adults)	Cannabis use	Car events
General population (adults)	THC	Driving impairment, cognitive impairment
General population (adults < 50)	Cannabis use, current	Testicular cancer, non-seminoma
HCV + NAFDL (adults)	Marijuana	Liver fibrosis
General population (adolescents, young adults)	Cannabis use	Physical dating violence

Table 32.1 (cont.)

Population	Cannabis type exposure	Outcomes
Mixed conditions (chronic neuropathic pain) (adults)	Cannabis (inhaled)	Pain
Mixed conditions (adults)	CBM	Pain, AEs
Mixed conditions (adults)	CBM	Pain, spasticity, nausea and vomiting, AEs
Multiple sclerosis (adults)	CBM	Pain, spasticity, bladder disfunction
Mixed conditions (chronic neuropathic pain, adults)	CBM	Pain, psychological distress, sleep problems
Mixed conditions (chronic pain, non-cancer, adults)	Cannabinoids	Pain
Mixed conditions (adults)	Cannabis	AEs
Cancer (adults)	Nabiximol, THC	Pain, maintenance of opioid dosage, daily breakthrough opioid dosage
Dravet syndrome (children)	CBD	Seizure, acceptability, AEs
Dravet syndrome, Lennox-Gastaut (children)	CBD	Seizure
Lennox-Gastaut syndrome (children)	CBD	Seizure, tolerability, AEs
Treatment-resistant Dravet syndrome, Lennox-Gastaut (children)	CBD	Seizure, acceptability, tolerability, AEs
Epilepsy (any age)	CBM	Seizure, quality-of-life, AEs, tolerability
Cancer (chemotherapy, adults)	Cannabinoids	Nausea, vomit, AEs
Multiple sclerosis (adults)	Cannabinoids	Spasticity, pain, AEs
Multiple sclerosis (adults)	Cannabinoids	Spasticity, AEs

Observational and interventional studies have been pooled in a number of meta-analyses. However, most meta-analytic findings originate from observational evidence and are subject to several sources of bias.

This chapter serves to review meta-analyses published on the association between cannabis, cannabinoids, and cannabis-based medicines and health outcomes. We did not put any restrictions in terms of outcomes of interest, nor in terms of definition of exposure to cannabis. The reader is directed to other chapters of this book for a more detailed exposition of specific topics.

32.2 Cognition

As detailed in Chapter 9, the short- and long-term impact of cannabis on cognition is widely discussed in the literature. It is important to clarify which domains

are possibly affected; whether the risk involves chronic users only, or also impacts occasional users; the duration of impairment; and whether there are some particularly susceptible sub-groups of individuals (e.g., youth, or people with schizophrenia).

Evidence on this topic can be drawn from observational studies conducted over the last two decades. A 2003 meta-analysis of studies investigating non-acute effects of cannabis on cognition in the general population found a small negative effect on learning and forgetting domains in some individuals, notably chronic users. Importantly, studies that tested people who had been at least 25 days abstinent did not find a significant enduring negative effect on cognition (Grant et al., 2003). A subsequent large meta-analysis was published in 2012 and reported a small negative effect on global neurocognitive performance associated with chronic cannabis use, but methodological

Table 32.2 Summary of main evidence

Observational studies

Acute cognitive impairment after cannabis use, including driving skills; IQ decline in chronic non-psychotic cannabis users and several domain impairments; direction of cognitive impairment in psychosis patients.

Alterations in brain regions such as the hippocampus and orbitofrontal cortex; greater activation of the default mode network.

THC use with or without CBD elicits psychiatric symptoms; cannabis use is associated with psychotic symptoms, psychosis-like experiences, and psychotic disorders; cannabis use has a causal association with schizophrenia and risk of transition from FEP to schizophrenia.

Possible association between cannabis use and depression, suicidality, and (preliminary) to mania symptoms.

Cannabis and tobacco use are associated with alterations in newborn's weight, head circumference, intensive care admission.

Motor vehicle accident risk is associated with cannabis use; acute driving skills impairment lasts at least 5–7 hours.

Suggestive evidence of association between cannabis use and physical dating violence.

RCTs

Medical cannabis is effective in chronic neuropathic pain, non-cancer pain conditions; efficacy in cancer-pain has conflicting evidence.

CBD is an effective adjunctive treatment for epilepsy in children.

Moderate evidence of THC and/or CBD in treatment of nausea and vomiting during chemotherapy, alone or as adjunctive treatment to antiemetics.

Medical cannabis improves spasticity in multiple sclerosis.

Preliminary findings in treatment of anxiety disorders and sleep disorders with CBD.

Adverse events in CBD treatment (high certainty): lower acceptability, tolerability, and increased serious adverse events, abnormal liver function tests, pneumonia, decreased appetite, somnolence.

Adverse events in THC treatment (moderate certainty): emerging psychiatric symptoms, increased adverse events, sedation/somnolence, lower tolerability, diarrhoea, dizziness, central nervous system adverse events, gastrointestinal adverse events, nausea/vomiting, disorientation/confusion, dry mouth, euphoria/dysphoria, feeling high, lower acceptability, and numerous additional outcomes including impaired attention, visual disturbance, problems with balance, vertigo.

Mendelian Randomization Studies

Risk-increasing effect of cannabis use disorder on liability to schizophrenia.

---

limitations of individual studies precluded any conclusions regarding the effect of abstinence.

Interestingly, a meta-analysis conducted to interrogate the effects of cannabis use in schizophrenia patients found better cognitive performance in cannabis-using patients than non-users (Rabin et al., 2011). Those authors proposed an explanatory model suggesting endocannabinoid system involvement in neurocognition but posited a possible sub-group of patients who are prone to cannabis use but have a better neurocognitive baseline profile. However, that meta-analysis was based on a relatively small number of studies, and one of the studies excluded from the analyses showed a detrimental dose-related effect of intravenous administration of THC in patients with no cannabis use disorder history.

Schoeler et al. (2016b) explored these controversial findings further, with their meta-analysis concluding that cannabis use is associated with impairment in global and prospective memory, verbal and immediate recall, and visual cognition in non-psychiatric subjects, but with better global memory, visual immediate recall and recognition in people with schizophrenia. Interestingly, lower depression scores and younger age moderated effects of cannabis; cannabis using schizophrenia patients had lower levels of depression and were younger than non-using schizophrenia patients, whilst non-psychiatric cannabis-users had higher depression scores than age-matched non-psychiatric non-users. Moreover, longer duration of abstinence was associated with improved memory in both patients and healthy subjects (Schoeler et al., 2016a). These findings corroborate that cannabis has a detrimental effect on cognition in healthy individuals and suggest the presence of a less cognitively impaired sub-group of psychotic patients who are differentially prone to cannabis use. Further evidence comes from studies of first episode psychosis patients, which have reported no significant differences in cognitive impairment between users and non-users (Sánchez-Gutiérrez et al., 2020). However, that meta-analysis did find several moderators of effect size variability, including frequency of cannabis use, first-generation antipsychotic use, and country where the study was carried out.

The impact of cannabis consumption on cognition in adolescents and young adults is particularly important from a public health standpoint. Scott et al. (2018) reviewed this topic and concluded that cognitive impairment is evident in heavy cannabis users, irrespective of current age or age of onset of cannabis use. It was not possible to examine individual differences in susceptibility (Scott et al., 2018). A subsequent meta-analysis of longitudinal data measuring IQ in young frequent or dependent cannabis users found an association with IQ decline (around 2 points). Studies included in that meta-analysis had low heterogeneity and moderate-to-high quality, but studies with longer follow-up periods are required, in order to assess the magnitude of developmental impact (Power et al., 2021).

A further important public health issue is whether the acute negative cognitive impacts of cannabis lead to impairment in skills such as driving. McCartney et al. (2021) performed a meta-analysis on this topic and showed that, in regular cannabis users, acute cognitive impairment was less marked than in occasional users. Also, the magnitude of the impairment was related to various factors, including whether the

cannabis was smoked or eaten and the THC potency. Duration of impairment was also dependent upon dose and route of administration; smoking 20 mg of THC predicted total recovery of driving-related cognitive skills within five to seven hours, whilst impairments associated with eaten product may take longer to subside (McCartney et al., 2021).

32.3 Neuroimaging

In order to understand and corroborate hypothetical long-term effects of cannabis and cannabinoids on brain function, investigations of morphology are helpful, but do not necessarily reflect functional differences. Generally, evidence from observational studies of associations between cannabis exposure and brain structural aberrations are weak, limited, and inconsistent, in part due to intrinsic limitations of neuroimaging techniques and the necessity for correcting for multiple testing.

Rocchetti et al. (2013) investigated effects of cannabis on brain structure in non-psychotic samples, and found a smaller hippocampal volume in cannabis users compared to non-users, suggesting that chronic and long-term cannabis exposure may affect brain regions rich in cannabinoids receptors. This finding has been confirmed in more recent MRI studies, along with findings of smaller orbitofrontal cortical volumes (Lorenzetti et al., 2019), implicating the parts of the brain involved in reward, learning and memory, and motivation circuitry. Interestingly – and perhaps reflecting high heterogeneity of the included studies – volume changes were not correlated with cannabis duration or dosage.

Functional neuroimaging studies have also investigated the impact of cannabis on brain function. Considering the robust evidence of acute effects of cannabis on cognitive impairment, along with the more controversial literature on chronic cognitive detrimental effects (see Chapter 9), structural and functional MRI studies are important to assess whether there are structural and functional changes in cannabis users after discontinuation. The most recent meta-analysis on this topic, conducted in adolescents, found significantly greater activation of executive and the default mode network in cannabis abstinent users compared to non-users, suggesting a persistence of neurofunctional alterations even after cannabinoids and their metabolites have been cleared from the brain (Blest-Hopley et al., 2019).

However, these studies all have to contend with the fact that multiple potential confounders might impact results, not least the use of substances other than cannabis. Further large-scale longitudinal neuroimaging studies are required.

32.4 Psychotic Symptoms, Psychosis Disorders, and Schizophrenia

The relationship between cannabis and psychosis is one of the central questions addressed in this book (see Chapters 14–17). It is well known that THC elicits psychotic and mood-related symptoms in vulnerable individuals. Cannabis use is of particular concern in adolescents, whose brain developmental processes are ongoing, increasing their risk of detrimental effects. Cannabis might have a specific role in the onset of psychotic chronic disorders, in particular schizophrenia: certainly it appears to 'bring forward' the initial episode of illness in vulnerable individuals and worsen the outcome in people with established schizophrenia (Chapter 23). It is thus important to establish whether – and how – cannabis use could increase absolute risk of first episode psychosis and/or schizophrenia itself.

Experimental administration of THC with or without CBD elicits positive and negative psychotic symptoms, and other psychiatric symptoms (including depression and anxiety) with a high evidence level of certainty (Hindley et al., 2020). Further, exposure to cannabis in adolescence is associated with psychotic symptoms, psychosis-like experience, and ultimately psychotic disorders in vulnerable individuals (Kiburi et al., 2021). Development of psychosis and earlier onset of first episode of psychosis in this population is further influenced by cannabis use frequency, exposure to childhood trauma, concurrent use of other substances, as well as genetic factors.

Sophisticated MR studies have confirmed a relationship between cannabis use disorder and schizophrenia, with a significant risk-increasing effect of cannabis use disorder on liability to schizophrenia, above and beyond tobacco smoking (Johnson et al., 2021). This evidence is consonant with previous data that excluded tobacco and other factors as confounders in the association between cannabis and age at onset of psychosis (Myles et al., 2012). The dose–response pattern of the relationship between cannabis and psychotic outcomes further supports a causal link

(Moore et al., 2007), as do data showing an increased risk of transition to psychosis in those with ultra-high risk of psychosis in the presence of cannabis use disorder (Kraan et al., 2016).

The impact of cannabis on mental health has also been studied within people with an established psychotic illness. For instance, cannabis use seems to be associated with increased risk for relapse in people with schizophrenia (Schoeler et al., 2016a). This relationship might be mediated to some extent by problems with adherence to antipsychotic treatments in those who use cannabis (Foglia et al., 2017), suggesting a particular therapeutic role for long-acting injectable antipsychotics in this group of individuals (see Chapter 24).

32.5 Affective Symptoms and Disorders

The associations between cannabis and affective symptoms and disorders have been reviewed in Chapters 12 and 13. The evidence base is generally less robust compared to the compelling and converging evidence from multiple sources, regarding links with psychotic disorders.

One of the first meta-analyses that investigated the cannabis/affective disorders connection reported a significant association between heavy cannabis use and depression but there was substantial heterogeneity as well as numerous sources of bias (Lev-Ran et al., 2014). A subsequent meta-analysis specifically tested whether use of cannabis increases risk of later depression in adolescents and young adults and confirmed both the association and the directionality (Esmaeelzadeh et al., 2018). Another meta-analysis found an association between chronic cannabis use and suicidality and specifically with both suicidal ideation and suicide attempt; however, studies did not comprehensively control for known risk factors for suicidality and also showed marked heterogeneity (Borges et al., 2016). The issues of confounding and reverse causality bedevil this literature and firm conclusions are difficult to draw, as discussed in Chapter 12.

As for the opposite polarity of mood, some studies have demonstrated an association between cannabis and the precipitation of manic symptoms in bipolar disorder patients (Gibbs et al., 2015) but, as detailed in Chapter 13, the literature is sparse and any conclusions should be considered preliminary.

32.6 Maternal and Neonatal Outcomes

Cannabinoids are lipophilic and cross the placenta into the developing foetus where they can potentially impact development. Several studies have investigated the effect of cannabis use during pregnancy on neonatal and maternal health (Conner et al., 2016; see Chapter 25). When considering health outcomes associated with cannabis exposure during pregnancy, life-style factors and in particular tobacco smoking need to be considered, as smoking tobacco is an established risk factor for poor foetal development. Indeed, it is virtually impossible to rule out the role of smoking in these analyses, as the vast majority of cannabis is smoked, sometimes mixed with tobacco. The review of Conner et al. (2016) suggested an association between cannabis use and pre-term delivery and low birth weight, but controlling for the confounding effect of tobacco smoking obviated this finding. Further studies have reported an association between cannabis use and low birth weight (Gunn et al., 2016), and a recent meta-analysis confirmed this association (less than 2,500 g at birth and lower mean birth weight); there is also meta-analytic evidence of an greater likelihood of the child requiring intensive-care unit care, having a low Apgar score, as well as smaller head circumference (Marchand et al., 2022). Again, these associations are likely strongly confounded by concomitant smoking and other substance use in the mothers.

In sum, cannabis use during pregnancy has been associated with a number of adverse markers in the offspring. As outlined in Chapter 25, there are also emerging indicators of an elevated risk of certain childhood psychopathologies in children exposed to cannabis *in utero*. Further evidence is required to disentangle the impact of genetic and environmental confounders, but it seems appropriate to advise pregnant women to refrain from the use of cannabis.

32.7 Driving

As described in Chapter 9, cannabis use can impact learning, short-term memory, and other cognitive functions, both during acute intoxication and – to a lesser extent – after discontinuation. It is thus perhaps not surprising that cannabis has been implicated in an increased risk of motor vehicle accidents (MVA). Indeed, increased MVA risk with acute cannabis consumption was identified a decade ago (Asbridge et al.,

2012). Meta-analytic evidence confirms that individuals testing positive for THC have a higher risk of MVA as well as MVA culpability (Rogeberg, 2019). A subsequent meta-analysis confirmed the association between cannabis use and MVA, as well as risk of sustaining an injury as a consequence (Hostiuc et al., 2018). Driving-skills tend to recover within five-to-seven hours after last inhaled cannabis consumption, which would imply that smoking cannabis any time of the day would compromise safe driving throughout the same day (McCartney et al., 2021). However, appropriate road-side testing of THC intoxication, as opposed to THC consumption, have yet to be developed.

32.8 Cancer

Associations between cannabis consumption and cancers have generally not been demonstrated, apart from weak evidence of association between lifetime cannabis and non-seminoma testicular cancer (Gurney et al., 2015). While the presence of cannabinoid receptors in the testicles is known, the hypothetical pathway is unclear and no causal association can be inferred.

32.9 Liver Fibrosis

There is moderate evidence from studies investigating liver disease in HIV and HCV patients that liver fibrosis progression is not worsened by cannabis consumption. Conversely, there seems to be a lower than expected risk of non-alcoholic fatty liver disease in cannabis users, possibly correlated with CBD use (Farooqui et al., 2019). Again, the mechanistic pathway is unclear and no causal inference can be made.

32.10 Pain Control

Interest in the potential effects of cannabis on acute and chronic pain stems in part from the association between the cannabinoid and opiate systems in the brain. Moreover, cannabinoids might play a role in reducing pain distress, decoupling painful peripheral stimuli and signalling cascades *per se* from central pain perception and related suffering.

Meta-analyses have confirmed the efficacy of inhaled cannabis-based medicines in particular in ameliorating neuropathic pain (Allan et al., 2018; Andreae et al., 2015). While a possible bias related to funding sources (i.e., industry) in some of these studies has been raised (Torres-Moreno et al., 2018), several additional meta-analyses have largely confirmed the findings. For instance, a Cochrane review found an effect on chronic neuropathic pain, across different types of cannabis administration and different conditions (Mücke et al., 2018). Isolated RCTs have reported on CBD alone, dronabinol, CT-3, and cannabidivarin in treating pain syndromes, but replication studies are needed (Sainsbury et al., 2021).

In terms of chronic non-cancer pain conditions, studies have generally confirmed the efficacy of a range of cannabis-based medicines (Wong et al., 2020). A recent meta-analysis of RCTs showed moderate-to-high certainty evidence that non-inhaled medical cannabis or cannabinoids result in a small to very small improvement in pain relief (Wang et al., 2021). Evidence regarding the effects of cannabis on cancer pain is more controversial. A recent meta-analysis found no significant effect of oromucosal nabiximols (Häuser et al., 2019), while in previous findings cannabis-based medicines outperformed control interventions (Aviram and Samuelly-Leichtag, 2017). Finally, a recent meta-analysis found low certainty evidence in observational studies that cannabis could allow reduction in opioid use in cancer pain treatment, but this was not confirmed for RCTs (Noori et al., 2021).

32.11 Epilepsy

Stockings et al. (2018) and Lattanzi et al. (2018a, 2018b, 2020a, 2020b) have produced important meta-analytic evidence summarizing cannabidiol efficacy in the treatment of epilepsy. In sum, adjunctive treatment with CBD has been associated with a significant reduction in seizure frequency in Lennox-Gastault syndrome and Dravet's syndrome (Lattanzi et al., 2018a, 2018b, 2020a); results were robust when clobazam concomitant therapy was treated as a confounder (Lattanzi et al., 2020b). Analogous results come from the review of Stockings et al. (2018) in a population including adults.

The most frequent adverse effects associated with CBD in treating epilepsy are somnolence, decreased appetite, diarrhoea, and increased aminotransferase. Further studies are needed in order to better assess anticonvulsant efficacy in other epilepsies and other age groups, as well as monotherapy versus augmentation of ongoing anticonvulsants.

32.12 Nausea and Vomiting

The antiemetic effects of cannabis are well described, albeit the mechanisms are unclear. Meta-analyses confirm THC and/or CBD to be effective in controlling nausea and vomiting in oncological patients as adjunctive therapy to other antiemetics (Corsi and Peña, 2017). A further meta-analysis reported that cannabinoids outperformed both placebo and other antiemetics, but further studies in diverse populations are required (Allan et al., 2018).

32.13 Spasticity in Multiple Sclerosis

An initial meta-analysis found no significant beneficial effect of cannabis treatments for spasticity in multiple sclerosis (Meza et al., 2017), but subsequent meta-analyses have shown benefits on measures such as the percentage of improved patients (Fu et al., 2018), and on a continuous measure of spasticity (Torres-Moreno et al., 2018). The tolerability profile was favourable, with no statistically significant excess in serious adverse events.

32.14 Adverse Events in Medical Cannabis Treatments

Across meta-analyses of RCTs of medical use of cannabis, the most important adverse events, with high certainty, were abnormal liver function tests, pneumonia, decreased appetite, and somnolence (all referring to children treated with CBD). Moderate certainty evidence emerged across various populations including emerging psychiatric symptoms, including euphoria/dysphoria and feeling high; sedation/somnolence, central nervous system adverse events, including disorientation/confusion, impaired attention, visual disturbance, problems with balance, dizziness and vertigo; and gastrointestinal adverse events, including nausea/vomiting and diarrhoea.

32.15 Conclusion

Cannabis is a complex plant with numerous constituent chemicals, and much work continues to be required to elucidate the positive and negative impacts on physical and mental health parameters. Such studies can inform how medicinal cannabis is deployed in clinical practice and how potential risks are weighed, at an individual patient level.

References

Allan, G. M., Finley, C. R., Ton, J., et al. (2018). Systematic review of systematic reviews for medical cannabinoids. *Can Fam Physician*, **64**, e78–e94.

Andreae, M. H., Carter, G. M., Shaparin, N., et al. (2015). Inhaled cannabis for chronic neuropathic pain: A meta-analysis of individual patient data. *J Pain*, **16**, 1221–1232.

Asbridge, M., Hayden, J. A., and Cartwright, J. L. (2012). Acute cannabis consumption and motor vehicle collision risk: Systematic review of observational studies and meta-analysis. *BMJ*, **344**, e536.

Aviram, J., and Samuelly-Leichtag, G. (2017). Efficacy of cannabis-based medicines for pain management: A systematic review and meta-analysis of randomized controlled trials. *Pain Physician*, **20**, E755–E796.

Bhattacharyya, S., Morrison, P. D., Fusar-Poli, P., et al. (2010). Opposite effects of Δ-9-tetrahydrocannabinol and cannabidiol on human brain function and psychopathology. *Neuropsychopharmacology*, **35**, 764–774.

Blest-Hopley, G., Giampietro, V., and Bhattacharyya, S. (2019). Regular cannabis use is associated with altered activation of central executive and default mode networks even after prolonged abstinence in adolescent users: Results from a complementary meta-analysis. *Neurosci Biobehav Rev*, **96**, 45–55.

Borges, G., Bagge, C. L., and Orozco, R. (2016). A literature review and meta-analyses of cannabis use and suicidality. *J Affect Disord*, **195**, 63–74.

Conner, S. N., Bedell, V., Lipsey, K., et al. (2016). Maternal marijuana use and adverse neonatal outcomes: A systematic review and meta-analysis. *Obstet Gynecol*, **128**, 713–723.

Corsi, O., and Peña, J. (2017). Are cannabinoids effective for the management of chemotherapy induced nausea and vomiting? *Medwave*, **17**, e7119.

Esmaeelzadeh, S., Moraros, J., Thorpe, L., et al. (2018). Examining the association and directionality between mental health disorders and substance use among adolescents and young adults in the U.S. and Canada: A systematic review and meta-analysis. *J Clin Med*, **7**, 543.

Farooqui, M. T., Khan, M. A., Cholankeril, G., et al. (2019). Marijuana is not associated with progression of hepatic fibrosis in liver disease: A systematic review and meta-analysis. *Eur J Gastroenterol Hepatol*, **31**, 149–156.

Foglia, E., Schoeler, T., Klamerus, E., et al. (2017). Cannabis use and adherence to antipsychotic medication: A systematic review and meta-analysis. *Psychol Med*, **47**, 1691–1705.

Fu, X., Wang, Y., Wang, C., et al. (2018). A mixed treatment comparison on efficacy and safety of treatments for spasticity caused by multiple sclerosis: A systematic review and network meta-analysis. *Clin Rehab*, **32**, 713–721.

Gibbs, M., Winsper, C., Marwaha, S., et al. (2015). Cannabis use and mania symptoms: A systematic review and meta-analysis. *J Affect Disord*, **171**, 39–47.

Grant, I., Gonzalez, R., Carey, C. L., et al. (2003). Non-acute (residual) neurocognitive effects of cannabis use: A meta-analytic study. *J Int Neuropsychol Soc*, **9**, 679–689.

Gunn, J. K., Rosales, C. B., Center, K. E., et al. (2016). Prenatal exposure to cannabis and maternal and child health outcomes: A systematic review and meta-analysis. *BMJ Open*, **6**, e009986.

Gurney, J., Shaw, C., Stanley, J., et al. (2015). Cannabis exposure and risk of testicular cancer: A systematic review and meta-analysis. *BMC Cancer*, **15**, 897.

Häuser, W., Welsch, P., Klose, P., et al. (2019). Efficacy, tolerability and safety of cannabis-based medicines for cancer pain. *Der Schmerz*, **33**, 424–436.

Hindley, G., Beck, K., Borgan, F., et al. (2020). Psychiatric symptoms caused by cannabis constituents: A systematic review and meta-analysis. *Lancet Psychiatry*, **7**, 344–353.

Hostiuc, S., Moldoveanu, A., Negoi, I., et al. (2018). The association of unfavorable traffic events and cannabis usage: A meta-analysis. *Front Pharmacol*, **9**, 99.

Johnson, E. C., Hatoum, A. S., Deak, J. D., et al. (2021). The relationship between cannabis and schizophrenia: A genetically informed perspective. *Addiction*, **116**, 3227–3234.

Kiburi, S. K., Molebatsi, K., Ntlantsana, V., et al. (2021). Cannabis use in adolescence and risk of psychosis: Are there factors that moderate this relationship? A systematic review and meta-analysis. *Subst Abuse*, **42**, 527–542.

Kraan, T., Velthorst, E., Koenders, L., et al. (2016). Cannabis use and transition to psychosis in individuals at ultra-high risk: review and meta-analysis. *Psychol Med*, **46**, 673–681.

Lattanzi, S., Brigo, F., Cagnetti, C., et al. (2018a). Efficacy and safety of adjunctive cannabidiol in patients with Lennox–Gastaut Syndrome: A systematic review and meta-analysis. *CNS Drugs*, **32**, 905–916.

Lattanzi, S., Brigo, F., Trinka, E., et al. (2018b). Efficacy and safety of cannabidiol in epilepsy: A systematic review and meta-analysis. *Drugs*, **78**, 1791–1804.

(2020a). Adjunctive cannabidiol in patients with Dravet Syndrome:

A systematic review and meta-analysis of efficacy and safety. *CNS Drugs*, **34**, 229–241.

Lattanzi, S., Trinka, E., Striano, P., et al. (2020b). Cannabidiol efficacy and clobazam status: A systematic review and meta-analysis. *Epilepsia*, **61**, 1090–1098.

Lev-Ran, S., Roerecke, M., Le Foll, B., et al. (2014). The association between cannabis use and depression: A systematic review and meta-analysis of longitudinal studies. *Psychol Med*, **44**, 797–810.

Lorenzetti, V., Chye, Y., Silva, P., et al. (2019). Does regular cannabis use affect neuroanatomy? An updated systematic review and meta-analysis of structural neuroimaging studies. *Eur Arch Psychiatry Clin Neurosci*, **269**, 59–71.

Marchand, G., Masoud, A. T., Govindan, M., et al. (2022). Birth outcomes of neonates exposed to marijuana in utero: A systematic review and meta-analysis. *JAMA Netw Open*, **5**, E2145653.

McCartney, D., Arkell, T. R., Irwin, C., et al. (2021). Determining the magnitude and duration of acute Δ9-tetrahydrocannabinol (Δ9-THC)-induced driving and cognitive impairment: A systematic and meta-analytic review. *Neurosci Biobehav Rev*, **126**, 175–193.

Meza, R., Peña, J., García, K., et al. (2017). Are cannabinoids effective in multiple sclerosis? *Medwave*, **17**, e6865.

Moore, T. H., Zammit, S., Lingford-Hughes, A., et al. (2007). Cannabis use and risk of psychotic or affective mental health outcomes: a systematic review. *Lancet*, **370**, 319–328.

Mücke, M., Phillips, T., Radbruch, L., et al. (2018). Cannabis-based medicines for chronic neuropathic pain in adults. *Cochrane Database Syst Rev*, **3**, CD012182.

Myles, N., Nielssen, O., and Large, M. (2012). The association between cannabis use and earlier age at onset of schizophrenia and other psychoses: Meta-analysis of possible confounding factors. *Curr Pharm Des*, **18**, 5055–5069.

Noori, A., Miroshnychenko, A., Shergill, Y., et al. (2021). Opioid-sparing effects of medical cannabis or cannabinoids for chronic pain: A systematic review and meta-analysis of randomised and observational studies. *BMJ Open*, **11**, e047717.

Power, E., Sabherwal, S., Healy, C., et al. (2021). Intelligence quotient decline following frequent or dependent cannabis use in youth: A systematic review and meta-analysis of longitudinal studies. *Psychol Med*, **51**, 194–200.

Rabin, R. A., Zakzanis, K. K., and George, T. P. (2011). The effects of cannabis use on neurocognition in schizophrenia: A meta-analysis. *Schizophr Res*, **128**, 111–116.

Rocchetti, M., Crescini, A., Borgwardt, S., et al. (2013). Is cannabis neurotoxic for the healthy brain? A meta-analytical review of structural brain alterations in non-psychotic users. *Psychiatry Clin Neurosci*, **67**, 483–492.

Rogeberg, O. (2019). A meta-analysis of the crash risk of cannabis-positive drivers in culpability studies: Avoiding interpretational bias. *Accid Anal Prev*, **123**, 69–78.

Sainsbury, B., Bloxham, J., Pour, M. H., et al. (2021). Efficacy of cannabis-based medications compared to placebo for the treatment of chronic neuropathic pain: A systematic review with meta-analysis. *J Dental Anesthesia Pain Med*, **21**, 479.

Sánchez-Gutiérrez, T., Fernandez-Castilla, B., Barbeito, S., et al. (2020). Cannabis use and nonuse in patients with first-episode psychosis: A systematic review and meta-analysis of studies comparing neurocognitive functioning. *Eur Psychiatry*, **63**, e6.

Schoeler, T., Kambeitz, J., Behlke, I., et al. (2016a). The effects of cannabis on memory function in users with and without a psychotic disorder: Findings from a combined meta-analysis. *Psychol Med*, **46**, 177–188.

Schoeler, T., Monk, A., Sami, M. B., et al. (2016b). Continued versus discontinued cannabis use in patients with psychosis: A systematic review and meta-analysis. *Lancet Psychiatry*, **3**, 215–225.

Scott, J. C., Slomiak, S. T., Jones, J. D., et al. (2018). Association of cannabis with cognitive functioning in adolescents and young adults A systematic review and meta-analysis. *JAMA Psychiatry*, **75**, 585–595.

Stockings, E., Zagic, D., Campbell, G., et al. (2018). Evidence for cannabis and cannabinoids for epilepsy: A systematic review of controlled and observational evidence. *J Neurol Neurosurg Psychiatry*, **89**, 741–753.

Torres-Moreno, M. C., Papaseit, E., Torrens, M., et al. (2018). Assessment of efficacy and tolerability of medicinal cannabinoids in patients with multiple sclerosis. *JAMA Netw Open*, **1**, e183485.

Wang, L., Hong, P. J., May, C., et al. (2021). Medical cannabis or cannabinoids for chronic non-cancer and cancer related pain: A systematic review and meta-analysis of randomised clinical trials. *BMJ*, **374**, n1034.

Wong, S. S. C., Chan, S. C., and Cheung, C. W. (2020). Analgesic effects of cannabinoids for chronic non-cancer pain: A systematic review and meta-analysis with meta-regression. *J Neuroimmune Pharmacol*, **15**, 801–829.

Index

Printed in Great Britain
by Amazon

35989837R00209